MW01201549

Non-Neoplastic Pulmonary Pathology

An Algorithmic Approach to Histologic Findings in the Lung

Sanjay Mukhopadhyay
Staff Pathologist, Department of Pathology, Cleveland Clinic, Cleveland, OH, USA

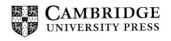
CAMBRIDGE
UNIVERSITY PRESS

CAMBRIDGE
UNIVERSITY PRESS

University Printing House, Cambridge CB2 8BS, United Kingdom

Cambridge University Press is part of the University of Cambridge.

It furthers the University's mission by disseminating knowledge in the pursuit of education, learning and research at the highest international levels of excellence.

www.cambridge.org
Information on this title: www.cambridge.org/9781107443501

© Sanjay Mukhopadhyay 2016

First published 2016
Reprinted 2018

Printed and bound in Great Britain by Clays Ltd, Elcograf S.p.A.

A catalogue record for this publication is available from the British Library

ISBN 978-1-107-44350-1 Hardback

To Mila, Ava, Erika and Kshama

Contents

Preface

This book is intended to be practical rather than encyclopedic. The focus is primarily on common non-neoplastic lung diseases likely to be encountered by surgical pathologists in lung biopsies and resections, such as granulomatous lung disease, infections and interstitial lung disease. A few uncommon entities are also addressed, but given the mission of the book, "zebras" are discussed briefly or omitted. Rare pediatric lung diseases are not included.

The text serves as a simple introduction to the complex world of non-neoplastic lung pathology for pathology residents, fellows and practising surgical pathologists. Pulmonary pathologists will be familiar with much of this material, but will find several helpful tips regarding difficult diagnoses and problem areas. Pulmonary clinical fellows, practising pulmonologists and thoracic radiologists who wish to enhance their understanding of lung pathology will find this book helpful and easy to read.

Although pertinent clinical and radiologic aspects of non-neoplastic lung disease are briefly discussed, the emphasis is on pathologic features, especially microscopic findings. I have found over the years that gleaning practical diagnostic information (microscopic features) from encyclopedic pathology textbooks requires wading through several pages of historic, epidemiologic and clinical information, akin to looking for a needle in a haystack. When microscopic findings are discussed, it is often unclear which findings are critical for a pathologic diagnosis and which ones are variable. This book attempts to simplify the diagnostic process for pathologists by separating the wheat from the chaff, i.e., by listing key pathologic features and variable pathologic features in separate sections. Microscopic findings are profusely illustrated, and there are many side-by-side comparisons of entities in the differential diagnosis.

Unlike other books on lung pathology, this book is organized by pathologic findings rather than etiology in order to facilitate diagnosis. Algorithms at the beginning of each chapter guide the reader from a particular microscopic finding to a specific diagnosis. The reader can then find further details about each individual diagnosis in the main body of the chapter.

Each entity is accompanied by a short list of 10 references that can be used as a starting point for more in-depth reading. The references are a mix of seminal pathology studies, recent articles in major pathology journals, large clinical series, smaller case series or case reports with clear illustrations of pathologic findings, and useful reviews of pathologic, clinical or radiologic features.

Another unique feature of this book is that it provides examples of actual terminology used by the author in surgical pathology reports. These examples illustrate the differences between diseases (tuberculosis) and pathologic diagnoses (necrotizing granuloma - AFB present), or in some cases between a clinical diagnosis (idiopathic pulmonary fibrosis) and the corresponding pathologic diagnosis (usual interstitial pneumonia). Examples of descriptive diagnoses in difficult situations are also provided.

It is my sincere hope that pathologists will find this book useful while struggling with cases of "medical lung disease" in their daily sign-out.

Sanjay Mukhopadhyay

Acknowledgements

First and foremost, greatest thanks are due to my wife Erika Doxtader for her support, advice, encouragement and patience during the several years that it took to write this book, and for encouraging me at the many points that I doubted my judgment in taking on a work of this magnitude. An excellent pathologist in her own right, Erika proof-read and corrected every chapter in this book and provided valuable advice along each stage of its preparation. I am also grateful to my mother, Kshama Mukhopadhyay, for donating her free time to painstakingly double-check reference formatting. Thanks are also due to my colleagues Dr. Carol Farver and Dr. A.V. Arrossi, who allowed me to take pictures from some of their cases.

Finally, I would like to express my appreciation to the wonderful editorial staff of Cambridge University Press. Nisha Doshi gave me the opportunity to write this book, helped define its scope, provided her unwavering support, and gave me time to get it right. I also owe a debt of gratitude to Jane Seakins for her tireless hard work, patience, attention to detail and guidance, which have improved the quality of this book.

Chapter

Introduction to lung pathology

This chapter aims to provide surgical pathologists with basic background knowledge that will prove helpful in the interpretation of pathologic findings in lung specimens. It includes the following:

1. Brief summary of normal lung histology.
2. Glossary of common terms used in non-neoplastic lung pathology.
3. Summary of the microscopic approach to lung biopsies with non-neoplastic pathologic findings.
4. Descriptions and illustrations of common artifacts and incidental findings in lung specimens.
5. Practical tips for interpretation and reporting of transbronchial and core needle biopsies.
6. Tables with menus of non-neoplastic lung diseases that can be diagnosed in small lung biopsies.

Normal lung histology

The most important features of normal lung histology are summarized in Table 1.1. The focus is on structures that can be seen with a light microscope in routine practice.

Airways (bronchi and bronchioles)

The main function of the airways is to bring air to and from the alveoli, where gas exchange occurs. Bronchi are branching, tube-like structures that contain cartilage and smooth muscle in their walls. They are lined by pseudo-stratified epithelium containing ciliated columnar cells and non-ciliated mucin-laden goblet cells (Figure 1.1). Ciliated cells in this epithelium push unwanted debris up the bronchial tree and out of the lungs so that it can be swallowed or spit out. Goblet cells produce mucin. As

Table 1.1. Normal lung histology

Structure	Notes
Bronchi and bronchioles (airways)	Bronchi contain cartilage, bronchioles do not Airways run with pulmonary arteries in "bronchovascular bundles" Respiratory bronchioles are the smallest, most distal bronchioles, continuous with alveoli Respiratory bronchioles do not appear round on cross section. Their ciliated lining gradually merges with cuboidal cells and alveolar pneumocytes
Alveoli	Lined by flat cells known as pneumocytes Alveolar walls = alveolar septa = **interstitium** Spaces within alveoli = **airspaces**
Blood vessels	In the lung, distinction between pulmonary arteries and veins is based on location (arteries run with airways, veins run in interlobular septa) Lymphatics run in bronchovascular bundles, interlobular septa and pleura Arterioles and venules run in the interstitium. They are intermediate in size between pulmonary arteries and capillaries Capillaries are the smallest blood vessels, found in alveolar septa
Pleura	Visceral pleura covers the lung It contains loose connective tissue with collagen and elastic fibers. Elastic fibers are much better seen with elastic stains The pleura contains lymphatics
Interlobular septa and lobules	Interlobular septa are cleft-like, linear connective tissue sheaths that dip down from the pleura They contain lymphatics and veins The lung between two adjacent interlobular septa is a lobule

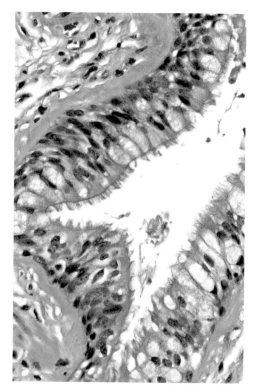

Figure 1.1. Bronchial epithelium. Ciliated columnar cells with interspersed goblet cells.

the bronchi branch and become smaller, goblet cells decrease in number and eventually disappear. At the base of the airway epithelium is a row of small, inconspicuous cells known as basal cells. These cells have very scant cytoplasm and are difficult to appreciate on H&E. They are beautifully highlighted by immunohistochemical stains for p63, p40 or CK5/6 (Figure 1.2). Scattered neuroendocrine cells known as Kulchitsky cells are also present at the base of the epithelium. They are inapparent on H&E but can be highlighted by synaptophysin or chromogranin staining. The bronchial epithelium rests on an eosinophilic basement membrane that is normally thin and indistinct. The epithelial cells in large bronchi are generally negative for TTF-1, but positivity can be seen in smaller bronchi, and progressively increases in intensity as bronchioles decrease in size.

The epithelium and subepithelial stroma of the bronchi is often referred to as *bronchial mucosa*, although, unlike the gastrointestinal tract, the line of demarcation between mucosa and submucosa is not always clearly defined since smooth muscle fibers are present in some areas but absent in others (Figure 1.3). In bronchioles, there is no precise boundary between mucosa and submucosa. It is therefore practical to refer to the entire subepithelial connective tissue in an airway as *bronchial wall* or *bronchiolar wall*. The bronchial wall also contains lymphatics, nerve twigs, salivary-type glands and cartilage (Figure 1.4). Salivary-type glands include

acini with mucinous and serous cells, and salivary-type ducts. They are usually located in the submucosa, but may intermingle with smooth muscle fibers, and occasionally extend superficial to the smooth muscle layer. Bronchial artery branches also run in and adjacent to the bronchial wall, but are seldom prominent.

The bronchi branch into bronchioles, which decrease in diameter with each generation. Unlike bronchi, bronchioles lack cartilage (Figure 1.5). Like bronchi, they contain smooth muscle and are lined by ciliated columnar epithelium. In the normal state, there is very little stroma between the epithelium and the underlying smooth muscle.

The nomenclature of bronchioles is confusing. Respiratory bronchioles, which constitute an important anatomic landmark in pulmonary pathology, are frequently misinterpreted as "terminal bronchioles". A practical system that can be used by practising surgical pathologists classifies small airways as respiratory bronchioles and non-respiratory (membranous) bronchioles. Non-respiratory (membranous) bronchioles have a well-defined, complete lumen lined entirely by ciliated columnar cells (Figure 1.5). In contrast, respiratory bronchioles are not lined entirely by ciliated cells since they merge into alveoli. Respiratory bronchioles represent the junction of the conducting system and the gas-exchange system. They are lined partially by ciliated columnar cells and partially by non-ciliated cuboidal cells (club cells, previously known as Clara cells), which in turn transition into flat cells lining the alveoli (Figure 1.6). Respiratory bronchioles contain smooth muscle fibers, which extend out for a short distance even after ciliated cells are no longer present, forming alveolar ducts (Figure 1.7).

The term *terminal bronchiole* refers to the portion of the non-respiratory bronchiole just proximal to the respiratory bronchiole. In practice, terminal bronchioles are difficult to identify in routine surgical pathology unless they can be seen in direct continuity with respiratory bronchioles. Their identification is of no special significance. In contrast, respiratory bronchioles are very important to recognize because some forms of lung disease show a predilection for their lumens (smoker's macrophages, hot tub lung, organizing pneumonia) or walls (hypersensitivity pneumonitis, coal workers' pneumoconiosis).

Bronchi and bronchioles run in bundles with the pulmonary artery and its branches like wires in an electrical cord. This airway–artery pairing starts at the main bronchi and remains constant all the way down to the most distal respiratory bronchioles. These pairs are known as *bronchovascular bundles* (Figure 1.8). Recognizing this relationship is important in lung pathology because bronchiolocentric pathologic processes often destroy or obscure the involved bronchioles, and the presence of an adjacent unaffected artery is often a clue to the correct interpretation. Bronchovascular bundles additionally contain lymphatics

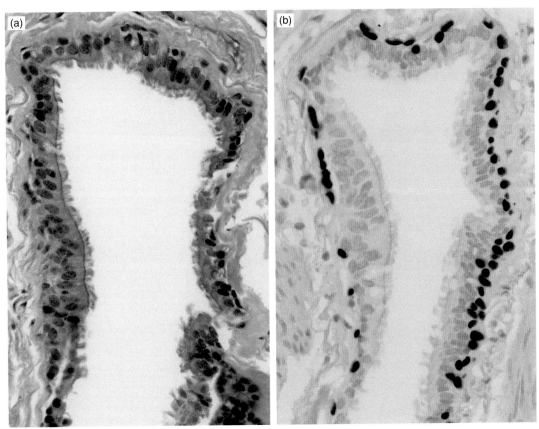

Figure 1.2. Basal cells in bronchial epithelium. (a) Basal cells lie at the base of the epithelium but are difficult to see on H&E. **(b)** p40, a basal cell marker.

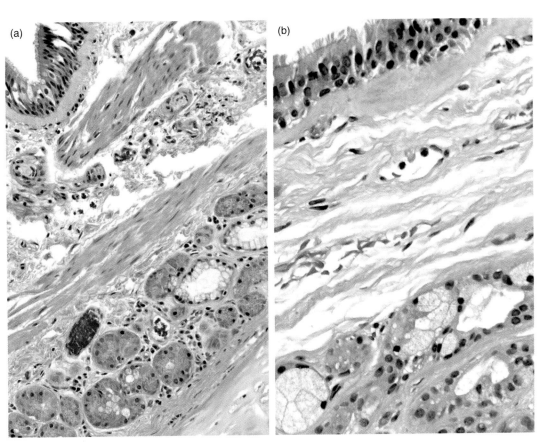

Figure 1.3. Bronchial mucosa. (a) Smooth muscle fibers separate bronchial mucosa from submucosa in this example. Note salivary-type glands in submucosa. **(b)** In this area from the same bronchus, there is no clear-cut demarcation between the mucosa and submucosa.

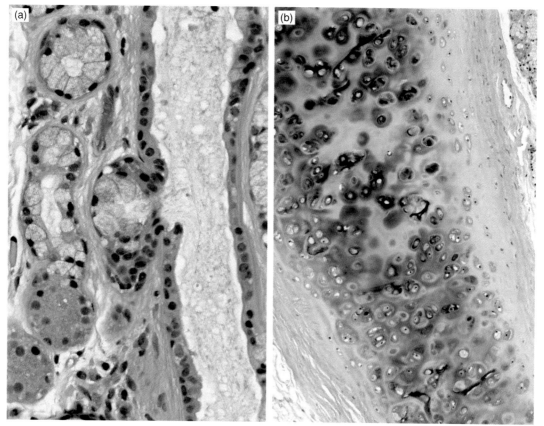

Figure 1.4. Bronchial wall. (a) Salivary-type glands containing mucinous and serous cells. A salivary-type duct is seen in the right half of the picture. **(b)** Bronchial cartilage, sandwiched between salivary-type glands (top right) and adventitia (bottom left).

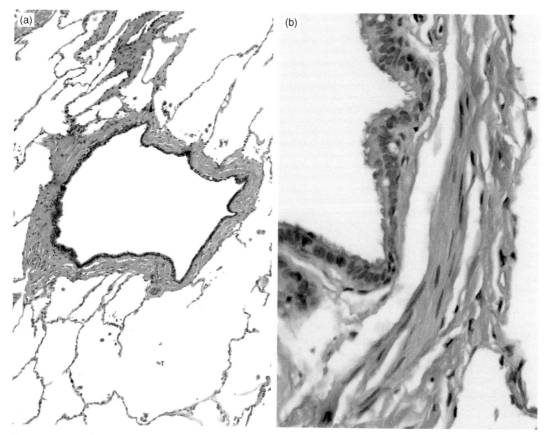

Figure 1.5. Bronchioles, non-respiratory. (a) Note absence of cartilage. **(b)** Higher magnification shows a ciliated columnar epithelial lining and smooth muscle bundles in the wall. There is very little tissue between the epithelium and the underlying smooth muscle.

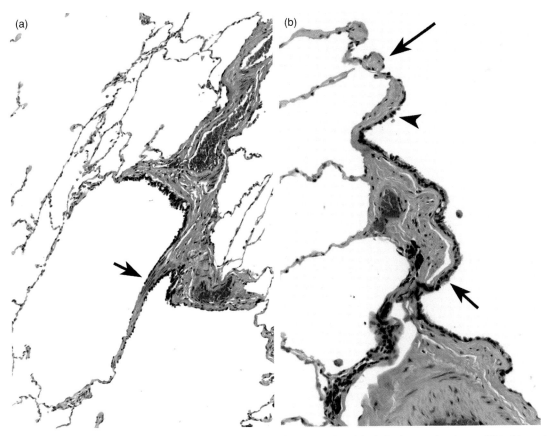

Figure 1.6. Respiratory bronchioles. (a) Note smooth muscle fibers (arrow) and the lack of a complete lumen. **(b)** In this respiratory bronchiole, the lining changes from ciliated epithelium (short arrow) to cuboidal non-ciliated cells (club cells, arrowhead) to flat alveolar pneumocytes (long arrow). Partner arteries are present in both images.

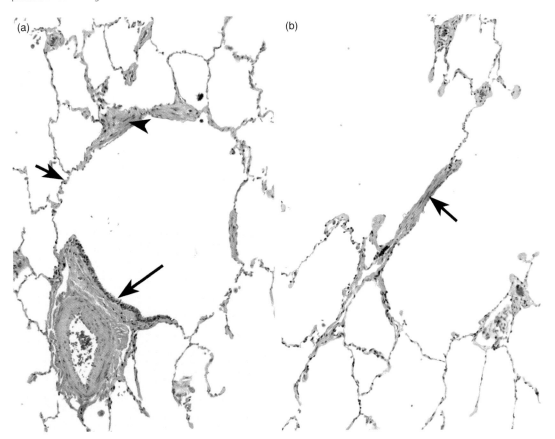

Figure 1.7. Alveolar ducts. (a) Transition between respiratory bronchiole (long arrow), alveolar duct (arrowhead) and alveoli (short arrow). Note artery adjacent to respiratory bronchiole. **(b)** Alveolar duct, characterized by the presence of smooth muscle fibers (arrow) in the absence of ciliated epithelium.

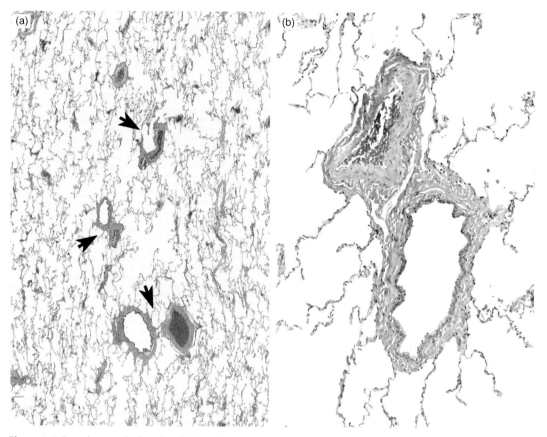

Figure 1.8. Bronchovascular bundles. (a) Bronchovascular bundles of various sizes (arrows). The first bundle from top contains a respiratory bronchiole and its partner artery. **(b)** Non-respiratory bronchiole and its partner artery. This bundle also contains lymphatics, but they are difficult to see unless dilated by pathologic processes.

and bronchial arteries, although these are seldom prominent in normal lungs. Lymphatics are especially easy to miss on H&E, because they are lined by flat cells and are often collapsed, mimicking alveoli. Their identification is greatly facilitated by immunohistochemical staining for D2–40 (Figure 1.9).

Alveoli

Respiratory bronchioles merge into alveoli lined by flat cells with minimal cytoplasm. These alveolar lining cells, known as *type 1 pneumocytes*, are inconspicuous on H&E (Figure 1.10). So-called *type 2 pneumocytes* are cuboidal in shape and produce surfactant. They are inconspicuous and relatively few in number in normal lungs but can become strikingly enlarged and prominent in interstitial lung disease and acute lung injury. Each alveolus contains a lumen and a wall. The alveolar lumens are referred to as *airspaces*. The alveolar walls, or *alveolar septa*, are exceedingly thin in order to facilitate gas exchange. They contain capillaries, minimal elastic tissue, little or no collagen, and rare fibroblasts. For practical purposes, alveolar septa constitute the **interstitium** of the lung, and the term **interstitial lung disease** refers to diseases that affect this compartment. In addition to the alveolar septa, the interstitial compartment of the lung also includes peribronchovascular connective tissue, interlobular septa and the pleura.

Normal alveolar epithelium is positive for cytokeratin stains such as keratin AE1/AE3, CAM 5.2 and CK7, as well as epithelial membrane antigen (EMA). It is negative for CK20. Type 1 and type 2 pneumocytes are additionally positive for TTF-1 (nuclear) and napsin A (granular, cytoplasmic). The latter antibody also stains alveolar macrophages.

Blood vessels

The main pulmonary artery divides into smaller and smaller branches that eventually become arterioles and capillaries. The pulmonary artery is an elastic-type artery at the hilum of the lung. It contains multiple elastic layers with several fragmented layers of interspersed smooth muscle (Figure 1.11). As bronchi turn into bronchioles, pulmonary artery branches turn into muscular-type arteries characterized by two layers of elastic tissue sandwiching a smooth muscle layer (Figure 1.12). The location of pulmonary arteries adjacent to airways is a more useful identifying feature in practice than the number and morphology of the elastic layers.

Small blood vessels intermediate in size between arteries and capillaries are found within the interstitium, without a partner airway. These vessels are *arterioles* and *venules*. Since

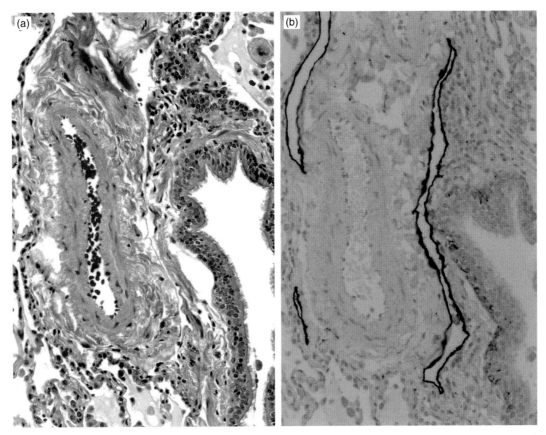

Figure 1.9. Lymphatics in bronchovascular bundle. (a) Lymphatics are present but are very difficult to see on H&E because they appear similar to alveoli. **(b)** They are clearly highlighted by D2–40.

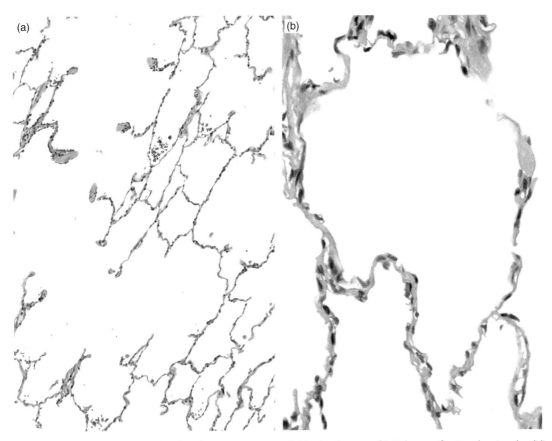

Figure 1.10. Alveoli. (a) Normal alveoli with empty airspaces and thin alveolar septa. **(b)** High magnification, showing alveoli lined by indistinct type 1 pneumocytes. These cells can be difficult to distinguish from capillary endothelium.

7

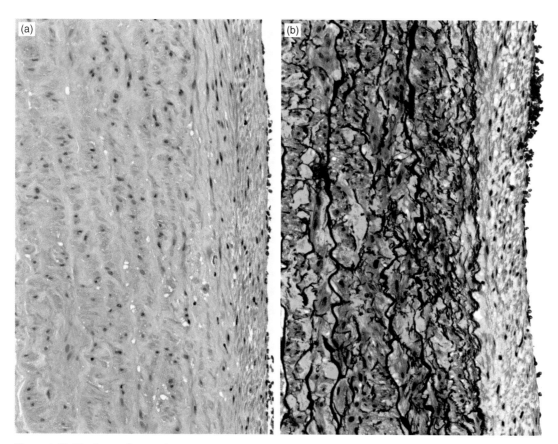

Figure 1.11. Elastic-type large pulmonary artery. (a) Main pulmonary artery from the vascular margin of a lobectomy specimen. There are multiple layers of elastic tissue, with interspersed smooth muscle fibers. **(b)** Movat pentachrome stains elastic tissue black.

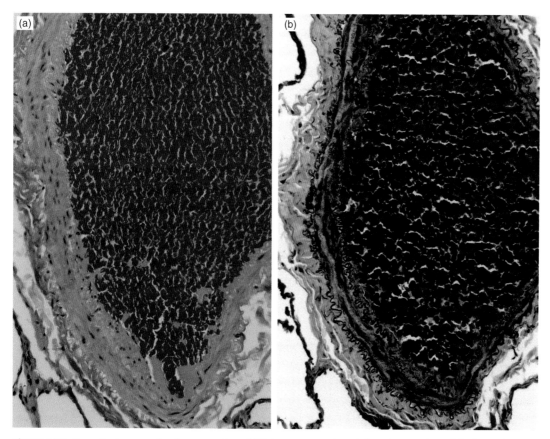

Figure 1.12. Muscular-type small pulmonary artery. (a) Pulmonary artery branch from the periphery of the lung. There are two elastic tissue layers sandwiching a single layer of smooth muscle. Elastic tissue stains very faintly on H&E and is difficult to see. **(b)** Movat pentachrome stains the squiggly elastic tissue layers black.

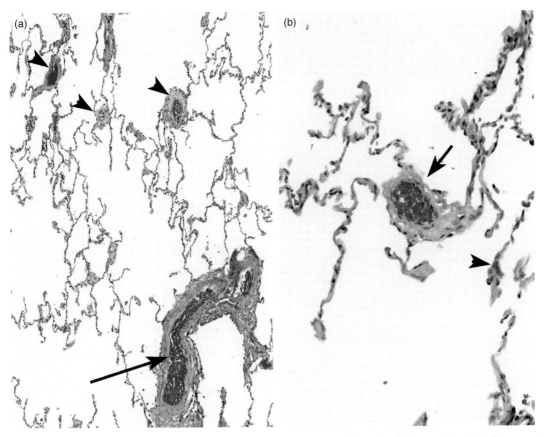

Figure 1.13. Arterioles/venules. (a) Small blood vessels within the interstitium (arrowheads), intermediate in size between arteries and capillaries. Compare with artery (arrow). **(b)** Small blood vessel (arteriole/venule) at high magnification (arrow). Compare with capillary (arrowhead).

there is only one elastic tissue layer in most blood vessels of this size, arterioles and venules cannot be reliably distinguished (Figure 1.13). Finally, and most importantly, the alveolar septa contain numerous capillaries lined by endothelial cells.

Pulmonary veins run in the interlobular septa. In contrast to pulmonary arteries, they contain a single elastic layer (lamina), or fragmented elastic tissue that does not form two well-defined layers. The appearance of pulmonary veins and their elastic laminae is illustrated later in this chapter, in the section on interlobular septa and lobules. Differentiating between arteries and veins on the basis of elastic layers can be problematic since elastic laminae are often fragmented and pathologic conditions can alter their morphology considerably.

Lymphatics in the lung are often collapsed, and are lined by flat endothelial cells, mimicking the appearance of alveoli. Unlike arteries and veins, their endothelium is positive for D2-40. Lymphatics course within the pleura, in interlobular septa, and along bronchovascular bundles. In the context of lung disease, this distribution is referred to as *peri-lymphatic* or *lymphangitic*. It is characteristic of a handful of lung diseases including sarcoidosis, low-grade lymphomas (most commonly extranodal marginal zone B-cell lymphoma or MALT lymphoma), primary or metastatic carcinomas with predominant intra-lymphatic spread (lymphangitic carcinomatosis),

IgG4-related lung disease, Erdheim–Chester disease and Rosai–Dorfman disease. Lymphatics are also seen adjacent to small blood vessels (arterioles/venules) in the interstitium but are not found in alveolar septa. They occasionally contain valves.

Pleura

A sheet-like layer of connective tissue known as *visceral pleura* covers the lung (Figure 1.14). The pleura lining the chest wall is known as *parietal pleura*. On H&E, visceral pleura is light pink because it contains collagen and elastic fibers. The latter are difficult to see on H&E, where they are only faintly visible as pale, squiggly lines. They are easier to appreciate on stains for elastic tissue such as Verhoeff–Van Gieson (VVG) or the Movat pentachrome stain (Figure 1.14). The pleura may contain one or several layers of elastic tissue, with a tendency towards multiple layers in pathologic conditions. Mesothelial cells line the outside of the visceral pleura *in vivo* but they are usually sloughed off in tissue processing and are only occasionally encountered in routine histologic sections.

Interlobular septa and lobules

An important structure that can be recognized in surgical lung biopsies and other resections is the *interlobular septum*.

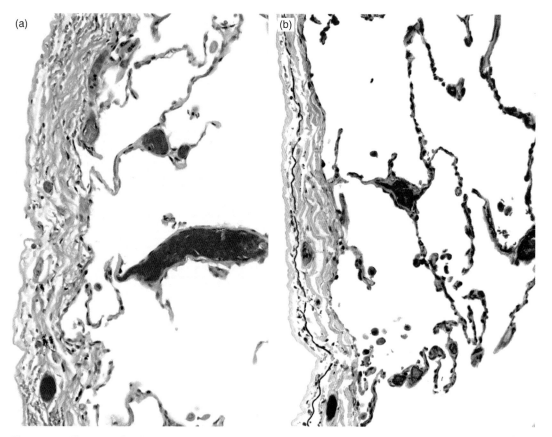

Figure 1.14. Pleura. (a) The pleura is readily identifiable on H&E (left), but elastic layers are not. **(b)** A Movat pentachrome stain highlights a single layer of elastic tissue. Collagen stains yellow. Note the absence of significant collagen deposition in the alveolar septa.

Interlobular septa are connective tissue sheaths that can be viewed as downward invaginations of the pleural connective tissue into the underlying lung. They appear as pale, cleft-like linear spaces extending down from the pleura into the underlying lung (Figure 1.15). They contain loose connective tissue, lymphatics (Figure 1.16) and veins (Figure 1.17). Interlobular septa divide the lung into compartments known as lobules (Figure 1.18). In general, each lobule contains a bronchovascular bundle in its center. Therefore, radiologists use *centrilobular* as a synonym for *peribronchovascular*. However, histologic examination shows that this is not necessarily the case – in fact, small bronchovascular bundles are randomly scattered throughout the lobule, including the periphery of the lobule adjacent to interlobular septa.

Glossary of common terms used in lung pathology

- Airspaces: The spaces within alveoli, normally empty (air-filled).
- Airways: Bronchi and bronchioles.
- Architectural distortion: Distortion of lung architecture by scarring or honeycomb change.
- Bulla: Air-filled space within lung, greater than 1 cm.

- Bleb: Air-filled space within pleura or subpleural lung, 1 cm or less.
- Bronchoscopic biopsy: A small biopsy of the bronchus or lung obtained with a bronchoscope.
- Central: Away from pleura, close to hilum.
- Centrilobular: In the center of a lobule. Considered equivalent to *peribronchovascular* by radiologists.
- CT: Computed tomogram. A more sensitive imaging method than conventional chest X-ray. CT scans are expensive and involve greater exposure to radiation than chest X-rays.
- Consolidation: In radiology, an infiltrate or opacity that obscures bronchial or vascular margins. In pathology, an area of lung that feels solid. The look and feel of a consolidated area may overlap with a mass, but is less well defined.
- Endobronchial biopsy: A bronchoscopic biopsy that aims to sample lesional tissue in a bronchial lumen or wall. It does not sample alveolated lung parenchyma. Contrast with *transbronchial biopsy*, below.
- Fibroblast focus (plural – fibroblast foci): A minute, microscopic focus of fibroblast proliferation within the interstitium, embedded in a pale-staining,

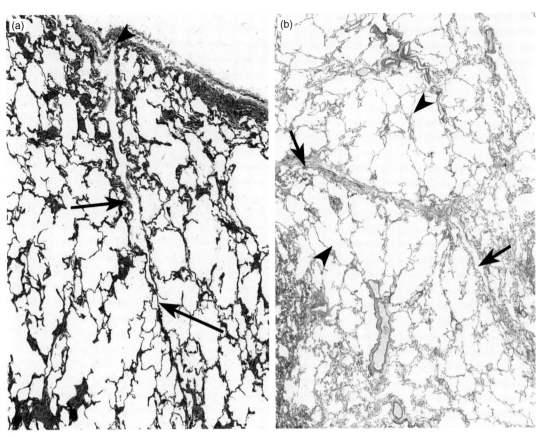

Figure 1.15. Interlobular septa. (a) Low magnification, showing an interlobular septum (arrows). Arrowhead: junction of interlobular septum with pleura. **(b)** Interlobular septum (arrows) separating two lobules (arrowheads).

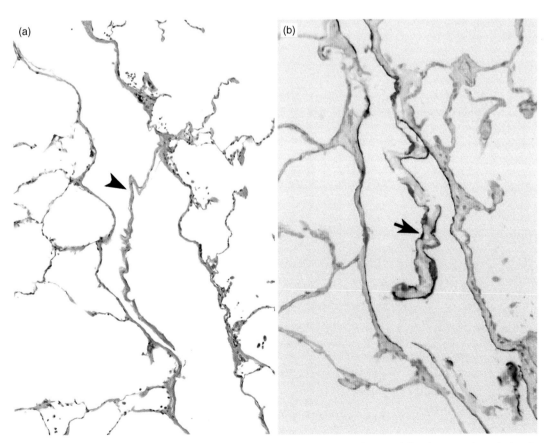

Figure 1.16. Lymphatics in interlobular septa. (a) Interlobular septum courses from top left to bottom right, with alveoli on either side. A lymphatic vessel is present, but it appears similar to adjacent alveoli on H&E. A valve is apparent (arrowhead). **(b)** D2–40 highlights lymphatic endothelium, including the valve (arrow). Alveolar epithelium is negative.

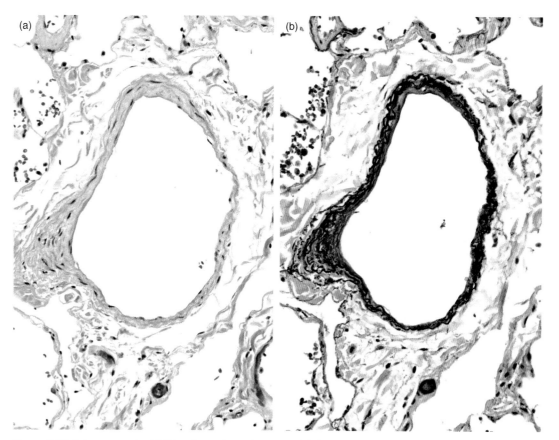

Figure 1.17. Pulmonary vein. (a) This vein was located in an interlobular septum. Note that there is no partner airway. **(b)** Movat pentachrome, showing single, fragmented elastic lamina (black). Despite the fragmentation, the elastic fibers do not form two well-defined layers. Compare to pulmonary artery, Figure 1.12.

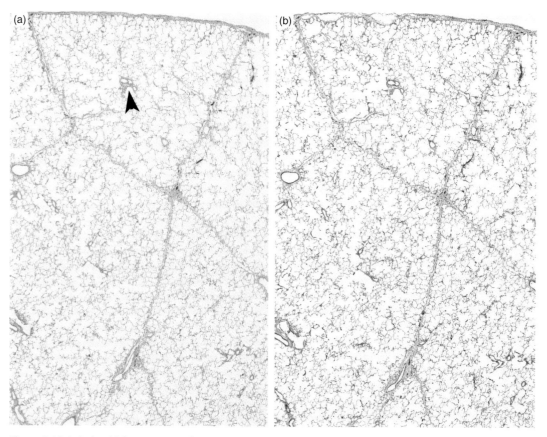

Figure 1.18. Lobules. (a) Scanning magnification of a near-normal lung, showing lobules demarcated by interlobular septa. A bronchovascular bundle is present in the center of a lobule (arrowhead). The tip of the arrowhead is in the lumen of a respiratory bronchiole. The partner artery is seen just above. **(b)** Same section, Movat pentachrome (collagen stains yellow).

myxoid-appearing stroma. Contrast with *fibroblast plug*. See Chapter 5 for detailed discussion.

- Fibroblast plug (synonym – Masson body): Minute, polyp-like plug of fibroblasts within the airspaces or the lumens of small bronchioles. The stroma is pale and myxoid-appearing, and usually contains inflammatory cells. Contrast with *fibroblast focus*. See Chapter 5 for detailed discussion.
- Fibrosis: Excessive, abnormal collagen deposition. Excessive fibroblast proliferation is also regarded as a form of early fibrosis.
- Ground-glass opacities: Blurry white hazy opacities on chest CT that represent abnormalities below the spatial resolution of the scan. Unlike consolidation, ground-glass opacities do not obscure bronchial or vascular margins. They are caused by a wide variety of pathologic changes, including interstitial or airspace inflammation, mild interstitial fibrosis, hemorrhage, edema and diffuse alveolar damage.
- High-resolution CT: A CT scan of the chest that uses a narrow slice width (1 to 2 mm) and a high-spatial-frequency reconstruction algorithm to provide greater detail than conventional CT and chest radiography. High-resolution CT is the ideal imaging study for evaluation of interstitial lung disease.
- Honeycomb change: Dilated and haphazardly clustered airspaces lined at least partially by ciliated columnar epithelium. When visible grossly, these dilated airspaces resemble a honeycomb. They are filled with mucin and located in fibrotic lung. Honeycomb change is a consequence of advanced fibrosis.
- Infiltrate: Radiologic term equivalent to opacity.
- Interlobular septum: Sheath of connective tissue that runs down from the pleura into the lung parenchyma. Contains lymphatics and veins. Interlobular septa divide the lung into lobules.
- Interstitium: Mainly alveolar septa. Also includes connective tissue in the walls of bronchovascular bundles, pleura and interlobular septa.
- Interstitial: Involving alveolar septa.
- Interstitial pneumonia: Any abnormality that predominantly involves the alveolar septa.
- Lobule: Portion of lung between two adjacent interlobular septa.
- Lymphangitic: Preferentially distributed within or around lymphatics.
- Macrophage: Histiocyte.
- Mass: In the lung, a localized solid lesion greater than 3 cm.
- Masson body: See *fibroblast plug*.
- Miliary: Innumerable, widespread, randomly distributed lung nodules, 3 mm or less.
- Mosaic attenuation: Radiologic term for patchwork of regions of differing attenuation on chest CT.

- Mycetoma: Fungus ball.
- Needle biopsy: Any biopsy performed with a needle, including percutaneous CT-guided core needle biopsies and fine-needle aspirates (FNA).
- Nodule: In the lung, a localized solid lesion measuring 3 cm or less.
- Opacity: In radiology, a descriptive term for an abnormal area that appears more opaque than the surrounding areas. Equivalent to *infiltrate*.
- Organizing: Involving fibroblasts. Usually denotes the stage following an acute process.
- Parenchyma (parenchymal): Involving the gas-exchanging substance of the lung, mainly the alveoli. This term is used to distinguish the substance of the lung from structures such as the pleura, airways or lymph nodes. Thus, a *parenchymal* nodule is located within the lung, and peribronchiolar *parenchyma* refers to alveoli adjacent to bronchioles.
- Peripheral: Close to pleura, away from hilum.
- Pneumonia: Lung abnormality. The term *pneumonia* is generally used to denote a lung infection in lay usage and general medical practice, but it is used in a broader sense by lung pathologists as an all-encompassing term for *lung abnormality*, whether infectious or non-infectious, interstitial or airspace. It is commonly used to describe non-infectious processes such as idiopathic interstitial pneumonia, usual interstitial pneumonia (UIP), non-specific interstitial pneumonia (NSIP), organizing pneumonia, desquamative interstitial pneumonia (DIP) and lymphoid interstitial pneumonia (LIP). In the context of interstitial lung disease, the word pneumonia has been used since 2002 in joint statements of the American Thoracic Society (ATS) and the European Respiratory Society (ERS).
- Pneumonitis: Some physicians and pathologists use the term "pneumonitis" to imply a non-infectious or interstitial process. The term is equivalent to *pneumonia*, which is currently the term of choice in interstitial lung disease terminology. The one entity where the word pneumonitis persists is hypersensitivity pneumonitis, and this is the only condition where the word pneumonitis is used in this book. Even for this entity, some authors use the equivalent term hypersensitivity pneumonia.
- Scarring: Confluent fibrosis that distorts or obliterates lung architecture.
- Small-airways disease: Any abnormality affecting the bronchioles.
- Spiculated: In radiology, a nodule or mass with irregular edges.
- Surgical biopsy: Any lung biopsy requiring a surgical procedure, also known as *wedge biopsy*. This includes traditional open lung biopsies that require thoracotomy, and less invasive biopsies

performed by video-assisted thoracoscopic surgery (VATS).

- Transbronchial lung biopsy: A bronchoscopic biopsy that aims to sample small bits of alveolated lung parenchyma through the airways.
- Tree-in-bud pattern: In radiology (on CT scans), centrilobular branching structures that resemble a budding tree. Indicates abnormalities involving bronchioles.

Microscopic approach to lung specimens

- Assess the histologic findings first, before viewing clinical information. This is the most valuable step in assessing a lung biopsy.
- Consider the specimen type. Is the biopsy a small bronchoscopic biopsy, a needle biopsy, a surgical lung biopsy or a lobectomy or other resection? The clinical question or setting can often be inferred by the type of specimen.
- Is the lesion a nodule/mass or an infiltrate? What is the clinical question?
- Are malignant cells present? If the pathologic findings are non-neoplastic, do they involve the airspaces, the interstitium, or both?
- Did you examine the pleura and blood vessels?
- Are the lymphatics dilated? Do they contain abnormal cells?
- Do the pathologic findings explain the radiologic findings?
- Will it help to obtain additional H&E-stained sections (recuts) from the paraffin block?
- Will special stains help in the diagnosis?
- What is the main pathologic finding? Does it fit into one of the major categories in this book? If so, review the algorithm for that chapter. The first figure in each chapter shows four examples of the types of lesions that are discussed.
  - Is the lesion granulomatous? (see Chapter 2)
  - Is the lesion an infection, but not granulomatous? (see Chapter 3)
  - Are the abnormalities predominantly within airspaces? (see Chapter 4)
  - Are the abnormalities predominantly within the interstitium? (see Chapter 5)
  - Is the lesion a nodule? (see Chapter 6)
  - Is the lesion cystic? (see Chapter 7)
  - Is the lesion mainly dust-related? (see Chapter 8)
  - Is the lesion in the bronchi or bronchioles? (see Chapter 9)
  - Is the lesion in the blood vessels? (see Chapter 10)
  - Is the biopsy from a lung transplant recipient? (see Chapter 11)

Common artifacts and incidental findings in lung specimens

Apparent hypercellularity due to collapse

Artifactual collapse is one of the most common artifacts in lung specimens, seen in transbronchial biopsies as well as surgical biopsies and resections. In resected lungs or surgical biopsies, it is probably a consequence of overzealous palpation, hence the admonition "palpate with thine eyes". In transbronchial biopsies, it probably results from undue squeezing with forceps. Since the alveoli are squeezed together, collapsed lung appears abnormal and hypercellular (Figure 1.19). Observers unfamiliar with this appearance often mistake it for interstitial fibrosis. Examination at high magnification usually resolves the problem by showing that the alveolar septa are closely spaced but otherwise normal. The presence of normal alveoli in adjacent, non-collapsed lung can also be helpful (Figure 1.19). Since collapse is almost always an artifact, "atelectasis" should not be used as a pathologic diagnosis.

Artifactual hemorrhage

Artifactual biopsy- or surgery-related hemorrhage within the alveoli is very common, and is often misinterpreted as pathologic. When bleeding is caused by a procedure, red blood cells fill the alveoli but are not associated with hemosiderin-laden macrophages, neutrophilic infiltrates, karyorrhectic debris, alveolar septal destruction or reactive type 2 pneumocytes. The presence of these findings should be a tip-off that the hemorrhage is pathologic (Figure 1.20). Since pathologic alveolar hemorrhage is very uncommon, the threshold for diagnosing it should be high. In the vast majority of cases, red blood cells within alveoli should be ignored.

Blue bodies

Blue bodies are small, light blue, laminated concretions found within intra-alveolar macrophages (Figure 1.21). They stain positive with von Kossa, iron, Periodic acid-Schiff (PAS) and Alcian blue. They are not birefringent. Blue bodies have been shown to contain calcium carbonate, and are thought to represent endogenous products of macrophage metabolism. They can be seen in any form of chronic lung disease that features numerous intra-alveolar macrophages, including smoking-related diseases. Blue bodies are morphologically similar to Schaumann bodies but the latter are larger, are found within granulomas or multinucleated giant cells, and do not occur within alveoli.

Bone marrow emboli

Bone marrow emboli are common within pulmonary arteries at autopsy, and may also be seen in surgical lung biopsies. They

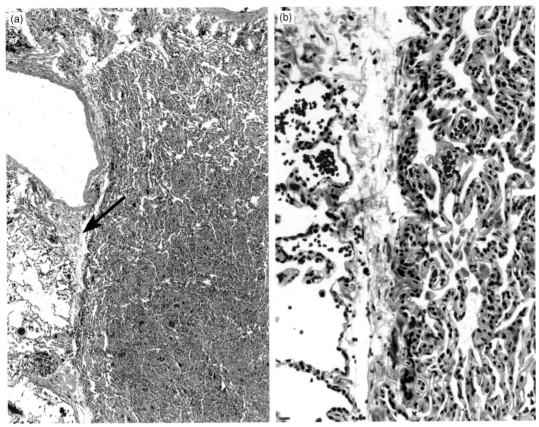

Figure 1.19. Artifactual collapse. (a) Lung parenchyma to the right of the interlobular septum (arrow) appears abnormal and hypercellular. Lung to the left is normal. **(b)** At high magnification, it is apparent that the abnormal area is collapsed, with normal alveolar septa identical to adjacent non-collapsed lung.

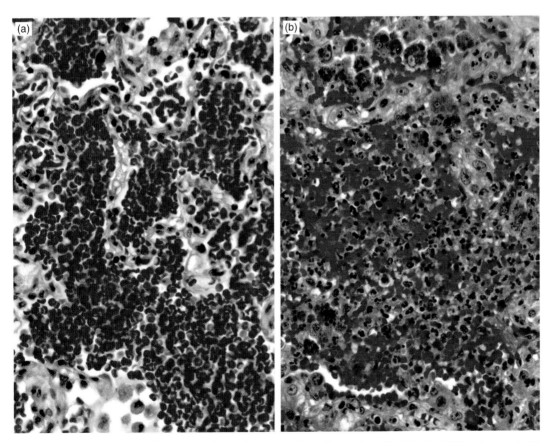

Figure 1.20. Artifactual hemorrhage vs. true hemorrhage. (a) Artifactual hemorrhage. Red blood cells fill the airspaces, but there is no hemosiderin, and alveolar septa are normal. **(b)** True alveolar hemorrhage from a case of necrotizing capillaritis. Hemosiderin-laden macrophages, neutrophilic infiltrates with karyorrhectic debris and reactive type 2 pneumocytes are tip-offs to the correct diagnosis.

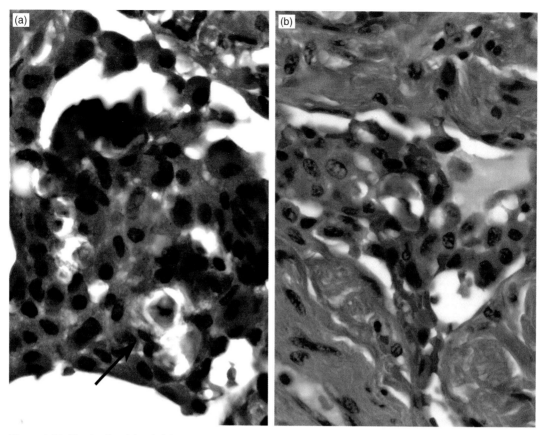

Figure 1.21. Blue bodies. (a) Light blue concretions within intra-alveolar macrophages. Concentric lamination is faintly visible (arrow). **(b)** Another example of a blue body. The patient was a cigarette smoker with severe respiratory bronchiolitis and interstitial fibrosis.

are thought to be an artifact resulting from trauma to the ribs caused by thoracic surgery or chest compression during cardiopulmonary resuscitation. They contain normal bone marrow elements including fat, megakaryocytes, myeloid precursors and nucleated red blood cells (Figure 1.22). Occasionally, numerous arteries may be involved.

Calcification and ossification

Calcification is a fairly common finding in the lung. It typically occurs as an incidental finding within necrosis or scars. Necrotizing granulomas caused by *Histoplasma* and mycobacteria appear particularly susceptible. When calcification in such lesions is extensive, it may be visible on CT scans, and serves as a clue to a benign diagnosis. Healed *Varicella* pneumonia, rarely seen by pathologists, is also characteristically associated with calcification. Lung calcification occurring within necrosis or scarring is termed *dystrophic calcification*. It is a degenerative change unrelated to serum calcium levels.

A more diffuse form of calcification occasionally occurs in lungs devoid of necrosis or scarring, and is termed *metastatic calcification*. It is characterized by extensive basophilic linear calcium deposits within alveolar septa and the walls of blood vessels (Figure 1.23). This distribution likely reflects the affinity of calcium deposits for elastic tissue. This type of calcification may elicit a foreign-body-type giant cell reaction. Superimposed features of organizing acute lung injury or organizing pneumonia may be present in the background lung. Metastatic calcification is most commonly seen in hypercalcemic individuals. Underlying causes of hypercalcemia include chronic renal failure with secondary hyperparathyroidism, primary hyperparathyroidism, multiple myeloma and leukemia. Metastatic calcification is seldom apparent on radiographs but can be visualized in a majority of CT scans as multiple diffuse calcified nodules, ground-glass opacities or consolidation. Centrilobular nodular ground-glass opacities with a fluffy appearance are characteristic. Rarely, metastatic calcification may occur in patients without an obvious underlying cause, preserved renal function and normal serum calcium levels.

Ossification in the lung is usually seen in the form of tiny foci of metaplastic bone, most commonly in usual interstitial pneumonia or organizing pneumonia (Figure 1.24). Focal ossification is also common in amyloidosis, apical caps and in the bronchial cartilage of older individuals. Most cases develop from prior calcification. Widespread interstitial ossification of unknown etiology is a rare entity, termed *dendriform pulmonary ossification*.

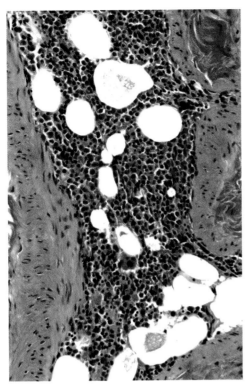

Figure 1.22. Bone marrow embolus. Bone marrow embolus within a pulmonary artery.

Carcinoid tumorlets

Carcinoid tumorlets are discussed in detail in Chapter 6. They are minute nodular proliferations of cytologically bland neuroendocrine cells, almost invariably located in the walls of small bronchioles (Figure 1.25). In most cases, they are an incidental finding in the background of small airway disease, scars or fibrosing lung disease.

Corpora amylacea

These are peculiar round eosinophilic spherules similar to corpora amylacea of the prostate (Figure 1.26). They are invariably intra-alveolar and may be few in number or numerous. Some have a laminated structure with faint concentric rings, while others contain lines radiating out from the center. A crack often develops within the structure. Dark central particles may occasionally be present. Adherent macrophages or foreign-body-type giant cells are sometimes identifiable. Corpora amylacea can be birefringent, and stain positive with PAS and Congo red. They are incidental findings of no significance and unknown origin. They should not be mistaken for aspirated material, parasites or foreign bodies.

Inclusions, endogenous (macrophage-related)

Endogenous inclusions are addressed in detail in the discussion on sarcoidosis in Chapter 2. They include asteroid bodies, Schaumann bodies, cholesterol clefts and calcium oxalate crystals (Figure 1.27). They are all thought to be endogenous products of macrophage metabolism. Asteroid bodies are tiny pink star-like structures. Schaumann bodies (conchoidal bodies) are purple, concentrically laminated microcalcifications. Cholesterol clefts are biconvex empty spaces with broad centers and tapered ends. Calcium oxalate crystals are colorless birefringent crystalline particles found within multinucleated giant cells. None of these inclusions is specific for any disease. They must not be mistaken for foreign particles.

Intra-alveolar macrophages (smoker's macrophages, respiratory bronchiolitis)

The lungs of cigarette smokers commonly contain lightly pigmented macrophages within the airspaces (Figure 1.28). The cytoplasm of these macrophages contains finely granular light-brown pigment with a few black specks. The pigment is presumably derived from particles present in cigarette smoke. In the vast majority of cases, the presence of these macrophages within the alveoli is an incidental finding. Smoker's macrophages can persist in the alveoli for many years, even if the individual quits smoking. In one study that carefully correlated pathologic findings with the history of cigarette smoking, smoker's macrophages were found in 15 ex-smokers more than 3 years after they had quit, 10 individuals with more than 5 years of smoking cessation, and in one person who had quit smoking 32 years before surgery! See Chapter 4 for a detailed discussion of this finding, the reason for the odd term *respiratory bronchiolitis*, and situations in which identification of these macrophages is clinically significant.

Dust-filled macrophages, interstitial

Macrophages laden with black carbonaceous dust are often present within the interstitium (Figure 1.29). The dust is generally assumed to be derived from polluted urban environments but it is also common in cigarette smokers. It is commonly referred to as "anthracotic pigment", a widely used but dubious term. Dust-filled macrophages differ from smoker's macrophages in that the intracytoplasmic pigment is coarse and black rather than fine and brown. For unclear reasons, dust-filled macrophages accumulate in the interstitium rather than the airspaces, while the reverse is true for smoker's macrophages (Figure 1.29).

Mallory hyalin

Droplets of dense eosinophilic intracytoplasmic material resembling Mallory hyalin are occasionally seen within the cytoplasm of type 2 pneumocytes in diffuse alveolar damage, organizing pneumonia, other forms of interstitial

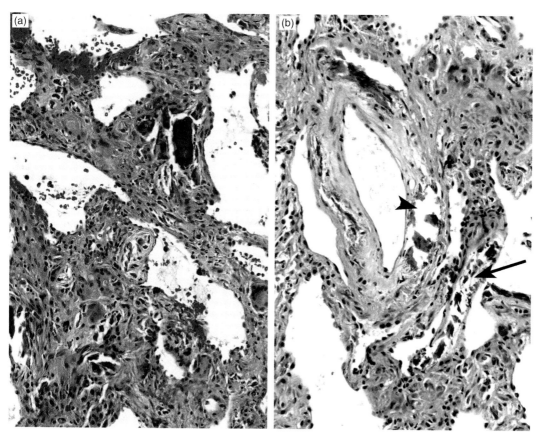

Figure 1.23. Calcification in the lung. (a) Diffuse alveolar septal calcification in a patient with hypercalcemia and renal failure. Note foreign-body giant cells. **(b)** Metastatic calcification. Calcific deposits are present in alveolar septa (arrow) and wall of a blood vessel (arrowhead).

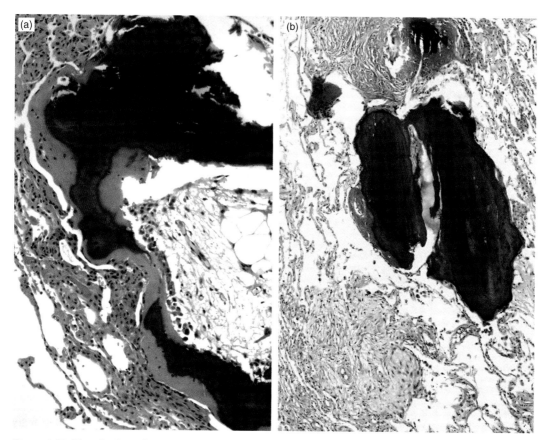

Figure 1.24. Metaplastic ossification. (a) Focus of metaplastic bone in a transbronchial biopsy. **(b)** Foci of metaplastic bone in a surgical lung biopsy with organizing pneumonia.

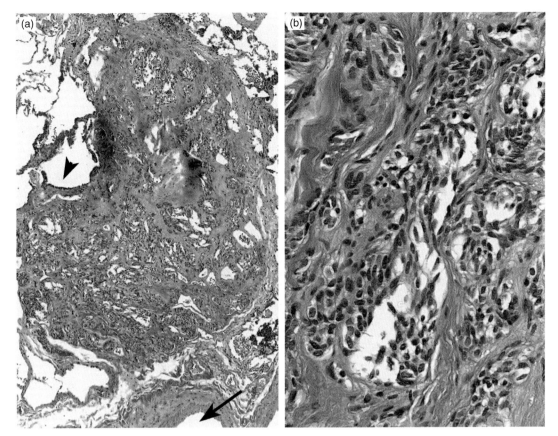

Figure 1.25. Carcinoid tumorlet. (a) Nodule in bronchiolar wall. Respiratory epithelium (arrowhead) and adjacent pulmonary artery (arrow) are clues to the location of the lesion. **(b)** The nuclei of the cells in the nodule are oval and cytologically bland.

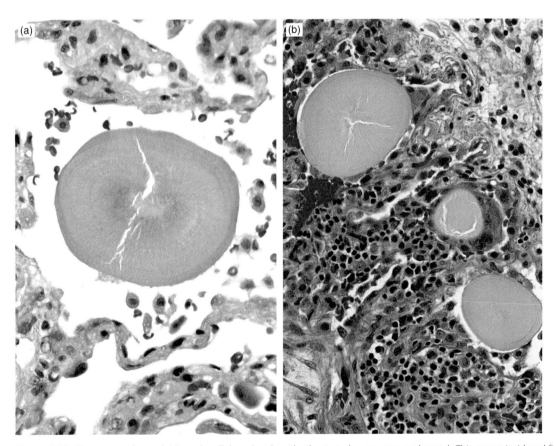

Figure 1.26. Corpora amylacea. (a) Round acellular spherule with a laminated appearance and a crack. This was an incidental finding in a case of organizing pneumonia from a 77-year-old woman. **(b)** Three corpora amylacea, from another case of organizing pneumonia. A multinucleated giant cell is attached to the smallest structure.

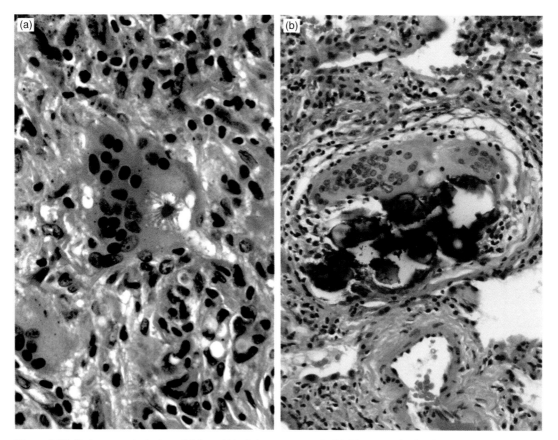

Figure 1.27. Endogenous inclusions. (a) Asteroid body in cryptococcosis. **(b)** Schaumann body in hypersensitivity pneumonitis.

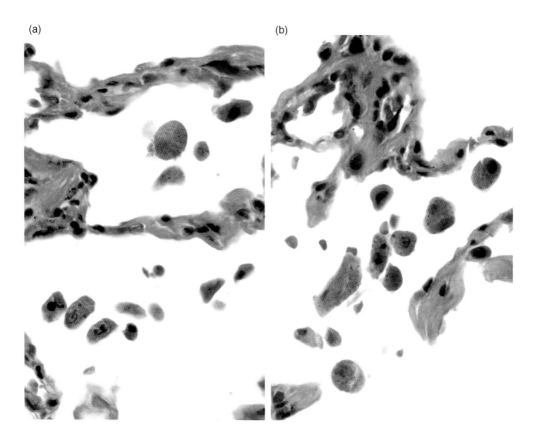

Figure 1.28. Intra-alveolar smoker's macrophages (respiratory bronchiolitis). (a) Lightly pigmented macrophages within the airspaces. **(b)** The intracytoplasmic pigment is light brown and finely granular, with a few black specks.

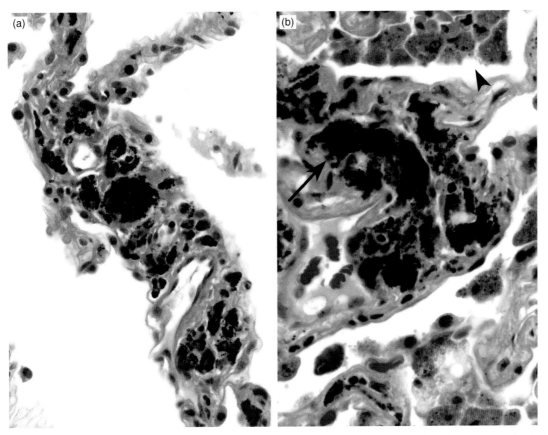

Figure 1.29. Dust-filled macrophages in the interstitium. (a) Macrophages laden with coarse black dust are seen within the interstitium. **(b)** Contrast the appearance and location of dust-filled macrophages (arrow) to smoker's macrophages (arrowhead).

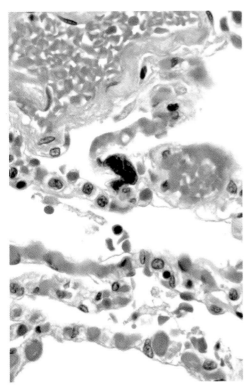

Figure 1.30. Megakaryocyte in lung. These cells have enlarged, irregular and hyperchromatic nuclei that should not be misinterpreted as malignant.

pneumonia, and asbestosis. They have been shown to contain the protein ubiquitin, and are thought to represent pneumocyte injury.

Megakaryocytes

A few scattered megakaryocytes are commonly found within alveolar septal capillaries in the lung. They can be numerous on occasion. They have enlarged, hyperchromatic, irregular nuclei and can appear quite bizarre (Figure 1.30). They have been reported in a variety of settings, including fever, sepsis, cardiovascular diseases and metastatic malignancies. They are of no clinical significance, and should not be mistaken for malignant cells, viral inclusions or parasites (see Chapter 3, Figure 3.18 for an image showing a parasite alongside a megakaryocyte).

Meningothelial-like nodules

Meningothelial-like nodules are minute cellular proliferations within the alveolar septa, often mistaken for granulomas or tumorlets (Figure 1.31). In the pre-immunohistochemistry era, they were erroneously interpreted as chemodectomas. The cells resemble meningothelial cells on H&E, and have an immunophenotype identical to meningiomas (Figure 1.32). Why cells with the morphology and

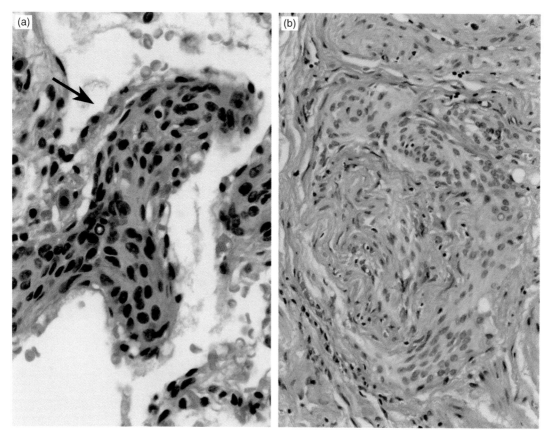

Figure 1.31. Meningothelial-like nodules. (a) A cellular proliferation expands the alveolar septa. The airspaces (arrow) are uninvolved. **(b)** The cells in this example resemble meningothelial meningioma.

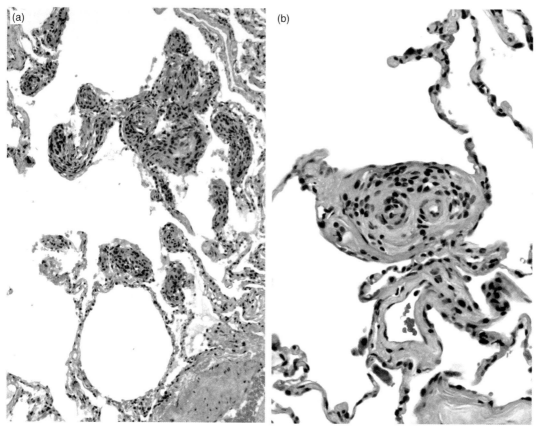

Figure 1.32. Meningothelial-like nodules. (a) This meningothelial-like nodule involves several alveolar septa. **(b)** This tiny lesion is confined to a single alveolar septum.

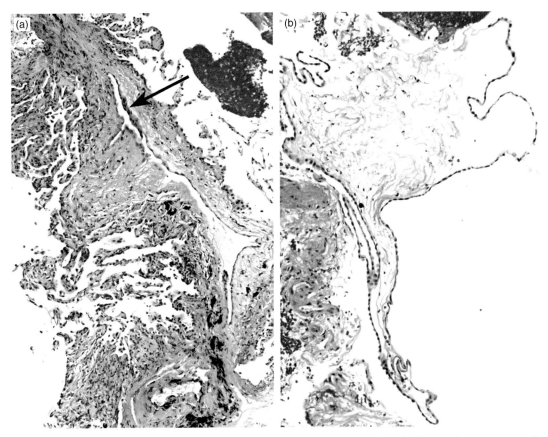

Figure 1.33. Pleura and mesothelial cells in a transbronchial biopsy. (a) In this transbronchial biopsy, pleura appears as a cleft lined by a row of cuboidal-to-flat cells. **(b)** This detached fragment of pleura has a folded configuration.

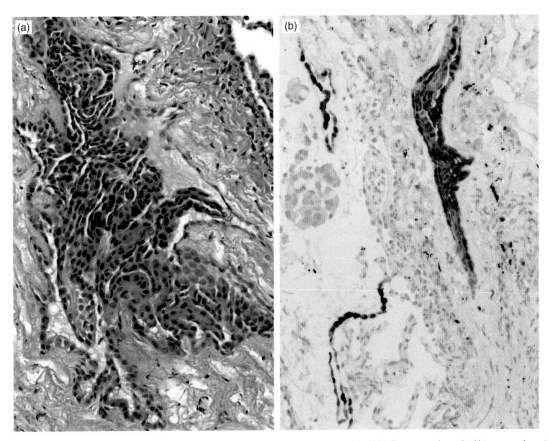

Figure 1.34. Mesothelial cells in transbronchial biopsies. (a) Hyperplastic mesothelial cells in a transbronchial biopsy can be misinterpreted as tumor. Alveolated lung is at top right. **(b)** Calretinin positivity in mesothelial cells.

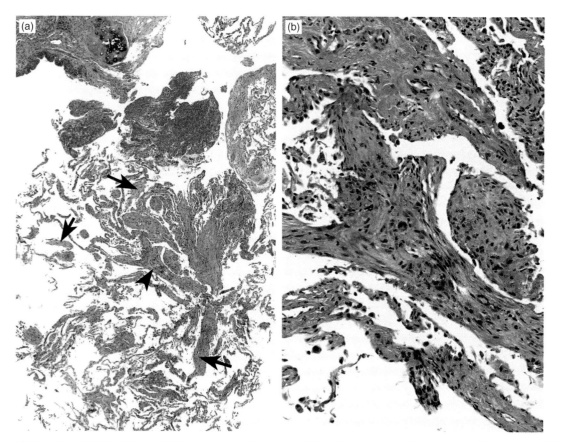

Figure 1.35. Organizing pneumonia in a transbronchial biopsy. (a) Fibroblast plugs are visible at low magnification (arrows). The branching plug indicated by the arrowhead is shown at high magnification in part b. The location of the plugs adjacent to an artery is a clue that they involve peribronchiolar parenchyma. **(b)** Fibroblast plug composed of fibroblasts in a pale-staining stroma. It also contains a few pigment-laden macrophages. The branched shape is a clue that this is not a fibroblast focus.

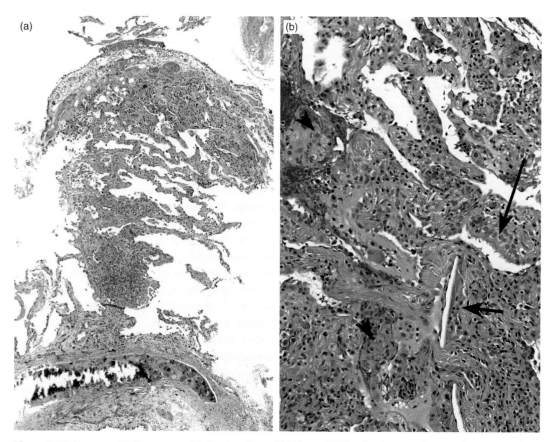

Figure 1.36. Hypersensitivity pneumonitis in a transbronchial biopsy. (a) The alveolar septa show patchy expansion by an inflammatory infiltrate. **(b)** The infiltrate consists predominantly of lymphocytes. A multinucleated giant cell containing a cholesterol cleft (short arrow) is seen in the interstitium adjacent to a small bronchiole (long arrow). Foamy macrophages are present in a few airspaces (arrowheads). These findings are consistent with hypersensitivity pneumonitis. The patient had a macaw and bilateral ground-glass infiltrates.

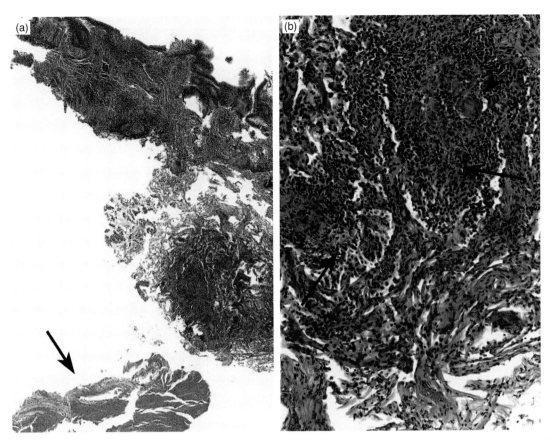

Figure 1.37. Non-tuberculous mycobacterial infection in a transbronchial biopsy. (a) Low magnification shows a heavily inflamed fragment of bronchial wall (top), alveolated lung with an inflammatory infiltrate (middle) and a detached fragment of exudate (arrow). Several acid-fast bacteria were identified within the exudate on an acid-fast bacteria (AFB) stain. **(b)** High magnification of the alveolated lung. The interstitium shows chronic inflammation but the airspaces are also filled with a lymphocytic infiltrate (arrows) containing an occasional poorly formed granuloma (arrowhead). Despite the absence of necrosis, the airspace location of the granulomatous inflammation is a clue to an infectious etiology. The patient was a 68-year-old woman with a right middle lobe infiltrate. *Mycobacterium avium–intracellulare* (MAI) grew on cultures.

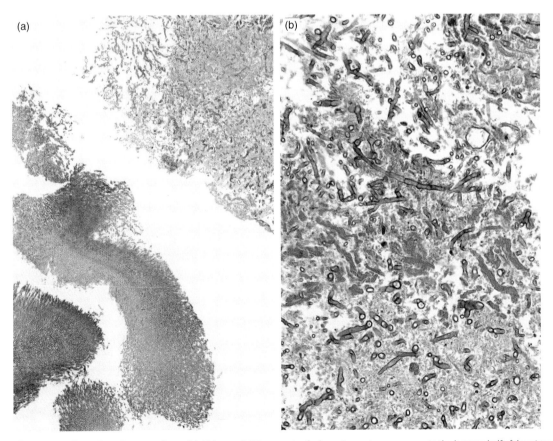

Figure 1.38. Organisms in a transbronchial biopsy. (a) Fragments of a fungal mycetoma are seen in the bottom half of the picture. However, the fragment at top right is different in appearance (shown at high magnification in b). **(b)** Septate fungal hyphae in a necrotic background. Several acid-fast bacteria were found within the necrosis. The patient had a history of cavitary *Mycobacterium xenopi* infection and cultures from the bronchial washings yielded *Aspergillus fumigatus*. The findings were interpreted as aspergilloma developing within a mycobacterial cavity.

(a)

(b)

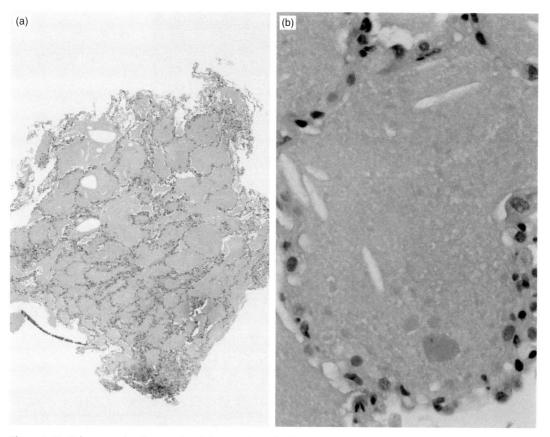

Figure 1.39. Pulmonary alveolar proteinosis in a transbronchial biopsy. (a) Eosinophilic material fills the airspaces. **(b)** The material is granular. It contains pink blobs and acicular spaces (see Chapter 4 for details).

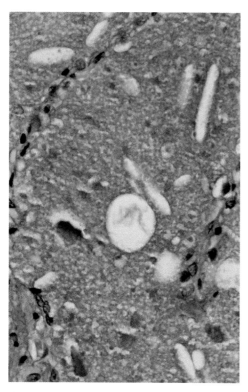

Figure 1.40. PAS stain of PAP in a transbronchial biopsy. The granular intra-alveolar material is usually PAS-positive.

immunophenotype of meningothelial cells occur in the lung is unknown. In the vast majority of cases, they are incidental findings of no significance. See Chapter 6 for a more detailed discussion.

Pleura and mesothelial cells in transbronchial and needle biopsies

Fragments of pleura are commonly seen in small lung biopsies. Although the presence of pleura in transthoracic core needle biopsies is not unexpected, small pleural fragments are surprisingly common in transbronchial biopsies of the lung. They are a testament to the ability of bronchoscopists to sample peripheral lung parenchyma as the bronchoscope is pressed against the lung parenchyma. In some cases their presence may indicate that the procedure was performed incorrectly, or that the patient coughed during the procedure.

Pleural tissue appears as infolded clefts within alveolated lung, or as detached fragments of fibrous tissue. The tip-off to the correct interpretation is the presence of mesothelial cells, which usually appear as a single row of cytologically bland, uniform cuboidal cells (Figure 1.33). Occasionally, there may be mild mesothelial hyperplasia (Figure 1.34). Mesothelial cells may also desquamate in the form of strips, and can be mistaken for malignant cells. Calretinin shows

(a)

(b)

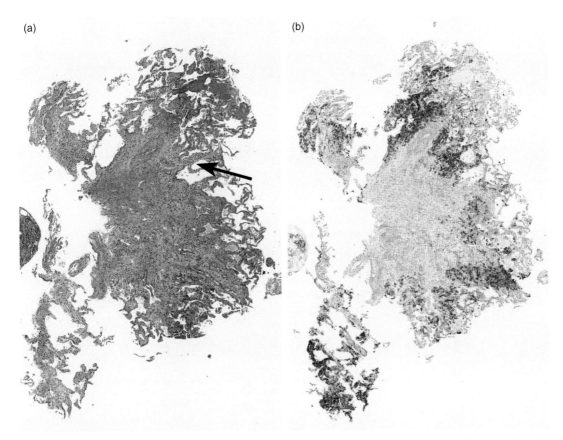

Figure 1.41. Pulmonary Langerhans cell histiocytosis in a transbronchial biopsy. (a) An irregular, stellate area of interstitial thickening is seen at low magnification. A high magnification view of the areas indicated by the arrow is shown in Figure 1.42. **(b)** CD1a stain, showing numerous Langerhans cells at the edges of the lesion. Note that the areas corresponding to CD1a positivity have a pale-staining background in part a.

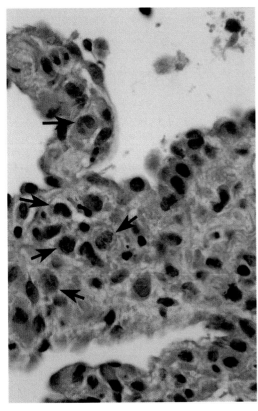

Figure 1.42. Pulmonary Langerhans cell histiocytosis in a transbronchial biopsy. Cluster of Langerhans cells with convoluted nuclei within the interstitium (arrows). Note the pale background, and single eosinophil at bottom right.

nuclear and cytoplasmic positivity in mesothelial cells, facilitating identification. Interestingly, the presence of pleural fragments in transbronchial biopsies is seldom associated with pneumothorax.

Transbronchial lung biopsies

The objective of transbronchial lung biopsies in the setting of non-neoplastic lung disease is to sample pathologic changes in the alveolated lung parenchyma. The pathologic diagnosis should be brief and to the point. However, clinicians often appreciate additional pertinent information in a comment. It is helpful to start the comment with a description of the biopsied tissue to give the clinician an estimate of what she has sampled. For example, one could state: "This biopsy consists of five fragments of alveolated lung parenchyma and two of bronchial wall". Fragments that contain bronchial wall as well as alveolated lung are counted as alveolated lung.

Pathologists should resist the urge to over-interpret minor findings of questionable significance. Biopsies without significant abnormalities should be diagnosed as such. We use the phrase "no significant pathologic changes". Clinicians are familiar with the fact that most transbronchial biopsies are non-diagnostic. The phrase "clinical correlation is recommended" is of no practical utility to

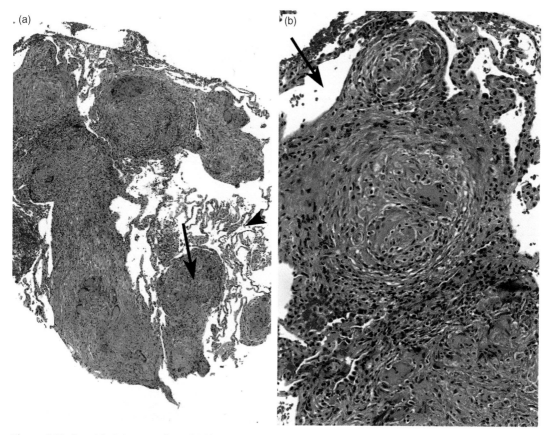

Figure 1.43. Sarcoidosis in a transbronchial biopsy. (a) Multiple non-necrotizing granulomas (arrow). An important feature is that lung away from the granulomas is normal (arrowhead). **(b)** The granulomas are well-formed and are located exclusively within the interstitium. There is concentric fibrosis around the granuloma in the center of the image. Airspaces are uninvolved (arrow).

clinicians, and can be construed as an attempt by the pathologist to deflect responsibility for the diagnosis. If the pathologic features are non-specific or non-diagnostic, this can be stated in a comment. If specific clinical, radiologic or laboratory features might be helpful in making or supporting the diagnosis, these should be specified. For example, one might state, "ANCA testing may be helpful" or "results of cultures will be important".

A helpful step in working up non-neoplastic transbronchial lung biopsies is to obtain additional H&E-stained recuts or deeper levels when the initial sections are non-diagnostic. A surprising number of such cases show unexpected diagnostic findings on deeper levels. This is especially true for cases of suspected sarcoidosis.

Since transbronchial lung biopsy is a relatively blind sampling method, the practical reality is that the majority of biopsies are non-diagnostic or show non-specific findings. However, the few cases that do yield a specific diagnosis are valuable because they help to avoid surgical lung biopsy or additional invasive testing. The yield of transbronchial biopsies is greatest in diseases in which the diagnostic findings are peribronchiolar or diffuse, but occasionally random pathology may be sampled. Pathologists who interpret transbronchial lung biopsies should become familiar with the entities that can be diagnosed on these biopsies, so that they can expand their repertoire beyond "no evidence of malignancy or granulomas". The non-neoplastic lung diseases that can be diagnosed in transbronchial lung biopsies are listed in Table 1.2. Diagnoses that cannot or should not be made on the basis of a transbronchial biopsy are listed in Table 1.3. Examples of specific diagnoses that can be made in transbronchial biopsies are shown in Figures 1.35 to 1.43.

Core needle biopsies of lung nodules

The objective of core needle biopsies is to provide a diagnosis for peripheral lung nodules or masses. Once malignancy has been ruled out, a variety of non-neoplastic causes of lung nodules enter the differential diagnosis. Granulomas are the most common finding, but a variety of other entities can be recognized, a surprising proportion of which are specific diagnoses that obviate the need for a surgical lung biopsy or further testing (see Table 1.4). Examples of core needle biopsies with specific diagnoses are shown in Figures 1.44 to 1.49.

Table 1.2. Non-neoplastic diagnoses that can be made in transbronchial lung biopsies

Diagnosis	Key findings and notes	Where to find more details in this book
Sarcoidosis	Well-formed non-necrotizing granulomas in interstitium Hyalinized fibrosis Lung away from granulomas is normal	Chapter 2 Also see Figure 1.43
Mycobacterial infections	Granulomatous inflammation, necrosis Acid-fast bacteria	Chapter 2 Also see Figure 1.37
Fungal infections	Granulomatous inflammation, necrosis Fungi: *Pneumocystis, Aspergillus, Histoplasma, Cryptococcus, Blastomyces, Coccidioides, Nocardia*	Chapter 2 Also see Figure 1.38
Viral infections	Cytomegalovirus, adenovirus, herpes, measles	Chapter 3
Hypersensitivity pneumonitis	Lymphocytic infiltrate within interstitium and airway walls, occasional multinucleated giant cells or loose clusters of histiocytes	Chapter 5 Also see Figure 1.36
Particulate matter aspiration	Food or vegetable matter (intact or degenerating); occasionally pill fillers Multinucleated giant cells around aspirated material Organizing pneumonia	Chapter 2
Talc granulomatosis	Filler materials (microcrystalline cellulose, crospovidone or talc) in alveolar septa, surrounded by a foreign-body giant cell reaction	Chapter 2
Pulmonary Langerhans cell histiocytosis	Stellate interstitial nodules containing sheets of Langerhans cells Smoker's macrophages within airspaces in background lung	Chapter 5 Also see Figures 1.41 and 1.42
Pulmonary alveolar proteinosis	Granular eosinophilic material within airspaces	Chapter 4 Also see Figures 1.39 and 1.40
Eosinophilic pneumonia	Eosinophils within airspaces	Chapter 4
Organizing pneumonia	Fibroblast plugs within airspaces	Chapter 5 Also see Figure 1.35
Diffuse alveolar damage	Hyaline membranes and/or diffuse alveolar septal fibroblast proliferation	Chapter 5
Usual interstitial pneumonia	Interstitial fibrosis in a "patchwork pattern", fibroblast foci, scarring, honeycomb change[a] Typical clinical and radiologic context: elderly individual, bilateral reticular infiltrates	Chapter 5
Drug-related lung disease	Interstitial expansion by chronic inflammation or fibroblast proliferation History of drug therapy (amiodarone, nitrofurantoin, methotrexate) No other obvious cause for pathologic findings	Chapter 5
Alveolar hemorrhage	Hemosiderin-laden macrophages (heart failure or capillaritis)	Chapter 4
Chronic bronchiolitis	Inflammation in bronchiolar or bronchial walls	Chapter 9
Acute bronchopneumonia	Acute inflammatory exudate (neutrophils, fibrin, debris) within alveoli	Chapter 4
Lymphangioleiomyomatosis	Cysts with scattered abnormal smooth muscle bundles in their wall	Chapter 7
Metastatic calcification	Diffuse calcification within alveolar septa; no obvious underlying cause	Chapter 1 Also see Figure 1.23
Acute cellular rejection	Exquisitely perivascular lymphoid infiltrates in lung transplant biopsies	Chapter 11
Chronic allograft rejection (constrictive bronchiolitis)	Constriction of bronchiole by extrinsic fibrosis, or complete obliteration of bronchiolar lumen by fibrous scar	Chapter 11

[a] In practice, the full spectrum of changes is seldom seen.

Table 1.3. Non-neoplastic diagnoses that should not or cannot be made in transbronchial lung biopsies

Diagnosis	Key findings and notes	Where to find more details in this book
Non-specific interstitial pneumonia (NSIP)	Alveolar septal chronic inflammation and fibrosis is very common and non-specific. It is impossible to confidently exclude UIP on a transbronchial lung biopsy Surgical biopsy required	Chapter 5
Respiratory bronchiolitis-interstitial lung disease (RBILD)	Smoker's macrophages are very common in cigarette smokers. It is impossible to confidently exclude other possibilities on a transbronchial lung biopsy Surgical biopsy required	Chapter 4
Lymphoid interstitial pneumonia (LIP)	This vanishingly rare diagnosis requires a surgical lung biopsy	Chapter 5
Desquamative interstitial pneumonia (DIP)	This conceptually incorrect diagnosis requires surgical lung biopsy; even in surgical biopsies, most cases of "DIP" are misdiagnosed examples of other entities	Chapter 4

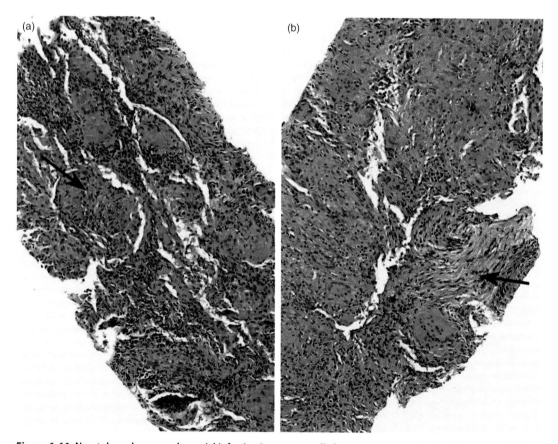

Figure 1.44. Non-tuberculous mycobacterial infection in a core needle biopsy. (a) This predominantly non-necrotizing granulomatous inflammation was misinterpreted as sarcoidosis. The airspace location of the granulomas is a tip-off to the correct diagnosis. **(b)** Organizing pneumonia (arrow) is another feature that argues against sarcoidosis. A solitary acid-fast bacterium was found on an AFB stain. The patient had a solitary lung nodule. Cultures grew MAI.

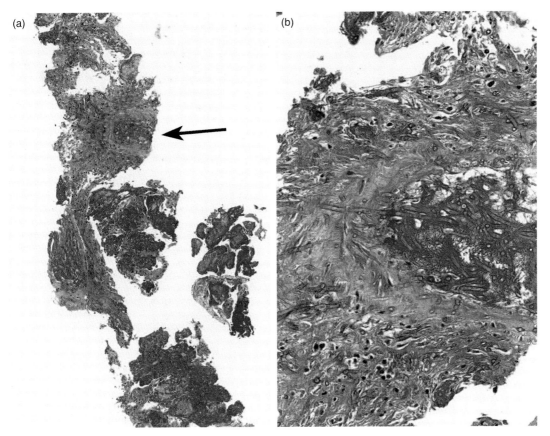

Figure 1.45. Invasive aspergillosis in a core needle biopsy. (a) At first glance, these cores appear to show only hemorrhage or hemorrhagic necrosis. The area indicated by the arrow is shown at high magnification in part b. **(b)** Fungal hyphae invade the wall of a blood vessel and plug its lumen. The patient was a 53-year-old woman with refractory acute myeloid leukemia and a large lung mass with a surrounding halo of ground-glass opacities. Cultures from the biopsy were negative but an *Aspergillus* galactomannan assay was positive.

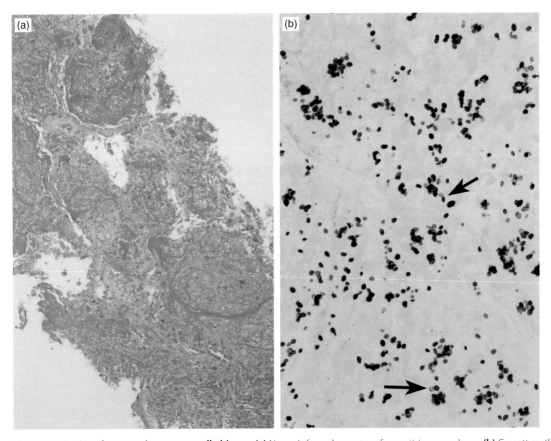

Figure 1.46. Histoplasmoma in a core needle biopsy. (a) Necrosis from the center of necrotizing granuloma. **(b)** Grocott methenamine silver (GMS) stain, showing small, uniform *Histoplasma* yeasts. Note narrow-based budding (arrows).

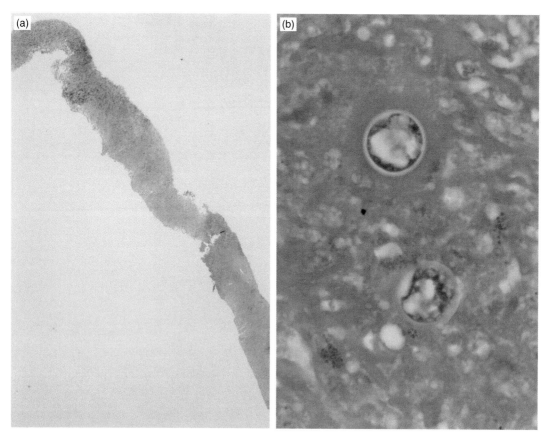

Figure 1.47. Coccidioidoma in a core needle biopsy. (a) Necrosis is at bottom right and granulomatous inflammation at top left. **(b)** Coccidioides spherules are visible within the necrosis. Note necrotic eosinophils in the background.

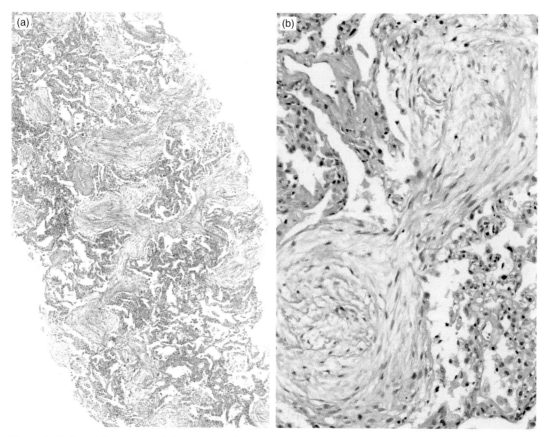

Figure 1.48. Organizing pneumonia in a core needle biopsy. (a) Numerous serpiginous, pale-staining fibroblast plugs fill the airspaces. A small artery, slightly left of center, is a clue that the process is involving peribronchiolar alveoli. **(b)** The dumbbell shape of this fibroblast plug is characteristic of organizing pneumonia. This shape is not seen in fibroblast foci of UIP.

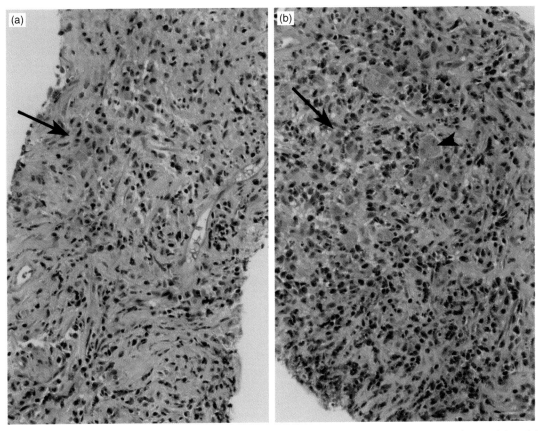

Figure 1.49. Pulmonary Langerhans cell histiocytosis in a core needle biopsy. (a) Interstitial infiltrate of eosinophils and clusters of Langerhans cells (arrow). **(b)** Eosinophils are innumerable in some areas. The admixture of eosinophils, Langerhans cells (arrow) and smoker's macrophages (arrowhead) is diagnostic.

References

Bejarano PA, Garcia MT, Ganzei-Azar P. Mesothelial cells in transbronchial biopsies. A rare complication with a potential for a diagnostic pitfall. *Am J Surg Pathol* 2007;**31**:914–8.

Chan ED, Morales DV, Welsh CH, McDermott MT, Schwarz MI. Calcium deposition with or without bone formation in the lung. *Am J Respir Crit Care Med* 2002;**165**:1654–69.

Colby TV, Yousem SA. Pulmonary histology for the surgical pathologist. *Am J Surg Pathol* 1988;**12**:223–39.

Doxtader EE, Mukhopadhyay S, Katzenstein AL. Core needle biopsy in benign lung lesions: pathologic findings in 159 cases. *Hum Pathol* 2010;**41**:1530–5.

Hansell DM, Bankier AA, MacMahon H, McLoud TC, Müller NL, Remy J. Fleischner society: glossary of terms for thoracic imaging. *Radiology* 2008;**246**:697–722.

Katzenstein AL, Askin FB. Interpretation and significance of pathologic findings in transbronchial lung biopsy. *Am J Surg Pathol* 1980;**4**:223–34.

Koss MN, Johnson FB, Hochholzer L. Pulmonary blue bodies. *Hum Pathol* 1981;**12**:258–66.

Mukhopadhyay S, Gal AA. Granulomatous lung disease. An approach to the differential diagnosis. *Arch Pathol Lab Med* 2010;**134**:667–90.

Mukhopadhyay S. Utility of small biopsies for diagnosis of lung nodules: doing more with less. *Mod Pathol* 2012;**25** Suppl 1:S43–57.

Mukhopadhyay S, Eckardt S, Scalzetti EM. Diagnosis of pulmonary Langerhans cell histiocytosis by CT-guided core biopsy of lung: a report of 3 cases. *Thorax* 2010;**65**:833–5.

Table 1.4. Specific non-neoplastic diagnoses that can be made in core needle biopsies of lung nodules

Diagnosis	Key findings and notes	Where to find more details in this book
Mycobacterial infections	Granulomatous inflammation, necrosis Acid-fast bacteria	Chapter 2 Also see Figure 1.44
Fungal infections	Granulomatous inflammation, necrosis *Aspergillus, Histoplasma, Cryptococcus, Blastomyces, Coccidioides, Nocardia*	Chapter 2 Also see Figures 1.45, 1.46, 1.47
Sarcoidosis	Non-necrotizing granulomas in interstitium Hyalinized fibrosis Special stains negative Appropriate clinical context	Chapter 2
Particulate matter aspiration	Food or vegetable matter, intact or degenerating; occasionally pill fillers Organizing pneumonia Multinucleated giant cells	Chapter 2
Wegener's granulomatosis/GPA	Necrotizing granulomas with "dirty necrosis" Necrotizing vasculitis ANCA positive	Chapter 2
Pulmonary Langerhans cell histiocytosis	Stellate interstitial nodules containing clusters of Langerhans cells	Chapter 5 Also see Figure 1.49
Scar	Fibrosis that obliterates lung architecture; may be collagenous or fibroelastotic	Chapter 6
Organizing pneumonia	Fibroblast plugs within airspaces	Chapter 5 Also see Figure 1.48
Abscess	Aggregates of neutrophils associated with necrosis or cellular debris	Chapter 4
Nodular amyloidosis	Amorphous eosinophilic material with multinucleated giant cells; Congo red positive	Chapter 6
Light chain deposition disease	Amorphous eosinophilic material with multinucleated giant cells; Congo red negative	Chapter 6
Pulmonary hyalinizing granuloma	Dense lamellated keloid-like fibrosis **No** granulomatous inflammation	Chapter 6
Intrapulmonary lymph node	Lymphoid tissue containing numerous dust-filled macrophages	

Granulomatous lung disease

This chapter addresses the approach to the differential diagnosis of granulomatous inflammation in the lung. Granulomas are a common pathologic finding in lung specimens, and the differential diagnosis is wide (Figure 2.1). An algorithmic approach to the diagnosis is suggested in Figure 2.2. Pearls and pitfalls related to granulomatous lung disease are summarized in Table 2.1.

A granuloma is a compact aggregate or cluster of histiocytes (macrophages). By definition, recognition of granulomatous inflammation requires microscopic examination. Although clinical and radiologic features can be quite suggestive of specific granulomatous lung diseases, only pathologic examination can confirm the presence of granulomas. The histiocytes that form granulomas have a distinctive morphology described as *epithelioid*. In contrast to ordinary histiocytes that contain round, oval or kidney-shaped nuclei and distinct cell borders, epithelioid histiocytes have elongated nuclei with a shape reminiscent of a cucumber or the sole of a shoe, and lack distinct cell borders (Figure 2.3). Epithelioid histiocytes are thought to be an activated form of ordinary histiocytes. The adjective *epithelioid* refers to their resemblance to epithelial cells – specifically, their occurrence in clusters and the abundance of cytoplasm. It is not surprising, therefore, that epithelioid histiocytes are occasionally mistaken for neoplastic epithelial cells and vice versa. Epithelioid histiocytes are also commonly misinterpreted as fibroblasts because of their elongated nuclei.

Contrary to common belief, neither lymphocytes nor multinucleated giant cells are mandatory for a diagnosis of granulomatous inflammation. The misconception that granulomas are composed of multinucleated giant cells surrounded by concentric layers of lymphocytes stems from standard medical school pathology textbooks. In practice, granulomas often deviate from this stereotypic image. While some granulomas are indeed surrounded by lymphocytes, others contain few or none ("naked" granulomas). Similarly, multinucleated giant cells may or may not be present in granulomas. These points are important to remember, especially for pathology residents, who often fail to identify granulomas when they lack giant cells or lymphocytes.

Granulomatous inflammation can manifest as a ball-like aggregate of epithelioid histiocytes or as a relatively thin rim of tightly clustered epithelioid histiocytes surrounding a fairly large zone of central necrosis (Figure 2.4). The latter type of granuloma is occasionally missed or misinterpreted since the bulk of the lesion consists of necrosis. Recognition of subtle granulomatous foci can be even more challenging in small biopsies.

Not all collections of histiocytes are granulomatous. In some diseases, histiocytes are arranged in sheets or loose clusters rather than compact or "organized" aggregates. One example is *Nocardia* pneumonia, which often has a vaguely granulomatous appearance caused by the presence of large numbers of histiocytes arranged in sheets (Figure 2.5). Another is lymphomatoid granulomatosis, a rare Epstein-Barr virus (EBV)-driven T-cell rich B-cell lymphoproliferative disorder, which mimics granulomatous inflammation due to the presence of large numbers of admixed histiocytes (Figure 2.5) associated with necrosis. Features that favor a true granulomatous process in these situations include compact or *organized* aggregates of histiocytes, epithelioid morphology and multinucleated giant cells. When in doubt, it is advisable to err on the side of caution and obtain special stains for microorganisms since poorly formed granulomas are common in immunodeficient persons and may contain numerous organisms.

Once granulomatous inflammation has been identified, the task of the surgical pathologist is to identify key morphologic findings of specific granulomatous diseases, perform appropriate special stains, and identify an etiology, if possible. The most important histologic feature that drives the differential diagnosis is *necrosis* (Figure 2.2). Granulomas containing necrosis are known as *necrotizing granulomas* while those lacking it are termed *non-necrotizing granulomas*. The outdated term "caseating granuloma" refers to gross rather than microscopic findings, and should be avoided. Specific granulomatous lung diseases are discussed below.

Tuberculosis

Worldwide, tuberculosis is the most common and best known cause of granulomatous inflammation in the lung. However, the historical emphasis on this disease has caused other common granulomatous infections to be overlooked. Specifically, it is not widely appreciated that in many geographic settings, tuberculosis is *not* the most common cause of granulomas – or even necrotizing granulomas – in the lung. Tuberculosis is prevalent in much of the developing world, with particularly large numbers of cases in South-East Asia and Africa. The largest numbers of patients are seen in India, China, Pakistan, Indonesia, Nigeria and South Africa. The disease is uncommon in Europe and North America.

These epidemiologic trends are reflected in pathology practice. While many surgical pathologists in the developing world see multiple cases of tuberculosis on a daily basis, tuberculosis is

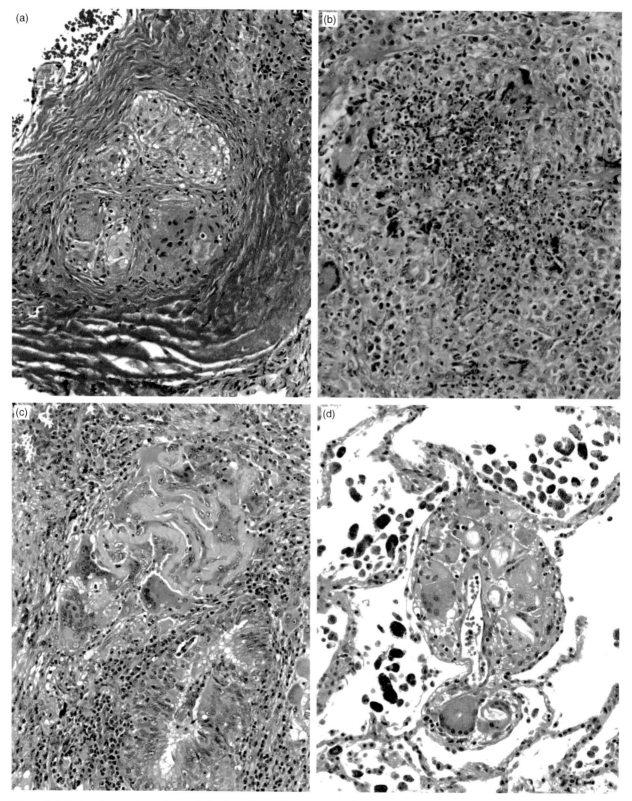

Figure 2.1. Various types of granulomas in the lung, illustrating the range of etiologies. (a) Sarcoidosis. **(b)** Granulomatosis with polyangiitis (GPA; Wegener's granulomatosis). **(c)** Particulate matter aspiration. **(d)** Talc granulomatosis. All images are shown at identical magnification.

an uncommon cause of pulmonary granulomas in the United States and Europe, where it is encountered mainly in at-risk populations such as immigrants from tuberculosis-endemic countries, drug and alcohol abusers, prisoners, residents of large urban centers, health care workers and the elderly. Immunosuppressed individuals such as those with HIV/AIDS or patients being treated with tumor necrosis factor-alpha (TNF-α) inhibitors are at high risk for tuberculosis.

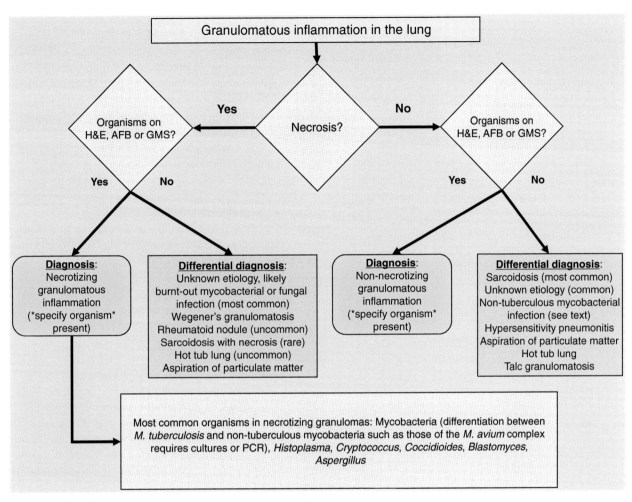

Figure 2.2. Algorithm for pathologic approach to granulomas in the lung.

In the United States, tuberculosis is currently at an all-time low. In large swaths of the country that are endemic for histoplasmosis and coccidioidomycosis, these fungal infections greatly outnumber bona fide culture-proven cases of pulmonary tuberculosis.

Pathologists may encounter tuberculosis in small lung biopsies as well as surgical biopsies and resections. Since tuberculosis is usually diagnosed on clinical grounds, cases seen by pathologists tend to be weighted towards clinically unsuspected cases, or those with atypical clinical or radiologic findings such as acute presentation, minimal symptoms, negative sputum smears or cultures, or lung infiltrates unresponsive to medical therapy.

Major diagnostic findings

- *Necrotizing granulomatous inflammation* is the classic histologic finding in tuberculosis. It typically consists of a relatively large zone of central eosinophilic necrosis surrounded by a granulomatous rim containing epithelioid histiocytes with or without multinucleated giant cells (Figure 2.6). The necrosis of tuberculosis is often described as "caseating", an outmoded term that refers to the cheese-like gross appearance of the necrosis. The term

dates back to the days when any necrotizing granuloma was presumed to be tuberculous in etiology. Despite extensive published literature describing identical gross and histologic features in non-tuberculous mycobacterial infections and fungal infections, the inordinate emphasis on caseation as a feature of tuberculosis persists. The necrosis of tuberculosis is actually quite variable, ranging from pink (eosinophilic or coagulative) to "dirty", characterized by a basophilic hue caused by nuclear debris derived from dead cells. Some tuberculous granulomas are frankly suppurative, i.e., they are rich in neutrophils ("liquefactive") and mimic abscesses. Eosinophilic necrosis is the most common type of necrosis in tuberculosis, but it can also be seen in virtually any other granulomatous mycobacterial or fungal infection. Langhans-type giant cells (multinucleated giant cells with nuclei arranged along the periphery of the cell in a wreath-like arrangement) (Figure 2.6), and "tuberculoid granulomas" or "tubercles" (micronodular collections of tightly knit epithelioid histiocytes and multinucleated giant cells) are similarly non-specific since they can be found in other granulomatous infections. To summarize, there are no pathognomonic histologic features on H&E that reliably

Table 2.1. Pearls and pitfalls in granulomatous lung disease

Always consider the possibility of a necrotizing granuloma when you see necrosis in a lung biopsy; a few epithelioid histiocytes at the edge of the necrosis are sufficient for diagnosing granulomatous inflammation

Necrotizing granulomatous inflammation is frequently missed, or misinterpreted as "necrosis", "abscess" or "hyalinized granuloma"

Multinucleated giant cells are not mandatory to diagnose granulomatous inflammation

Granulomas can develop hyalinized fibrosis: do not diagnose this as "hyalinizing granuloma". *Pulmonary hyalinizing granuloma* is a distinctive non-granulomatous keloid-like lesion (see Chapter 6)

Avoid a diagnosis of sarcoidosis when there is extensive necrosis or organizing pneumonia associated with granulomatous inflammation. Granulomatous infections are very common, but necrotizing sarcoidosis is very rare

Avoid the term *non-necrotizing granulomas* in the diagnosis unless you think sarcoidosis is the most likely diagnosis

Inclusions such as asteroid bodies and Schaumann bodies are **not** specific for sarcoidosis, or any other disease

Birefringent particles are not always exogenous (foreign). An example of an endogenous birefringent particle is calcium oxalate

Aspirated food and vegetable particles are seldom birefringent

Aspiration of food or particulate matter is one of the most frequently missed causes of lung granulomas

Special stains for microorganisms (AFB and GMS) should be routinely performed in immunocompromised patients and carefully examined, regardless of the tissue reaction. Lung transplant biopsies are a notable exception

Do not call a special stain for microorganisms negative unless you have examined the slide with a 40× objective

In granulomas, organisms are most commonly found within necrosis

Severe lymphocytic vasculitis has a limited differential diagnosis, including granulomatous mycobacterial and fungal infections, lymphomatoid granulomatosis, other lymphomas and IgG4-related lung disease

distinguish tuberculous granulomas from granulomas seen in other mycobacterial and fungal infections.

- Acid-fast bacteria. See *diagnostic work-up*, below, for detailed tips on identifying acid-fast bacteria in granulomas.

Variable pathologic findings

- Several lesions fall under the broad umbrella of necrotizing granulomatous inflammation. In the past, a range of descriptive terms have been used to describe these lesions in the lung, including *tubercles* ("soft" or "hard"), *nodules* (small, large, or "healed"), *fibrocaseous lesions* (with or without cavitation), and *miliary nodules*. Although these terms had some merit in emphasizing the wide spectrum of pathologic findings and their clinical, radiologic and microbiologic correlates, they have little or no bearing on the diagnosis of tuberculosis. Necrotizing granulomas of various sizes and morphologies often co-exist in the same lung.

- A mix of necrotizing and non-necrotizing granulomas is common in tuberculosis (Figure 2.7). However, it is uncommon to encounter pure non-necrotizing granulomatous inflammation, especially in surgical specimens where sampling error is not an issue. Even in small biopsies, at least focal necrosis is present in most cases.

- The term *tuberculoma* refers to a solitary necrotizing granuloma caused by tuberculosis. As in other infections, such nodules can mimic lung cancer radiologically and may be biopsied or resected to rule out malignancy.

- Varying degrees of fibrosis may supervene in tuberculous granulomas of all sizes, accounting for the terms "fibrous capsule", "fibrocaseous" and "fibrocavitary". Old, healed tuberculous granulomas presumably burn out as scarred nodules, leaving behind no trace of a residual granulomatous component.

- Calcification and ossification are common in old lesions. This is a metaplastic phenomenon.

- Histiocytes laden with black carbonaceous dust may be deposited around tuberculous granulomas. Knowledge of this possibility is important in the differential diagnosis with silicotic nodules.

- Granulomatous inflammation in tuberculosis can be subtle and poorly formed, especially in biopsies from immunocompromised patients, where acid-fast bacteria tend to be numerous (Figure 2.8). This type of lesion can be missed since its granulomatous nature is not obvious. This highlights the importance of maintaining a low threshold for performing special stains when faced with a histiocyte-rich inflammatory infiltrate.

- Tuberculous tracheobronchitis refers to granulomatous inflammation predominantly involving the tracheobronchial tree, with associated acute and/or chronic inflammation.

- Bronchiectasis is a well-known complication of long-standing tuberculosis. It is characterized by destruction and dilatation of bronchi by necrotizing granulomatous inflammation. Lungs with tuberculous bronchiectasis may be resected if medical therapy fails. Grossly, they show extensive bronchial dilatation extending out to the periphery of the lung (in contrast to normal bronchi, which are not grossly visible in the periphery of the lung). The walls of the dilated bronchi are thick, and their lumens often contain a mix of mucin and necroinflammatory debris. Microscopically, the main finding is severe chronic inflammation in the bronchial wall, accompanied by necrotizing granulomatous inflammation.

- A form of bronchopneumonia similar to bacterial bronchopneumonia can occur in tuberculosis. It is

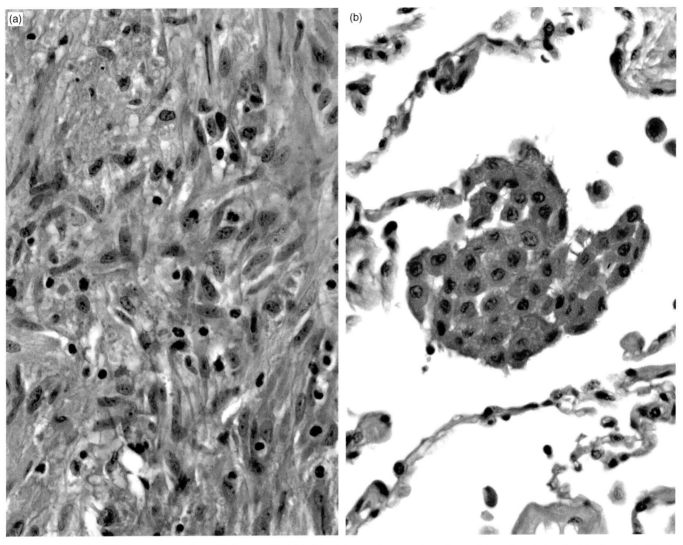

Figure 2.3. Epithelioid histiocytes vs. ordinary histiocytes. (a) Epithelioid histiocytes in a granuloma. The nuclei are elongated and cell borders are indistinct. **(b)** Ordinary histiocytes in an alveolus. This loose cluster is not a granuloma.

characterized by the presence of neutrophils within the airspaces, accompanied by fibrin, histiocytes and variable degrees of granulomatous inflammation.

- Miliary tuberculosis (disseminated tuberculosis) is characterized by the presence of innumerable tiny tuberculous nodules distributed throughout the lungs in a random distribution. This form of tuberculosis can usually be recognized radiologically, but the characteristic millet-seed-like tiny nodules can also be identified by pathologists in surgical lung biopsies or at autopsy. The nodules consist of tiny granulomas which may be necrotizing, non-necrotizing or poorly formed. Necrotizing granulomas predominate in most cases. Organisms tend to be numerous. Miliary tuberculosis is a consequence of hematogenous dissemination of organisms, often accompanied by widespread secondary involvement of lung parenchyma, analogous to lung involvement in disseminated histoplasmosis. This form of tuberculosis may also disseminate to the spleen, liver, bone marrow, kidneys, adrenals, choroid (eye), thyroid, breast, pancreas,

heart, prostate, testis and pituitary, in decreasing order of frequency.

- Striking vasculitis can occasionally be seen in tuberculosis, especially in immunocompromised patients, and may mimic lymphomatoid granulomatosis. Similar lymphocytic infiltrates in blood vessels have been described in acute pulmonary histoplasmosis. The cells in the vascular infiltrate are predominantly lymphocytes, with fewer numbers of histiocytes. Necrotizing vasculitis is not a feature of tuberculosis, however.
- Mycobacterial spindle cell tumors have been described in tuberculosis in immunocompromised individuals.
- Pleural involvement is common in tuberculosis. It is characterized by granulomatous inflammation accompanied by numerous lymphocytes. Tuberculous empyema, characterized by the presence of necrotic debris within the pleural cavity, is also a well-known complication of pleural involvement.
- Pulmonary tuberculosis has been traditionally associated with several eponyms, the best known being the Ghon

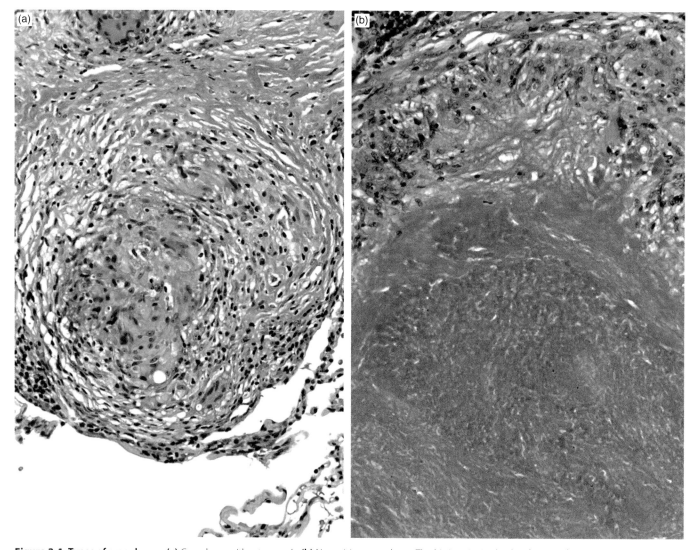

Figure 2.4. Types of granulomas. (a) Granuloma without necrosis. **(b)** Necrotizing granuloma. The histiocytic rim (top) is the granulomatous component.

focus (initial focus of infection in the lung), Ranke complex (Ghon focus plus affected draining hilar lymph node) and Simon focus (focus of disseminated infection). These eponyms were coined to highlight various findings or combinations of findings in tuberculosis. They are of historical significance and help to understand the natural history of the disease, but are irrelevant for diagnostic purposes.

Diagnostic work-up

- Special stains for acid-fast bacteria (AFB) and fungi (GMS) should be performed when granulomatous inflammation is identified in the lung. Organisms are far more likely to be found in necrotizing granulomas than in non-necrotizing granulomas. Also, the greater the amount of necrosis, the higher the likelihood of finding an organism. Well-formed non-necrotizing granulomas with hyalinized fibrosis, such as those typically seen in sarcoidosis, have a near-zero yield on acid-fast stains. Similarly, AFB stains are almost never positive in histologically normal lungs or in lungs with non-specific chronic inflammation or reactive changes.

- Ziehl-Neelsen is the standard AFB stain in most surgical pathology laboratories in the United States. The Fite stain (a modified AFB stain that uses less xylene in the staining and mounting process) is used in some labs as an alternative, but there are no reliable data on its sensitivity for tuberculosis compared to the Ziehl-Neelsen stain.

- If multiple blocks contain necrotizing granulomas, at least two should be stained for organisms. It has been shown that staining multiple blocks increases the likelihood of finding an organism, up to three blocks. The value of staining additional blocks is unclear.

- AFB are tiny rod-shaped bacteria that cannot be seen on H&E but stain red on acid-fast stains (Figures 2.8 and 2.9). The background is typically counterstained blue. Mycobacteria may be straight, slightly curved, beaded or non-beaded. Most measure less than 5 μm in length. *Mycobacterium tuberculosis* is usually 2 to 3 μm. Many clinicians and pathologists incorrectly assume that identification of AFB in a granuloma confirms the diagnosis of tuberculosis. In many geographic locations (including the United States), AFB in pulmonary

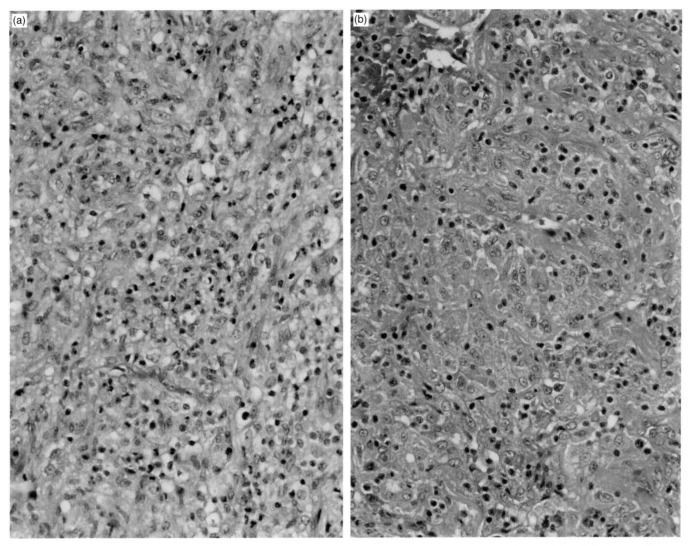

Figure 2.5. Mimics of granulomatous inflammation. (a) Sheets of histiocytes in *Nocardia* pneumonia. Note occasional neutrophils, and the absence of compact or well-formed histiocyte aggregates. **(b)** Lymphomatoid granulomatosis. Lymphohistiocytic infiltrate mimicking a granulomatous process.

granulomas are more likely to be non-tuberculous mycobacteria such as *M. avium* complex than *M. tuberculosis*. Although acid-fast stains are valuable for identifying mycobacteria, they do not allow differentiation of *M. tuberculosis* from non-tuberculous mycobacteria. The morphology of *M. tuberculosis* and non-tuberculous mycobacteria on acid-fast stains is similar or identical. Although subtle differences in length and beading have been described, they cannot be relied upon for a definitive diagnosis of tuberculosis. Morphologic features such as serpentine *cording* (*M. tuberculosis*), broad rods with cross-barring ("ladders" or "candy canes", *M. kansasii*) and long beaded forms (*M. gordonae*) have been described by microbiologists in AFB-stained smears prepared from positive liquid cultures. However, even in this setting – which cannot be extrapolated to histologic slides – morphologic features are neither perfectly sensitive nor specific for tuberculosis.

- A common mistake is to assume that AFB will be numerous and easy to find, a misconception that perhaps stems from

the large numbers of organisms seen in positive control slides for AFB stains. Although granulomas in immunocompromised patients may indeed contain numerous AFB, in immunocompetent individuals mycobacteria are usually few in number and difficult to find (Figure 2.9). We have seen several cases over the years in which only a single AFB was found in a necrotizing granuloma. Screening with a low-power objective lens may miss organisms in such cases. If organisms are not readily visible at low power, pathologists should begin their search in the necrotic center of the granuloma with a 40× objective lens or a 100× oil immersion lens (Figure 2.9). Constant adjustment of the fine focus is helpful so as not to miss organisms that may be visible in only one plane. This process is painstaking, tedious and time-consuming, but can be rewarding and clinically significant. Mycobacteria are most commonly found within the necrotic center of necrotizing granulomas, but they can also be found within viable histiocytes and multinucleated giant cells in the granulomatous rim. Acute inflammatory exudate or

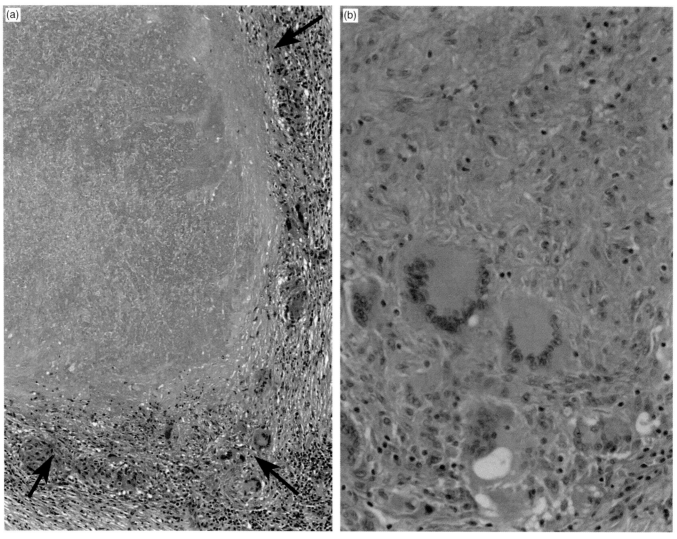

Figure 2.6. Tuberculosis. (a) Necrotizing granuloma with abundant pink necrosis and a relatively thin granulomatous rim (arrows). **(b)** Langhans-type multinucleated giant cells.

necrotic exudates within the lumens of airways may also contain organisms. Lung parenchyma outside the granulomatous areas virtually never contains organisms.

- The auramine-rhodamine fluorescence stain is an alternative to AFB stains. Some studies claim that this is a more sensitive procedure than the Ziehl-Neelsen stain, and some institutions have adopted it in part because it can be interpreted by a microbiology technician, saving time for the pathologist. However, the need for specialized equipment makes this a cumbersome process that is not widely utilized. Another approach is to use the fluorescence stain as a screen, and the AFB stain as a confirmatory test.

- A Grocott methenamine silver (GMS) stain for fungi should be requested in tandem with the acid-fast stain, since some fungi can cause granulomatous reactions identical to mycobacterial infections. Acid-fast bacteria stain black on silver stains. Finding rod-shaped GMS-positive bacteria of the appropriate size can be a valuable tip-off to the presence of mycobacteria, and should prompt careful re-examination of the AFB stain.

- In the ideal scenario, AFB stains on pathologic material will be confirmed by positive microbiologic cultures. However, it is well documented that special stains on histologic material can be negative in culture-positive tuberculosis, and vice versa. Therefore, a negative AFB stain does not exclude tuberculosis. Sampling error is the most plausible explanation for this phenomenon.

- Pathologists must anticipate the next step when they find and report AFB in a granuloma. In most cases, including all cases where infection is an unexpected finding, the presence of AFB should be rapidly communicated to the treating physician, especially in non-endemic countries where isolation procedures may be initiated based on this finding. In addition, pathologists will often receive calls from infectious disease specialists and other clinicians anxious to confirm the diagnosis of tuberculosis prior to starting therapy.

- Pathologists should be prepared to explain to their clinical colleagues that microbiologic cultures are the most reliable means for distinguishing between

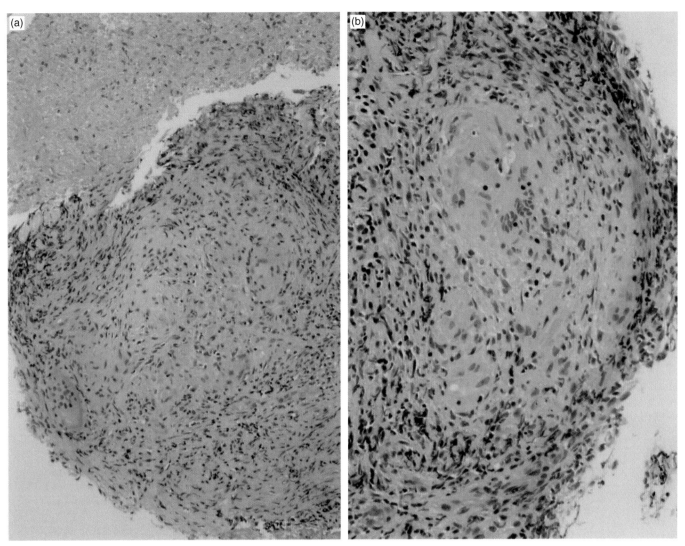

Figure 2.7. Necrotizing and non-necrotizing granulomas in tuberculosis. (a) Necrotizing granuloma in a lung biopsy from a patient with culture-confirmed tuberculosis. Necrosis is at top. **(b)** Focus of non-necrotizing granulomatous inflammation from the same case.

M. tuberculosis and non-tuberculous mycobacteria. Waiting for cultures for definitive identification of *M. tuberculosis* has traditionally delayed the diagnosis for intervals ranging from 2 to 6 weeks, although the application of polymerase chain reaction (PCR) to microbiologic specimens has decreased this interval. Currently, some microbiology labs automatically perform PCR for tuberculosis and non-tuberculous mycobacteria on smear-positive specimens and results can potentially be available within 24 hours. In smear-negative cases, the interval between receipt of a sample in the microbiology laboratory and definitive identification of *M. tuberculosis* can be as long as 6 weeks. Since cultures are crucial for definitive identification and antibiotic sensitivity testing, clinicians must be encouraged to submit tissue for cultures from any lesion where infection enters the differential diagnosis. Unfortunately, in practice, tissue in small specimens such as core needle biopsies of lung nodules is often prioritized for histopathology if the main clinical concern is malignancy, and no material is submitted for cultures. In such cases, PCR for mycobacteria can be attempted on formalin-fixed paraffin-embedded tissue. Although this test has been touted as a magic bullet for several years, its yield is very low in practice, especially when organisms are few in number. It is more helpful when numerous organisms are present. Availability of the test is also a significant practical issue, since most laboratories do not offer PCR testing on formalin-fixed paraffin-embedded tissue.

• Pathologists who encounter necrotizing granulomas at the time of frozen section should attempt to submit a piece of the granuloma for cultures. Tissue sampled at frozen section is seldom, if ever, handled in an aseptic fashion, and concerns regarding contamination are valid. However, the tissue can still be submitted for cultures and may yield valuable information, especially since it directly samples the center of the granuloma. Surgeons may also be able to send additional tissue in an aseptic fashion for cultures intraoperatively, and should be urged by pathologists to do so.

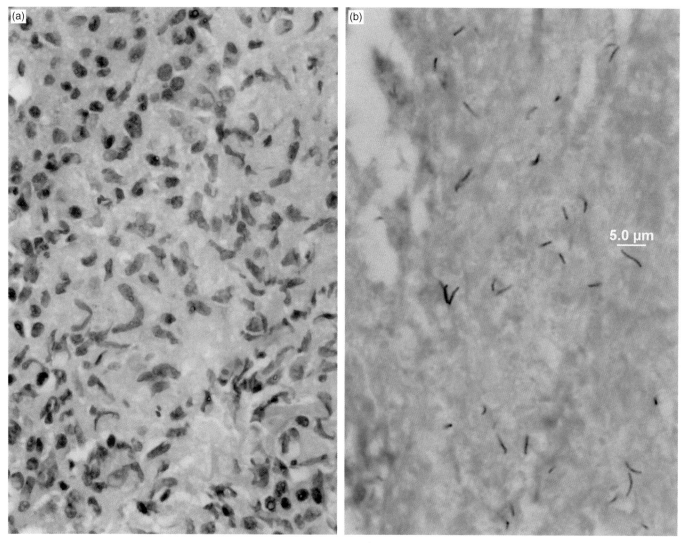

Figure 2.8. Ill-defined granulomatous inflammation in culture-positive tuberculosis. (a) This granulomatous infiltrate is poorly formed and easy to miss. **(b)** Numerous acid-fast bacteria (Ziehl-Neelsen stain).

- In the United States, many surgical pathology laboratories shut down and decontaminate cryostats in which potentially infectious tissue has been cut.

Clinical profile

Tuberculosis can occur at any age and affects both sexes. The classic symptoms of advanced, active tuberculosis include fever, chills, night sweats, cough, hemoptysis, profound weight loss, fatigue and cachexia. The onset is typically indolent. The tuberculin skin test, also known as the purified protein derivative (PPD) test or Mantoux test, is usually positive. However, infected individuals may be completely asymptomatic, or can present with a wide range of atypical features including mild self-limited illness, isolated lymphadenopathy and PPD negativity. Individuals with a solitary lung nodule (tuberculoma) tend to be asymptomatic. This type of lesion is presumably the pathologic basis of *latent tuberculosis*, defined as tuberculin skin test positivity (PPD positivity) in the absence of signs or symptoms of active disease.

Miliary tuberculosis, which occurs in debilitated or immunocompromised individuals, is a dreaded form of tuberculosis with a notoriously wide spectrum of atypical clinical manifestations. Although some patients present with fever, cough, dyspnea, lethargy, weight loss or anorexia, pulmonary symptoms and constitutional symptoms are absent in others. Symptoms may appear acutely, or patients may present with acute hypoxemic respiratory failure. A wide variety of laboratory findings, including pancytopenia and leukemoid reactions, can be attributed to extrapulmonary involvement. Elderly individuals with miliary tuberculosis can present with progressive wasting without fever, mimicking malignancy. The tuberculin skin test is frequently negative. Chest radiographs may be normal.

Tuberculosis is a clinical diagnosis, not a histologic one. Ideally, the diagnosis is confirmed by microbiologic identification of *M. tuberculosis* in cultures of sputum, bronchial washings, bronchial brushings, biopsied lung tissue or other tissues. Growth in cultures is well accepted as the gold standard for diagnosis.

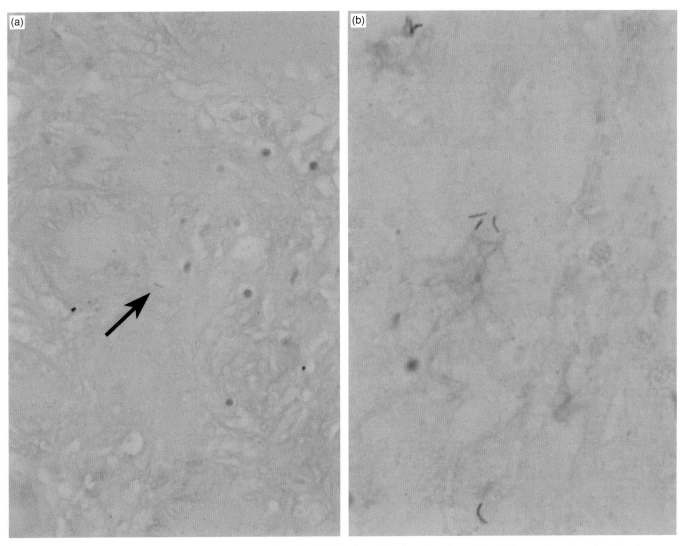

Figure 2.9. Variation in numbers of acid-fast bacteria in tuberculosis. (a) Single acid-fast bacterium (arrow) in a histiocyte adjacent to a Langhans-type giant cell (Ziehl-Neelsen stain, 40x objective). **(b)** Organisms are easier to see in this case, especially with an oil-immersion lens (Ziehl-Neelsen, 100x objective).

However, in practice, tuberculosis is often diagnosed without culture confirmation. The degree of stringency utilized by clinicians in making the diagnosis varies greatly depending on the degree to which tuberculosis is endemic. Even in affluent Western countries in modern times, the diagnosis is often made presumptively without culture confirmation. According to the 2013 United Kingdom annual tuberculosis report, only 60% of cases of tuberculosis diagnosed in the United Kingdom were culture-confirmed. The rate of culture confirmation was 69% in pulmonary tuberculosis and 50% in extrapulmonary tuberculosis. A presumptive diagnosis of tuberculosis is usually based on clinical and radiologic features, tuberculin skin testing, the QuantiFERON® assay (a blood test that measures the release of interferon-gamma in whole blood in response to stimulation by mycobacterial antigens), or adenosine deaminase levels in pleural fluid. The role of the surgical pathologist is to exclude alternative diagnoses, identify granulomatous inflammation, and find AFB. Granulomatous inflammation and acid-fast bacteria can be identified in cytology specimens, transbronchial or endobronchial biopsies, core needle biopsies and surgical lung biopsies.

Radiologic findings

The classic radiologic finding in tuberculosis is an upper lobe cavitary infiltrate with hilar lymphadenopathy. Chest CT shows unilateral or bilateral patchy cavitary consolidation in the upper lung zones with multiple small ill-defined nodules. A range of other radiologic presentations have been described, including unilateral or bilateral nodules, and infiltrates of various types, including cavitary, tree-in-bud (branching linear and nodular opacities indicative of small airway involvement) or miliary. Miliary tuberculosis features innumerable tiny (1 to 3 mm) bilateral nodules randomly distributed throughout the lungs. It is occasionally associated with clinical and radiologic features of the acute respiratory distress syndrome (ARDS).

Other radiologic features in tuberculosis include bronchial wall thickening or narrowing, bronchiectasis and airspace consolidation. Pleural effusions are usually unilateral. Unilateral hilar lymphadenopathy manifesting as a unilateral hilar mass or paratracheal lymphadenopathy is common, especially in children. Central areas of low attenuation within the enlarged nodes are thought to represent necrosis. None of these findings is specific for tuberculosis. Patients with atypical findings such as large masses or atypical infiltrates are less likely to be diagnosed clinically and are consequently more likely to be biopsied.

Differential diagnosis

- Non-tuberculous mycobacterial infection. Differentiation of *M. tuberculosis* from non-tuberculous mycobacteria such as organisms of the *Mycobacterium avium* complex (MAC) is clinically important, since treatment regimens are different. There may also be important implications for respiratory isolation and follow-up. Unfortunately, as detailed in the preceding sections, *M. tuberculosis* and non-tuberculous mycobacteria are histologically indistinguishable. Pathologists should be prepared to have a discussion with their clinicians regarding the fact that mycobacterial speciation is best performed by microbiologic cultures. If, as is often the case, cultures were not performed or are negative, polymerase chain reaction (PCR) assays for *M. tuberculosis* and non-tuberculous mycobacteria can be performed on formalin-fixed paraffin-embedded tissues. In practice, however, this test is unavailable for clinical use in most laboratories. Another problem is that PCR, being highly sensitive, may detect mycobacterial DNA from non-viable organisms. Tissue blocks can be sent to reference labs in difficult cases. In some instances, definitive identification may require a repeat biopsy so that additional material can be submitted for cultures.
- Fungal infections. *Histoplasma, Cryptococcus* and *Coccidioides* can cause necrotizing granulomatous inflammation in the lung histologically indistinguishable from tuberculosis. The distinction rests on identification of the causative organism, either by histology or by cultures.
- Other bacteria such as *Nocardia, Rhodococcus* and *Legionella micdadei* have been reported to be acid-fast. This is rarely a problem in practice, since these organisms are uncommon, do not cause necrotizing granulomas and are morphologically distinctive. *Nocardia* is a long, slender, filamentous organism that causes mixed neutrophilic-histiocytic inflammatory infiltrates but not true granulomas. *Rhodococcus* is a tiny coccobacillus seen in the rare condition known as malakoplakia; necrotizing granulomas are not a feature.
- Granulomatosis with polyangiitis (GPA, Wegener's granulomatosis). Necrotizing granulomatous inflammation is a key histologic feature of GPA. In most cases, the granulomas are distinctive, with irregular ("geographic") contours, "dirty" necrosis rich in neutrophils and small palisaded suppurative granulomas resembling microabscesses. However, similar features can also be seen in granulomatous infections, including tuberculosis. Non-necrotizing lymphocytic infiltrates can be seen within vessel walls in tuberculosis as well as in GPA. The histologic features that most reliably separate the two entities are necrotizing vasculitis (seen in GPA but not in infections)

and necrotizing granulomas in lymph nodes (seen in infections but not in GPA). Of course, identification of organisms will settle the issue. In cases that are difficult to resolve by histology, results of cultures or anti-neutrophil cytoplasmic antibody (ANCA) testing can be helpful.
- Sarcoidosis is usually easy to distinguish from tuberculosis since the granulomas are non-necrotizing. However, there is scope for overlap, since necrosis is occasionally seen in sarcoidosis. The necrosis in such cases is usually focal and minimal. Extensive necrosis should prompt careful examination of special stains and should not be labeled as "necrotizing sarcoidosis" unless cultures are negative. The diagnosis of *necrotizing sarcoid granulomatosis* should be reserved for the rare cases in which necrosis is present in a background of otherwise typical non-necrotizing granulomas, along with negative stains and cultures, in a surgical lung biopsy. The presence of hyalinized fibrosis or a lymphangitic distribution of the granulomas favors sarcoidosis. Identification of an organism excludes sarcoidosis.

Treatment and prognosis

Treatment of tuberculosis requires multi-drug anti-tubercular therapy for several months. The most commonly used drugs are isoniazid (INH), rifampicin (rifampin), streptomycin, ethambutol and pyrazinamide. The World Health Organization (WHO) currently recommends a 6-month regimen in immunocompetent individuals involving four drugs (INH, rifampicin, ethambutol, pyrazinamide) for 2 months, followed by two drugs (INH and rifampicin) for 4 months. Directly observed therapy (DOT) is ideal for monitoring compliance. However, the precise regimen used depends on the patient's immune status and the presence of symptoms. INH monotherapy is recommended for latent tuberculosis. Immunocompromised individuals such as those with HIV/AIDS require therapy for a longer duration. Multi-drug-resistant (MDR) and extensively drug-resistant (XDR) tuberculosis are increasingly significant clinical problems but are seldom relevant for surgical pathologists.

Tuberculosis is responsive to appropriate therapy, with a cure rate of approximately 90% in HIV-negative patients. In the United Kingdom, only 5% of patients diagnosed in 2011 died within 12 months. The prognosis depends on the extent of disease, the organs involved and the degree of compliance to therapy. Cure rates are lower in drug-resistant tuberculosis. The mortality of miliary tuberculosis is very high, ranging from 57% to 89%.

Sample diagnosis on pathology report

Lung, right upper lobe, transbronchial biopsy – Necrotizing granulomatous inflammation (few mycobacteria present) (See comment).

or

Lung, right middle lobe, endobronchial biopsy – Necrotizing granulomatous inflammation (numerous acid-fast bacteria present) (See comment).

Non-tuberculous mycobacterial infection

The term *non-tuberculous mycobacteria* (NTM) is currently used for mycobacterial organisms other than *M. tuberculosis*. In the past, these organisms have been referred to as "atypical mycobacteria" or "mycobacteria other than tuberculosis (MOTT)". In pulmonary granulomas, the most common organisms of this group are *M. avium* and *M. intracellulare*, once grouped together as *M. avium–intracellulare* (MAI) and now referred to as *M. avium* complex (MAC). Other common species isolated from respiratory tract specimens in the United States are *M. kansasii* and *M. abscessus*. Other less common species include *M. chelonae*, *M. fortuitum*, *M. scrofulaceum*, *M. xenopi*, *M. microti*, *M. porcinum* and *M. llatzerense*.

Most pathologists and clinicians instinctively associate granulomatous inflammation in the lung (especially necrotizing granulomas) with tuberculosis. Non-tuberculous mycobacteria are seldom considered in the differential diagnosis, especially outside the setting of HIV/AIDS. Reasons for the lack of inclusion of non-tuberculous mycobacteria in the differential diagnosis of granulomatous lung disease include the strong historic emphasis on tuberculosis, the prominence accorded to tuberculosis in classic textbooks, the highly infectious, high-profile nature of tuberculosis, lingering doubts in the minds of many clinicians regarding the pathogenic potential of non-tuberculous mycobacteria (they are ubiquitous in the environment, especially in natural or treated water), the difficulty in distinguishing contamination from true infection, the low virulence and pathogenicity of non-tuberculous mycobacteria compared to *M. tuberculosis*, and confusing changes in nomenclature over the years. Perhaps the most important factor that leads to under-recognition of non-tuberculous mycobacteria in granulomatous lung disease is the strong historic link between HIV/AIDS and non-tuberculous mycobacterial disease. A combination of these factors obscures the fact that these organisms frequently cause significant granulomatous lung disease in immunocompetent hosts.

Non-tuberculous mycobacterial infections may be encountered in transbronchial lung biopsies, endobronchial biopsies and core needle biopsies, or may be seen in larger specimens such as surgical lung biopsies or even explant pneumonectomies. Larger samples increase the likelihood of finding an organism.

Major diagnostic findings

- Necrotizing granulomatous inflammation. Well-formed classic necrotizing granulomas identical to tuberculosis are common in non-tuberculous mycobacterial infections (Figure 2.10). Several studies have demonstrated that such granulomas can be positive for non-tuberculous mycobacteria by microbiologic cultures, PCR or both. A radiologically solitary nodule may correspond to a large solitary necrotizing granuloma or the confluence of multiple small necrotizing granulomas. As in tuberculosis, each necrotizing granuloma is composed of a zone of central necrosis surrounded by one or more layers of epithelioid histiocytes. The necrosis may be pink ("caseous") or basophilic ("dirty"). Multinucleated giant cells, Langhans-type or foreign-body type, may be present in the granulomatous rim. In older lesions, the granulomatous periphery may be difficult to recognize as it is gradually replaced by fibrosis.

- Organisms may be demonstrable within the necrotic centers of the granulomas by AFB stains, but many cases are negative. It is well documented that cases negative for organisms by histology can be culture-positive, and vice versa. Indeed, in practice cultures are often diagnostic in stain-negative cases.

- Non-necrotizing granulomas are common in non-tuberculous mycobacterial infections, especially in lung parenchyma adjacent to necrotizing granulomas. The granulomas can be well-formed, mimicking sarcoidosis. However, they lack the concentric layers of hyalinized, "cracked" fibrosis usually seen in sarcoidosis. Instead, they are often associated with dense chronic inflammation or embedded within fibromyxoid plugs of organizing pneumonia, an appearance that has been termed *organizing granulomatous pneumonia* (Figure 2.11). The presence of organizing pneumonia in association with granulomas argues strongly against sarcoidosis.

- The granulomas of non-tuberculous mycobacterial infection can be small and poorly formed, and may be present in the walls of densely inflamed bronchioles, mimicking hypersensitivity pneumonitis. The granulomas may contain non-specific endogenous inclusions similar to those seen in sarcoidosis, such as polarizable calcium oxalate crystals. Organisms are seldom found in histologic specimens in such cases, although we have seen rare examples in which AFB were detectable in detached fragments of acute inflammatory exudate presumably originating from an airway lumen. Definitive diagnosis and speciation of non-tuberculous mycobacteria requires microbiologic cultures.

- The image that most pathologists associate with non-tuberculous mycobacterial infection is that of *M. avium-intracellulare* infection in HIV/AIDS patients. This form of the infection is characterized by sheets of foamy and/or epithelioid histiocytes laden with innumerable organisms (Figure 2.12). This histologic picture, most prevalent at the peak of the HIV/AIDS epidemic in the late twentieth century prior to the introduction of HAART, is no longer common in lung biopsies.

Variable pathologic findings

- Non-necrotizing granulomas may be found within the lumens of respiratory bronchioles, alveolar ducts and airspaces (contrast to hot tub lung, page 105 of this chapter).

- Organizing pneumonia is common at the periphery of granulomatous inflammation in non-tuberculous mycobacterial infection. It is characterized by plugs of

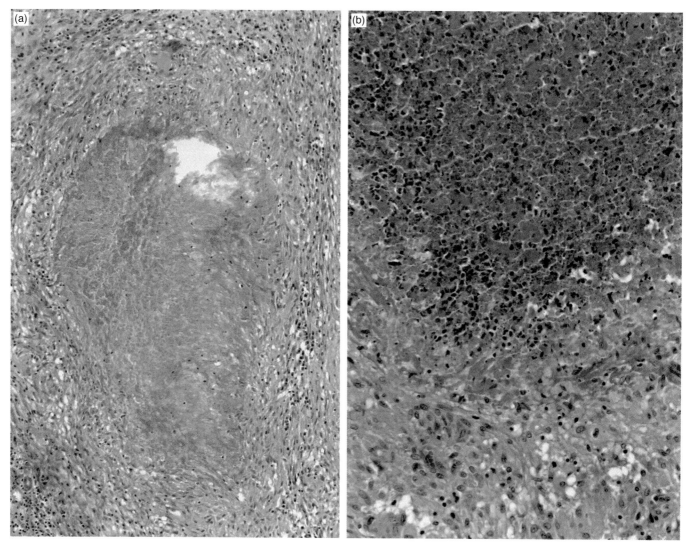

Figure 2.10. Necrotizing granulomas in non-tuberculous mycobacterial infection. PCR on this surgical lung biopsy was negative for *M. tuberculosis* but positive for *M. intracellulare*. A sputum sample subsequently grew *M. chelonae-abscessus*. **(a)** A necrotizing granuloma from the case shows pink necrosis, identical to tuberculosis. **(b)** Another necrotizing granuloma from the same case shows "dirty" necrosis rich in nuclear debris.

fibroblasts within a pale-staining matrix. The plugs often have a snake-like configuration because they fill airspaces as they extend from one alveolus to the next.

- Non-specific chronic bronchitis and bronchiolitis may be a prominent finding in some cases. It is characterized by an inflammatory infiltrate composed mainly of lymphocytes within the walls of bronchi and bronchioles. There may be associated bronchiolar dilatation. Mucin with admixed acute inflammatory exudates may be present within the lumens. Ulceration of the airway epithelium may occur. The surrounding lung may show post-obstructive changes such as organizing pneumonia and sheets of foamy macrophages. A clue to the diagnosis in such cases is the presence of an occasional granuloma within the inflammatory infiltrate in the airway walls. In contrast to hypersensitivity pneumonitis, the infiltrate does not extend significantly into the alveolar septa (interstitium).
- Spindle cell pseudotumors have been reported in HIV-positive patients. This histologic picture is not pathognomonic, since it can also occur in tuberculosis in immunosuppressed patients.
- As in other infections, necrotizing granulomas may develop microcalcifications.
- Histiocytes laden with carbonaceous black dust may accumulate at the periphery of necrotizing granulomas.
- Fibrous or fibroelastotic parenchymal scars may be found adjacent to granulomas. These presumably represent burnt-out granulomatous inflammation.

Diagnostic work-up

- Acid-fast stains. The Ziehl–Neelsen stain is most commonly used. As with tuberculosis, special stains on histologic material can be negative in culture-positive cases, and cultures may be negative in stain-positive cases. In some cases, tissue may not have been submitted for cultures.
- As in tuberculosis, non-tuberculous mycobacteria can be GMS-positive (Figure 2.13).

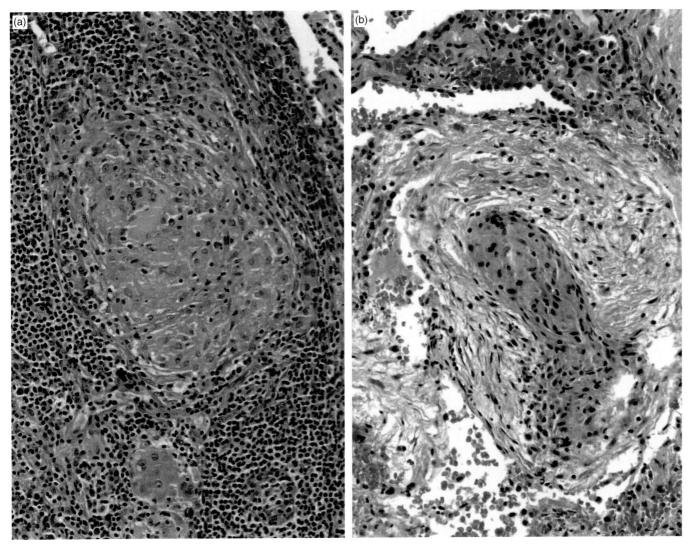

Figure 2.11. Non-necrotizing granulomas in non-tuberculous mycobacterial infection. Same case as Figure 2.10. **(a)** Well-formed non-necrotizing granuloma, similar to sarcoidosis. **(b)** Non-necrotizing granuloma embedded within a plug of organizing pneumonia. This finding is also seen in other granulomatous infections, particulate matter aspiration and hot tub lung, but argues strongly against sarcoidosis.

- The most important criterion for the diagnosis of a non-tuberculous mycobacterial infection is the exclusion of tuberculosis, best accomplished by isolating and identifying non-tuberculous mycobacteria by microbiologic techniques. Non-tuberculous mycobacteria are commonly isolated and speciated in cultures of respiratory tract specimens such as sputum (at least three samples are recommended), bronchial washings, bronchoalveolar lavage, lung biopsies and lung resections. The most common organism by far is *Mycobacterium avium-intracellulare* (MAI), currently known as *Mycobacterium avium* complex (MAC). Since non-tuberculous mycobacteria are common in the environment (especially water), the clinical question is often whether the organisms are causative or merely contaminants. There is no easy answer to this question, but clinical criteria to aid in this issue are available (Griffith *et al* (2007)). As in tuberculosis, the role of histology is to exclude malignancy, identify granulomatous inflammation, and find organisms on acid-fast stains. For a complete discussion on

examination of acid-fast stains and mycobacterial speciation, see the preceding section on tuberculosis.
- PCR for mycobacteria on formalin-fixed paraffin-embedded specimens is very helpful, and may be the only way to speciate organisms when cultures are negative. This test is available only in a few specialized laboratories in large centers, destroys the paraffin block, and has a long turnaround time (1 to 2 weeks or longer). Some laboratories differentiate between *M. tuberculosis* and non-tuberculous mycobacteria but do not speciate the latter, whereas others perform speciation. Results do not always correlate with cultures, which remain the gold standard.

Clinical profile

Non-tuberculous mycobacterial infection can occur at any age and involve either gender. The most common symptoms are cough and shortness of breath. Many cases seen by surgical pathologists are discovered incidentally in asymptomatic

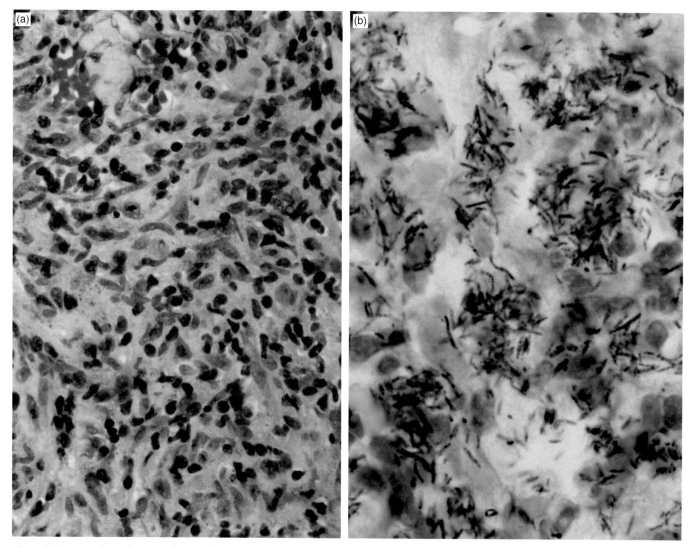

Figure 2.12. Non-tuberculous mycobacterial infection in HIV/AIDS (*M. avium* grew in cultures). (a) Inflammatory infiltrate composed of sheets of histiocytes and lymphocytes. Some of the histiocytes are epithelioid, but well-formed granulomas are absent. **(b)** Innumerable acid-fast bacteria within histiocytes (Ziehl–Neelsen stain).

individuals or in persons being investigated for unrelated symptoms. The archetypal phenotype of an immunocompetent individual with a non-tuberculous mycobacterial infection is that of a tall and lean middle-aged or elderly woman with low body mass index, kyphoscoliosis, pectus excavatum and mitral valve prolapse. These women may have mutations of the cystic fibrosis transmembrane regulator (CFTR). The risk of pulmonary non-tuberculous mycobacterial disease is also high in individuals with underlying chronic respiratory disease, particularly chronic obstructive pulmonary disease (COPD) on inhaled corticosteroids. The typical immunocompromised individual with non-tuberculous mycobacterial infection is an HIV-positive patient with AIDS and a low CD4 count.

Radiologic findings

The most common radiologic findings in non-tuberculous mycobacterial infections are multiple small nodules (often centrilobular and bilateral) with or without cavitation, multifocal bronchiectasis, small airway disease characterized by centrilobular or "tree-in-bud" opacities, or multiple nodules in the right middle lobe or lingula. The findings can mimic tuberculosis, especially when the causative agent is *M. kansasii*. Some cases present with a solid or cavitary solitary lung nodule. Lung nodules caused by non-tuberculous mycobacteria can occur in smokers, rapidly increase in size, and be PET-positive, mimicking malignancy. The presence of waxing and waning nodules is a clue to a benign diagnosis.

Differential diagnosis

* Tuberculosis is the main consideration in the differential diagnosis when acid-fast bacteria are identified in a pulmonary granuloma. Although there are many differences between tuberculosis and non-tuberculous infection in terms of epidemiology, pathogenesis and virulence, for practical purposes in an individual case, tuberculosis is indistinguishable from non-tuberculous infection on histologic grounds. As mentioned in the section on tuberculosis, morphologic differences between

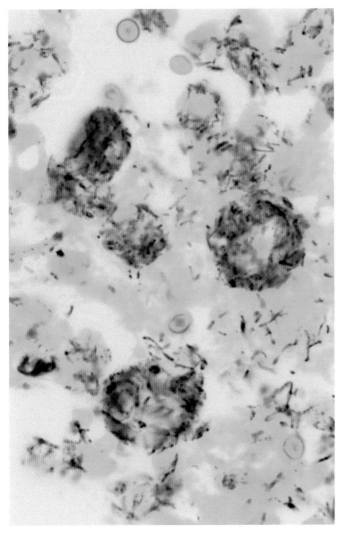

Figure 2.13. GMS staining in non-tuberculous mycobacterial infection. The mycobacteria are GMS-positive. Same case as Figure 2.12.

M. tuberculosis and non-tuberculous mycobacteria have been described in the setting of AFB-stained smears prepared from positive cultures, but they have never been shown to be valid on AFB-stained tissue sections. The only definitive means of separating *M. tuberculosis* and non-tuberculous mycobacteria are microbiologic cultures, or PCR on formalin-fixed paraffin-embedded tissue. For further details, please see the section on tuberculosis.

- Fungal infections such as histoplasmosis or coccidioidomycosis can cause granulomas identical to non-tuberculous mycobacterial infection. Identification of AFB or fungi settles the issue in most cases.
- Sarcoidosis can be difficult to differentiate from non-tuberculous mycobacterial infection because non-necrotizing granulomas may occur in both. The distinction can be especially challenging in small biopsies. The presence of hyalinized fibrosis or granulomas distributed along peri-lymphatic routes favors sarcoidosis. Features that favor an infectious etiology include necrosis, granulomas within airspaces and granulomas embedded within organizing pneumonia.

Treatment and prognosis

Treatment of non-tuberculous mycobacterial infection of the lung is not trivial, and differs significantly from regimens used for tuberculosis. Immunocompetent individuals are treated with a multi-drug regimen (typically two or three antimicrobials) for at least 12 months. The most commonly used drugs for *M. avium* complex-related lung disease are macrolides (clarithromycin or azithromycin), ethambutol and rifamycin. Treatment is associated with considerable toxicity and compliance can be an issue. Rifampin-containing regimens have been shown to be effective for the treatment of *M. kansasii*. There are no drug regimens with proven efficacy for *M. abscessus*. A special situation with particular relevance to surgical pathologists is that of a solitary lung nodule that is resected to rule out malignancy and found to be a necrotizing granuloma containing non-tuberculous mycobacteria. In such cases, it is thought that surgical resection is curative without antibiotic therapy, provided that there is no evidence of MAC-related disease elsewhere in the lungs radiologically.

Other than solitary lung nodules, which have an excellent prognosis, the outcome of non-tuberculous mycobacterial pulmonary disease is poor. The overall cumulative death rate is 34%. Untreated disseminated MAC disease is a life-threatening condition, with a 1-year survival rate of 13% without therapy.

Sample diagnosis on pathology report

Lung, right middle lobe, surgical biopsy – Necrotizing granulomatous inflammation (mycobacteria present) (See comment).

Histoplasmosis

Histoplasmosis is the most common cause of necrotizing granulomas of the lung in large swaths of the United States. Well-known endemic areas include several states along the Ohio and Mississippi river valleys, but the infection is also common in lesser known regions such as the St. Lawrence River Valley in northern New York State. The causative agent is the dimorphic fungus *Histoplasma capsulatum*. The term dimorphic refers to the formation of yeasts in tissue and hyphae in cultures. Other *Histoplasma* species have been described but are rare.

Histoplasmosis is acquired by inhalation of spores into the lungs from the environment. Initial infection is often asymptomatic but occasionally causes a flu-like illness of variable severity known as *acute pulmonary histoplasmosis*. In immunocompetent individuals, the organisms are eventually destroyed or rendered non-viable by necrotizing granulomatous inflammation, and may be contained within localized granulomatous foci that represent the residuum of past infection. The high incidence of asymptomatic infection and spontaneously resolving mild acute pulmonary histoplasmosis explains why most patients have no recollection of an antecedent illness. When localized foci of walled-off infection form tumor-like nodules in the lung, the term *histoplasmoma* can be used. As in the Ghon complex of tuberculosis, organisms frequently drain from the lung to hilar or mediastinal lymph nodes, resulting in the formation of necrotizing granulomas in those locations.

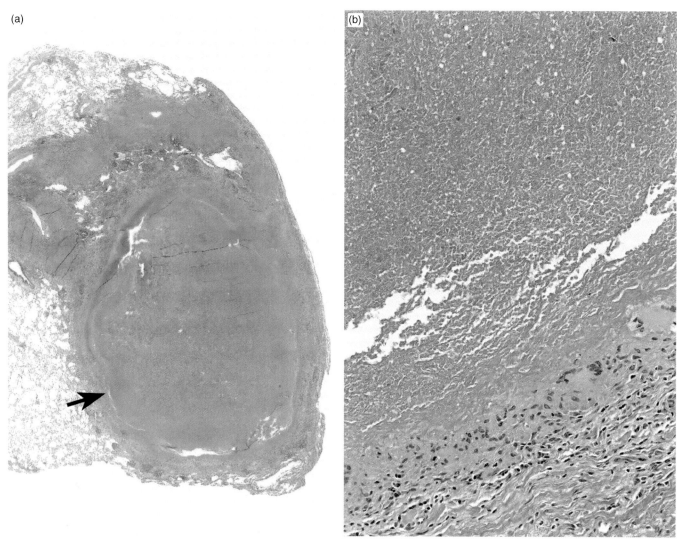

Figure 2.14. Pulmonary histoplasmoma. (a) Typical necrotizing granuloma. The lesion was surgically resected to rule out a neoplasm. The area indicated by the arrow is flipped 90 degrees counterclockwise and shown at high magnification in **(b)**. Note the pink necrosis at the top and the granulomatous rim composed of epithelioid histiocytes at the bottom.

The clinical form of histoplasmosis known as *chronic pulmonary histoplasmosis* is currently defined subjectively on the basis of symptoms "compatible with pulmonary histoplasmosis" occurring for 6 weeks or greater, along with microbiologic or serologic evidence of histoplasmosis. Pathology is seldom required for diagnosis. The pathologic features are not well described, especially in the modern era, and it is unclear whether the findings differ from those of histoplasmomas.

The most dreaded form of histoplasmosis occurs in immunocompromised hosts, in whom the initial infection progresses unchecked and disseminates within macrophages to extrapulmonary tissues in a well-known syndrome known as *disseminated histoplasmosis*.

Major diagnostic findings

• Necrotizing granulomatous inflammation is the hallmark of pulmonary histoplasmosis in immunocompetent individuals. Most cases manifest as solitary or multiple lung nodules. The term *histoplasmoma* refers to the fact that

these lesions may mimic a neoplasm radiologically. Such nodules are thus commonly biopsied or resected to rule out malignancy, and represent the most common form of histoplasmosis seen by surgical pathologists in the United States. The typical necrotizing granuloma of histoplasmosis is a well-demarcated nodule with a large zone of central necrosis surrounded by a relatively thin rim of epithelioid histiocytes and variable numbers of multinucleated giant cells (Figure 2.14). The necrosis is usually eosinophilic but may be "dirty", especially at the edges. Suppurative necrosis is uncommon. Both Langhans-type and foreign-body-type giant cells may be present. Similar necrotizing granulomas may be found in the draining hilar lymph nodes. The overall histologic picture is remarkably similar to tuberculosis.

• In necrotizing granulomas, *Histoplasma* yeasts are invariably located within the necrotic center but cannot be seen on H&E. Organisms are typically absent in histiocytes in the granulomatous rim. The concept that *Histoplasma* is

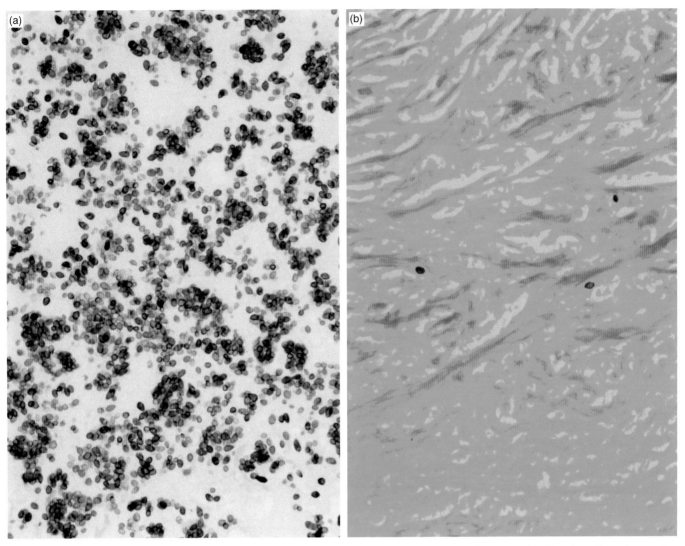

Figure 2.15. *Histoplasma* yeasts on GMS. **(a)** Numerous yeasts are seen in this example of a necrotizing granuloma caused by *Histoplasma* (histoplasmoma). They are small, uniform, round to oval, and often have tapered ends. Narrow-based budding is present. **(b)** Only three yeasts are seen in this example. This type of case can be easily missed at low magnification. The tapered shape and small, uniform size facilitates the diagnosis.

an intracellular organism is therefore misleading in this setting, and can lead to misdiagnosis. Visualization of *Histoplasma* in a necrotic background requires GMS staining, where the organisms appear as small, uniform, oval yeasts that are often tapered at one or both ends (Figure 2.15). Occasional narrow-based budding is characteristic but not pathognomonic since it is also a feature of *Cryptococcus*. Budding may not be identifiable when organisms are few in number, as is often the case (Figure 2.15). The morphologic features of the yeasts are best appreciated at high magnification, using a 40× objective. Measuring the sizes of fungal yeasts is not practical with most standard microscopes. Having said this, it is important to recognize that *Histoplasma* yeasts are the smallest of the four major fungi that cause necrotizing granulomas in the lung. It is usually 3 μm in size, with a range of 1 to 5 μm.

- Disseminated histoplasmosis is the best known form of the disease, but unlike the necrotizing granulomas described

above, it is a rare finding in lung biopsies and resections. It occurs mainly in immunocompromised hosts. A pathognomonic feature of this form of the disease is the presence of numerous enlarged histiocytes engorged with large numbers of fungal yeasts. In contrast to necrotizing granulomas, the organisms in disseminated histoplasmosis are easily seen on H&E within the cytoplasm of the infected histiocytes. With a 40× objective lens, the organisms appear as tiny dots or rings, but greater detail becomes apparent under oil immersion, where an eccentric dot or crescent can be seen within each ring-shaped yeast form (Figure 2.16). This is the classic morphology of histoplasmosis that Samuel Darling described in 1906 and that the literature has referred to ever since as "intracellular yeasts". Granulomas are typically absent in the lung in disseminated histoplasmosis, but may be present in some cases. Other histologic findings include tiny ill-defined nodular lymphohistiocytic infiltrates, poorly formed non-necrotizing granulomas within airspaces (Figure 2.17)

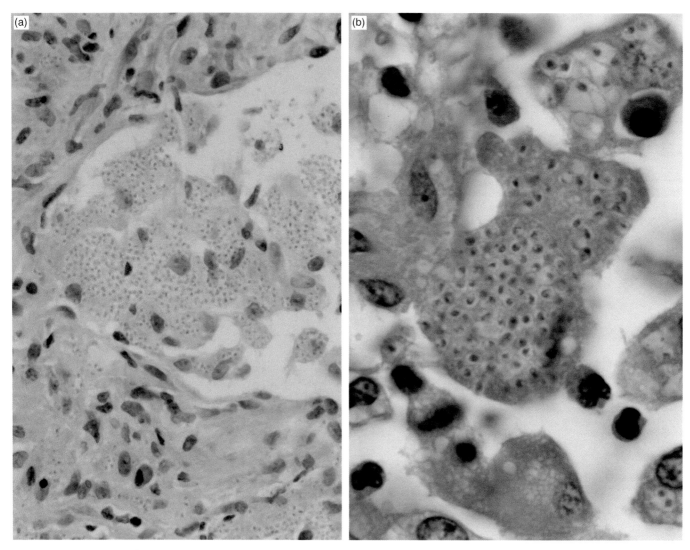

Figure 2.16. Disseminated histoplasmosis involving the lung. (a) With a 40x objective lens, the organisms appear as numerous tiny dots or rings within histiocytes. **(b)** Under oil immersion, an eccentric dot or crescent is usually visible within each ring.

and palisaded histiocytes rimming irregular zones of necrosis. The presence of *Histoplasma*-laden histiocytes within which organisms are readily visible on H&E is the only pathognomonic feature of disseminated histoplasmosis. The value of this finding is that it allows a diagnosis of disseminated disease on a lung biopsy several days before clinical or microbiologic evidence of extrapulmonary involvement becomes evident. The organism-laden histiocytes may be only focally present and difficult to find. In some cases, they may be absent.

Variable pathologic findings

- Necrotizing granulomas containing *Histoplasma* yeasts are commonly found in mediastinal, hilar and peribronchial lymph nodes, either incidentally during pathologic examination of lymph nodes in lobectomy or pneumonectomy specimens for lung cancer, or in the course of mediastinal staging for lung cancer. The histologic appearance is identical to necrotizing granulomas in the lung (Figure 2.18).

- Non-specific chronic inflammation is common around the main necrotizing granuloma. The inflammatory cells are predominantly lymphocytes but plasma cells are also common. The inflammatory infiltrate may be located within the walls of bronchioles, alveolar septa or airspaces. Importantly, blood vessels may show a lymphocytic infiltrate in the media or even the intima. This type of secondary lymphocytic vasculitis is a common finding in histoplasmosis and other mycobacterial and fungal granulomatous infections, and should not be mistaken for a true primary vasculitis such as granulomatosis with polyangiitis (Wegener's).

- As in other infections, there may occasionally be plugs of fibroblasts within airspaces (organizing pneumonia) surrounding the main necrotizing granuloma.

- Dense bundles of hyalinized collagen arranged in a lamellated pattern are often present at the periphery of necrotizing granulomas caused by *Histoplasma*, especially in hilar and mediastinal lymph nodes (Figure 2.18). As the necrotizing granulomas "burn out", dense hyalinized

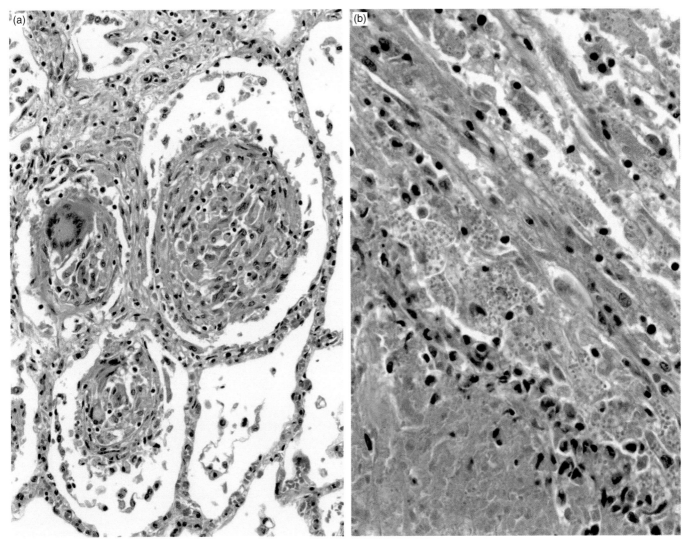

Figure 2.17. Granulomas in the lung in disseminated histoplasmosis. (a) Granulomas are present within airspaces in this example of disseminated histoplasmosis encountered at autopsy. **(b)** Section from an adrenal gland from the same case, showing characteristic histiocytes laden with *Histoplasma* yeasts. The organisms are clearly visible on H&E. No *Histoplasma*-laden histiocytes were identified in the lungs.

fibrosis eventually replaces the granulomatous infiltrate, leaving behind a residual mass of fibrosis and chronic inflammation. The end-result of this process in the hilar and mediastinal region is known as sclerosing mediastinitis (fibrosing mediastinitis) (Figure 2.19). The term is somewhat misleading since it implies that the lesion is primarily inflammatory when in fact the defining feature is fibrosis. The lesion is characterized by lamellated bundles of dense hyalinized collagen with a characteristic "cracked" appearance. Although fibrosis predominates, variable numbers of lymphocytes and plasma cells are often present (Figure 2.19). In some cases, lymphoid aggregates, numerous plasma cells or eosinophils may be seen. Nerves and blood vessels may be entrapped within the dense fibrosis (Figure 2.20). The antecedent necrotizing granulomas are identifiable in some but not all cases. In the absence of necrotizing granulomas, there are no organisms. Cultures are invariably negative.

- Calcification and ossification. The necrotic centers of *Histoplasma* granulomas frequently contain microcalcifications. These tiny pleomorphic basophilic structures are commonly misinterpreted as fungi on H&E, but a negative GMS stain easily refutes this impression. Occasionally, very old *Histoplasma* nodules can be extensively calcified or ossified. Surprisingly, organisms can occasionally be demonstrated on GMS even within completely calcified lesions that harbor no trace of residual necrosis or granulomatous inflammation. As with the vast majority of necrotizing granulomas in the lung in immunocompetent hosts, the organisms in such lesions are non-viable and culture-negative.

- Acute pulmonary histoplasmosis is rarely seen by pathologists since it is usually diagnosed on clinical grounds. The histologic features have been described in a recent small series of surgical lung biopsies. The findings are more pneumonia-like than histoplasmomas, i.e., the alveoli are filled with an inflammatory infiltrate composed

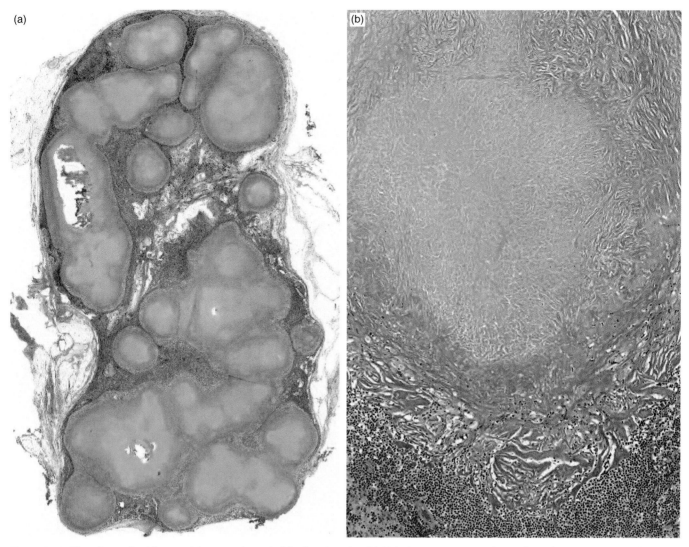

Figure 2.18. Histoplasmosis with necrotizing granulomas in hilar lymph nodes. (a) Multiple necrotizing granulomas identical to "caseating granulomas" of tuberculosis. *Histoplasma* yeasts were identified within the necrosis on GMS (not shown). **(b)** Higher magnification of one of the granulomas shows a necrotic center (top) and an ill-defined granulomatous rim merging into dense lamellar hyalinized fibrosis (bottom).

of lymphocytes, histiocytes and fibrin. Adjacent alveolar septa are also expanded by the infiltrate. The infiltrate may form multiple tiny nodules or a single large nodular mass. Within this background, there are occasional tiny foci of parenchymal necrosis, large zones of parenchymal necrosis or palisaded necrotizing granulomas (Figure 2.21). *Histoplasma* yeasts can be found within the necrotic areas, and may be numerous. Severe lymphocytic vasculitis is common and may be sufficiently striking so as to mimic lymphomatoid granulomatosis (Figures 2.21 and 2.22). Misinterpretation can be avoided by careful examination of GMS-stained slides.

- Diffuse alveolar damage has been described in disseminated histoplasmosis. In such cases, a clue to the correct diagnosis is the presence of patchy lymphohistiocytic infiltrates or enlarged histiocytes. The diagnosis of disseminated histoplasmosis is confirmed by the identification of *Histoplasma*-laden histiocytes on H&E. As is the case with other fungal infections, far

greater numbers of organisms become apparent on GMS staining.

Diagnostic work-up

- Grocott methenamine silver (GMS) stain. As *Histoplasma* organisms may be few in number and present in some granulomas but not in others, it is important to stain multiple blocks. Staining two to three blocks is adequate in most cases. The features of *Histoplasma* on GMS are described in detail in the previous section. It is important to remember that GMS also stains mucin and dust particles. This is a frequent source of difficulty for those inexperienced with the organism. Dust particles are smaller, darker and more pleomorphic than *Histoplasma* yeasts. They also lack the characteristic tapered shape and budding.
- Periodic acid-Schiff (PAS) is a fairly good fungal stain in general, but is unreliable for identifying *Histoplasma*. In general, GMS is superior to PAS for this purpose. PAS

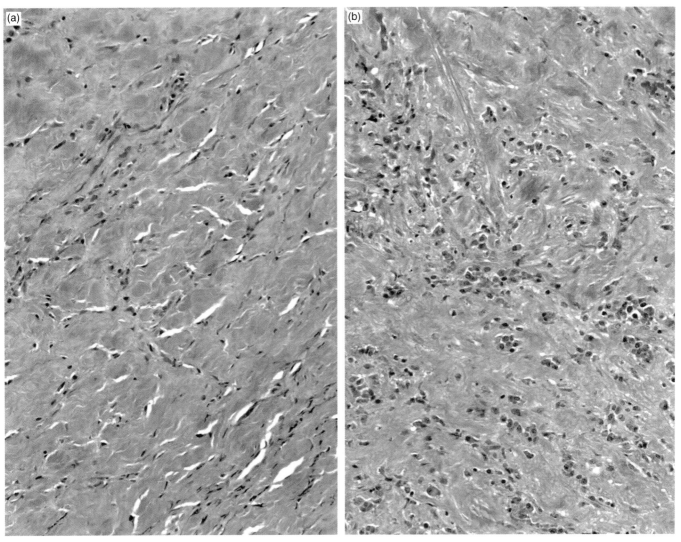

Figure 2.19. Sclerosing mediastinitis (fibrosing mediastinitis) caused by histoplasmosis. (a) Dense bundles of paucicellular eosinophilic hyalinized collagen with a lamellated appearance are seen in this biopsy of a mediastinal mass in a young man. Necrotizing granulomas containing *Histoplasma* were identified in a concurrent lung biopsy, and also in other areas in the mediastinal lymph nodes. **(b)** This area from the same case contains several plasma cells in addition to dense fibrosis.

staining may be strong in some cases, but in others *Histoplasma* yeasts stain weakly or may be completely negative. PAS is especially unhelpful in cases where organisms are few in number.

- Histology is the most accurate means – and usually the only means – of definitively diagnosing lung nodules caused by *Histoplasma* since cultures are negative in the majority of cases in this form of histoplasmosis. Serology is helpful only if it is positive. However, serology is often negative in histologically-proven cases. In many cases, serology is not performed since malignancy is the primary clinical consideration. Definitive diagnosis therefore rests on histologic identification of organisms.
- Histology is also helpful in diagnosing the disseminated form of the disease that occurs in the immunocompromised. This form is usually diagnosed clinically by identification of *Histoplasma* by cultures, cytology or histology in extrapulmonary sites in

immunocompromised patients with signs and symptoms of systemic disease. However, some patients present with signs and symptoms of pulmonary disease, prompting lung biopsy. The pathologic finding of organism-laden histiocytes on H&E is highly characteristic of the disseminated form of the disease, and must be reported as such, since cultures often take weeks to become positive.

Clinical profile

The most common form of histoplasmosis seen by surgical pathologists is a solitary lung nodule or mass biopsied or resected to rule out malignancy. This type of nodule can occur at any age, but most cases are seen in adults. In the vast majority, the nodule is discovered incidentally on a radiologic study performed for an unrelated reason such as surveillance for breast cancer or colon cancer. In many cases, a nodule is discovered in the lung base on abdominal imaging. This finding raises concern for a neoplasm (primary or metastatic),

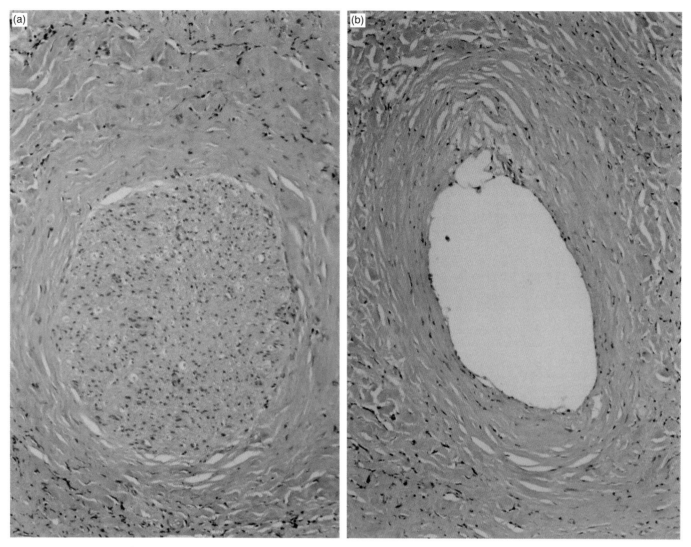

Figure 2.20. Entrapment of nerves and blood vessels in sclerosing mediastinitis (fibrosing mediastinitis). (a) Nerve entrapped in dense hyalinized fibrosis. (b) Entrapped blood vessel.

prompting biopsy or resection. Radiologic studies may be performed for a wide variety of other unrelated conditions, including trauma, abdominal pain and chest pain. Even when imaging is performed for a respiratory complaint, the symptoms are often unrelated to the nodule.

Mediastinal lymph node involvement by histoplasmosis is also common. As with solitary lung nodules, such lesions are typically found incidentally on chest X-rays or CT scans performed for other reasons. When such lesions are found in smokers or in those with a prior history of malignancy, they are likely to be considered suspicious for malignancy on clinical grounds.

Acute pulmonary histoplasmosis presents as an acute flu-like illness. The duration of symptoms varies from a few days to a few weeks. Common presenting symptoms include fever, cough, dyspnea and malaise. Clinical clues to the diagnosis are a history of exposure and the presence of other acutely ill individuals exposed at the same time as the index patient. Activities that predispose to acute pulmonary histoplasmosis include construction, and any pastime or occupation that involves exposure to bat guano, chicken coops, soil or caves (spelunking).

Disseminated histoplasmosis is uncommon. Most patients are immunosuppressed. However, it is well documented that a small proportion of cases occurs in apparently immunocompetent individuals. Common settings in which the disease is seen include HIV/AIDS, organ transplantation and immunosuppressant therapy with corticosteroids or TNF-α inhibitors such as infliximab, adalimumab or etanercept. Patients present with a wide range of non-specific pulmonary and constitutional symptoms such as fever, chills, night sweats, weakness, dyspnea and cough. Most cases are diagnosed on the basis of clinical and radiologic evidence of multi-organ involvement and the demonstration of *Histoplasma* by histology or cultures in an extrapulmonary site such as bone marrow or liver. Since extrapulmonary involvement is a key feature, pathologists are rarely called upon to make this diagnosis in lung specimens. Thrombocytopenia and elevation of hepatic transaminases are clues to the presence of disseminated disease.

The role of microbiologic cultures in the diagnosis of histoplasmosis is well documented but frequently misunderstood. Although cultures have been alluded to in prior sections,

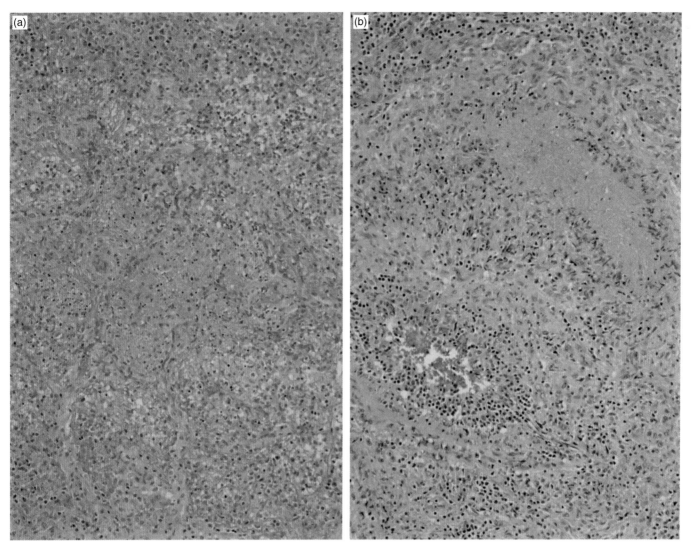

Figure 2.21. Acute pulmonary histoplasmosis. (a) Lymphohistiocytic inflammatory infiltrate with a tiny, poorly demarcated focus of parenchymal necrosis. **(b)** Lymphohistiocytic inflammatory infiltrate with a tiny palisaded necrotizing granuloma (top right) and an inflamed blood vessel (bottom left).

several points are worth re-emphasizing. Microbiologic cultures, if positive, are the gold standard for fungal identification. However, cultures can be negative in every form of histoplasmosis, the yield varying on the form of disease. Even in disseminated histoplasmosis, where cultures are of high yield, up to 60% of cases can be negative. Cultures are almost invariably negative in solitary necrotizing granulomas of the lung in which organisms are found by histology, supporting the contention that the organisms are non-viable in this setting. Mediastinal histoplasmosis is also usually culture-negative. Acute pulmonary histoplasmosis may be culture-positive, but some cases are negative. In many cases of histoplasmosis seen by pathologists, tissue is not submitted for cultures. *Histoplasma* is a notoriously slow-growing fungus, taking several weeks (usually 1 to 5 weeks) to grow in cultures. Therefore, in most cases, pathologists will see this organism several days to weeks before culture results become available, and should be prepared to make a diagnosis in the absence of culture results. In disseminated histoplasmosis, timely identification of *Histoplasma* by pathologists allows initiation of potentially life-saving anti-fungal therapy.

Radiologic findings

The most common radiologic finding that prompts biopsy or resection in histoplasmosis is a solitary lung nodule or mass. This represents a localized focus of walled-off histoplasmosis in the lung (necrotizing granuloma/ histoplasmoma) and is usually seen in immunocompetent individuals. Multiple nodules are also common. Tiny satellite nodules are often present around a dominant solitary nodule. The nodule may grow in size, prompting concern for malignancy. On the other hand, a decrease in size, or a waxing and waning course favors a benign interpretation. Other radiologic features of *Histoplasma* granulomas that raise concern for malignancy include cavitation, spiculated borders, abnormal uptake on positron emission tomography (PET) and PET-positive hilar lymph node enlargement. Doxtader *et al* (2010) reported positive PET scans in 36% of lung nodules that underwent core needle biopsy and were confirmed to be necrotizing granulomas. We have seen standardized uptake values (SUV) as high as 7.8 in histologically confirmed histoplasmomas of the lung. Although

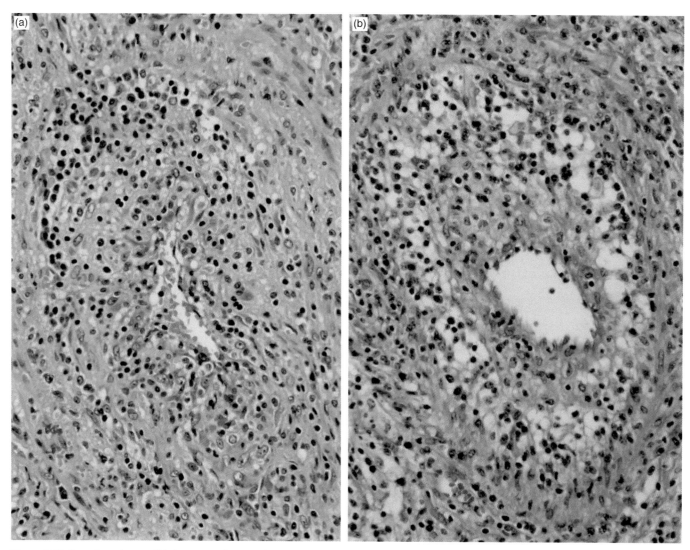

Figure 2.22. Lymphocytic vasculitis in acute pulmonary histoplasmosis. (a) Striking lymphocytic infiltrate within the wall of a blood vessel. **(b)** Numerous lymphocytes expand the media and intima of this pulmonary artery, mimicking lymphomatoid granulomatosis.

many nodules are correctly identified as granulomas by radiologists on the basis of slow growth, calcification and hilar adenopathy, it is the enlarging, non-calcified nodules that are most likely to be biopsied.

Histoplasmosis involving hilar or mediastinal lymph nodes presents as hilar or mediastinal masses or adenopathy, commonly found on imaging performed for other reasons.

Acute pulmonary histoplasmosis is characterized radiologically by bilateral reticulonodular infiltrates. Solitary lung masses have also been reported.

Radiologic findings in disseminated histoplasmosis involving the lungs include diffuse bilateral reticulonodular infiltrates, bilateral airspace opacities, centrilobular nodules, and bilateral hilar and mediastinal adenopathy. Rarely, a solitary nodule may be present in a background of interstitial infiltrates.

Differential diagnosis

- In lung specimens, *Cryptococcus* is the closest mimic of *Histoplasma* (see next section in this chapter). Both are

small yeasts associated with granulomatous inflammation in the lung, and can be found within necrotizing granulomas. The features that help to differentiate the two are visibility on H&E, the shape of the yeasts and uniformity of yeast size (Table 2.2). *Cryptococcus* is usually visible on H&E, both within necrotic areas as well as within histiocytes. The yeasts are round, with considerable size variation. In contrast, *Histoplasma* yeasts cannot be seen within a necrotic background, are oval to tapered, and relatively uniform in size. Mucicarmine is often touted as a useful stain in this situation, but it is commonly negative in *Cryptococcus* in necrotizing granulomas in the lung. The gold standard in difficult cases is growth of the organisms in cultures. However, although *Cryptococcus* may occasionally grow in cultures from lung granulomas, *Histoplasma* seldom does.

- *Pneumocystis* pneumonia seldom enters the differential diagnosis of histoplasmosis, since most cases of the former present as bilateral infiltrates in immunocompromised individuals, while the latter commonly manifests as lung

Table 2.2. Differential diagnosis of the major fungal yeasts and yeast-like fungi found in lung granulomas

	Histoplasma	Cryptococcus	Blastomyces	Coccidioides
Visible on H&E	No (in necrotizing granulomas) Yes (in disseminated histoplasmosis)	Yes	Yes	Yes
Typical morphology of organisms on H&E	Not visible in necrotizing granulomas In disseminated histoplasmosis, numerous small dots within histiocytes at low magnification, tiny rings with eccentric crescent or dot under oil immersion	Round yeasts with light gray cell walls surrounded by a halo	Round yeasts with thick cell wall and basophilic nuclear material	Large thick-walled spherules, filled with endospores or ruptured
Location of organism	Necrotizing granuloma: in necrosis (extracellular) Disseminated histoplasmosis: within histiocytes (intracellular)	Within multinucleated giant cells and histiocytes (intracellular), and in necrosis (extracellular)	Within multinucleated giant cells and histiocytes (intracellular), and in necrosis (extracellular)	Within multinucleated giant cells and histiocytes (intracellular), and in necrosis (extracellular)
Typical granuloma[a]	Necrotizing granuloma with pink necrosis	Non-necrotizing granuloma with prominent multinucleated giant cells	Suppurative granuloma	Necrotizing granuloma with pink necrosis
Usual size	Small 1 to 5 μm	Small 4 to 10 μm	Large 8 to 15 μm	Large 30 to 60 μm (spherules) 2 to 5 μm (endospores)
Shape	Round to oval, often tapered at one or both ends	Round	Round	Spherules: round or fragmented Endospores: round
Size variation	Minimal	Marked	Moderate	Moderate
Budding	Narrow-based	Narrow-based	Broad-based	Absent
Nuclear material in yeast	Usually none (in necrotizing granulomas) Single purple dot or crescent (in disseminated histoplasmosis)	None	Present, basophilic	None
GMS	Positive	Positive	Positive	Positive
Mucicarmine	Negative	Usually positive, but may be negative	Occasional weak staining	Negative
Fontana-Masson	Negative	Positive (nearly all cases)	Positive (50%)	Positive (nearly all cases, both spherules and endospores)

[a] See text for full range of tissue reactions

nodules in immunocompetent hosts. However, on the GMS stain, *Pneumocystis* is a small, thin-walled fungus that can appear very similar to *Histoplasma*. Histologically, *Histoplasma* is a far more common cause of necrotizing granulomas in the lung than *Pneumocystis*, which usually manifests as an intra-alveolar exudate ("froth-with-dots") or mild interstitial chronic inflammation. However, *Pneumocystis* can occasionally cause a granulomatous reaction in the lung, including (rarely) well-formed necrotizing granulomas. On GMS, the features that help to identify *Histoplasma* in this situation include budding and tapered shapes. In contrast, helmet-shaped forms, collapsed, crescent-shaped forms and intra-cystic bodies (capsular dots) are features of *Pneumocystis*. On H&E, the presence of a frothy intra-alveolar exudate associated with the granuloma is a clue to the presence of *Pneumocystis*. Immunohistochemistry for *Pneumocystis* can also be helpful if available.

- *Candida glabrata* (*Torulopsis glabrata*) yeasts can enter the differential diagnosis of *Histoplasma*, especially in cases of disseminated histoplasmosis. Similarities to *Histoplasma* include the small size, round to oval shape, the presence of budding and GMS positivity. The organisms may be located within histiocytes or extracellularly. In contrast to *Histoplasma*, they are basophilic or amphophilic on H&E, may be Gram-positive, bud more frequently and do not form granulomas. Fortunately, clinically significant pulmonary involvement by this organism is extremely rare.

- *Leishmania*. Disseminated leishmaniasis is frequently cited as being in the differential diagnosis of disseminated histoplasmosis since it features histiocytes laden with tiny organisms. However, well-documented cases of pulmonary involvement in disseminated leishmaniasis are vanishingly rare. This possibility does not pose a problem in practice, since *Leishmania* is GMS-negative.

- Hodgkin lymphoma can be very difficult to distinguish from fibrosing mediastinitis, since both entities feature fibrosis and polymorphous mixed inflammatory infiltrates in young individuals. Eosinophils may be present in both entities. The diagnosis of Hodgkin lymphoma rests on the identification of neoplastic Reed–Sternberg cells.

- IgG4-related disease enters the differential diagnosis of fibrosing mediastinitis because the two share the presence of fibrosis and mixed inflammatory infiltrates containing plasma cells. The presence of sheets of IgG4-positive plasma cells favors the former, while dense, lamellated fibrosis favors the latter.

- Acute histoplasmosis can be misdiagnosed as lymphomatoid granulomatosis because of the combination of lymphohistiocytic infiltrates, necrosis and striking lymphocytic vasculitis. In this setting, the presence of true necrotizing granulomas argues against lymphomatoid granulomatosis, and identification of organisms in the necrotic zones on GMS will usually establish the correct diagnosis. In situ hybridization for Epstein–Barr virus encoded RNA (EBER) is positive in most cases of lymphomatoid granulomatosis.

Treatment and prognosis

- Legitimate grounds for anti-fungal therapy in pulmonary histoplasmosis include overt immunosuppression, respiratory symptoms related to multiple progressive nodules and positive cultures. The most urgent and unequivocal need for anti-fungal therapy is in patients with clinical, microbiologic or histologic evidence of disseminated histoplasmosis.

- No treatment is required for pulmonary necrotizing granulomas containing *Histoplasma* yeasts, especially if they present as an incidentally discovered solitary pulmonary nodule in an immunocompetent patient. Such nodules are usually small, radiologically stable and slow-growing, and most do not cause significant symptoms. The prognosis is excellent. Long-term follow-up (up to 7 years) of resected pulmonary histoplasmomas without additional medical therapy has shown no evidence of progressive disease. Since the organisms in such cases are non-viable and cultures are almost invariably negative, there is no rationale for anti-fungal agents. Itraconazole is sometimes prescribed in this setting by clinicians unfamiliar with the benign nature of this lesion. Response to such therapy is impossible to assess in a lesion whose natural history is stability or spontaneous resolution. Further, although itraconazole is generally well-tolerated, it is not completely benign. Side effects include nausea, vomiting, abdominal discomfort, diarrhea and rashes. Drug interactions with other medications have also been reported.

- For the reasons discussed above, anti-fungal treatment is also unnecessary for most histoplasmomas involving hilar or mediastinal lymph nodes. Such lesions are almost invariably culture-negative, and the prognosis is excellent.

- Fibrosing (sclerosing) mediastinitis is a fibrosing process that is invariably culture-negative and does not benefit from anti-fungal therapy, even when it is associated with histologically documented histoplasmomas. The prognosis is variable. Some patients live for several years without symptoms whereas others suffer considerable morbidity due to compression of mediastinal structures such as arteries, veins and nerves. Obstruction of the pulmonary vein can cause striking congestion in the lung associated with hemosiderin-laden macrophages, thick pulmonary arteries and venous infarcts, mimicking pulmonary veno-occlusive disease. Surgical resection of fibrosing mediastinitis can be very difficult or impossible due to the presence of extensive fibrotic adhesions to major blood vessels. Stenting of compressed blood vessels is currently the only effective therapeutic option.

- Most cases of acute pulmonary histoplasmosis are self-limited and do not require therapy. Patients with severe symptoms may benefit from a short course of itraconazole. The prognosis is excellent, with complete resolution in most cases.

- Disseminated histoplasmosis is fatal without aggressive anti-fungal therapy. Amphotericin B is the drug of choice, although itraconazole can be used in some circumstances. Liposomal preparations reduce renal toxicity associated with amphotericin B. Some patients with disseminated histoplasmosis recover completely with appropriate therapy, whereas others die even after aggressive treatment with amphotericin B.

Sample diagnosis on pathology report

Lung, right middle lobe, needle biopsy – Necrotizing granuloma (*Histoplasma* yeasts present).

or

Lymph node, subcarinal, biopsy – Necrotizing granuloma (*Histoplasma* yeasts present).

or

Lung, right lower lobe, surgical biopsy – Necrotizing granulomatous inflammation and lymphohistiocytic inflammatory infiltrate consistent with acute pulmonary histoplasmosis.

or

Lung, right middle lobe, surgical biopsy – Disseminated histoplasmosis (See comment).

Cryptococcosis

Pulmonary cryptococcosis is an uncommon fungal infection caused by *Cryptococcus neoformans* and *Cryptococcus gattii*. The epidemiology of these species is of interest, since *C. neoformans* seems to be the most common species in patients with HIV/AIDS, whereas *C. gattii* has been associated with lung nodules in immunocompetent individuals in the United States and Canada. However, speciation is only possible by microbiologic techniques, and does not fall within the purview of surgical pathologists. In contrast to other major fungal yeasts, *Cryptococcus* is encountered worldwide without specific endemic areas. It is classified as an invasive, opportunistic, yeast-like fungus. It is not dimorphic, i.e., it forms yeasts in tissue as well as in cultures. It is thought to be acquired by inhalation of spores from soil and bird droppings.

The diagnosis can be made in fine-needle aspirates, bronchioalveolar lavage fluid, pleural fluid, core needle biopsies, transbronchial biopsies and surgical lung biopsies. Unfortunately, some cases are diagnosed only at autopsy.

Major diagnostic findings

- *Cryptococcus* yeasts are visible on H&E, where they appear as small, round pale-staining structures with light gray or light blue-gray cell walls within histiocytes, necrotic debris, granulomas or multinucleated giant cells (Figure 2.23, also see book cover, first image from left). Individual yeasts or clusters of yeasts are surrounded by a clear space ("halo"), which often imparts a "bubbly" appearance to the infected tissue at low magnification. Some authors claim that the halo is an artifact caused by retraction of the organism from the histiocyte that engulfs it, whereas others feel that it represents the capsule.
- *Cryptococcus* yeasts are usually 4 to 10 μm in size, but can vary from 2 to 15 μm. Although yeast size is commonly cited as a helpful feature in the identification of fungal yeasts, precise measurement of such tiny organisms is not practical with most standard microscopes. However, it is important to broadly recognize small yeasts (*Histoplasma* and *Cryptococcus*) and differentiate them from larger fungi (*Blastomyces* and *Coccidioides*).

Variable pathologic findings

- *Cryptococcus* yeasts are easy to identify if they are numerous and well stained. However, they often stain lightly and are easy to miss at low magnification. Even at high magnification, pale-staining organisms can be difficult to find, emphasizing the value of careful examination of granulomatous infiltrates for fungal organisms at high magnification on H&E.
- Non-necrotizing granulomatous inflammation with numerous and prominent multinucleated giant cells is a common tissue reaction in pulmonary cryptococcosis (Figure 2.23). *Cryptococcus* is by far the most common fungal organism found in non-necrotizing granulomas. Unlike sarcoidosis, where individual granulomas are well formed and associated with hyalinized fibrosis, the granulomas of cryptococcosis tend to occur in confluent ill-defined sheets rather than as individual well-formed granulomas. A variation on this theme is an inflammatory pattern in which a granulomatous infiltrate containing organisms fills the alveoli in the distribution of a bronchopneumonia. This reaction has been termed "granulomatous pneumonia".
- Another frequent inflammatory reaction in pulmonary cryptococcosis is the presence of organizing pneumonia containing non-necrotizing granulomas within fibroblast plugs, a pattern known as *organizing granulomatous pneumonia*. The organizing pneumonia is characterized by polypoid plugs of fibroblasts located within airspaces, accompanied by varying degrees of interstitial chronic inflammation composed of lymphocytes and plasma cells. Non-necrotizing granulomas rich in multinucleated giant cells are embedded within the fibroblast plugs (Figure 2.24). The presence of tiny holes within the granulomas and giant cells is a clue to the presence of organisms.
- *Cryptococcus* can occasionally be found in necrotizing granulomas identical to those seen in tuberculosis and histoplasmosis (Figure 2.25). The necrosis can be pink ("caseous") or, less commonly, suppurative (neutrophil-rich). In a necrotic background, the organisms are particularly easy to miss at low magnification.
- Large numbers of fungal yeasts without a significant inflammatory response ("yeast lakes") were described frequently in patients with HIV/AIDS prior to the widespread use of highly active antiretroviral (HAART) therapy, as well as in patients with hematologic malignancies. This pathologic picture is now uncommon. It corresponds to the gross appearance referred to in the older literature as "gelatinous" or "slimy". In this form of the disease, large numbers of fungal yeasts proliferate unchecked within the airspaces and interstitium, including extracellular spaces such as the lumens of alveolar septal capillaries, with little or no granulomatous inflammation. This histologic pattern has been shown to correspond to disseminated cryptococcosis.
- Pleural involvement occurs in a subset of cases, and is often accompanied by subpleural giant cells and fibrosis.

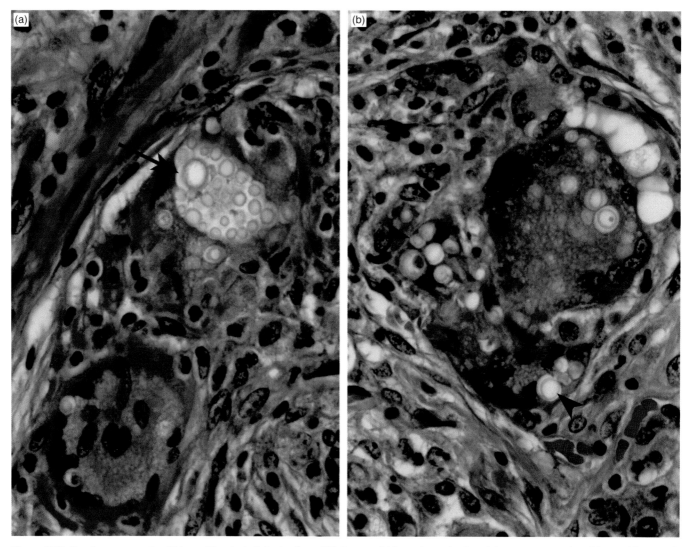

Figure 2.23. *Cryptococcus* **yeasts within multinucleated giant cells and histiocytes. (a)** Several round, pale-staining yeasts are easily visible on H&E, especially at high magnification. Multiple yeasts appear to float within a clear space (arrow). **(b)** Numerous *Cryptococcus* yeasts within a multinucleated giant cell. Note the light gray cell walls, haloes surrounding individual yeasts and the size variation (arrowheads).

- Hilar lymph nodes may be involved. Total obliteration of lymph nodes by organisms has been described in HIV/AIDS. The combination of pulmonary and hilar involvement is known as a "cryptococcal complex", analogous to but less common than similar lung–lymph node complexes in tuberculosis and histoplasmosis.
- In severely immunocompromised individuals, co-infection with other organisms is not uncommon, and may be overlooked. The most common organism in this setting is *Pneumocystis*, but *Histoplasma, cytomegalovirus* and mycobacteria may also be found in the same biopsy.

Diagnostic work-up

- The distinctive appearance of *Cryptococcus* on H&E is the mainstay of the diagnosis. Special stains are not necessarily required, although GMS and mucicarmine stains can be helpful.
- GMS stains highlight far greater numbers of organisms than are apparent on H&E. Some characteristic features,

such as size variation and fragmented forms, are better appreciated on GMS than on H&E (Figure 2.26).
- Mucicarmine stains the polysaccharide capsule of *Cryptococcus* pink (i.e., the capsule is *carminophilic*) and can be helpful in confirming the diagnosis (Figure 2.26). In practice, however, many cases of pulmonary cryptococcosis are mucicarmine-negative (Figure 2.27). Proposed reasons for this phenomenon include the presence of capsule-deficient cryptococci or degradation of the capsule by phagocytic histiocytes. The latter hypothesis may explain why many cases of cryptococcal lung infection associated with a granulomatous response are mucicarmine-negative while those lacking a significant host response are often mucicarmine-positive. Mucicarmine staining is quite specific for *Cryptococcus*, although *Blastomyces* can be weakly positive.
- The Fontana-Masson (modified Fontana-Masson silver) stain exploits the fact that the cell wall of *Cryptococcus* contains a melanin precursor (phenyl oxidase), which causes the wall to stain black due to silver deposition

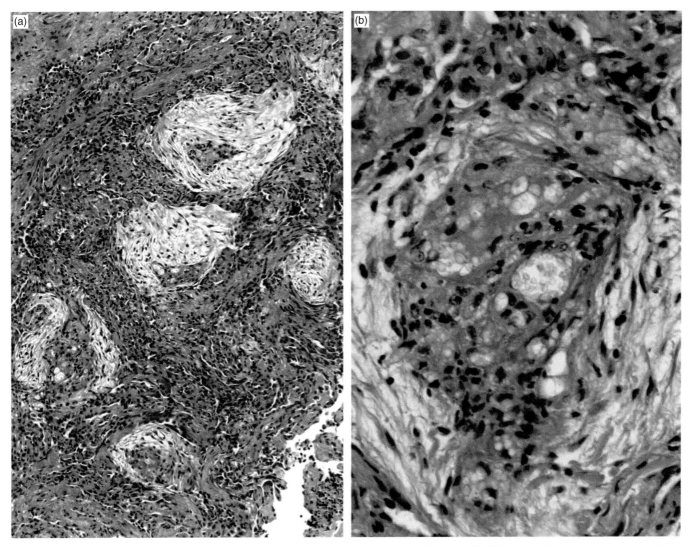

Figure 2.24. Organizing granulomatous pneumonia in cryptococcosis. (a) Granulomas are visible within fibroblast plugs of organizing pneumonia at low magnification. Some have a "bubbly" appearance. **(b)** Higher magnification shows *Cryptococcus* yeasts within histiocytes, surrounded by haloes.

(Figure 2.27). Based on this observation, several authors have touted the utility of Fontana-Masson for the diagnosis of mucicarmine-negative (or capsule-deficient) cryptococcosis. Although the reported sensitivity of this stain is high, in practice not all cases stain positive. Further, Fontana-Masson is not specific for *Cryptococcus*; it also stains *Blastomyces*, *Coccidioides* and *Sporothrix*. However, since *Histoplasma* is Fontana-Masson-negative, the stain may play a role in differentiating *Histoplasma* from *Cryptococcus*.

- India ink, well known as a stain for *Cryptococcus* in cerebrospinal fluid, is not suitable for use in formalin-fixed paraffin-embedded material.
- Other specialized techniques such as electron microscopy and direct immunofluorescence are not widely available.

Clinical profile

- Cryptococcosis can occur at any age and sex, but is rare in children. The reported age range is 2 to 89 years.

Fever, malaise, chest pain, weight loss, dyspnea, night sweats and cough are common. Many cases are found incidentally in asymptomatic individuals. The clinical impression often includes pneumonia, tuberculosis or malignancy. Due to the non-specific presentation, the possibility of cryptococcosis is infrequently considered in the clinical differential diagnosis prior to biopsy. In patients with pre-existing conditions, the lung findings are often mistakenly attributed to the underlying disease.

- Many – but not all – patients with pulmonary cryptococcosis are immunocompromised. Common settings in which pulmonary cryptococcosis is encountered include HIV/AIDS, corticosteroid (prednisone) therapy and hematologic malignancies (various leukemias, Hodgkin lymphoma and various non-Hodgkin lymphomas). In leukemias and lymphomas, cryptococcosis can occur even in the absence of prior chemotherapy. Other settings include organ transplantation, diabetes, renal failure, liver cirrhosis and carcinomas of various sites.

65

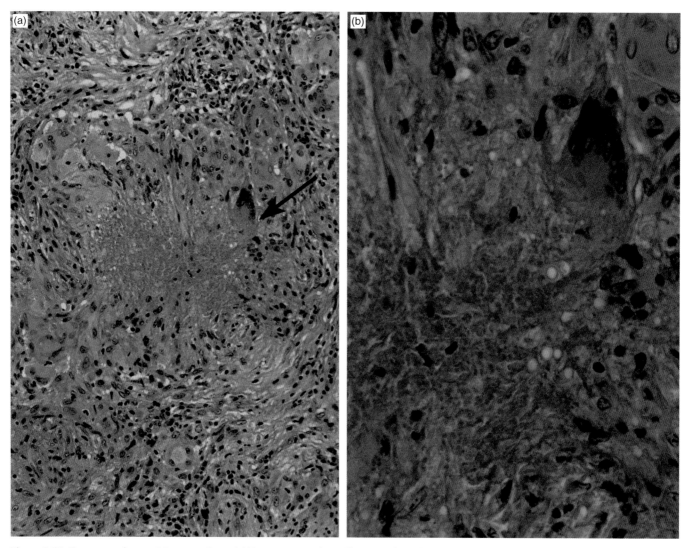

Figure 2.25. Cryptococcal necrotizing granuloma. (a) Necrotizing granuloma. The area indicated by the arrow is shown at high magnification in part b. **(b)** Small yeasts with light gray cell walls typical of *Cryptococcus* are visible within the necrosis on H&E.

Immunosuppressed patients often show evidence of disseminated disease concomitant with pulmonary disease.

- Disseminated (extrapulmonary) cryptococcosis occurs more commonly in immunocompromised individuals than in immunocompetent hosts. Central nervous system involvement (cryptococcal meningitis) is the most dreaded manifestation of cryptococcosis, and carries a high mortality without therapy. Skin involvement is also common, usually manifesting as nodules with or without ulceration. Less common sites of dissemination include liver, spleen, bone marrow, kidneys and adrenal glands.

- Although disseminated cryptococcosis in severely immunocompromised patients receives the most attention in the clinical literature, it is important to remember that isolated pulmonary cryptococcosis can occur in both immunocompetent and immunocompromised individuals, and may occasionally be asymptomatic. Solitary lung nodules (*cryptococcomas*) mimic lung cancer clinically, and

may be biopsied to rule out cancer, analogous to histoplasmomas.

- Microbiologic cultures remain the gold standard for the identification and speciation of *Cryptococcus*. Cultures typically become positive within 36 to 72 hours. Specimens that may yield positive cultures include biopsied lung tissue, other respiratory tract specimens (sputum, bronchoalveolar lavage (BAL), bronchial washings), blood, cerebrospinal fluid, urine and pleural fluid. In the absence of positive cultures, histology provides a reliable diagnosis in the majority of cases. It is well documented that histologically typical cases of cryptococcosis can be culture-negative, and there is some evidence to suggest that this phenomenon is more common in granulomatous lesions in immunocompetent individuals.

- Serologic evidence of cryptococcosis may be obtained by detecting cryptococcal antigen or antibody in the serum (latex agglutination test).

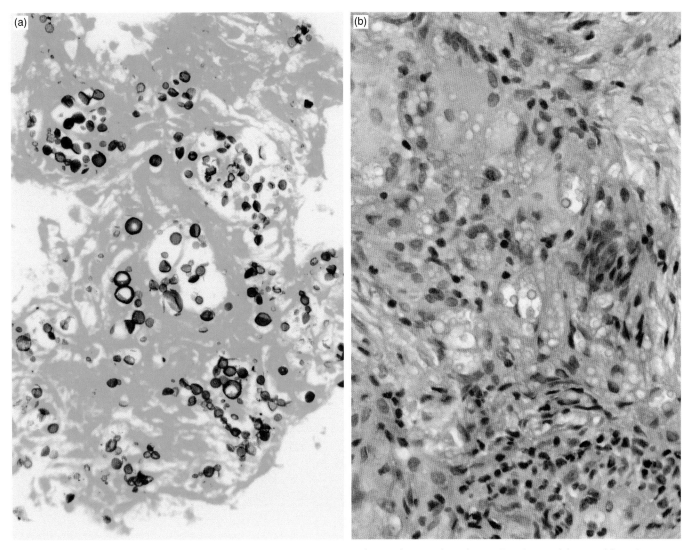

Figure 2.26. GMS and mucicarmine in pulmonary cryptococcosis. (a) GMS stain showing large numbers of yeasts. Note the round shape and the wide variation in size. Narrow-based budding is present. **(b)** Mucicarmine stains the yeasts pink. Staining intensity varies considerably.

- In cases with disseminated disease, organisms may be detectable in the CSF using the India ink stain.

Radiologic findings

In immunocompetent individuals, the most common radiologic finding is a solitary pulmonary nodule (coin lesion) or multiple lung nodules. Solitary nodules are uncommon in immunocompromised hosts. The reported size of cryptococcal nodules ranges from 0.5 to 5.2 cm. They may be smoothly marginated or spiculated. Cavitation is common; the cavities may have thin or thick walls. Lesions with air-fluid levels mimicking abscesses have been described. There is no predilection for any side or lobe. Lung infiltrates or areas of consolidation (single or multiple, often with cavitation) are also common. Infiltrates range from segmental to lobar, and have been described as interstitial, alveolar, airspace, reticulonodular and miliary. Hilar lymphadenopathy and pleural effusion have been reported but are uncommon. Some studies report that these manifestations are more common in immunocompromised individuals.

Differential diagnosis

- *Histoplasma* is the main consideration in the differential diagnosis (Table 2.2). Both fungi are small yeasts that may show narrow-based budding, and can be found in necrotizing granulomas. The most reliable differentiating features are the oval or tapered shape of *Histoplasma* yeasts (*Cryptococcus* is round), the lack of visibility of *Histoplasma* within necrosis on H&E (*Cryptococcus* is visible on H&E) and the uniform size of *Histoplasma* (*Cryptococcus* shows significant size variation on GMS, as well as fragmentation). Mucicarmine is helpful if positive, but negative staining is common and does not exclude *Cryptococcus*, as discussed above. Positive staining for Fontana-Masson also favors *Cryptococcus*, since *Histoplasma* is negative. *Histoplasma* is visible within histiocytes on H&E in disseminated histoplasmosis (which can involve the lung), but the morphology of the organisms on H&E in this setting differs from *Cryptococcus* in that the organisms are tiny rings with an eccentric purple crescent or dot. The morphologic differences on GMS (discussed

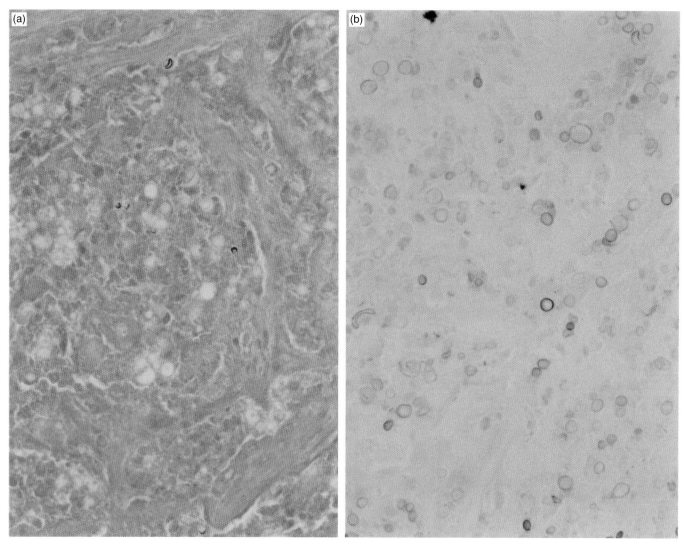

Figure 2.27. Mucicarmine-negative *Cryptococcus*. (a) Mucicarmine is negative in this example of cryptococcosis. **(b)** A Fontana-Masson stain is positive.

above) are also helpful in this situation. Rarely, these two organisms can be impossible to differentiate on histologic grounds.

- *Blastomyces* is larger than *Cryptococcus* and is characteristically found within suppurative granulomas. However, both are fungal yeasts and are visible within histiocytes on H&E. Additionally, there may be some size overlap between small *Blastomyces* yeasts and large *Cryptococcus* yeasts. Broad-based budding and basophilic nuclear material are seen only in *Blastomyces*, whereas narrow-based budding and strong mucicarmine staining are indicative of *Cryptococcus*.
- *Pneumocystis*. This small fungus is usually easy to differentiate from *Cryptococcus* because of the pathognomonic frothy exudate. However, cases lacking the dots-in-froth appearance can cause problems, especially on the GMS stain. Although the findings on GMS are helpful (size variation in *Cryptococcus*, intra-cystic dots and helmet-shaped forms in *Pneumocystis*), the H&E findings are most helpful. Visibility of yeasts on H&E supports

Cryptococcus since the cysts of *Pneumocystis* cannot be seen on H&E.
- There is a theoretical risk of mistaking *Coccidioides* endospores for *Cryptococcus* yeasts. Finding large spherules or endospore-filled spherules should resolve the issue. Narrow-based budding and mucicarmine positivity are seen in *Cryptococcus* but not in *Coccidioides* endospores.

Treatment and prognosis

- Pulmonary cryptococcosis in *immunocompromised* patients carries a high risk of disseminated disease, and is an indication for lumbar puncture to exclude cryptococcal meningitis. Treatment options include fluconazole (for non-disseminated, non-severe disease) or amphotericin B (for severe disease or CNS dissemination).
- Symptomatic pulmonary disease requires anti-fungal therapy, even in *immunocompetent* individuals. Oral fluconazole for 6 to 12 months is recommended for non-disseminated, non-severe disease. For severe disease or pulmonary disease accompanied by CNS dissemination,

primary/induction therapy with intravenous amphotericin B is followed by consolidation and maintenance therapy with fluconazole.

- The need for anti-fungal therapy in solitary lung nodules (cryptococcal granulomas/cryptococcomas) in asymptomatic *immunocompetent* individuals is controversial. Some authors advocate observation without treatment in this setting, whereas others argue that observation without anti-fungal therapy carries a small but unacceptable risk of disseminated disease. Fluconazole therapy and lumbar puncture is an alternative approach in such patients.

- The well-known proclivity of *Cryptococcus* for the central nervous system, especially the meninges, is a leading cause of death in the subset of patients with pulmonary cryptococcosis in whom death is attributable to cryptococcosis. In immunocompromised patients, the interval between pulmonary disease at presentation and subsequent central nervous system dissemination ranges from 2 to 48 weeks. Rarely, death occurs due to disseminated disease without central nervous system involvement. Some deaths are attributable primarily to the underlying immune-suppressing disease, or other infections.

- There are a few reports of isolated pulmonary cryptococcosis in immunocompetent individuals followed without anti-fungal therapy for prolonged periods. Most of these patients have shown no evidence of disseminated disease.

Sample diagnosis on pathology report

Lung, right lower lobe, needle biopsy – Necrotizing granulomatous inflammation (*Cryptococcus* yeasts present).
   or
Lung, right lower lobe, transbronchial biopsy – Cryptococcal pneumonia (See comment).

Blastomycosis

Blastomyces is the least common of the four major fungal yeasts that cause necrotizing granulomatous inflammation in the lung. It is caused by *Blastomyces dermatitidis* and is thought to be acquired from soil or rotting wood. Like *Histoplasma*, *Blastomyces* is a dimorphic fungus that forms yeasts in tissue and hyphae in cultures. Blastomycosis is classified as an endemic mycosis, i.e., most cases occur in a limited geographic distribution. The endemic area for blastomycosis parallels that of histoplasmosis. It includes the Ohio and Mississippi river valleys and most areas in the Midwestern United States and Canada surrounding the Great Lakes. The southeast is also considered a high-incidence area. The greatest numbers of cases are reported from Illinois, Wisconsin, Mississippi, Minnesota and Kansas. As with other endemic mycoses, cases occasionally occur outside traditional endemic regions, such as the St. Lawrence River Valley in the northern part of New York State.

As with histoplasmosis, blastomycosis is a disease with a wide range of clinical presentations, including asymptomatic infection, self-limited pulmonary disease, acute pneumonia, fulminating acute respiratory failure resembling ARDS, chronic pulmonary infection, localized mass-like lesions in the lung mimicking malignancy, and disseminated infection. Blastomycosis can occur in immunocompromised hosts, but many cases occur in immunocompetent individuals.

Most cases of blastomycosis involve the lungs, but disseminated disease can involve the skin, bones, brain and head and neck sites, often without overt evidence of antecedent pulmonary disease. The skin is the best known site of extrapulmonary disease. Blastomycosis should always be considered in patients with a combination of pulmonary and dermatologic disease, especially when raised lesions are found on the face.

Major diagnostic findings

- Of the four fungi that commonly cause granulomas in the lung, *Blastomyces* forms the most distinctive granulomas, classically referred to as "pyogranulomas". These are *suppurative* granulomas, characterized by a necrotic, neutrophil-rich center that resembles an abscess (Figure 2.28). The central zone of suppurative necrosis is surrounded by a granulomatous rim composed of epithelioid histiocytes and variable numbers of multinucleated giant cells.

- Organisms may be found in the suppurative center or the granulomatous rim, including within multinucleated giant cells. *Blastomyces* is large, round and thick-walled, and is visible on H&E as well as GMS. Its most distinctive characteristics are the presence of a single broad-based bud and basophilic nuclear material. The latter is appreciated on H&E but not on GMS, emphasizing the importance of examining H&E-stained sections in fungal identification (Figures 2.28 and 2.29). The size of the organism ranges from 8 to 15 μm.

Variable pathologic findings

- Organizing pneumonia (plugs of fibroblasts within airspaces) may be found at the edge of the granulomatous inflammation. Non-necrotizing granulomas may be embedded within fibroblast plugs.

- Diffuse alveolar damage can occur in patients with severe infection, especially at the edge of the granulomatous infiltrate. This finding is the pathologic correlate of ARDS in severe pulmonary blastomycosis.

- Varying degrees of chronic inflammation are common in and around the granulomas.

Diagnostic work-up

- In classic cases, the identification of large yeasts with broad-based budding in suppurative granulomas is sufficient for the diagnosis and no further testing is required.

- A special stain for fungi (GMS or PAS) is not necessarily required since *Blastomyces* is visible on H&E. As with other fungi, GMS staining brings out far greater numbers of organisms than is apparent on H&E, and is superior to the

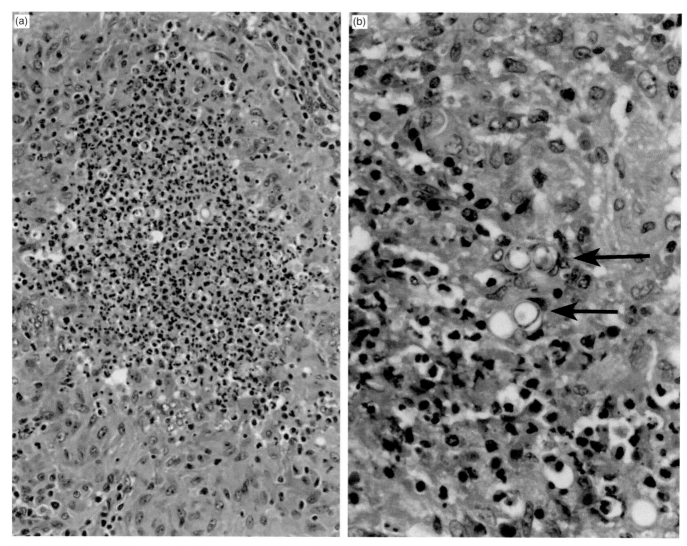

Figure 2.28. Pulmonary blastomycosis. (a) Suppurative granuloma. Abscess-like center rich in neutrophils is characteristic of blastomycosis. **(b)** *Blastomyces* organisms at high magnification (arrows). Note broad-based budding and basophilic nuclear material.

PAS stain. Mucicarmine is generally negative in *Blastomyces*, but weak positivity has been reported.

Clinical profile

Blastomycosis occurs in immunocompetent as well as immunocompromised individuals. Most patients are immunocompetent. Cases have been reported in patients with HIV/AIDS, transplant recipients and diabetics. There is a predilection for men, perhaps related to the association with outdoor activities involving extensive contact with soil and wood.

Many cases of blastomycosis are asymptomatic. Among symptomatic patients, most initially present with features resembling bacterial pneumonia and are presumptively treated as such. Some patients present with a combination of pulmonary and cutaneous manifestations.

Pathologists looking for epidemiologic clues to confirm their diagnosis will seldom find useful information in the clinical chart. Blastomycosis is associated with outdoor activities, construction and other hobbies that involve contact with wood and soil, but most patients have no relevant exposure history.

Cultures may or may not be positive. As with other fungi, when culture results are available, they are the gold standard. A well-recognized pitfall in the laboratory diagnosis of blastomycosis is that urine tests for *Histoplasma* antigen can be falsely positive.

Radiologic findings

Blastomycosis may present as solitary or multiple lung nodules or as patchy, ill-defined infiltrates or opacities. Airspace consolidation is the most common finding, followed by masses. Air bronchograms may be present within the consolidated areas. The radiologic appearance is not distinctive, and commonly mimics malignancy. Unlike histoplasmosis, calcification is rare. Lymphadenopathy and pleural effusions are uncommon.

Differential diagnosis

- Coccidioidomycosis. The most difficult differential diagnosis is with *Coccidioides* spherules, whose large size,

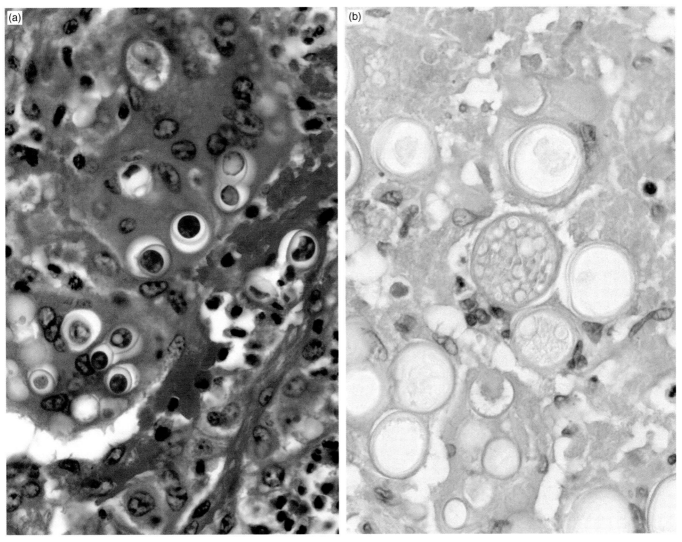

Figure 2.29. Blastomyces vs. Coccidioides. (a) *Blastomyces.* Note broad-based budding and basophilic nuclear material. **(b)** *Coccidioides.* Note spherule and endospores. Both pictures were taken at identical magnification, using a 60x objective lens.

thick cell wall and internal endospores can closely mimic *Blastomyces* (Figure 2.29). As seen in Figure 2.29, large *Blastomyces* yeasts that lack nuclear material are identical to small *Coccidioides* spherules that lack endospores. The key features that differentiate between the two are broad-based budding and nuclear material, seen in *Blastomyces*, and spherules filled with endospores, which are a feature of *Coccidioides* (Table 2.2). In cases that lack these diagnostic features, the organisms cannot be confidently differentiated by histology, and definitive identification must await culture confirmation.

- Cryptococcosis. *Cryptococcus* yeasts are smaller than *Blastomyces* but can be morphologically similar when organisms are few in number. Both can be found on H&E within histiocytes and multinucleated giant cells, and are often surrounded by a halo. Suppurative granulomas are much more common in blastomycosis than cryptococcosis. Broad-based budding and nuclear material are features of *Blastomyces* but not *Cryptococcus*. Conversely, narrow-based budding and strong

mucicarmine positivity are features of *Cryptococcus* but not *Blastomyces*.

- Other causes of neutrophil-rich granulomas include particulate matter aspiration and granulomatosis with polyangiitis (Wegener's). Identification of diagnostic features such as food particles or necrotizing vasculitis should settle the issue.

- *Paracoccidioides* enters the differential diagnosis in South America but is seldom a serious consideration in the United States. The characteristic feature of *Paracoccidioides* is the presence of multiple narrow-necked buds.

Treatment and prognosis

Anti-fungal treatment is almost always indicated in blastomycosis. The most commonly used drugs are itraconazole or ketoconazole for mild infections, and amphotericin B for severe life-threatening infections.

The prognosis is variable. Individuals with low organism burden may recover completely with adequate therapy while those with bilateral diffuse lung infiltrates or ARDS at presentation do poorly, with death occurring despite aggressive anti-fungal therapy. However, cases of severe pulmonary blastomycosis and even disseminated blastomycosis with complete resolution after amphotericin B therapy have been reported. Overall, the introduction of amphotericin B has reduced the mortality rate from 80% to 20%.

Sample diagnosis on pathology report

Lung, right middle lobe, core needle biopsy – Necrotizing (suppurative) granulomatous inflammation (*Blastomyces* organisms present).

Coccidioidomycosis

Coccidioidomycosis is a fungal infection caused by *Coccidioides immitis* and the histologically identical species *Coccidioides posadasii. Coccidioides* is a dimorphic fungus, but unlike other dimorphic fungi that cause granulomatous inflammation in the lung (*Histoplasma* and *Blastomyces*) it forms endosporulating spherules in tissue rather than budding yeasts. Occasionally, hyphae may also be present in tissues. In the microbiology laboratory, cultures positive for *Coccidioides* are highly infectious and pose a significant hazard to laboratory personnel. Therefore, pathologists who encounter this organism in tissue specimens must inform microbiology laboratory personnel so that appropriate precautions can be taken.

There are many clinical, radiologic and histologic similarities between coccidioidomycosis and the other major granulomatous fungal infections of the lung (histoplasmosis, blastomycosis and cryptococcosis). Coccidioidomycosis is acquired by inhalation of airborne spores derived from the soil in dry and dusty environments. The endemic zone includes the southwestern United States, northern Mexico and some areas in central and South America such as Venezuela and northeastern Brazil. Endemic areas in the United States include California (extending from the southern San Joaquin valley in central California to southern California), southern Arizona, New Mexico, Nevada, Utah and west Texas. It is helpful for pathologists, when faced with equivocal or atypical fungal morphology, to inquire whether the patient is from or has visited these endemic areas. Pathologists outside these locations will occasionally encounter coccidioidomycosis, since some individuals infected in endemic areas travel and subsequently seek medical attention in a non-endemic area.

Coccidioidomycosis can be diagnosed by surgical pathologists in a variety of lung specimens, including transbronchial, endobronchial and needle biopsies, as well as surgically resected specimens.

Major diagnostic findings

- Necrotizing granulomatous inflammation. The typical histologic reaction to *Coccidioides* is a necrotizing granuloma containing a necrotic center surrounded by a rim of epithelioid histiocytes (Figure 2.30). This lesion, known as a *coccidioidoma*, is histologically identical to

similar lesions in tuberculosis (tuberculoma) and histoplasmosis (histoplasmoma). The granulomas can be solitary or multiple. Small non-necrotizing granulomas are frequently present at the periphery of the main necrotizing granuloma. The granulomatous inflammation may be missed when it takes the form of palisading epithelioid histiocytes with few or no giant cells in the wall of a cavity.

- *Coccidioides* is the largest of the four common fungi that cause granulomas in the lung in the United States. In tissues, it forms large round structures known as spherules, which contain tiny round yeast-like structures known as endospores (Figures 2.30 and 2.31). Spherules usually range from 30 to 60 μm in size, but can occasionally be as small as 10 μm. They can be found within necrosis or in the granulomatous rim within histiocytes or multinucleated giant cells. They may be empty (ruptured), filled with endospores, distorted or collapsed. Budding is absent.

Variable pathologic findings

- Hyphae may be present. In cavitary coccidioidomycosis, they have been found in up to 60% of cases. They are composed of barrel-shaped structures known as arthroconidia, arranged back-to-back. Most hyphae of this type appear septate but do not branch in the regular, dichotomous fashion typical of *Aspergillus*. However, branching may occur in some cases.
- Eosinophils, when present, can be a clue to the diagnosis. They may be present in large numbers, forming eosinophil "abscesses" surrounded by epithelioid histiocytes. Alternatively, necrotic eosinophils may be present within the necrotic centers of granulomas. There may also be florid tissue eosinophilia in the lung parenchyma surrounding the granulomatous inflammation, occasionally in the form of eosinophilic pneumonia. Eosinophils may also be prominent in the pleura. The main diagnostic utility of tissue eosinophilia associated with granulomatous inflammation is that its presence should prompt a careful search for *Coccidioides* organisms. Unfortunately, eosinophils are not a consistent finding, and can rarely be seen in other mycobacterial and fungal infections.
- In some cases, necrotizing granulomas of the "suppurative" type are seen, identical to the suppurative granulomas of blastomycosis. These have a neutrophil-rich, abscess-like center. It is hypothesized that spherules elicit a granulomatous tissue reaction whereas endospores (released by rupture of spherules) cause a neutrophilic response.
- The inflammatory reaction may be centered exclusively or predominantly on bronchi and bronchioles, mimicking so-called "bronchocentric granulomatosis".
- In immunocompromised patients, there may be numerous organisms and minimal granulomatous inflammation, which may be limited to a few multinucleated giant cells containing endosporulating spherules.
- Like other granulomatous infections, non-specific findings such as chronic inflammation, chronic bronchiolitis,

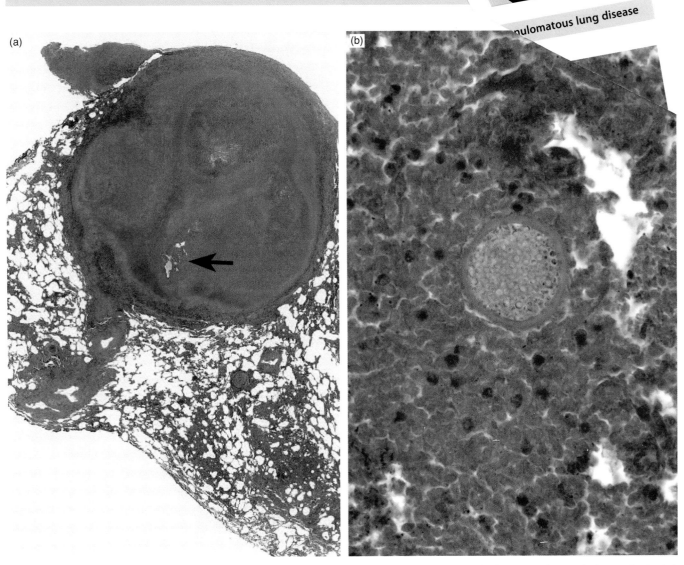

Figure 2.30. Pulmonary coccidioidoma. (a) Necrotizing granuloma identical to tuberculosis. The area indicated by the arrow is shown at high magnification in b. **(b)** Spherule with endospores. Case courtesy of Dr. Sanjay Lahiri.

lymphoid hyperplasia and organizing pneumonia may accompany or surround the granulomas.

- When hilar lymph nodes are sampled, granulomas containing *Coccidioides* spherules are found in a significant proportion of cases.

Diagnostic work-up

Special stains are not necessary if diagnostic spherules are identified on H&E. However, organisms may occasionally be few in number and difficult to see on H&E-stained sections. In such cases, GMS staining is very helpful to pick out organisms and highlight their morphologic features. Endospores stain consistently with GMS, whereas spherules may or may not be positive (Figure 2.31).

Clinical profile

Most cases of coccidioidomycosis occur in adults of either sex residing in endemic areas. Men are more commonly affected. Cases do occur in children but are uncommon. Pregnant women are vulnerable to infection and develop more severe disease.

The clinical diagnosis is hindered by a lack of specific symptoms or radiologic findings. Many cases are discovered incidentally in asymptomatic patients. When symptoms do occur, they are non-specific, including cough, fever, dyspnea and chest pain. Hemoptysis can occur in cavitary lesions. Systemic symptoms such as headache, weight loss and fatigue are not uncommon. Contrary to common misconception, most patients with coccidioidomycosis are immunocompetent. Immunocompromised hosts, such as transplant recipients, individuals with HIV/AIDS or patients receiving corticosteroids are susceptible to infection and are prone to severe and disseminated disease.

As in histoplasmosis, initial exposure may be completely asymptomatic or may result in a flu-like illness that is very common in endemic areas and is frequently misdiagnosed as community-acquired pneumonia. The disease is popularly known as "valley fever", after its high incidence in the hyper-endemic San Joaquin River Valley in California. The clinical

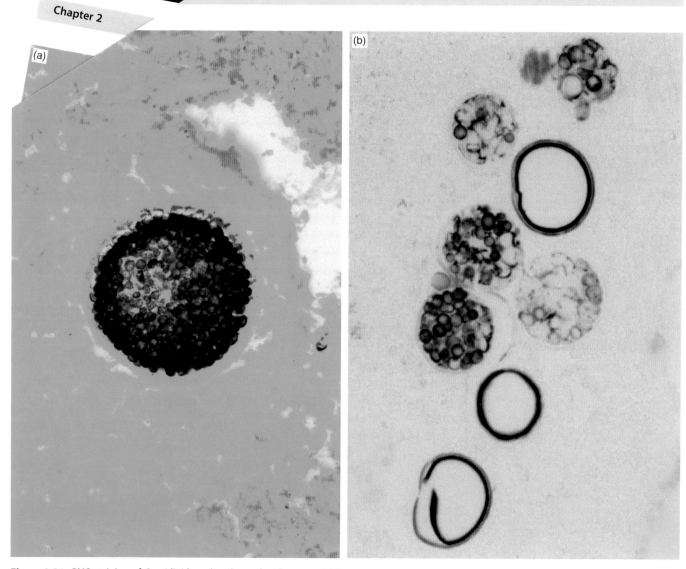

Figure 2.31. GMS staining of *Coccidioides* spherules and endospores. (a) Same case as Figure 2.30. Endospores are GMS-positive but spherule is negative. **(b)** Miliary coccidioidomycosis. Note consistent GMS staining of endospores and variable staining of spherules.

manifestations of "classic" valley fever include fever, chills, headache, non-productive cough, chest pain, erythema multiforme, erythema nodosum and polyarthralgia. Most cases are self-limited and resolve spontaneously without therapy.

A few individuals with pulmonary coccidioidomycosis present with hypoxemic acute respiratory failure causing the acute respiratory distress syndrome (ARDS). Chronic coccidioidomycosis is another uncommon form of the disease, characterized by persistent or progressive fever, weight loss and sputum production. Disseminated coccidioidomycosis is also uncommon. It usually occurs in immunocompromised individuals and may involve the bones and meninges.

In clinical practice, most patients in endemic areas are diagnosed on the basis of serology, and relatively few cases are confirmed by positive cultures or histology. Like blastomycosis and cryptococcosis, and *unlike* pulmonary histoplasmomas, cultures are often positive, even in solitary necrotizing granulomas. Cultures can be positive in cases that are negative by histology, and vice versa. In cavitary

lesions, sputum cultures are often negative, and serology has low sensitivity.

Radiologic findings

The radiologic features of coccidioidomycosis include consolidation, patchy infiltrates, nodules and peribronchial thickening. The abnormalities may be unilateral or bilateral, the former being more common. Pleural effusions can occur in isolation or in association with parenchymal disease. Many cases masquerade as bacterial pneumonia.

Lung nodules may be solitary or multiple, with or without cavitation. Cavitation occurs in 13 to 15% of cases. Hilar and mediastinal adenopathy may be present. Miliary nodules are seen in disseminated disease. As in histoplasmosis and other mycobacterial and fungal infections, a localized focus of walled-off infection may present as a solitary lung nodule (coccidioidoma) radiologically indistinguishable from a neoplasm. Most cases of coccidioidomycosis seen by surgical pathologists are diagnosed when such nodules are biopsied or resected to rule out malignancy.

Differential diagnosis

- Large *Blastomyces* yeasts can be similar in size and morphology to small *Coccidioides* spherules (Figure 2.29). Both organisms can cause suppurative granulomas. The nuclear material of *Blastomyces* can appear similar to the endospores of *Coccidioides*. The most reliable finding to differentiate the two is broad-based budding, which is pathognomonic of *Blastomyces* (Table 2.2). *Coccidioides* does not bud. The presence of ruptured spherules also favors *Coccidioides*. Differentiation between these organisms can be impossible in cases that lack definitive morphologic findings, and in such cases a descriptive diagnosis is appropriate. Microbiologic cultures may be productive in this setting.
- Fungal hyphae. Since *Coccidioides* can form hyphae in tissues, it may mimic fungi such as *Aspergillus*. The hyphae of *Coccidioides* are septate and occasionally branch, but they are invariably composed of barrel-shaped structures (arthroconidia), a feature that facilitates distinction from *Aspergillus*. Identification of spherules should resolve the question, and cultures can be helpful in difficult cases.
- Smaller yeasts such as *Histoplasma* and *Cryptococcus* are hardly ever in the differential diagnosis, since endospores are seldom found in the absence of spherules.

Treatment and prognosis

Standard management involves fluconazole or itraconazole for mild symptomatic infection and amphotericin B for severe or disseminated disease, with a subsequent transition to azoles. As with histoplasmosis, incidentally detected solitary pulmonary nodules do not require therapy, especially if they have been resected.

Most individuals with acute coccidioidomycosis recover completely. The prognosis is likewise excellent for incidentally discovered solitary nodules in immunocompetent individuals. The prognosis of ARDS and disseminated coccidioidomycosis is very poor, with high mortality rates.

Sample diagnosis on pathology report

Lung, right middle lobe, core needle biopsy – Necrotizing granulomatous inflammation (*Coccidioides* present).

Chronic necrotizing pulmonary aspergillosis

The best known and perhaps most common forms of pulmonary aspergillosis (*mycetomas* and *invasive aspergillosis*) are not associated with granulomatous inflammation. They are addressed in Chapter 3 (Table 3.3 of Chapter 3 compares the main features of all four major forms). However, necrotizing granulomatous inflammation does occur in an uncommon but distinctive form of pulmonary aspergillosis known as *chronic necrotizing pulmonary aspergillosis*. Granulomas are also seen in another uncommon form of aspergillosis known as *allergic bronchopulmonary aspergillosis* (ABPA), which is discussed in the next section in this chapter.

Chronic necrotizing pulmonary aspergillosis was initially described as a clinically and radiologically distinctive form of aspergillosis in the 1980s. In contrast to invasive aspergillosis, which affects severely immunocompromised neutropenic hosts, and mycetomas, which colonize pre-existing lung cavities, chronic necrotizing pulmonary aspergillosis is characterized by the development of persistent and progressive cavitary nodules or infiltrates in individuals with either mild or no immunosuppression, or underlying structural but non-cavitary lung disease. Several other terms have been proposed for this type of aspergillosis, including "chronic cavitary pulmonary aspergillosis" and "complex aspergilloma". The term "chronic pulmonary aspergillosis" lumps aspergillomas and progressive chronic cavitary disease into one category.

An early hypothesis that has held up well over the years was that chronic necrotizing pulmonary aspergillosis is a form of *semi-invasive* aspergillosis. This observation is supported by the clinical and radiologic features as well as the pathologic findings in these lesions.

Major diagnostic findings

- Cavitary lesion with necrotizing granulomatous inflammation in its wall and fungal hyphae in the lumen (Figures 2.32 and 2.33). The necrotic center of the lesion can vary from less than a millimeter to several centimeters in size. The appearance of the granulomatous inflammation is similar to necrotizing granulomas caused by other fungi and mycobacteria. The necrosis may be pink, dirty, suppurative or infarct-like.
- *Aspergillus* forms fungal hyphae that are typically septate and show dichotomous narrow-angle branching. By histology, the organisms cannot be reliably differentiated from other morphologically similar fungal hyphae such as *Pseudallescheria*, *Fusarium* and *Scedosporium*. Definitive identification requires microbiologic cultures. The umbrella term *fungal hyphae* can be used in pathology reports when culture confirmation is not available.
- Fungal hyphae are typically found within the necrotic center of the lesion. They are often arranged in a streaming pattern in which individual hyphae are splayed apart in a necrotic background, in contrast to the tightly packed, haphazard arrangement seen in mycetomas (Figure 2.33).
- The presence of fungal hyphae within necrosis and granulomatous inflammation at the edge of the lesion supports the concept of limited tissue invasion, accounting for the term *semi-invasive*. The hyphae may penetrate focally into the granulomatous rim but do not usually extend into the surrounding lung parenchyma. True vascular invasion by fungal hyphae is indicative of *invasive aspergillosis*.

Variable pathologic findings

- Features of the underlying lung disease may be prominent. Most commonly, this takes the form of emphysema and other smoking-related abnormalities.

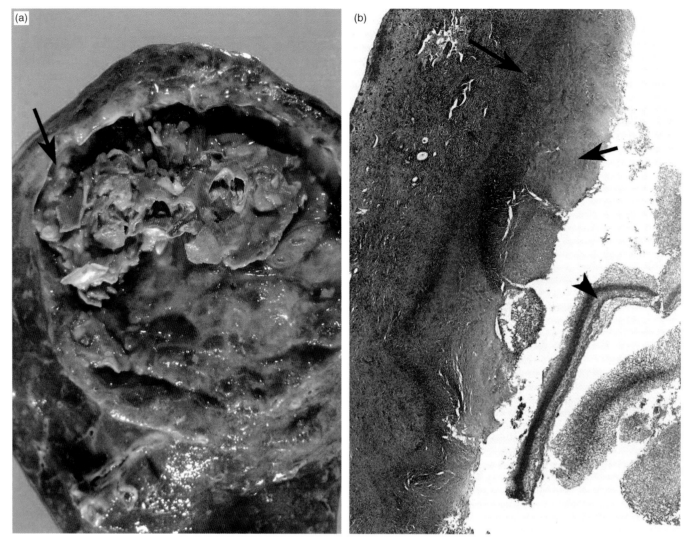

Figure 2.32. Chronic necrotizing pulmonary aspergillosis. (a) Lobectomy specimen containing a large cavitary mass with necrotic-appearing, putty-like contents. The area indicated by the arrow is shown at low magnification in b. **(b)** Wall and contents of the cavitary lesion. The wall contains a cellular granulomatous rim (long arrow). The putty-like luminal contents consist of necrosis (short arrow) and fungi (arrowhead).

- A few cases have been described in which necrotizing granulomas containing *Aspergillus* are located exclusively in a bronchocentric distribution. These have been termed "bronchocentric mycosis" or "pulmonary aspergillosis with bronchocentric granulomas". The best nomenclature for these rare lesions remains unclear, but they likely represent a variant of chronic necrotizing pulmonary aspergillosis or invasive aspergillosis.
- Necrotizing granulomas containing *Aspergillus* may be found incidentally in lung resections performed for other reasons. It is unclear whether such lesions should be classified as chronic necrotizing pulmonary aspergillosis based solely on the pathologic features, even if the clinical presentation is discordant. These lesions have been referred to in the clinical literature as "*Aspergillus* nodules". The prognosis is generally excellent.

Diagnostic work-up

- Since *Aspergillus* is visible on H&E, GMS staining is not mandatory. However, it does help to find organisms when they are few in number.
- Knowledge of the clinical and radiologic findings helps to determine whether the term *chronic necrotizing pulmonary aspergillosis* is appropriate.

Clinical profile

Chronic necrotizing pulmonary aspergillosis has traditionally been defined clinically as a syndrome of progressive cavitary lung disease. Typical symptoms include fever, weight loss and malaise. The diagnosis requires the presence of radiographic infiltrates that persist or progress over time resulting in cavitary lesions. Severely immunocompromised patients such as those with leukemia, transplantation or intensive chemotherapy have been excluded from this definition. The reported age range of

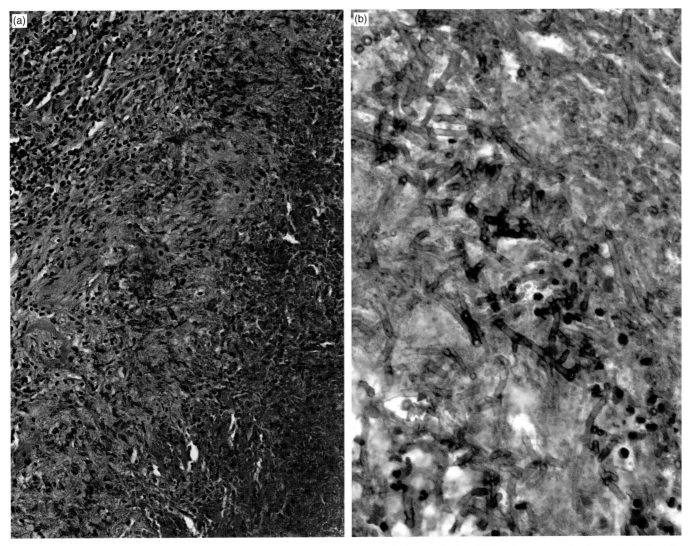

Figure 2.33. Chronic necrotizing pulmonary aspergillosis. Same case as Figure 2.32, at high magnification. **(a)** Granulomatous wall and necrosis. **(b)** Fungal hyphae in a necrotic background. Cultures grew *Aspergillus fumigatus*.

clinically defined cases is 34 to 79 years. Most patients are cigarette smokers. The most common underlying structural lung disease is emphysema. Many patients have a history of prior treatment with inhaled, oral or intravenous corticosteroids.

In practice, a history of progressive cavitary disease is usually unavailable in cases in which *Aspergillus* is identified within necrotizing granulomas by surgical pathologists. Such cases can be seen in adults of both sexes, but may also rarely be seen in children. Many patients have evidence of underlying structural (but not cavitary) lung disease, most commonly emphysema. There is often some degree of immune dysfunction that falls short of overt immunocompromise. Necrotizing granulomatous inflammation associated with *Aspergillus* rarely occurs in the setting of acute leukemia, HIV infection, oral corticosteroid therapy or severe malnutrition.

From a clinical perspective, chronic necrotizing pulmonary aspergillosis can often be diagnosed without a lung biopsy. Laboratory evidence of *Aspergillus* infection may come from cultures of sputum or BAL fluid, positive serologic studies for *Aspergillus*-specific IgG or enzyme immunoassays that measure galactomannan derived from the cell wall of the organism. *Aspergillus fumigatus* is the most commonly isolated organism.

Radiologic findings

Chronic necrotizing pulmonary aspergillosis usually presents as multiple pulmonary nodules or masses. The nodules may be solid or cavitary, but cavitation is the most characteristic radiologic finding. Progressive development and enlargement of a cavitary lesion was a cardinal feature of the earliest cases described in the literature.

Differential diagnosis

- Aspergilloma (mycetoma) is a fungus ball that develops within a pre-existing cavity. It shows several features that overlap with chronic necrotizing pulmonary aspergillosis, including the presence of fungal hyphae, lack of vascular invasion, the presence of a localized lung lesion, and the absence of severe immunosuppression or profound neutropenia (Chapter 3, Table 3.3). In contrast to chronic necrotizing pulmonary aspergillosis, the wall of mycetomas contains chronic inflammation and fibrosis but not granulomatous inflammation. The fungal hyphae are typically matted together with alternating tight and loose areas resulting in a characteristic lamellated pattern at low magnification. Although there may be an acute inflammatory exudate at the periphery of the fungus ball, hyphae are not usually dispersed in a background of necrosis (see Figures 3.8 and 3.9).

- Invasive aspergillosis overlaps in several ways with chronic necrotizing aspergillosis (Chapter 3, Table 3.3). Both entities are associated with varying degrees of immune dysfunction, can show cavitation radiologically and are characterized pathologically by necrosis containing fungal hyphae. To complicate matters, granulomatous inflammation may occasionally occur in invasive aspergillosis. However, invasive aspergillosis typically affects overtly immunocompromised, severely neutropenic individuals, and features vascular invasion by fungal hyphae (see Figure 3.6). In contrast, chronic necrotizing pulmonary aspergillosis usually occurs in the setting of minimal or no immune dysfunction and does not feature vascular invasion.

- Rarely, fungi such as *Rhizopus* or *Mucor* may elicit a granulomatous inflammatory response in the lung. These fungi are usually aseptate and show wide-angle branching. However, histology is unreliable for definitive identification of these uncommon organisms, and cultures must be considered the gold standard.

Treatment and prognosis

Long-term anti-fungal therapy with orally administered itraconazole is recommended for chronic necrotizing pulmonary aspergillosis. Other commonly used drugs are voriconazole and posaconazole. Amphotericin B and voriconazole are used for severe disease. However, some cases with large cavities may require surgery. The prognosis is generally good, with no evidence of recurrence or progressive disease in most cases. However, not all patients improve with treatment. Progressive disease and death may occur in debilitated individuals despite adequate therapy.

Sample diagnosis on pathology report

Lung, right middle lobe, surgical biopsy – Necrotizing granulomatous inflammation (fungal hyphae present) (See comment).

or (if clinical features are consistent, and cultures are positive for *Aspergillus*)

Lung, left lower lobe, lobectomy – Chronic necrotizing pulmonary aspergillosis (See comment).

Allergic bronchopulmonary aspergillosis

Allergic bronchopulmonary aspergillosis is an uncommon form of non-invasive pulmonary aspergillosis, the clinical and pathologic manifestations of which are a consequence of a florid allergic tissue reaction (hypersensitivity) to fungal organisms rather than tissue invasion by fungal hyphae or saprophytic colonization by fungus balls. Thus, allergic bronchopulmonary aspergillosis is clinically and pathologically distinct from invasive aspergillosis and aspergillomas. The disease occurs mainly in asthmatics and is considered to be one of the "asthma-plus" syndromes, the other being eosinophilic granulomatosis with polyangiitis (Churg–Strauss syndrome). The asthma-plus syndromes are characterized clinically by worsening of pre-existing asthma, development of lung infiltrates and other distinctive clinical and pathologic findings that warrant their separation from uncomplicated asthma.

Cases in which fungi other than *Aspergillus* are cultured have been termed "allergic bronchopulmonary fungal disease". Fungi that have been implicated include *Pseudallescheria boydii*, *Bipolaris*, *Torulopsis glabrata*, *Curvularia* and *Lunata*. The practical implication is that pathologists must not use the label *allergic bronchopulmonary aspergillosis* unless there is microbiologic confirmation that the organism is *Aspergillus*. Cases where microbiologic confirmation is lacking can be termed *allergic bronchopulmonary fungal disease*.

With the development and refinement of clinical criteria, allergic bronchopulmonary aspergillosis is now usually diagnosed on the basis of clinical, radiologic and laboratory findings. Pathologists seldom see specimens from patients with this syndrome, unless clinical and radiologic findings are atypical. Lung biopsy or resection may be performed to exclude malignancy, often prompted by imaging or bronchoscopic findings suggesting bronchial obstruction. Unnecessary surgery is occasionally performed if clinical and radiologic clues to the correct diagnosis are missed. The full spectrum of pathologic changes is ideally recognized on surgical lung biopsies or larger resection specimens, but the diagnosis can also be suggested in transbronchial biopsies.

Major diagnostic findings

- The diagnostic triad of allergic bronchopulmonary aspergillosis consists of bronchocentric granulomatosis, mucoid impaction of bronchi (allergic mucin) and eosinophilic pneumonia. The pathologic diagnosis can be difficult because this triad is not always present, and each component of the triad can be seen in conditions other than allergic bronchopulmonary aspergillosis. In surgical specimens, however, all cases show either bronchocentric granulomatosis or mucoid impaction of bronchi (allergic mucin) or both, and eosinophils are always increased in number in the lung.

- Bronchocentric granulomatosis is the most common finding, seen in slightly more than half of all cases, especially in surgical lung biopsies. It is characterized by necrotizing granulomatous inflammation that is centered almost exclusively on bronchi and bronchioles (Figure 2.34). The granulomatous infiltrate either replaces the mucosa partially or completely destroys the affected airway. In the latter situation, the granulomas resemble ordinary necrotizing granulomas and the most reliable

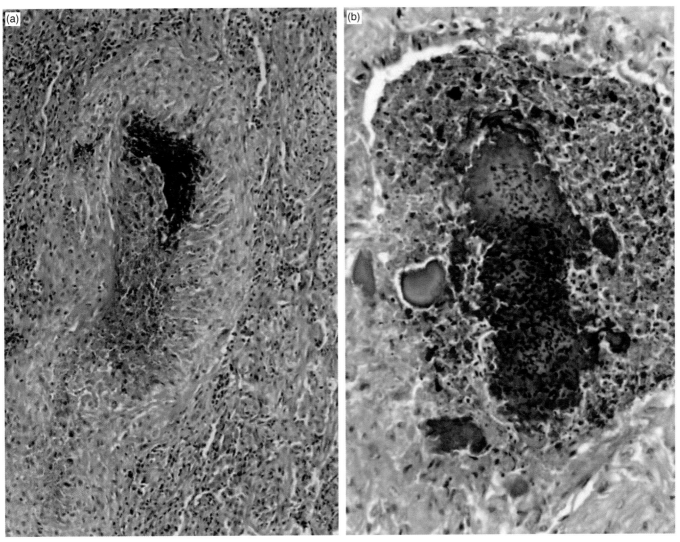

Figure 2.34. Allergic bronchopulmonary aspergillosis. (a) Necrotizing granuloma. Numerous eosinophils are present within the necrosis, as well as in the surrounding lung. **(b)** Lumen of a small bronchiole, containing a characteristic mix of degenerating fungi, necrotic debris and eosinophils.

clue to their bronchocentric nature is the presence of an adjacent partner pulmonary artery. The necrotic center of the lesion varies from less than a millimeter to several centimeters in size. The lesion may form a large cavity with abundant central necrosis but only a thin granulomatous rim, or tiny necrotizing granulomas, each with a small necrotic center. A key feature of bronchocentric granulomas in allergic bronchopulmonary aspergillosis is the presence of numerous eosinophils within the necrotic center, as well as around the granulomas. The eosinophils are usually necrotic, and are typically accompanied by numerous Charcot-Leyden crystals derived from the breakdown products of eosinophils (see below). Other necrotic inflammatory cells, amorphous debris and clumps of granular eosinophilic material may also be present in the necrotic center. The granulomas are surrounded by an inflammatory infiltrate containing lymphocytes and plasma cells. Fungal hyphae can be identified in the necrotic center in most but not all cases.

- Charcot-Leyden crystals are thought to be derived from a protein known as lysolecithin acylhydrolase, which is found in eosinophil granules. They are named after a French neurologist (Jean-Martin Charcot) and a German internist (Ernst Viktor von Leyden). It is thought that the Charcot-Leyden crystal protein aggregates into crystals when released from eosinophils into tissues. Charcot-Leyden crystals are a histologic hallmark of eosinophil-related disease. They are especially numerous in the presence of necrotic or degenerating eosinophils. On H&E, they appear on longitudinal section as pink bipyramidal crystals whose shape has been likened to a compass needle. On cross section, they appear hexagonal. In the lung, they are found in several conditions that feature large numbers of eosinophils, including allergic bronchopulmonary aspergillosis, mucoid impaction of bronchi, asthma and eosinophilic pneumonia.
- Mucoid impaction of bronchi is seen in 30 to 50% of cases. It is characterized by the presence of dilated segmental and subsegmental bronchi plugged with a histologically

distinctive form of mucin that has been termed *allergic mucin*. Allergic mucin is the histologic correlate of the "sputum plugs" illustrated by Hinson, Moon and Plummer in 1952. It has a layered appearance at low magnification that has been described as lamellated or laminated (Figure 9.7). It consists of alternating wavy concentric bands of light and dark (eosinophilic) material. At high magnification, the light bands are composed of mucin, but the dark bands contain large numbers of tightly packed, degenerating, necrotic or viable eosinophils, eosinophil granules, granular and amorphous debris, sloughed epithelial cells, fibrin and Charcot-Leyden crystals (Figure 9.8). Degenerating eosinophils often lack typical bilobed nuclei, and may be mistaken for macrophages.

- Eosinophilic pneumonia is present in nearly 50% of cases, but is very focal in most. It is characterized by the presence of eosinophils within the airspaces, usually accompanied by histiocytes and a fibrinous exudate. The alveolar septa are often expanded by eosinophils, lymphocytes, histiocytes and plasma cells. Eosinophils may form microabscesses.

- Although the disease is named after the presence of *Aspergillus* organisms, fungal hyphae are never numerous. Most often, only a few degenerated hyphae are scattered within allergic mucin, necrotic debris within bronchocentric granulomas or within exudative bronchiolitis. Their identification often requires GMS staining. Degenerative changes in the hyphae manifest as dilatation, irregularities of cell walls and fractured forms. Hyphae may occasionally be seen on H&E. Bronchial plugs, which are a hallmark of allergic bronchopulmonary aspergillosis, are thus composed predominantly of mucin and cell debris rather than fungi. As in other forms of aspergillosis, the hyphae are septate and show narrow-angle dichotomous branching. On occasion, they may be dilated or varicose. They cannot be reliably distinguished by histologic examination from other fungal hyphae that cause allergic bronchopulmonary fungal disease, including *Pseudallescheria*, *Fusarium*, *Curvularia* and *Dreschlera*. Definitive identification requires microbiologic cultures.

Variable pathologic findings

- Bronchioles are often filled with amorphous necrotic debris, necrotic acute inflammatory cells, eosinophils and clumps of dark eosinophilic debris (Figure 2.34). This lesion, termed exudative bronchiolitis, often co-exists with bronchocentric granulomatosis and is thought to represent spillage of the exudate generated by bronchocentric granulomatosis into contiguous small airways.

- Severe chronic bronchiolitis is a common finding. The inflammatory infiltrate is composed of lymphocytes, plasma cells and variable numbers of eosinophils.

- Large clumps of a brightly eosinophilic material may be present in the lumens of bronchioles and in the necrotic centers of bronchocentric granulomas. This material, which has been described as "conglutinated cellular

debris", is thought to be derived from necrotic eosinophils. It may be surrounded by a foreign-body giant cell reaction.

- Tissue invasion, either of the bronchial wall or blood vessels, does not occur in allergic bronchopulmonary aspergillosis. The identification of tissue invasion by fungal hyphae, especially vascular invasion, strongly suggests invasive aspergillosis.

- Vascular inflammation may be present in allergic bronchopulmonary aspergillosis and is thought to be a secondary phenomenon. It is characterized by the presence of a chronic inflammatory infiltrate in the media of pulmonary arteries, without necrosis.

- Histologic features of bronchial asthma are occasionally seen in the bronchi or bronchioles. They include goblet cell hyperplasia, basement membrane thickening, eosinophils in the bronchial mucosa and smooth muscle hypertrophy.

- Foci of organizing pneumonia may be present.

- Foamy macrophages may be present within the airspaces of distal lung parenchyma in association with bronchocentric granulomatosis.

Diagnostic work-up

Multiple sections should be examined with H&E and GMS stains, since organisms can be difficult to find. Elastic stains such as elastic Van Gieson (EVG) or Movat pentachrome can highlight blood vessels and bronchioles, facilitating recognition of bronchocentric granulomatosis in allergic bronchopulmonary aspergillosis.

Clinical profile

Allergic bronchopulmonary aspergillosis usually develops in young individuals, nearly all of whom have pre-existing asthma. In a few patients, asthma is discovered at the time of the pathologic diagnosis, and rarely asthma develops after a pathologic diagnosis. Allergic bronchopulmonary aspergillosis is rare in non-asthmatics, but the absence of asthma does not exclude the diagnosis.

The average age in histologically well-documented series is in the 20s, with a range from 9 to 81 years. Occurrence in children is not uncommon. Both sexes are affected. Cough, fever and asthma exacerbations are common presenting symptoms. Other symptoms include anorexia, weight loss, malaise, recurrent pneumonia, shortness of breath, pulmonary infiltrates, blood-streaked sputum, flu-like symptoms and chest pain. Patients may cough up sputum plugs containing *Aspergillus*. Some individuals are completely asymptomatic, even in the presence of radiologic abnormalities. Peripheral blood eosinophilia is frequent, seen in nearly all cases of allergic bronchopulmonary aspergillosis. In most cases, the peripheral eosinophil count is at least 8%.

Other tests that can be used to support a clinical diagnosis of allergic bronchopulmonary aspergillosis include skin testing for immediate cutaneous reactivity to *Aspergillus*, serology for precipitating antibodies to *A. fumigatus*, elevated serum total IgE level, and elevated *Aspergillus*-specific IgG and IgE levels. *Aspergillus* may be cultured from coughed up sputum plugs.

Conversely, negative serology or skin tests do not exclude the diagnosis.

Radiologic findings

The most characteristic radiologic finding is central bronchiectasis, especially in the upper and middle lobes, along with perihilar mucus plugging. Radiologically, mucus plugs appear highly opaque or hyperattenuated. Finger-in-glove opacities usually involve the upper lobes. Mucoid impaction and bronchiectasis predominantly involve the segmental and subsegmental bronchi of the upper lobes. Mucoid impaction manifests as tubular areas of increased attenuation on chest CT. Other common findings include atelectasis, lobar or segmental collapse or consolidation, and transient or fleeting infiltrates involving different lobes at different points in time. The absence of central bronchiectasis does not exclude the diagnosis.

Differential diagnosis

- Eosinophilic granulomatosis with polyangiitis (Churg–Strauss syndrome) can be very difficult to differentiate from allergic bronchopulmonary aspergillosis on histologic grounds. Clinically, both occur in asthmatics and are associated with exacerbation of underlying disease. Histologically, both feature necrotizing granulomas, striking tissue eosinophilia, eosinophilic pneumonia and non-necrotizing eosinophil-rich infiltrates within blood vessels. The inflammatory infiltrate, necrosis and eosinophilic pneumonia are more extensive in eosinophilic granulomatosis with polyangiitis (Churg–Strauss syndrome) than in allergic bronchopulmonary aspergillosis, but without extensive experience with these entities, this assessment can be subjective. The finding of mucoid impaction of bronchi or fungal hyphae indicates allergic bronchopulmonary aspergillosis, while the identification of necrotizing vasculitis establishes a pathologic diagnosis of eosinophilic granulomatosis with polyangiitis (Churg–Strauss syndrome). Clinical features such as multi-organ involvement, evidence of systemic vasculitis or p-ANCA positivity may also help to establish a diagnosis of eosinophilic granulomatosis with polyangiitis (Churg–Strauss syndrome).
- Other forms of aspergillosis are easy to separate from allergic bronchopulmonary aspergillosis since they lack a florid eosinophil-rich infiltrate and Charcot-Leyden crystals (Chapter 3, Table 3.3).
- Bronchocentric granulomatosis is a term that was initially promulgated to differentiate conditions like Wegener's granulomatosis ("angiocentric" granulomatosis) from granulomas seen in allergic bronchopulmonary aspergillosis ("bronchocentric" granulomatosis). Over the years, it has become increasingly apparent that bronchocentric granulomas occur not only in asthmatics in the context of allergic bronchopulmonary aspergillosis but also in a wide variety of other fungal and mycobacterial infections including tuberculosis,

blastomycosis, chronic necrotizing aspergillosis and coccidioidomycosis, as well as other inflammatory conditions such as Wegener's granulomatosis and rheumatoid arthritis. Therefore, "bronchocentric granulomatosis" has virtually disappeared as a stand-alone diagnosis. Pathologists should consider the possibility of allergic bronchopulmonary aspergillosis as well as infections when they identify bronchocentric granulomas, and the former should be strongly favored if the granulomas are associated with striking tissue eosinophilia or allergic mucin.
- Mucoid impaction of bronchi can form an airway-occluding mass in the absence of other features of allergic bronchopulmonary aspergillosis. The pathologic findings in isolated mucoid impaction of bronchi are identical to the findings in mucoid impaction of bronchi occurring in allergic bronchopulmonary aspergillosis. Both conditions occur in asthmatics. However, the clinical and radiologic setting is different, in that most patients with isolated mucoid impaction of bronchi present with a solitary lung nodule rather than bilateral infiltrates with central bronchiectasis. At bronchoscopy, the pulmonologist typically encounters thick, tenacious plugs of mucus rather than a solid mass. The condition is self-limited.
- Mucoid impaction can occur in cystic fibrosis or chronic bronchitis but it is not composed of allergic mucin. Instead, the cells within the mucin are mainly necrotic neutrophils and epithelial cells.
- Eosinophilic pneumonia also occurs in a wide variety of other settings, and is often idiopathic. The presence of mucoid impaction of bronchi or bronchocentric granulomatosis readily differentiates allergic bronchopulmonary aspergillosis from these conditions.
- Clinically, bronchiectasis occurs in many other etiologic settings. The florid tissue eosinophilia seen in allergic bronchopulmonary aspergillosis is not a feature of usual forms of bronchiectasis caused by cystic fibrosis, tuberculosis or recurrent infection.

Treatment and prognosis

Corticosteroid therapy is effective. It ameliorates symptoms, results in rapid resolution of fever, hastens resolution of infiltrates and results in a decrease in total serum IgE levels. Patients who undergo surgery may do well without any additional medical therapy. Recurrences are common. Undiagnosed and untreated allergic bronchopulmonary aspergillosis can result in recurrent pneumonia, bronchiectasis, chronic sputum production, loss of lung function, ineffective control of asthma and respiratory failure.

Sample diagnosis on pathology report

If organism is known to be *Aspergillus* by cultures or serology:

Lung, right upper lobe, lobectomy – Changes consistent with allergic bronchopulmonary aspergillosis (fungal hyphae present) (See comment).

Without culture confirmation:

Lung, right middle lobe, surgical biopsy – Necrotizing bronchocentric granulomas, mucoid impaction of bronchi and eosinophilic pneumonia suggestive of allergic broncho-pulmonary fungal disease (See comment).

Dirofilariasis

Human pulmonary dirofilariasis is caused mainly by the filarial nematode (roundworm) *Dirofilaria immitis*. The organism is well known to veterinarians since it causes a potentially fatal parasitic infection in dogs known as canine heartworm disease. Another *Dirofilaria* species that infects dogs, *Dirofilaria repens*, mainly causes subcutaneous and ocular disease in humans (human ocular dirofilariasis).

Dogs are infected by mosquitoes, which serve as the vector for the disease. When mosquitoes bite dogs, they introduce the infective third-stage larvae into the bloodstream. The larvae travel to the right side of the heart, where they attach to the endocardium and turn into mature adult worms, eventually forming tangled masses of thread-like parasites with serious consequences. After reaching sexual maturity, adult worms mate and release microfilariae into the bloodstream. From the peripheral blood, microfilariae can be again ingested by mosquitoes, repeating the cycle.

Human pulmonary dirofilariasis is rare. Approximately 372 cases were reported worldwide by the year 2012, including 116 from the United States (Simón *et al*, see references). As is the case with dogs, humans are infected by mosquito bites. However, since humans are "unsuitable hosts", the worms fail to reach sexual maturity in the human heart and subsequently die without releasing microfilariae. Therefore, the form found in the human right ventricle is the *immature adult worm*, which differs from a mature worm in that it does not contain ova, spermatozoa or microfilariae. Eventually, the dead immature worm is swept into the pulmonary artery and from there embolizes into a small to medium-sized pulmonary artery branch, causing infarct-like necrosis. The necrosis eventually assumes a nodular configuration and develops a thin weakly granulomatous rim. It is at this stage that the lesion is discovered in the human lung.

In the United States, *Dirofilaria* is the most common parasite associated with a granulomatous reaction in the lung. Most reported cases have been from states along the Atlantic and Gulf coasts, especially Florida and Texas. The highest prevalence appears to be in the southeast, mirroring canine prevalence rates. However, sporadic cases have been reported from all over the country, including central and western states. Outside the USA, the next-largest numbers of cases have been reported from Japan, South America (mainly Brazil) and Australia. Sporadic cases have also been reported from Italy, France, Greece, Spain, Canada, Russia, Germany and many other countries.

Most cases of human pulmonary dirofilariasis are diagnosed in surgical resections of lung nodules.

Major diagnostic findings

- Nodular lesion containing a large zone of central necrosis, a thin weakly granulomatous rim, and a necrotic artery in the center containing an immature adult *Dirofilaria* worm (Figure 2.35). The worm is usually necrotic. It is often coiled and is thus seen in multiple cuts in transverse or oblique section. It has a thick, smooth, eosinophilic cuticle without spines. In relatively well-preserved worms, one may see thin-walled tube-like internal organs including uterine tubes or a gut. Muscle tissue may be prominent. The diameter of the worm ranges from 125 to 330 μm and the thickness of the cuticle ranges from 5 to 25 μm. Occasionally, the worm is found within necrotic lung parenchyma rather than an arterial lumen. It may be partially calcified. Subtle findings such as longitudinal ridges and layers in the cuticle have been described, but are difficult to appreciate in degenerated worms.

Variable pathologic findings

- The granulomatous rim usually contains a few epithelioid histiocytes, occasional multinucleated giant cells, lymphocytes and plasma cells. Eosinophils are found in 66% of cases. Discrete non-necrotizing granulomas may be present in the rim in a few cases.
- The central necrosis is usually pink and infarct-like. Charcot-Leyden crystals have been reported in up to 27% of cases.
- The lung adjacent to the necrotic nodule may show a wide variety of secondary pathologic changes, including chronic inflammation, intra-alveolar macrophages and organizing pneumonia. A secondary vasculitis composed of eosinophils or plasma cells occurs in almost half of all cases. Foci of eosinophilic pneumonia have been reported in 10%.

Diagnostic work-up

An elastic stain such as EVG or Movat pentachrome can be very helpful in highlighting the artery with two elastic layers in the center of the necrosis.

Clinical profile

Most cases of pulmonary dirofilariasis occur in adults 40 to 60 years of age, but the reported age range is 8 to 79 years. There is a male predilection. Most patients are immunocompetent. The infection is usually detected incidentally in asymptomatic individuals on radiographs performed for other reasons such as a routine health screen or radiologic follow-up for a malignancy. A wide range of non-specific symptoms have been reported in a minority (5 to 30%) of cases, including cough, chest pain, fever, hemoptysis, dyspnea, wheezing and malaise. Eosinophilia in the peripheral blood is unusual (10%). Serologic tests are unreliable because they cross-react with other helminths. The diagnosis is typically made by histologic examination of a surgically resected lung nodule.

Radiologic findings

The main radiologic finding is a solitary lung nodule or *coin lesion*, often in the periphery of the lung. Multiple nodules have also been reported in a few cases. The reported size range is

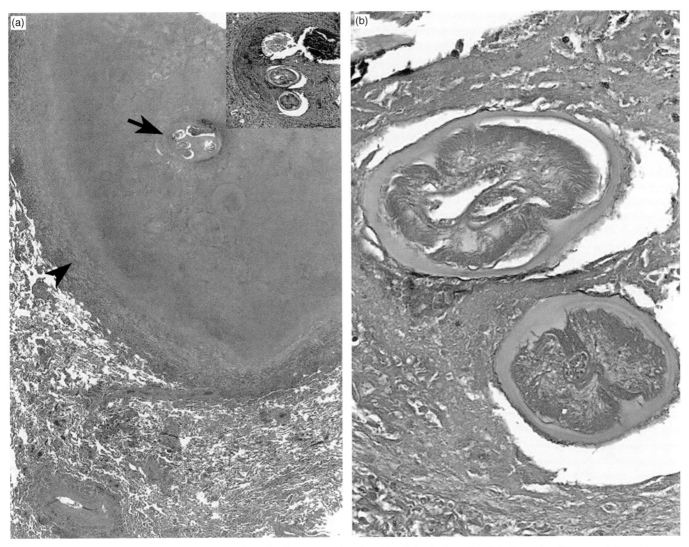

Figure 2.35. Dirofilariasis. (a) Lung nodule composed mainly of necrosis, with only a thin cellular rim (arrowhead). In the center of the necrosis is an artery (arrow), shown in the inset on a Movat pentachrome stain. Two elastic laminae can be appreciated, and a parasite is visible within the arterial lumen. **(b)** *Dirofilaria* worm with smooth pink cuticle. The organism is necrotic, and internal organs are not clearly identifiable. Case courtesy of Dr. Carol Farver.

0.5 to 4.5 cm; most nodules are 2 cm or less in diameter. Any lobe may be involved, but there appears to be a predilection for the right lower lobe. Unlike other granulomatous infections, calcification is uncommon (10%). PET positivity has been reported in some cases. Malignancy is the most common consideration in the differential diagnosis. There are no pathognomonic radiologic findings.

Differential diagnosis

The finding of a parasite with a smooth eosinophilic cuticle in a pulmonary artery surrounded by necrosis is virtually diagnostic of dirofilariasis. *Dirofilaria repens* can rarely cause pulmonary disease in humans, but in contrast to the smooth cuticle of *D. immitis*, its cuticle contains longitudinal ridges on the external surface that appear as tiny spines on cross section.

Treatment and prognosis

No specific medical therapy is required. The condition is self-limited, with an excellent prognosis. On radiologic follow-up,

most dirofilarial lung nodules remain stable, undergo calcification or resolve completely.

Sample diagnosis on pathology report

Lung, right lower lobe, wedge resection – Necrotizing granuloma (*Dirofilaria* worm present within pulmonary artery).

Paragonimiasis

Paragonimus is a trematode (flatworm/fluke) colloquially known as the *lung fluke*. *Paragonimus westermani* is the best-known species. Pleural and pulmonary paragonimiasis is endemic in Southeast Asia and China. There is only one indigenous species in the United States, known as *P. kellicotti*. Other species predominate in other geographic locations. Most cases of paragonimiasis occur in Asia, mainly in Japan, parts of China, the Philippines, South Korea, Taiwan, Laos, Thailand and Vietnam. Paragonimiasis is caused by consumption of raw, undercooked or alcohol-pickled seafood, especially crustaceans such as crayfish and crabs.

The disease is very rare in the United States. The few reported cases fall under one of three categories. First, individuals who have never traveled outside the United States may acquire *P. westermani* infection by consuming raw crustaceans imported from endemic areas. Second, the disease may be diagnosed in the United States in immigrants or returning travelers who contracted *P. westermani* infection in endemic areas. Third, the infection may rarely occur in individuals who acquire *P. kellicotti* infection within the United States by consuming raw crayfish, especially from rivers in the Missouri river basin.

After ingestion of contaminated seafood, the infective forms (metacercariae) invade the duodenal wall, crawl up the peritoneum and penetrate the diaphragm to gain access to the thoracic cavity. They then penetrate the lung parenchyma, causing pneumothorax, a characteristic clinical feature of the infection. In the lung, parasites migrate from the pleura into the parenchyma, forming *migration tracts*, a characteristic radiologic and pathologic feature of the disease. They then mature into adults and lay eggs within the airways, which are either coughed up in the sputum or swallowed into the gastrointestinal tract and excreted in the feces. Fecal contamination of water leads to ingestion of eggs by snails, which release infective cercariae that penetrate the soft tissues of crustaceans (usually crabs). Metacercariae develop within the crustacean host. This is the stage infective to humans when consumed.

Paragonimus eggs can be detected in stool samples, sputum specimens, bronchial brushings, bronchial washings, bronchoalveolar lavage fluid, pleural samples, needle biopsies of the lung, surgical lung biopsies and lobectomies.

Major diagnostic findings

- *Paragonimus* eggs are the most commonly found diagnostic form of the parasite in lung tissues. They are tiny round, oval or wrinkled structures with a thick yellow or golden brown cell wall (Figure 2.36). The average size is 85 × 55 μm

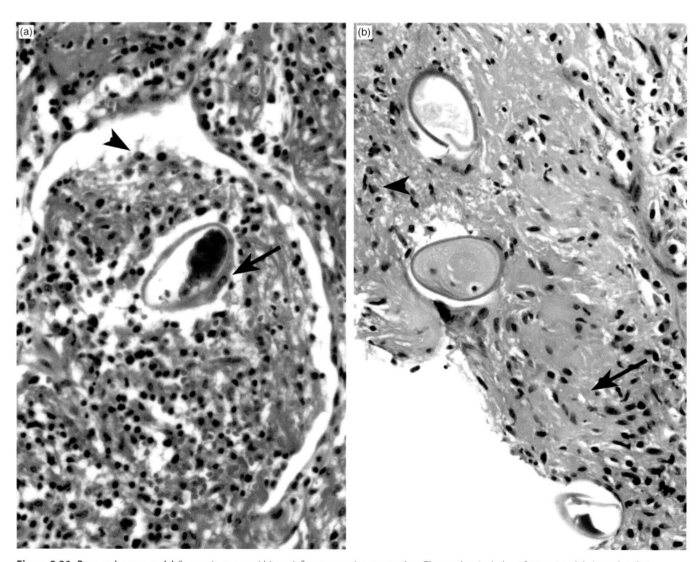

Figure 2.36. *Paragonimus* eggs. (a) *Paragonimus* egg within an inflammatory airspace exudate. The exudate includes a few eosinophils (arrowhead). A multinucleated giant cell is attached to the egg (arrow). The egg has a thick yellow cell wall. **(b)** *Paragonimus* eggs. A collapsed operculum is visible in the eggs at top and bottom. There is a subtle granulomatous response (arrow) with a few eosinophils (arrowhead). Images courtesy of Dr. Jennifer Boland.

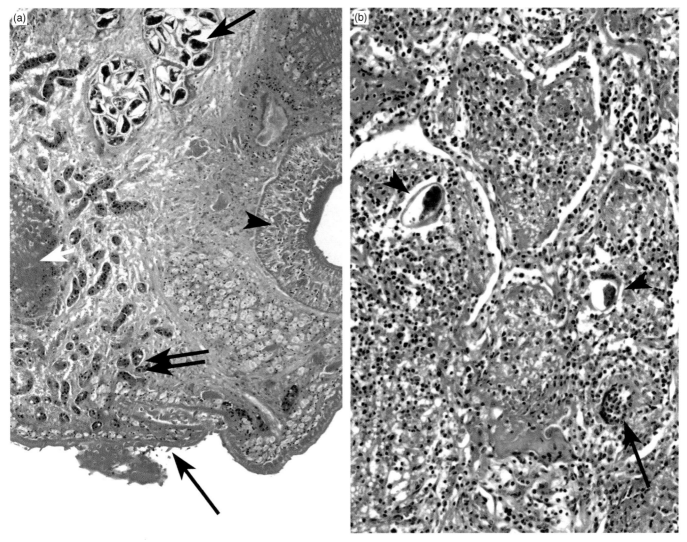

Figure 2.37. Paragonimiasis. (a) Adult fluke. Several structures can be identified in this image, including the acetabulum/sucker (arrowhead), uterus with eggs (top arrow), cecum (white arrow), vitelline glands (double arrows) and spines on the tegument (long arrow). **(b)** *Paragonimus* eggs (arrowheads) within a fibrinous exudate that fills the airspaces and contains eosinophils (arrow). Images courtesy of Dr. Jennifer Boland.

(length × width). They are often distorted or fractured in histologic sections. An important feature for the diagnosis is that the eggs are operculated, i.e., they have a "lid" at one end. The operculum is best seen in cytologic preparations. The cell wall (shell) is birefringent under polarized light. The eggs are usually found within non-necrotizing granulomas or multinucleated giant cells. A slight retraction artifact may be present between the eggs and the surrounding giant cells.

- Adult *Paragonimus* worms (flukes) are rarely seen in lung tissue. They may be found within the airways. They contain an acetabulum and spines. The acetabulum is the ventral sucker that appears in histologic sections as a hole surrounded by radiating spokes (Figure 2.37). Spines are minute needle-like structures on the wall (tegument) of the fluke. Other structures that may be visible in histologic sections include the uterus with eggs (*Paragonimus* is hermaphroditic), the intestinal cecum and vitelline glands (Figure 2.37).

- Differentiation between *P. westermani* and *P. kellicotti* is traditionally based on differences in adult worms and metacercariae. Subtle morphologic differences in the eggs have also been described, but these may not be appreciable in histologic sections and are irrelevant for therapy. In some cases reported in the literature, speciation has been based primarily on travel and dietary history rather than morphologic features.

- Eggs and flukes are not always present. In such cases, the diagnosis requires serologic confirmation.

Variable pathologic findings

- Eosinophilic pneumonia is a common finding in paragonimiasis, present in almost all cases. It is characterized by the presence of large numbers of eosinophils within the airspaces accompanied by a fibrinous exudate and variable number of macrophages (Figure 2.37). Focal organization may occur. The interstitium shows varying degrees of chronic inflammation containing mainly eosinophils and lymphocytes. Large abscess-like lesions composed of eosinophils have also been described. Admixed neutrophils and areas of acute pneumonia have been described in some cases.

- Granulomatous inflammation is present in virtually all cases. Variants of this process include serpiginous necrosis with a granulomatous rim, necrotizing granulomatous inflammation, non-necrotizing granulomas and scattered multinucleated giant cells. Giant cells have also been described within blood vessels. *Paragonimus* eggs are commonly found within granulomas or multinucleated giant cells.
- Vascular changes include granulomatous inflammation (granulomatous vasculitis), mural eosinophil-rich inflammatory infiltrates, thrombi and scattered giant cells.
- *Migration tracts* – linear or serpiginous zones of necrosis tracking from the pleura into the lung – may be present. These are thought to represent the path followed by the organism as it enters the lung.
- Pleural findings include acute fibrinous eosinophilic pleuritis, non-necrotizing granulomas containing eggs, fibrinous exudates, reactive mesothelial hyperplasia and hyalinizing fibrosis. The inflammatory infiltrate may include lymphocytes, plasma cells, eosinophils and neutrophils.
- Necrosis or an acute inflammatory infiltrate may be present. Eggs may be found within the necrosis.

Diagnostic work-up

There are no useful special stains or immunohistochemical markers. Multiple sections may be required to demonstrate an operculum in the eggs. The wall of the eggs is birefringent under polarized light.

Clinical profile

Most patients are adults. The infection has also been reported in children, and occurs in both sexes. Common presenting symptoms include cough, hemoptysis, chest pain, dyspnea and fever. Headache, fatigue and weight loss have also been reported. Many patients present with chest pain due to pneumothorax. Migratory skin nodules in the extremities (trematode larva migrans) are found in some cases. Some individuals are asymptomatic or have minimal symptoms.

Eosinophilia in the peripheral blood is a hallmark of paragonimiasis ("worms, wheezes and weird diseases"). Eosinophil counts are commonly elevated and may be as high as 25%. However, eosinophilia is not present in all cases. Pleural effusions are common. Pleural fluid analysis often shows evidence of an exudative process with eosinophilia, high lactate dehydrogenase (LDH) and low glucose levels.

Consumption of raw or undercooked seafood is the main risk factor for paragonimiasis. In the United States, the disease has been reported in people who ate at Sushi bars, especially after ingestion of imported live crabs. One case occurred in a person who drank a crab martini.

The diagnosis is confirmed on the basis of serologic studies or direct identification of the adult or eggs. Useful serologic tests include ELISA and immunoblot testing, which is performed at the Division of Parasitic Diseases of the Centers for Disease Control and Prevention (CDC). Operculated eggs may also be found in the sputum, stool, gastric washings, bronchoalveolar lavage fluid or pleural fluid. Sputum examination is a time-honored method that is highly specific but lacks sensitivity compared with serologic tests.

Radiologic findings

Radiologic abnormalities may involve the lung parenchyma, pleura or both; combinations of pleural and parenchymal disease are most suggestive. Non-specific linear streaks have been described on chest radiographs. Chest CT findings include pneumothorax (unilateral or bilateral), pleural effusions, lung cavities and nodules. Pleural effusions can be massive. They may be unilateral, but bilateral effusions are most characteristic. Occasionally, pleural effusions are the only radiologic manifestation of the disease. A solitary cavitary lung mass has been reported in several cases. Peripheral lung nodules with linear tracking (migration tracks) to pleural surfaces are characteristic. The right lower lobe is commonly involved, perhaps owing to its proximity to the diaphragm. Several reports have documented that lung cavities and nodules in paragonimiasis can be PET-positive, with SUVs ranging from 3.5 to 4.7.

Differential diagnosis

- The finding of operculate eggs with yellow cell walls in the respiratory tract is virtually pathognomonic of *Paragonimus*. *Schistosoma* eggs can appear similar but lack an operculum and are not birefringent.
- Eosinophilic pneumonia (whether due to other defined causes, or idiopathic) enters the pathologic differential diagnosis whenever numerous eosinophils are found within airspaces. However, the clinical setting in paragonimiasis is usually that of a lung mass, cavity or nodule rather than bilateral infiltrates, and the pathologic findings (granulomatous inflammation or eggs) should also help to exclude this possibility.
- The clinical differential diagnosis may include tuberculosis. Peripheral eosinophilia, bilateral lung involvement and bilateral pleural effusions are clues to the correct diagnosis. Pathologically, tuberculosis should not be a consideration given the striking tissue eosinophilia. Finding eggs will resolve the issue.

Treatment and prognosis

The drug of choice is oral praziquantel, with a cure rate approaching 100%. Successful therapy results in resolution of symptoms, clearing of radiologic abnormalities, improvement in peripheral eosinophilia and a decrease in serologic titers. Complications of paragonimiasis include recurrent pneumothoraces, pleural effusions, empyema and (rarely) cerebral involvement.

Sample diagnosis on pathology report

Lung, right lower lobe, surgical biopsy – Eosinophilic pneumonia and granulomatous inflammation (operculated ova present) (See comment).

Granulomatosis with polyangiitis (GPA, Wegener's)

Granulomatosis with polyangiitis (GPA, Wegener's) is the most common cause of non-infectious necrotizing granulomas in the lung. It is also the most common form of vasculitis involving the lung and one of the most common causes of small-vessel vasculitis (capillaritis) resulting in diffuse alveolar hemorrhage. In 2011, experts from three organizations recommended that the term *granulomatosis with polyangiitis* (GPA) with "Wegener's" in parentheses be used in order to gradually do away with the eponym *Wegener's granulomatosis*. The main reasons behind this recommendation were Dr. Friedrich Wegener's background (he was a member of the Nazi party before and during World War II) and the perceived need to shift from eponyms to disease-descriptive terminology. The abbreviation GPA will be used for the remainder of this chapter and throughout the rest of the book.

The widespread familiarity of clinicians and pathologists with anti-neutrophil cytoplasmic antibody (ANCA) testing has greatly aided the diagnosis of GPA. Most cases of GPA that present with multi-system involvement are positive for ANCA and are diagnosed on the basis of clinical features and serology without the need for a biopsy. However, surgical pathologists continue to play a role in the diagnosis, especially when the clinical setting is unusual. Examples include unusual age or presentation, disease localized to one organ (localized GPA), ANCA-negative cases or cases in which infection or malignancy is a strong consideration. Pathologists must therefore be prepared to recognize the histologic features of GPA in unusual settings and should not be deterred by the absence of multi-system involvement or a negative ANCA result. Pathologists may also be asked to rule out vasculitis in lung biopsies and evaluate biopsies for evidence of alveolar hemorrhage.

The pathologic features of GPA are best appreciated in surgical lung biopsies but occasionally can also be identified in transbronchial biopsies or core needle biopsies of the lung.

Major diagnostic findings

- *Necrotizing granulomatous inflammation.* Granulomatous inflammation in GPA is often distinctive, but since there is considerable overlap with mycobacterial and fungal granulomas, a definitive diagnosis cannot be based on the granulomatous component alone without necrotizing vasculitis or a positive ANCA test. The necrosis of GPA is often described as *geographic*, a term that refers to the map-like, irregular contours of the necrotic areas. However, this type of contour is not always present. A more helpful clue to the diagnosis is "dirty necrosis", which appears deeply basophilic, in contrast to the pink

appearance common in infectious granulomas. The basophilic appearance is caused by the presence of necrotic and karyorrhectic nuclear debris, derived mostly from necrotic neutrophils (Figure 2.38, Figure 2.1b). Another distinctive finding in GPA is the presence of suppurative granulomas with neutrophil-rich centers, resembling microabscesses (Figure 2.38, Figure 2.1b). Suppurative granulomas differ from true microabscesses in that they contain a rim of palisading histiocytes with variable numbers of multinucleated giant cells.

- *Necrotizing vasculitis* is the other major finding required for a pathologic diagnosis of GPA. Unfortunately, it is often difficult (and sometimes impossible) to demonstrate since the affected vessels may be completely destroyed. When demonstrable, it manifests as a mixed inflammatory infiltrate that destroys the vessel wall. It affects medium-sized arteries, veins or both. The inflammatory infiltrate in the involved blood vessels is composed of neutrophils and histiocytes, tiny necrotizing granulomas, or histiocytic infiltrates accompanied by tiny, subtle foci of fibrinoid necrosis. A characteristic feature of the vasculitis of GPA is that the inflammatory infiltrate frequently destroys one side of the affected vessel while sparing the remainder (*eccentric vasculitis*, Figure 2.39). Karyorrhectic nuclear debris is often present and should serve as a tip-off to the diagnosis. Findings that should not be misinterpreted as necrotizing vasculitis include vascular inflammation comprised entirely of lymphocytes and plasma cells (common in infections), non-necrotizing granulomas within vessels (common in sarcoidosis) and necrotic vessels within areas of parenchymal necrosis (innocent bystanders).

Variable pathologic findings

- Multinucleated giant cells with prominent hyperchromatic nuclei may be present. They often stand out at low magnification because of the striking hyperchromasia of their nuclei. They usually accompany necrotizing granulomas but in some cases they may be scattered singly or may be the predominant manifestation of the disease. Necrotic multinucleated giant cells, when present, have also been cited as a characteristic feature of GPA.
- Dense acute and chronic inflammation containing neutrophils, lymphocytes and plasma cells is seen in nearly every case. Plasma cells tend to be especially numerous.
- GPA can also manifest as capillaritis, which is a small-vessel vasculitis that destroys alveolar septal capillaries, causing diffuse alveolar hemorrhage. Capillaritis is discussed in detail in Chapter 10.
- Organizing pneumonia (plugs of fibroblasts within airspaces) is often seen at the edge of the main granulomatous infiltrate. Rarely, it is the most prominent pathologic finding, a condition that has been termed the "bronchiolitis obliterans-organizing pneumonia (BOOP)-like" variant of GPA.

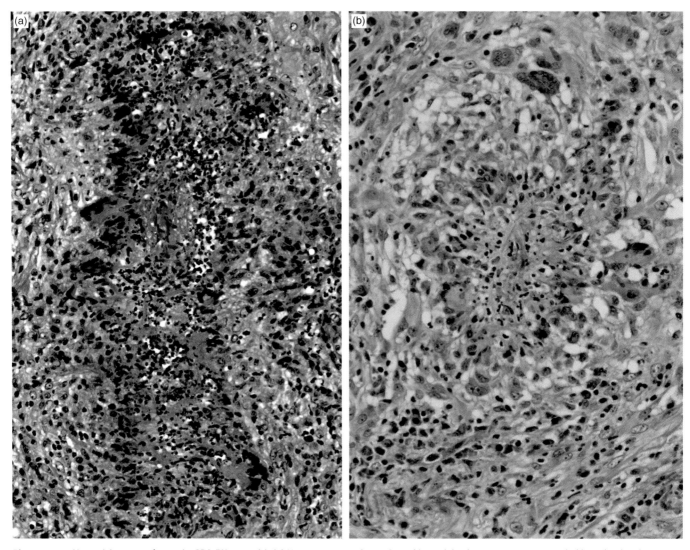

Figure 2.38. Necrotizing granulomas in GPA (Wegener's). (a) Necrotizing granuloma. Central basophilic dirty necrosis is surrounded by palisading histiocytes and occasional multinucleated giant cells with hyperchromatic nuclei. **(b)** Microabscess-like necrotizing granuloma. The prominent palisade of histiocytes distinguishes this lesion from an abscess.

- Hemosiderin-laden macrophages are often found in alveoli around the granulomatous process, and are indicative of prior hemorrhage.

Diagnostic work-up

A special stain for elastic tissue such as elastic Van Gieson (EVG), Verhoeff–Van Gieson (VVG) or Movat pentachrome can be very useful, provided that pathologists recognize the pitfalls involved (Figure 2.39). The main danger of using elastic stains to make the diagnosis of GPA is that innocent bystander vessels in necrotic lung tissue can be misinterpreted as necrotizing vasculitis. The best way to avoid this situation is to diagnose necrotizing vasculitis only in blood vessels that are located outside necrotic zones.

Clinical profile

GPA can occur at any age, although it is most common in adults between the ages of 35 and 55. There is a slight predilection for men. The disease is more common in Caucasians, and is rare in childhood. However, cases have been reported in children as young as 4 years, as well as in adults in their 90s.

Many patients describe a flu-like prodrome prior to the onset of other symptoms. Typical systemic symptoms include fever, migratory joint pain, malaise, anorexia and weight loss. The well-known triad of GPA comprises involvement of the upper respiratory tract, lungs and kidneys. Greater than 90% of patients seek medical attention for symptoms attributable to upper or lower respiratory tract disease. However, the complete triad seldom manifests at presentation. Upper respiratory tract disease presents as sinusitis, nasal crusting, epistaxis, otitis media, subglottic stenosis, sensorineural hearing loss, perforation of the nasal septum or saddle-nose deformity. Involvement of the lungs causes cough, dyspnea and hemoptysis. Renal involvement may cause only asymptomatic hematuria, or may lead to acute renal failure. Many other tissues, including the eyes, skin, joints and nervous system may be

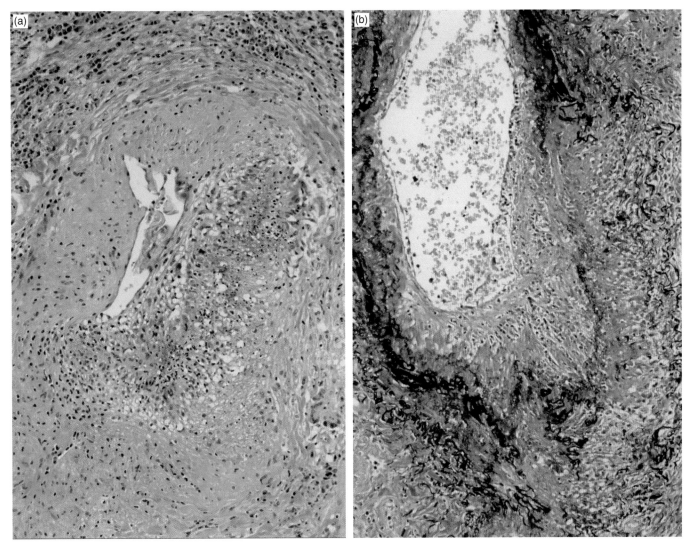

Figure 2.39. Vasculitis in granulomatosis with polyangiitis (GPA, Wegener's). (a) Necrotizing vasculitis. The right side of this artery is destroyed by necrotizing granulomatous inflammation. The left side of the vessel is spared ("eccentric vasculitis"). **(b)** Necrotizing vasculitis involving a blood vessel from a different case. Elastic stain (EVG) helps to demonstrate that the structure is a blood vessel, and highlights destruction of elastic laminae at bottom right.

involved, and the resultant range of clinical manifestations is bewildering.

Localized forms of GPA limited to the lungs or upper airways have been described in the pathology literature for several decades, and the clinical literature has gradually acknowledged the existence of this phenomenon. Such cases present a clinical challenge because they do not show evidence of multi-system involvement and have a lower frequency of ANCA positivity (approximately 50%). However, they do cause local destruction and inflammation, and a subset of cases requires immunosuppressant therapy. A small proportion (10%) of patients with localized GPA eventually go on to develop systemic generalized disease.

Anti-neutrophil cytoplasmic antibodies (ANCA) are directed against components of neutrophil and monocyte granules, and are thought to be important in the pathogenesis of the disease. Serologic tests for ANCA are currently the cornerstone of the clinical/laboratory diagnosis of GPA, as well as the two other ANCA-associated vasculitides, eosinophilic

granulomatosis with polyangiitis (Churg–Strauss syndrome), and microscopic polyangiitis. Most cases of severe multi-system GPA are positive for c-ANCA while most cases of eosinophilic granulomatosis with polyangiitis (Churg–Strauss syndrome) and microscopic polyangiitis are positive for p-ANCA. GPA can occasionally be positive for p-ANCA. The letters c and p refer to immunofluorescence patterns seen in alcohol-fixed neutrophils, which form the substrate for immunofluorescence testing (c-cytoplasmic, p-perinuclear). ANCA testing can also be performed by ELISA, which detects the specific protein against which the antibody is directed. ANCA antibodies directed against proteinase-3 (PR3-ANCA) are associated with the c-ANCA pattern by immunofluorescence and are generally seen in GPA. In contrast, ANCA antibodies directed against myeloperoxidase (MPO-ANCA) are associated with the p-ANCA pattern by immunofluorescence and are more common in eosinophilic granulomatosis with polyangiitis (Churg–Strauss syndrome). In general, ANCA testing by ELISA is thought to be more specific than

Table 2.3. ANCA-associated vasculitides in the lung

ANCA-associated vasculitis	Major clinical and pathologic features	ANCA positivity
Granulomatosis with polyangiitis (Wegener's)	Radiology: cavitary nodules or bilateral ground-glass opacities Necrotizing granulomas Necrotizing vasculitis, including capillaritis Asthma usually absent Blood eosinophilia usually absent Tissue eosinophilia rare	Any ANCA: 85 to 96% c-ANCA: 64 to 78% (generalized) c-ANCA: 50 to 60% (localized) p-ANCA: 5 to 21% PR3-ANCA: 76% MPO-ANCA: 5%
Eosinophilic granulomatosis with polyangiitis (Churg–Strauss syndrome)	Radiology: patchy airspace opacities Necrotizing granulomas can be seen, but infrequent Necrotizing vasculitis, difficult to find Asthma in 90% or more Blood eosinophilia, high Tissue eosinophilia, invariable	Any ANCA: 38 to 47% c-ANCA: 4 to 9% p-ANCA: 74 to 95% PR3-ANCA: 0 to 7% MPO-ANCA: 32 to 92%
Microscopic polyangiitis	Radiology: bilateral ground-glass opacities Capillaritis No necrotizing granulomas No asthma Blood eosinophilia absent Tissue eosinophilia absent	Any ANCA: 70 to 80% c-ANCA: 23% p-ANCA: 58%

immunofluorescence. The combined use of immunofluorescence and ELISA increases the sensitivity. The various ANCA-related vasculitides involving the lung and the frequency of ANCA positivity in these conditions are summarized in Table 2.3.

Radiologic findings

The usual radiologic findings in GPA are multiple and often bilateral cavitary nodules or nodular infiltrates. Capillaritis with diffuse alveolar hemorrhage causes bilateral ground-glass opacities or bilateral alveolar infiltrates. Localized GPA affecting the lung presents as solitary or multiple nodules. Solitary lung lesions are uncommon but are well documented in the literature. The solitary lesion may be a nodule or mass (with or without cavitation), or an infiltrate.

Differential diagnosis

- Granulomatous mycobacterial and fungal infections are the most important entity in the differential diagnosis. They may show necrotizing granulomas with dirty necrosis and multinucleated giant cells, as well as a non-necrotizing lymphocytic vasculitis. It is worth re-emphasizing that organisms may not always be demonstrable in necrotizing granulomas caused by mycobacteria or fungi. Therefore, the apparent absence of an infectious etiology should not be equated to a diagnosis of GPA. The most reliable pathologic finding that differentiates GPA from granulomatous infections is necrotizing vasculitis. Of course, identification of an organism by histology (special stains) or cultures will also resolve the problem.
- Abscess. The necrotizing granulomas of GPA are often misinterpreted as abscesses because they contain numerous neutrophils. However, true abscesses do not contain a rim of granulomatous inflammation. Therefore, the presence of epithelioid histiocytes or multinucleated giant cells should exclude this possibility.
- Aspiration of particulate matter can mimic GPA because it sometimes features a combination of acute inflammation and granulomatous inflammation rich in multinucleated giant cells. Finding degenerated particles of food or other particulate matter is diagnostic.
- Other ANCA-related vasculitides have overlapping clinical and pathologic findings, and may enter the differential diagnosis. The main features that help to separate these entities are listed in Table 2.3. It should be apparent to the reader that GPA overlaps considerably with microscopic polyangiitis. The distinction between these two entities is based primarily on the presence of necrotizing granulomatous inflammation, which excludes microscopic polyangiitis.

Treatment and prognosis

The management of GPA involves therapy with corticosteroids combined with methotrexate (for mild disease), cyclophosphamide or rituximab (for severe disease). Rituximab is also used for refractory cases. A remission rate of 90% is now achieved regularly, although some patients still die relatively soon after the diagnosis. The major current challenge in therapy is the high relapse rate after remission, seen in as many as 50% of patients at 5 years of follow-up.

If left untreated, GPA carries a mortality of 90% within 2 years. Prior to the introduction of cyclophosphamide, it was uniformly fatal and had a median survival of 5 months. However, the prognosis is now considerably better. Current estimates of mortality with therapy range from 12 to 13% at 7 years to 24 to 44% at 4 to 10 years. Morbidity and mortality are related to tissue damage by refractory disease as well as infectious complications of immunosuppression.

Sample diagnosis on pathology report

Lung, right middle lobe, surgical biopsy – Necrotizing granulomatous inflammation and necrotizing vasculitis consistent with granulomatosis with polyangiitis (Wegener's).

Eosinophilic granulomatosis with polyangiitis (EGPA, Churg–Strauss syndrome)

Churg–Strauss syndrome is a rare disease described by Jacob Churg and Lotte Strauss in 1951. In 2001, the same experts that proposed the change of nomenclature from Wegener's granulomatosis to *granulomatosis with polyangiitis* (GPA) also proposed that the eponym Churg–Strauss syndrome be changed to the descriptive term *eosinophilic granulomatosis with polyangiitis* (EGPA). The abbreviation EGPA will be used in place of Churg–Strauss syndrome for the remainder of this chapter.

EGPA is an ANCA-associated vasculitis that occurs almost exclusively in asthmatics (see previous section for a detailed discussion of ANCA, and Table 2.3 for a list of the main ANCA-associated vasculitides). It is mostly diagnosed on the basis of clinical findings. In lung pathology practice, EGPA is far less common than GPA. Pathologically, it is characterized by a unique triad of *tissue eosinophilia, vasculitis and granulomatous inflammation*. The number of eosinophils in affected tissues can be striking, and is one of the cardinal features of the disease. Unfortunately, the full histologic triad is only rarely seen in practice, making the pathologic diagnosis challenging. Histologic evidence for the diagnosis of EGPA usually comes from nerve, muscle or skin biopsies. However, lung biopsies are occasionally performed. The full histologic triad is best appreciated in surgical lung biopsies, but individual components, especially eosinophilic pneumonia, can be identified in transbronchial biopsies.

Major diagnostic findings

- Eosinophilic pneumonia is the most common but least specific histologic finding in EGPA (Figure 2.40). It is characterized by the presence of large numbers of eosinophils within the airspaces accompanied by variable numbers of macrophages and varying amounts of fibrin. As in eosinophilic pneumonia in any other setting, the alveolar septa are often expanded by a mixed inflammatory infiltrate composed mainly of eosinophils and lymphocytes. Parenchymal necrosis is not a feature of uncomplicated eosinophilic pneumonia. Therefore the presence of necrosis in association with eosinophilic pneumonia should raise the possibility of EGPA (Figure 2.40).
- Necrotizing vasculitis in the presence of marked tissue eosinophilia is the most helpful finding for the diagnosis, but is also the most difficult to identify. In full-blown examples, it is similar to the necrotizing vasculitis of GPA, the main difference being that eosinophils are the predominant inflammatory cell. The affected vessels are

small arteries and veins. As in GPA, the vascular destruction may be "eccentric", i.e., one side of the vessel is involved to a greater extent than the other (Figure 2.41). The media and intima are usually greatly expanded by large numbers of eosinophils. The necrosis is typically fibrinoid and may contain viable and necrotic eosinophils.

- Necrotizing granulomatous inflammation. Granulomas are the most variable of the three main pathologic findings in EGPA. They contain a central zone of pink fibrinous necrosis rich in eosinophils and debris derived from necrotic eosinophils (Figure 2.41). The necrotic zone is surrounded by epithelioid histiocytes and variable numbers of multinucleated giant cells. Numerous eosinophils are also present around the granulomas. As in GPA, some of the granulomas may be very tiny, resembling eosinophil microabscesses.

Variable pathologic findings

- An organizing fibrinous exudate may be present within the airspaces and bronchioles, or there may be plugs of organizing pneumonia within the airspaces.
- The bronchioles may be filled with large numbers of eosinophils admixed with necrotic debris and mucin, and numerous eosinophils may be present within airway walls. Histologic changes of asthma may be present in the airways, including thickened basement membranes, goblet cell hyperplasia, smooth muscle hypertrophy and increased eosinophils.
- A non-necrotizing vasculitis is often present and may be prominent, but this finding is common in eosinophilic pneumonia regardless of the underlying cause, and does not help to discriminate between uncomplicated idiopathic eosinophilic pneumonia and EGPA. It usually consists of large numbers of eosinophils within the intima and media of small arteries.

Diagnostic work-up

- Elastic stains can be helpful if vasculitis is suspected but they are not mandatory for the diagnosis.
- Before making the diagnosis, it is helpful to know whether the patient has asthma and peripheral eosinophilia, since EGPA is very uncommon outside this setting.
- Pathologists must understand their role in the diagnosis. Since the classic histologic triad is rare and formes frustes are so common, the possibility of EGPA should be communicated to the clinician in all cases with lung eosinophilia of unknown cause. Rare cases with the full histologic triad can be diagnosed on the basis of lung pathology alone if the findings are unequivocal.

Clinical profile

EGPA affects adults of both genders. The mean age at diagnosis is approximately 50 years, with a wide age range including children and the elderly. There is no sex predominance. The main clinical criteria for the diagnosis include asthma, evidence of eosinophilia in the peripheral blood and tissues,

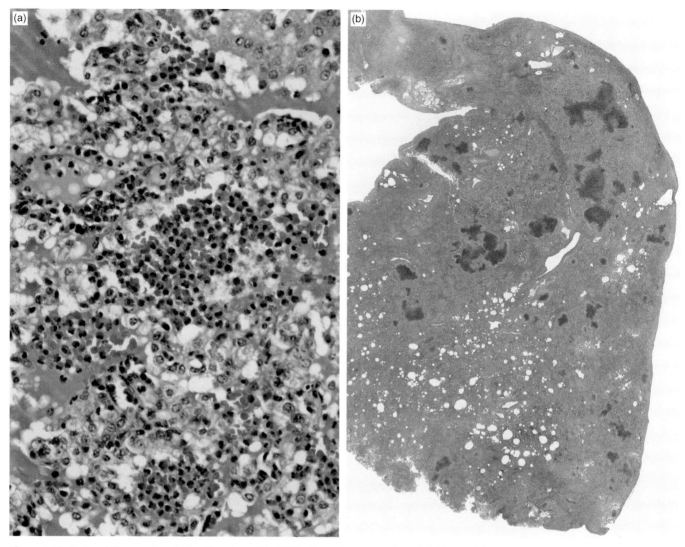

Figure 2.40. Eosinophilic granulomatosis with polyangiitis (EGPA, Churg–Strauss syndrome). **(a)** Eosinophilic pneumonia. Large numbers of eosinophils fill the alveoli. **(b)** Low magnification view of same case, showing multiple foci of parenchymal necrosis. This finding should serve as a tip-off to the diagnosis of Churg–Strauss syndrome.

fleeting pulmonary infiltrates and sinusitis. Patients with EGPA are almost invariably asthmatics. The frequency of asthma in most series is 100%, although 8 to 9% of patients in two recent large series were not asthmatics. In the vast majority of cases, the diagnosis of asthma is known at the time of presentation. Clinically, EGPA is one of two diseases associated with complications and unusual features in asthmatic patients, colloquially known as the *asthma-plus* syndromes; the other major entity in this group is allergic bronchopulmonary aspergillosis.

Patients with EGPA typically present with fever and hypereosinophilia. Other common presentations include weight loss, mononeuritis multiplex, nonerosive sinusitis or polyps, skin lesions and lung infiltrates. Recurrent episodes of pneumonia, abdominal pain, diarrhea, heart failure and constitutional symptoms may be present, reflecting the multi-system nature of the disease. Sites of extrapulmonary involvement include nerves (mononeuritis multiplex), skin (purpura), heart (cardiomyopathy), kidneys (glomerulonephritis) and the gastrointestinal tract. Compared to GPA, cardiac involvement is more

common and renal involvement is less common. Both can show inflammation in the upper respiratory tract, but ulcerative or erosive lesions are more often seen in GPA. Hemorrhagic or ischemic strokes occur in some patients.

Most patients with EGPA have eosinophilia in the peripheral blood unless they are being treated with corticosteroids. Serology for ANCA can also be useful for the diagnosis. Approximately 38 to 47% of patients are ANCA-positive (see Table 2.3). In contrast to GPA, in which c-ANCA with PR3 specificity predominates, in EGPA p-ANCA is the predominant pattern by immunofluorescence and MPO is the most common specificity by ELISA. As in GPA, patients are often biopsied when classic clinical features are absent or serologic studies for ANCA are negative.

Radiologic findings

The usual radiologic findings in the lung are bilateral infiltrates or nodules. The infiltrates tend to be patchy opacities that shift in location, and are generally less mass-like than in GPA.

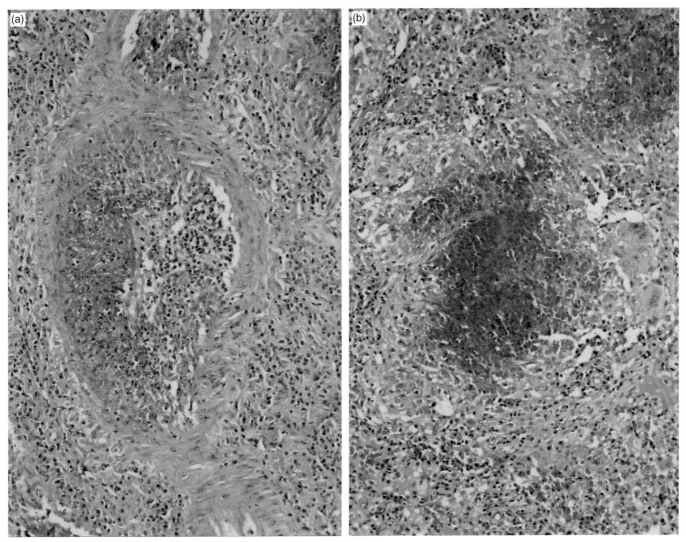

Figure 2.41. Eosinophilic granulomatosis with polyangiitis (EGPA, Churg–Strauss syndrome). (a) Necrotizing vasculitis. Note fibrinoid necrosis at left of vessel wall, and striking eosinophil infiltrate. **(b)** Necrotizing granuloma. This so-called *allergic granuloma* with central pink necrosis contains fibrin and numerous eosinophils.

Differential diagnosis

- Allergic bronchopulmonary aspergillosis can be very difficult to distinguish from EGPA. Both entities occur in asthmatics, and can feature eosinophilic pneumonia and necrotizing granulomas in the lung. Necrotizing vasculitis is a feature of EGPA but not allergic bronchopulmonary aspergillosis. Another helpful feature is that the granulomatous inflammation in EGPA is extensive and occurs in all compartments of the lung, whereas granulomas are confined to bronchioles and peribronchiolar parenchyma in allergic bronchopulmonary aspergillosis.
- Eosinophilic pneumonia. As mentioned above, eosinophilic pneumonia is one of the most common pathologic findings in EGPA. Unfortunately, it is far more commonly encountered as an isolated, idiopathic finding. A non-necrotizing eosinophil-rich vascular infiltrate can occur in idiopathic eosinophilic pneumonia as well as EGPA. Parenchymal necrosis and necrotizing vasculitis are tip-offs to the diagnosis of EGPA.

- GPA shares some features in common with EGPA, including necrotizing granulomas, necrotizing vasculitis, potential multi-system involvement and ANCA positivity. These conditions are usually easy to separate histologically since neutrophils are the most characteristic cells in GPA while eosinophils predominate in EGPA. However, an eosinophil-rich variant of GPA has been described and may cause diagnostic difficulties. In cases with tissue eosinophilia, a history of asthma or peripheral eosinophilia favors EGPA. Histologically, extensive parenchymal necrosis and the absence of eosinophilic pneumonia favor GPA.

Treatment and prognosis

Standard management of EGPA involves corticosteroids. Refractory cases may be treated with cyclophosphamide. The prognosis is good, with an overall 5-year survival of 89%. However, relapses occur in 25% of patients and deaths in approximately 10%. The most common causes of death are myocardial infarction, cardiac insufficiency and arrhythmias.

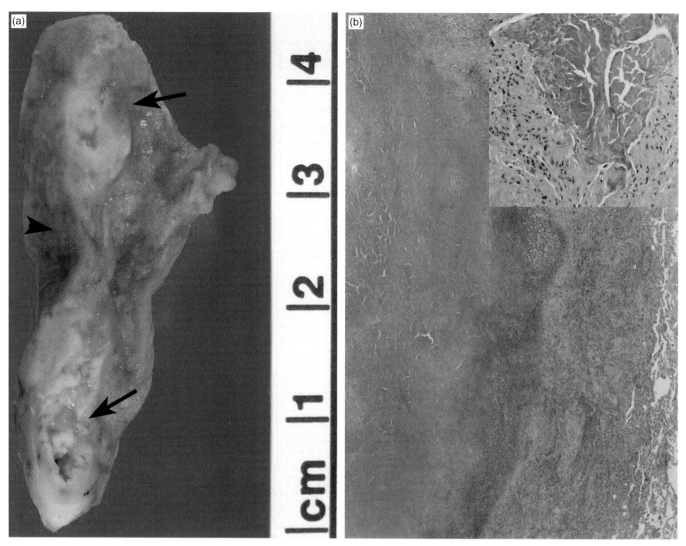

Figure 2.42. Rheumatoid nodule in the lung. (a) Two cavitary nodules are seen in the subpleural parenchyma (arrows). Arrowhead indicates pleura. The patient had seropositive rheumatoid arthritis with cavitary lung nodules. **(b)** Necrotizing granuloma. Necrotic center is at left and granulomatous rim at right. Note the basophilic hue at the periphery of the necrosis. Inset: subcutaneous rheumatoid nodule excised from the patient's thumb 2 years earlier.

Other causes include infection, malignancy and severe asthma attacks.

Sample diagnosis on pathology report

Lung, right middle lobe, surgical biopsy – Necrotizing granulomatous inflammation, necrotizing vasculitis and eosinophilic pneumonia consistent with eosinophilic granulomatosis with polyangiitis (Churg–Strauss syndrome) (See comment).

Rheumatoid nodules

Rheumatoid nodules are necrotizing nodules that occur in patients with rheumatoid arthritis, usually in the skin and soft tissues of the extremities. Less commonly, necrotic nodules also occur in the lungs. In contrast to the extremities, where the rheumatoid nodule is well-recognized and histologically distinctive, in the lungs rheumatoid nodule is a diagnosis of exclusion since the radiologic and pathologic appearance is identical to necrotizing granulomas caused by mycobacterial and fungal infections. Adding to the difficulty

is the fact that patients with rheumatoid arthritis are often treated with immunosuppressants that predispose them to granulomatous infections. Finally, although negative stains and cultures are used as a feature to exclude the possibility of infection, it is well known that burnt-out infectious necrotizing granulomas can be negative on special stains and cultures.

Major diagnostic findings

- Necrotizing granulomatous inflammation. The appearance of the necrotizing granulomas that form rheumatoid nodules in the lung is not distinctive, and overlaps with infectious necrotizing granulomas as well as GPA. Most rheumatoid nodules are located in subpleural lung parenchyma (Figure 2.42). As in other necrotizing granulomas, there is a cellular rim composed of epithelioid histiocytes surrounding a necrotic center. The necrosis may have a basophilic or "dirty" appearance, especially at the periphery near the junction between the necrosis and the surrounding granulomatous rim (Figure 2.42). The basophilic hue is caused by necrotic debris rich in nuclear material derived from necrotic neutrophils. The characteristic pink degenerative-appearing necrosis described as "necrobiosis" in rheumatoid nodules of the extremities is not usually seen in pulmonary rheumatoid nodules.

- Special stains for organisms (AFB and GMS) must be negative in order to exclude infection. Rigorous exclusion of infection is the mainstay of the diagnosis.
- There should be no evidence of necrotizing vasculitis, in order to exclude GPA.
- In most cases, patients should have an established diagnosis of seropositive rheumatoid arthritis with multiple lung nodules. In many cases, there is a history of prior rheumatoid nodules in the extremities.

Variable pathologic findings

Vasculitis (chronic inflammation within vessel walls) is common in rheumatoid nodules. The inflammatory infiltrate consists mainly of lymphocytes. In contrast to GPA, the vasculitis is non-necrotizing and does not destroy the affected blood vessel.

Diagnostic work-up

The most important step for the pathologist is to meticulously examine special stains for microorganisms (AFB and GMS) to rule out mycobacterial and fungal infections. Unfortunately, burnt-out infections may also be negative on special stains, and have a microscopic appearance identical to rheumatoid nodules. Therefore, there are no reliable pathologic features to differentiate burnt-out infectious necrotizing granulomas from rheumatoid nodules. Necrotizing granulomas of unclear etiology are assumed to be rheumatoid nodules when they occur as bilateral nodules in the context of seropositive rheumatoid arthritis with negative cultures, but this remains an assumption. It has been reported that pulmonary rheumatoid nodules contain CD20-positive cells in their periphery, but there is no evidence that this finding helps to differentiate rheumatoid nodules from their mimics.

Clinical profile

Pulmonary rheumatoid nodules are said to occur in 20 to 25% of patients with rheumatoid arthritis. The age at diagnosis ranges from 51 to 79 years. Both genders are affected. Many patients have had rheumatoid nodules in the soft tissues before the lung lesions are discovered. Most patients with pulmonary rheumatoid nodules are positive for anti-rheumatoid factor (anti-RF) and anti-cyclic citrullinated peptide (anti-CCP) antibodies at the time that they are diagnosed with pulmonary rheumatoid nodules. The nodules are often detected incidentally on chest imaging performed for other reasons.

Radiologic findings

The usual radiologic findings are multiple bilateral cavitary nodules in the subpleural lung parenchyma, but solitary nodules have also been reported. In series where the number of nodules has been documented, they vary in number from 1 to 6, and in size from 1.1 to 4.3 cm.

Differential diagnosis

- Necrotizing granulomas caused by mycobacterial or fungal infection. As mentioned above, granulomatous and fungal infections cause histologically identical necrotizing granulomas. Identification of an organism by histology or cultures solves the problem. However, if an organism is not found, clinical and radiologic features need to be taken into consideration before attributing the nodules to rheumatoid arthritis.
- GPA. The presence of necrotizing granulomatous inflammation, "dirty" necrosis or vasculitis can raise the possibility of GPA. The main histologic finding of value in this setting is necrotizing vasculitis, which is not a feature of rheumatoid nodules.

Treatment and prognosis

Responses to rituximab have been reported. The prognosis is good.

Sample diagnosis on pathology report

Lung, right middle lobe, surgical biopsy – Necrotizing granulomatous inflammation most consistent with rheumatoid nodule (See comment).

Sarcoidosis

Sarcoidosis is the most common cause of non-necrotizing granulomatous inflammation in the lung, and is one of the most common causes of interstitial lung disease seen by surgical pathologists. It is discussed here rather than in the chapter on interstitial lung disease since granulomatous inflammation is the most striking feature from the pathologist's perspective. However, the interstitial location of the granulomas is also a key and consistent feature of this disease.

Despite decades of hypotheses and research, the etiology of sarcoidosis remains unknown. The hallmark of the disease is the presence of non-necrotizing granulomas in a variety of organs and tissues, the most common being the lungs and hilar and mediastinal lymph nodes. Involvement of the skin, eyes, lymph nodes, liver and spleen is also common. However, almost any other organ or tissue can be involved, resulting in a wide array of possible clinical and radiologic manifestations. Sites that are rarely (if ever) involved by sarcoidosis include the adrenal glands, penis, scrotum, ovaries, fallopian tubes and cervix.

Pathologists will encounter sarcoidosis in a wide variety of specimens, including transbronchial lung biopsies, endobronchial biopsies, cytologic specimens including endobronchial ultrasound (EBUS)-guided fine-needle aspirates of hilar and mediastinal lymph nodes, surgical lung biopsies and explant pneumonectomies. Sarcoid granulomas can also be found in biopsies or resections of a wide range of extra-thoracic specimens including liver, skin, lymph nodes, dura, thyroid and bone marrow.

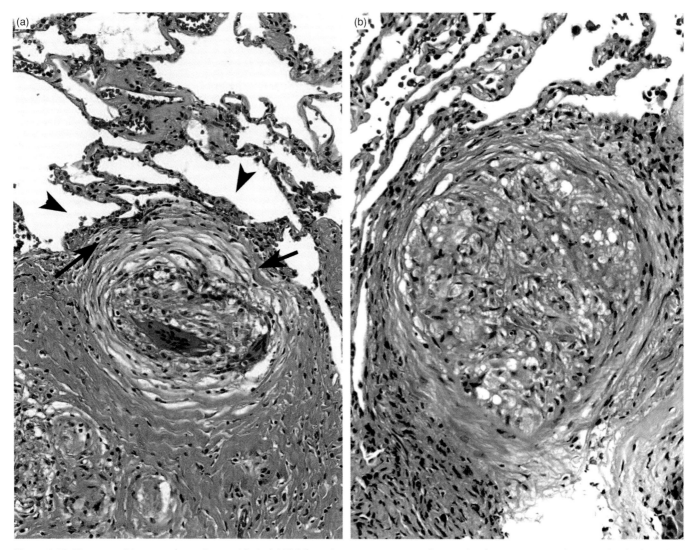

Figure 2.43. Non-necrotizing granulomas in sarcoidosis. (a) Well-formed non-necrotizing granuloma within the interstitium, with surrounding hyalinized fibrosis. Note the characteristic "cracked" appearance of the hyalinized collagen. Arrows indicate interstitium, arrowheads indicate airspaces. **(b)** Non-necrotizing granuloma with surrounding fibrosis. In this example, the fibrosis is composed of fibroblasts rather than hyalinized collagen. Note the interstitial location of the granuloma. In both photomicrographs, lung away from the granulomas is normal, a consistent feature in sarcoidosis.

Major diagnostic findings

- Non-necrotizing granulomas within alveolar septa (interstitium) or within the mucosa or walls of bronchi or bronchioles (Figure 2.43). The granulomas are usually well formed. They are located in the interstitium, including the mucosa and walls of the airways, alveolar septa, interlobular septa and the pleura.
- The characteristic distribution of sarcoid granulomas along the pleura, interlobular septa and bronchovascular bundles is referred to as *lymphangitic*, since this is the distribution in which lymphatics run in the lungs (Figure 2.44). Perhaps a more appropriate term would be *peri-lymphatic*. This distribution can only be fully appreciated in a surgical lung biopsy or larger resected or autopsied lung. The reason for this distribution is unknown. A lymphangitic distribution of pathologic abnormalities is also characteristically seen in MALT lymphomas and other low-grade B-cell lymphomas of the lungs, primary lung carcinoma or metastatic

carcinomas with predominant intra-lymphatic dissemination (lymphangitic carcinomatosis), Hodgkin lymphoma and Erdheim–Chester disease.
- Special stains for mycobacteria and fungi should be negative in all cases. Performing special stains on every case is currently standard practice, although the yield in morphologically classic cases with typical well-formed non-necrotizing granulomas and hyalinized fibrosis is close to zero.
- Lung away from the granulomas is normal.

Variable pathologic findings

- A distinctive form of hyalinized fibrosis is frequently seen in the interstitium adjacent to or around the granulomas of sarcoidosis (Figure 2.43, Figure 2.1a). It is a very helpful and characteristic finding, when present. It consists either of concentric layers of hyalinized, "cracked"-appearing collagen or concentric

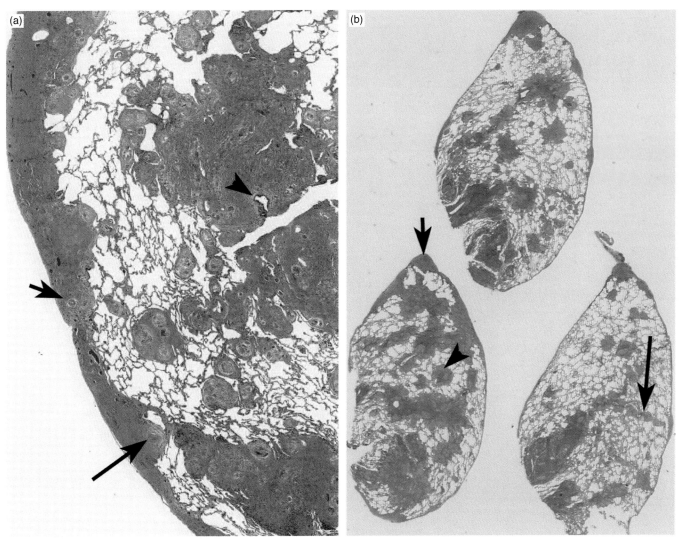

Figure 2.44. Lymphangitic distribution of granulomas in sarcoidosis. (a) Surgical lung biopsy, showing granulomas and associated fibrosis distributed along pleura (short arrow), interlobular septa (long arrow at junction of interlobular septum and pleura) and bronchovascular bundles (arrowhead). **(b)** The lymphangitic distribution in this case is best appreciated at the lowest magnification. Note granulomas in pleura (short arrow), interlobular septa (long arrow) and bronchovascular bundles (arrowhead).

layers of fibroblasts in a pale-staining background. The fibrosis may eventually replace the granulomas, giving rise to a dense, confluent mass of fibrous tissue. Confluent hyalinized fibrosis with few or no granulomas is common in explanted lungs with end-stage sarcoidosis. End-stage sarcoidosis in explanted lungs may also occasionally show features of usual interstitial pneumonia (UIP) such as fibrosis in a patchwork pattern, scarring, honeycomb change and fibroblast foci. It is likely that such cases represent two separate processes (sarcoidosis and UIP) rather than end-stage fibrosis attributable solely to sarcoidosis.

- In the bronchial mucosa, granulomas may be superficial or deep to smooth muscle bundles, or may interdigitate among smooth muscle fibers. Several granulomas may become confluent and form large nodules or masses.
- Granulomas may be present in the walls of blood vessels (Figure 2.45). Non-necrotizing granulomas and multinucleated giant cells are commonly present within the

walls of small and medium-sized arteries in the lung in sarcoidosis. This *granulomatous vasculitis* is best appreciated in surgical lung biopsies, but may also be sampled in a transbronchial biopsy, where it is a useful diagnostic finding. On the other hand, it can be misinterpreted as a true vasculitis and lead to an erroneous diagnosis of GPA. In contrast to GPA, however, the inflammatory infiltrate in the vessel walls in sarcoidosis consists exclusively of non-necrotizing granulomatous inflammation and does not feature neutrophils, necrosis or karyorrhectic debris.

- The presence of necrosis in a granulomatous infiltrate should always intensify the search for an organism. In most cases of sarcoidosis, necrosis is absent. When present, it is minimal, focal and punctate (Figure 2.46). It is usually eosinophilic, with a "fibrinoid" or "degenerative" appearance, and often contains a few pyknotic nuclei. In most cases, this type of necrosis affects only a minority of granulomas in a given specimen.

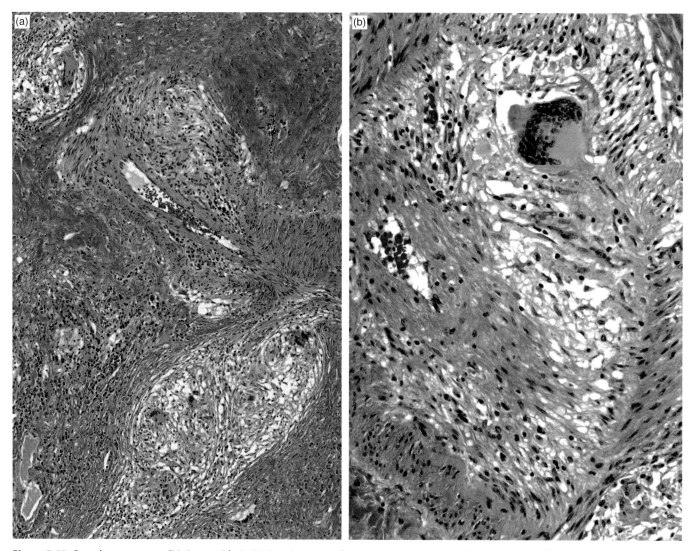

Figure 2.45. Granulomatous vasculitis in sarcoidosis. (a) Granulomatous inflammation in the wall of a pulmonary artery. **(b)** This artery was located adjacent to an area of non-necrotizing granulomatous inflammation. The granulomatous infiltrate expands and distorts the media and intima. Note multinucleated giant cell.

- Extensive necrosis is rare in sarcoidosis. So-called "necrotizing sarcoidosis" or "necrotizing sarcoid granulomatosis" receives an inordinate amount of attention in the literature, out of proportion to its extremely low incidence in practice. This causes many clinicians and pathologists to consider sarcoidosis in the differential diagnosis of necrotizing granulomas with negative special stains when in fact the main consideration should be a burnt-out mycobacterial or fungal infection. The diagnosis of necrotizing sarcoidosis requires the presence of non-necrotizing granulomas typical of sarcoidosis in lung parenchyma adjacent to the necrotic zone. Granulomas with extensive necrosis are far more likely to represent infections or GPA rather than necrotizing sarcoidosis.
- Multinucleated giant cells are often present in the granulomas of sarcoidosis, and may be large, numerous and prominent. However, they are not mandatory for the diagnosis. They may be of the Langhans type, with nuclei arranged along the periphery of the giant cell, or of the foreign-body type, with numerous nuclei bunched in the center of the cell.
- Non-specific inclusions of several types can be seen in sarcoidosis, all of which are thought to be endogenous products of macrophage metabolism.
- Asteroid bodies are tiny pink star-like or spider-like inclusions within histiocytes or multinucleated giant cells. They consist of a central pink core with thin radiating pink spokes (Figure 2.47). They are seen in a wide variety of lung diseases featuring granulomas or multinucleated giant cells, including non-tuberculous mycobacterial infections, histoplasmosis, cryptococcosis, talc granulomatosis, particulate matter aspiration pneumonia and even pulmonary alveolar proteinosis. Therefore, they should not be construed as supportive evidence for a diagnosis of sarcoidosis. We have seen a few cases in which misinterpretation of the significance of asteroid bodies has led to an incorrect diagnosis of sarcoidosis.
- Schaumann bodies are basophilic or purple concentrically laminated microcalcifications resembling psammoma

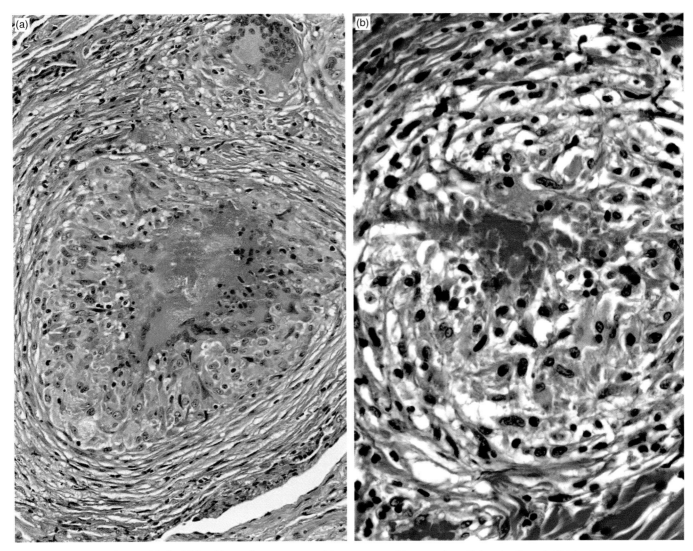

Figure 2.46. Necrosis in sarcoidosis. (a) Small focus of punctate necrosis in a non-necrotizing granuloma. Note pyknotic nuclei. **(b)** Another example of a tiny focus of necrosis in an otherwise classic non-necrotizing granuloma.

bodies, found within granulomas or multinucleated giant cells (Figure 2.47). They are also known as conchoidal bodies. They are found in up to 70% of cases of sarcoidosis in biopsy specimens. They may be numerous in sarcoidosis, but they are not specific since they may also be found in hypersensitivity pneumonitis, blastomycosis and other causes of granulomatous lung disease. They may or may not contain a birefringent center.

- Calcium oxalate crystals are colorless birefringent crystalline particles found within multinucleated giant cells (Figure 2.48). Despite the strong birefringence, they are not foreign particles. They are not specific for sarcoidosis.

Diagnostic work-up

- Special stains for microorganisms (AFB and GMS) are routinely performed in cases of suspected sarcoidosis, although the yield is extremely low, especially in the context of well-formed non-necrotizing granulomas with H&E features that strongly suggest the diagnosis. Nevertheless,

the potential impact of a positive special stain is so great that most pathologists prefer to err on the side of caution in this situation.

- Pathologists are rarely given a detailed account of the history and radiologic findings, but those with access to electronic medical records should familiarize themselves with the usual clinical and radiologic features of sarcoidosis. It is helpful to take these findings into account. The most pertinent features are the age of the patient, the radiologic findings (especially bilateral hilar adenopathy) and the clinical impression. Cases in young individuals with hilar adenopathy and a clinical diagnosis of sarcoidosis are very likely to represent sarcoidosis, unless the histologic features are extremely atypical. In contrast, unless the pathologic findings are unequivocal (such as in a surgical biopsy, or a transbronchial biopsy with classic findings), pathologists should be guarded in their interpretation of non-necrotizing granulomas in older (60s or older) or immunosuppressed individuals, cases that lack hilar adenopathy or when clinical or radiologic findings

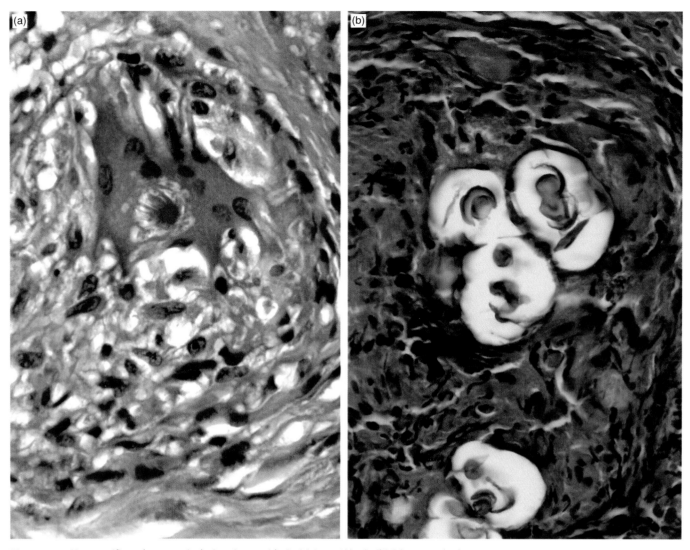

Figure 2.47. Non-specific endogenous inclusions in sarcoidosis. (a) Asteroid body. **(b)** Schaumann bodies.

suggest an alternative diagnosis. Such findings include fever, drenching night sweats, bilateral diffuse ground-glass opacities with a "head-cheese" appearance, a large solitary mass, bronchiectasis or tree-in-bud opacities.

- The role of the pathologist in the diagnosis of sarcoidosis is to identify granulomas, determine whether and how much necrosis is present and identify features that support a diagnosis of sarcoidosis. Even more important is the identification of pathologic features that suggest an alternative diagnosis, the most important being mycobacterial or fungal infection, chronic hypersensitivity pneumonitis, hot tub lung and lymphoma (see Table 2.4).

Clinical profile

Sarcoidosis usually occurs in young adults of either sex. Although the incidence in African-Americans is relatively high, the race of the patient is irrelevant to the diagnosis in an individual case. Most patients are between 20 and 55 years of age at the time of diagnosis, with a peak incidence in the 30s and 40s. In the ACCESS (A Case Control Etiologic Study of

Sarcoidosis) study, 46% of patients were less than 40 years old. The disease is uncommon before the age of 25 and after the age of 65, although well-documented cases do exist in these age groups. Many patients are asymptomatic at presentation, and come to clinical attention because of the incidental finding of hilar prominence in chest radiographs performed for unrelated reasons. Symptoms, when present, are often non-specific and are not always related to sarcoidosis. The most common symptoms attributable to pulmonary sarcoidosis are cough and shortness of breath.

Involvement of extrapulmonary organs leads to a wide variety of clinical presentations referable to the site of involvement. Many extrapulmonary tissues may be involved in sarcoidosis, although nearly half of all patients present with disease limited to the thorax (lungs and/or hilar lymph nodes). Common extrapulmonary sites include skin, lymph nodes, eyes and liver. Sarcoidosis can also involve the heart, brain, meninges, bones, bone marrow and thyroid.

Laboratory findings do not establish the diagnosis with any degree of certainty. Historically, angiotensin-converting enzyme (ACE) has been the most widely used test. The

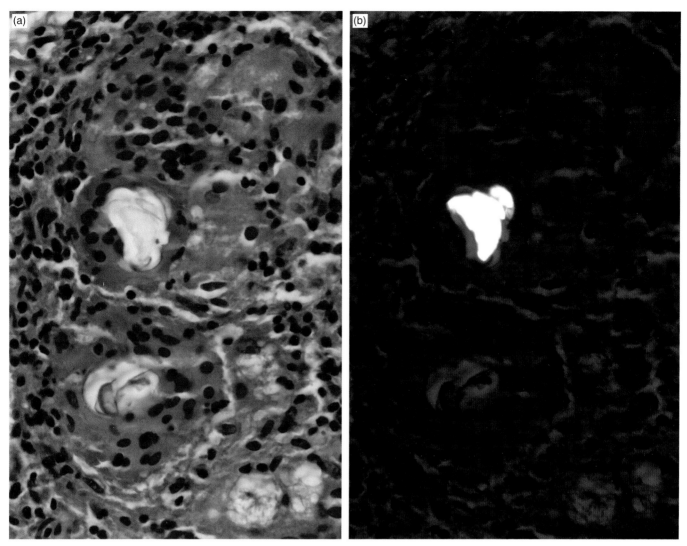

Figure 2.48. Non-specific birefringent inclusions in sarcoidosis. (a) Two inclusions are seen within multinucleated giant cells, one colorless, the other basophilic. **(b)** Under polarized light, the colorless inclusion (likely a calcium oxalate crystal) is strongly birefringent while the basophilic inclusion (probably a Schaumann body) is not. Neither structure is a foreign particle.

sensitivity of an elevated ACE level for sarcoidosis is 57% and the specificity is 90%. Therefore, a normal ACE level does not rule out sarcoidosis, and an elevated level, although helpful, is not specific enough to allow a confident diagnosis in an individual patient. The Kveim test is a skin test of extremely limited availability that is seldom used in practice.

Radiologic findings

The classic radiologic findings of sarcoidosis are multiple small bilateral lung nodules or infiltrates accompanied by bilateral and symmetric hilar and mediastinal lymphadenopathy. A "lymphangitic" (lymphatic/peri-lymphatic) distribution of the nodules along the pleura, interlobular septa and broncho-vascular bundles may be evident on chest CT.

Differential diagnosis

- Granulomatous mycobacterial and fungal infections enter the differential diagnosis of sarcoidosis since they

occasionally manifest as non-necrotizing granulomatous inflammation, or because necrosis may not be sampled in a small biopsy. Tuberculosis and histoplasmosis usually feature abundant necrosis, and there is at least focal necrosis in virtually all cases. However, some granulomatous infections such as cryptococcosis and non-tuberculous mycobacterial infections may not show any necrosis, even in surgical lung biopsies. Cryptococcosis should not be difficult to differentiate from sarcoidosis in most instances because the organisms are visible on H&E and are easily highlighted with a GMS stain. However, the granulomas of non-tuberculous mycobacterial infections can be very similar to those of sarcoidosis. Histologic features that are helpful in this differential diagnosis are granulomas within airspaces or in plugs of organizing pneumonia, which argue for an infectious etiology and against sarcoidosis. Needless to say, identification of an organism on special stains, or growth of organisms on cultures will resolve this problem. Similar considerations

Table 2.4. Histologic findings that argue against sarcoidosis

Histologic finding	Significance
More than minimal, degenerative-appearing necrosis	Should suggest an infection and prompt careful examination of special stains
Granulomas within airspaces, or organizing pneumonia containing granulomas	Should raise the possibility of infection (especially non-tuberculous mycobacterial infections) or hot tub lung
Diffuse interstitial chronic inflammation away from granulomas	Consider hypersensitivity pneumonitis
Scattered, isolated multinucleated giant cells without well-formed granulomas	Consider hypersensitivity pneumonitis
Organizing pneumonia (polyp-like fibroblast plugs within airspaces)	Consider infections, particulate matter aspiration, or GPA
Talc, microcrystalline cellulose or crospovidone	Drug abuse if present exclusively within interstitium
Vegetable fragments (intact or degenerated)	Particulate matter aspiration pneumonia
Atypical lymphoid cells, Reed-Sternberg cells, eosinophils	Consider Hodgkin lymphoma

apply to the entity known as hot tub lung, which is not a true infection, but is histologically similar to non-tuberculous mycobacterial infections. Airspace granulomas, positive AFB stains, positive cultures for MAC or a history of hot tub use aid in the diagnosis of hot tub lung, whereas a lymphangitic distribution of granulomas or the presence of dense hyalinized fibrosis favors sarcoidosis.

- Hypersensitivity pneumonitis is often included in the differential diagnosis of sarcoidosis, and occasionally interpretation can be challenging in a small biopsy. However, in most cases, the histologic appearance of hypersensitivity pneumonitis is easily distinguished from sarcoidosis (Figure 2.49). While the histologic picture in sarcoidosis is dominated by granulomas, the main pathologic finding in hypersensitivity pneumonitis is the presence of lymphocytes within alveolar septa; granulomas are inconspicuous. In most cases of hypersensitivity where granulomas are present, they are small, subtle, few in number and difficult to find. Often, the so-called granulomas consist only of rare multinucleated giant cells scattered within an interstitial lymphocytic infiltrate (Figure 2.49). In contrast, in sarcoidosis, alveolar septa away from the granulomas are entirely normal.
- Granulomatous-lymphocytic interstitial lung disease (GLILD) is a term used for a mixed bag of odd and

unexplained granulomatous and lymphocytic inflammatory infiltrates that occur in the lungs of patients with common variable immunodeficiency (CVID). Most patients are diagnosed in the teenage years or later, and the age at diagnosis may be similar to sarcoidosis. There may be no prior history of recurrent infection in childhood or known immunodeficiency. In most cases, although the clinical diagnosis may be challenging, the pathologic findings do not resemble sarcoidosis (Figure 2.50). The entity enters the differential diagnosis because of the presence of occasional unexplained non-necrotizing granulomas in the context of negative special stains and cultures. In most cases of this type, the primary pathologic finding is a lymphoid infiltrate in bronchiolar walls and peribronchiolar interstitium, variably accompanied by lymphoid aggregates and germinal centers (Figure 2.50). When present, granulomas are sparse and ill-defined, and lack the classic features of sarcoid granulomas such as hyalinized fibrosis or a lymphangitic distribution. The best way to confirm or exclude a diagnosis of GLILD is by measuring serum immunoglobulin levels. All patients have low IgG levels, and most also have low levels of IgA or IgM.

- "Sarcoid-like reactions" to tumor usually occur within malignant tumors such as seminoma and Hodgkin lymphoma, or in tissue immediately adjacent to neoplastic cells. Such granulomas seldom show features of classic sarcoidosis (well-formed granulomas with hyalinized fibrosis). In rare cases in which a neoplasm co-exists with lung or lymph node granulomas that appear histologically identical to sarcoidosis, it can be difficult to exclude the possibility that the patient has concurrent, coincidental sarcoidosis and neoplasia.
- GPA should not be difficult to distinguish from sarcoidosis because the granulomas are necrotizing, do not involve lymph nodes, and are associated with necrotizing vasculitis. However, there is some scope for confusion because both diseases can involve blood vessels. The vasculitis of GPA features necrosis, neutrophils and karyorrhexis, whereas the vasculitis of sarcoidosis is characterized by non-necrotizing granulomas and giant cells within vessel walls without necrosis, neutrophils or karyorrhexis.
- Silicosis can be difficult to differentiate from sarcoidosis on clinical and radiologic grounds because it causes bilateral upper lobe-predominant nodules along with hilar and mediastinal adenopathy (attributable to the presence of silicotic nodules in lymph nodes). An occupational history may not be forthcoming or is occasionally overlooked. However, on histologic grounds, silicosis is easy to distinguish from sarcoidosis because it does not feature granulomas. Instead, it is characterized by fibrous nodules containing lamellated collagen surrounded by dust-laden macrophages with birefringent, needle-shaped silica and silicate particles (see Chapter 8).
- Hodgkin lymphoma can sometimes mimic sarcoidosis of the hilar lymph nodes since it is occasionally associated with granulomatous inflammation. In most cases of this type, the granulomas are not well formed, and the presence

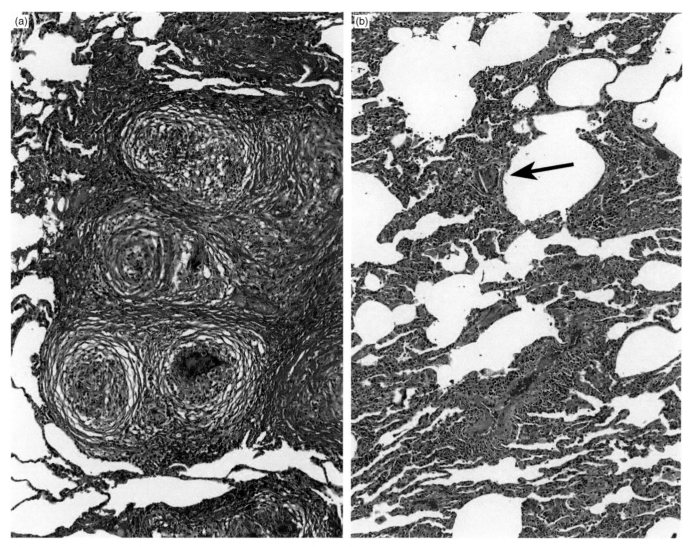

Figure 2.49. Sarcoidosis vs. hypersensitivity pneumonitis (identical magnification). (a) Sarcoidosis. Well-formed non-necrotizing granulomas and hyalinized fibrosis dominate the histologic picture. **(b)** Hypersensitivity pneumonitis. The main histologic finding is mild interstitial expansion by a lymphocytic infiltrate. There is only a single tiny multinucleated giant cell (arrow).

of large, atypical cells in a polymorphous background is a tip-off to the correct diagnosis. However, in rare cases atypical cells may not be prominent, making the identification of Hodgkin lymphoma extremely challenging. Well-formed non-necrotizing granulomas associated with hyalinized fibrosis argue against Hodgkin lymphoma, especially if they involve the entire lymph node in a wall-to-wall fashion. When only scattered non-necrotizing granulomas are present in a lymphoid background, a careful search for atypical cells should be performed, and immunohistochemistry for CD30 and CD15 should be considered.

Treatment and prognosis

The management of sarcoidosis varies depending on the presence and extent of symptoms. Most asymptomatic patients with minimal disease do not require therapy. On the other hand, most symptomatic patients receive corticosteroids (prednisone). Steroid-sparing agents such as methotrexate and TNF-alpha inhibitors such as infliximab are being increasingly used. The prognosis is good in most cases. It is well known that sarcoidosis often regresses or resolves spontaneously without therapy, especially in the early stages of the disease. A minority of patients progress and develop serious complications such as pulmonary fibrosis or life-threatening cardiac arrhythmias. Considerable morbidity and mortality is also caused by complications of immunosuppressive therapy, including drug toxicities, opportunistic infections such as tuberculosis and histoplasmosis, and lymphomas.

Sample diagnosis on pathology report

Lung, right middle lobe, transbronchial biopsy – Non-necrotizing granulomas (See comment).

or

Lung, right upper lobe, surgical biopsy – Non-necrotizing granulomas consistent with sarcoidosis (See comment).

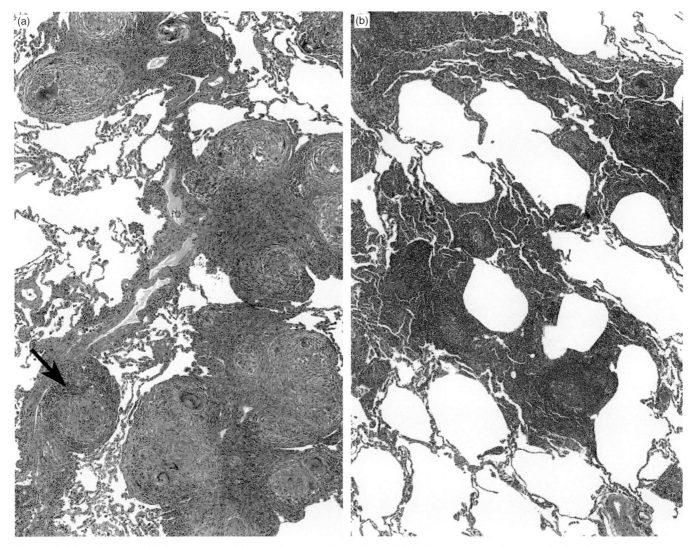

Figure 2.50. Sarcoidosis vs. GLILD. (a) Non-necrotizing granulomas consistent with sarcoidosis. Some of the granulomas are distributed along an interlobular septum (arrow). **(b)** Lymphoid infiltrate in a patient with common variable immunodeficiency, diagnosed as GLILD. A patchy lymphocytic infiltrate is present within the interstitium, including a few lymphoid aggregates with germinal centers. There are no granulomas. Case courtesy of Dr. Carol Farver.

Hot tub lung

Hot tub lung is a hypersensitivity pneumonitis-like syndrome characterized by a granulomatous response to inhaled non-tuberculous mycobacteria derived from warm water aerosols, most commonly hot tubs. Although the disease is caused by exposure to non-tuberculous mycobacteria, it is more akin to hypersensitivity pneumonitis than non-tuberculous mycobacterial infection, in that it resolves rapidly and completely (without antimycobacterial therapy) after cessation of exposure to the offending hot tub, with or without corticosteroid therapy. In contrast, non-tuberculous mycobacterial infections require prolonged antimycobacterial therapy and would be expected to worsen with steroids.

In most reported cases of hot tub lung, the organism isolated from respiratory samples and/or the offending hot tub belongs to the *Mycobacterium avium* complex (MAC, including *Mycobacterium avium* and *Mycobacterium intracellulare*). *Mycobacterium fortuitum* has been reported in rare cases. Although hot tubs are the usual source of MAC-contaminated

warm water aerosols, a similar disease can occur in susceptible individuals upon exposure to MAC derived from showerheads or therapy pools. Improper cleaning of hot tubs and poor personal hygiene predispose to contamination by MAC.

Major diagnostic findings

- Granulomatous inflammation. The granulomas of hot tub lung are usually non-necrotizing and well formed, but a few necrotizing granulomas may also be present. The most characteristic feature of the granulomas is that they are located predominantly within airspaces, including the lumens of bronchioles, alveolar ducts and alveoli (Figure 2.51). They are larger and more prominent than the granulomas of hypersensitivity pneumonitis, and may closely mimic the well-formed granulomas of sarcoidosis.
- There are no other constant or pathognomonic pathologic findings. In the absence of microorganisms or other obvious etiologies, the presence of well-formed granulomas within small bronchioles and alveoli should raise the

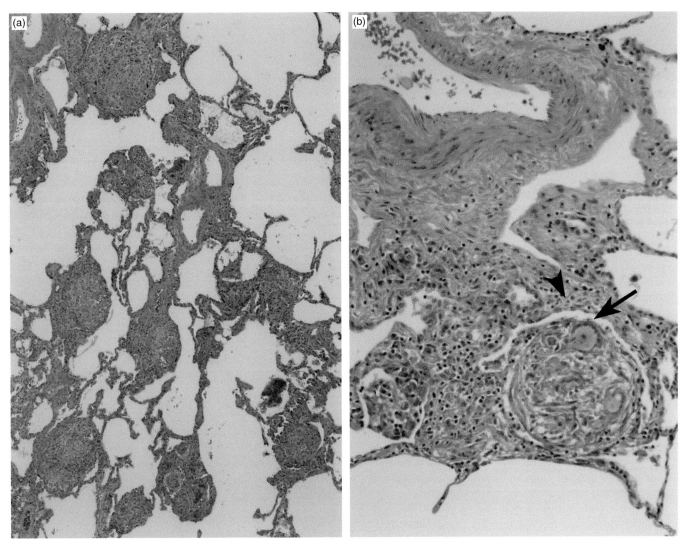

Figure 2.51. Hot tub lung. (a) Non-necrotizing granulomas. Note the superficial resemblance to sarcoidosis. The granulomas are prominent at low magnification, in contrast to hypersensitivity pneumonitis, where they are difficult to find. **(b)** Non-necrotizing granuloma within an airspace, accompanied by interstitial chronic inflammation (arrow – airspaces, arrowhead – interstitium). These pictures are from a woman with breast cancer, worsening shortness of breath and diffuse interstitial lung disease on chest radiographs. After the possibility of hot tub lung was raised based on the pathologic findings, additional history was obtained, revealing that her symptoms had begun after she had started using a hot tub.

possibility of hot tub lung and this should be communicated to the clinician. Identification of AFB in histologic specimens or isolation of MAC organisms from respiratory samples can be helpful but is not mandatory for the diagnosis. The key element is a history of hot tub use. The diagnosis is supported by resolution of symptoms and radiologic abnormalities after cessation of exposure to the contaminated hot tub.

Variable pathologic findings

- Organizing pneumonia often accompanies the granulomas of hot tub lung. It is characterized by fibroblast plugs that fill the airspaces, and is often closely admixed with the granulomatous infiltrate.
- Variable degrees of interstitial chronic inflammation are usually present. The inflammatory infiltrate typically involves small bronchioles and alveolar septa and is composed mainly of lymphocytes. In contrast to hypersensitivity pneumonitis, granulomas predominate over interstitial chronic inflammation in most cases.
- AFB may or may not be identifiable in histologic sections of lung biopsies, and are not mandatory for the diagnosis. MAC may be isolated in cultures in cases where no organisms are demonstrable by histology. The presence of AFB in tissue does not differentiate true infection from hot tub lung.

Diagnostic work-up

An AFB stain for mycobacteria must be performed if hot tub lung is suspected.

Clinical profile

Patients with hot tub lung are usually young adults with a mean age of 43 years, although the disease can occur at any age (9 to

70 years). There is a predilection for women. The most common symptom is dyspnea, followed by cough, fever and flu-like symptoms. Symptoms can be present for several months, or can come on acutely. Cleaning the dirty filter of a hot tub often precipitates symptoms. As in hypersensitivity pneumonitis, symptoms are exacerbated by contact with the contaminated hot tub, and ameliorated by cessation of exposure. The clinical features are essentially identical to those of hypersensitivity pneumonitis due to other causes.

Isolation of MAC from cultures of biopsied lung tissue, respiratory specimens or water from the offending hot tub is helpful in supporting the diagnosis. Hot tub lung is not a pure pathologic diagnosis. The role of the pathologist is to identify granulomatous inflammation, recognize its airspace location, raise the possibility of hot tub lung and encourage the clinician to obtain a history of hot tub use. In the appropriate clinical and radiologic context, the finding of airspace granulomas in an individual with hot tub exposure is sufficient to make the diagnosis. The diagnosis can also be made without the aid of pathology, if culture results are supportive.

Radiologic findings

Most cases of hot tub lung show bilateral ground-glass opacities with or without centrilobular nodules. The features are similar to hypersensitivity pneumonitis caused by exposure to other organic antigens.

Differential diagnosis

- Sarcoidosis. Hot tub lung can mimic sarcoidosis since the granulomas are numerous and often well formed. In contrast to sarcoidosis, the granulomas of hot tub lung are located within airspaces and do not show hyalinized fibrosis or a lymphangitic distribution (Figure 2.51). Identification of AFB excludes sarcoidosis.
- Non-tuberculous mycobacterial infections can be histologically identical to hot tub lung, and, as in hot tub lung, AFB may or may not be detected by special stains. In this situation, a history of hot tub use prior to the onset of symptoms is the key differentiating feature, and resolution of the disease upon cessation of exposure is confirmatory.
- It is not surprising that hypersensitivity pneumonitis caused by other exposures (bird fancier's lung, for example) is similar to hot tub lung, since the latter is essentially a variant of the former. Both entities feature a combination of interstitial chronic inflammation, granulomas and foci of organizing pneumonia. The distinction between the two rests on the relative prominence of interstitial inflammation and granulomas, the morphologic characteristics and location of the granulomas and a history of hot tub use. While alveolar septal expansion by chronic inflammation is the most striking feature in most cases of hypersensitivity pneumonitis, granulomas are the predominant finding in hot tub lung (see Figures 2.49 and 2.51). The granulomas of hot tub lung are well formed and located within airspaces, whereas in hypersensitivity pneumonitis they are mostly tiny, poorly formed and interstitial. A clinical history of hot tub use is essential for a diagnosis of hot tub lung.
- Other granulomatous infections. Granulomas can be found within airspaces in other mycobacterial and fungal infections, especially cryptococcosis. Identification of organisms other than non-tuberculous mycobacteria by histology or cultures excludes hot tub lung.

Treatment and prognosis

The most important step in the management is complete avoidance of the contaminated hot tub. In some cases, patients have sold their hot tubs or converted them into indoor gardens. Avoidance of hot tubs alone, even without additional medical therapy, can result in amelioration of symptoms. Other approaches include cleaning the hot tub or changing the filter type. Corticosteroids have been used in severe cases. Although anti-mycobacterial therapy has been used in some cases, there is no evidence of benefit and there is potential for considerable toxicity. Hot tub lung improves or resolves in most instances upon cessation of hot tub use combined with corticosteroid therapy.

Sample diagnosis on pathology report

Lung, left lower lobe, surgical biopsy – Organizing granulomatous pneumonia (See comment).
   or
Lung, left lower lobe, surgical biopsy – Granulomatous inflammation and organizing pneumonia (See comment).

Granulomatous lung disease caused by aspiration of food and other particulate gastric contents

The form of aspiration pneumonia that most clinicians are familiar with involves aspiration of oral flora (bacteria) into the right lower lobe, causing a bacterial bronchopneumonia. These patients are severely debilitated individuals, or suffer from clinically obvious neurologic problems such as cerebrovascular accidents or seizures that hinder adequate protection of the airway. Most physicians are also familiar with aspiration of foreign bodies into the tracheobronchial tree.

However, most clinicians and many pathologists are unfamiliar with aspiration of particulate matter from gastric contents (food or pills) into the lungs, especially in patients who do not report choking on food, lack severe gastro-esophageal reflux and are not severely debilitated. The diagnosis is often missed because clinicians and radiologists do not usually include aspiration in the differential diagnosis of nodular lesions on chest imaging, or in the differential diagnosis of infiltrates involving sites other than the right lower lobe. To compound the problem, most pathologists do not associate granulomas with aspiration, adding to under-recognition of this condition. The typical and predictable sequence of events associated with aspiration of food particles into the lungs (acute inflammation followed by foreign-body type granulomas and organization) has been described for several decades

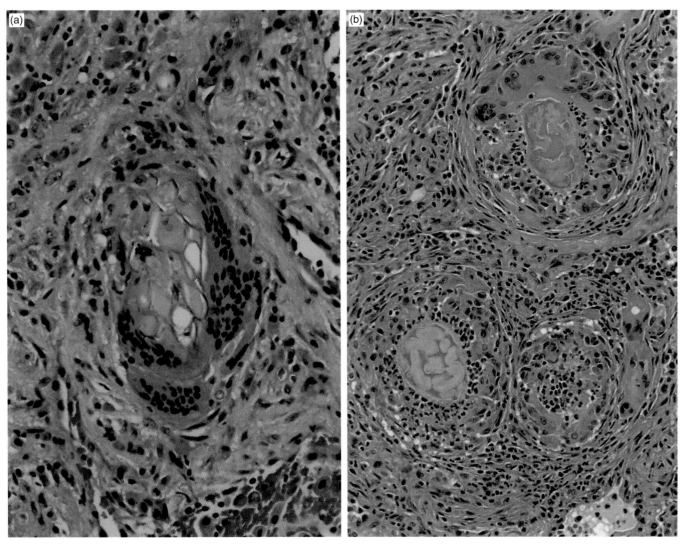

Figure 2.52. Organizing particulate matter aspiration pneumonia. (a) An intact, septate, well-preserved vegetable particle is surrounded by multinucleated giant cells in a background of organizing pneumonia. **(b)** Tiny round intact vegetable particles ("lentils") are surrounded by neutrophils, multinucleated giant cells (foreign-body granulomas) and organizing pneumonia.

in autopsy-based reports, but the recognition of these findings in lung biopsies is a relatively recent development.

Aspiration of gastric acid presumably causes diffuse alveolar damage (DAD), and will not be further addressed here. The following discussion pertains to the aspiration of food and pills from the gastric contents into the lungs.

Particulate matter aspiration can be diagnosed in transbronchial lung biopsies and surgical lung biopsies. It is occasionally encountered as an incidental finding in lobectomy specimens for lung cancer, or in explant pneumonectomy specimens. It can also be identified in surveillance transbronchial biopsies performed after lung transplantation.

Major diagnostic findings

- Aspirated particulate matter (Figures 2.52 to 2.54). In the vast majority of cases, this consists of food or vegetable particles. These may be easily identifiable septate vegetable fragments (Figure 2.52) or fragments

of skeletal muscle, but in our experience well-preserved particles are less common than vegetable particles in various stages of degeneration (Figure 2.53, Figure 2.1c). A common particle found in aspiration pneumonia is the so-called *lentil*, a tiny, eosinophilic, roughly spherical starch particle with curved internal septa derived from a variety of leguminous foods (see book cover, first image from right). Aspiration of this type of particle was well known in bygone days as "lentil pulse pneumonia" or "lentil aspiration pneumonia" and was often attributed to aspiration of lentil soup. Degenerating vegetable particles are difficult to identify because they are often few in number, irregular, smudgy, eosinophilic and nondescript, without septation or thick cuticles. The most degenerated particles have a wrinkled, collapsed appearance. The inflammatory reaction is often minimal, and when present is frequently misinterpreted. The presence of an attached multinucleated giant cell can be a valuable clue that a given nondescript particle

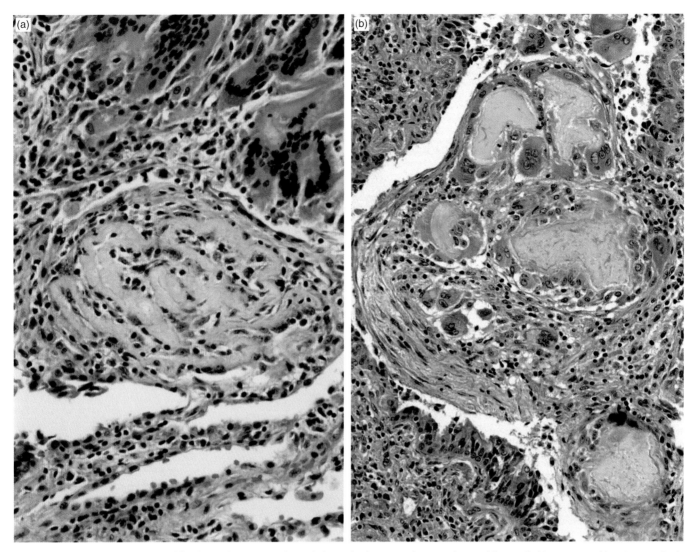

Figure 2.53. Degenerated aspirated food particles. (a) Typical morphology of a degenerated aspirated vegetable particle. Note interstitial location, attached histiocytes (pigmented) and adjacent multinucleated giant cells. This type of particle is frequently missed. **(b)** Degenerated food particles within a bronchiolar lumen. This photomicrograph is from the lung of a patient with a gastropleural fistula. The surgeon noted food particles in the lung. Note degenerating food particles surrounded by multinucleated giant cells in a background of organizing pneumonia. The particles lack the septated internal structure of intact vegetable fragments. Identical degenerative changes occur in aspirated food particles.

represents aspirated particulate matter rather than a normal structure or artifact (Figure 2.53, Figure 2.1c).

- An important feature of particulate matter aspiration is that the particles and the attendant tissue reaction are most commonly found in peribronchiolar lung parenchyma (Figure 2.54). Pathologists expect to see aspirated particles within bronchiolar lumens, but they are more often found in bronchiolar walls, alveolar septa (interstitium) or within the associated inflammatory infiltrate.

- If pills from the gastric contents are aspirated into the lungs, the material that evokes a granulomatous reaction is the filler or excipient. These insoluble substances are used in pills to provide bulk and other physical properties – they are not the active ingredient of the medication. The most common fillers seen in surgical pathology are microcrystalline cellulose, talc and crospovidone. The first two are colorless particles and are strongly birefringent,

while the last is purple, coral-like and non-birefringent (Figure 2.55). Most pathologists are aware of these particles only in the context of IV drug abuse (intravenous injection of crushed pills, see next section). Therefore, their presence in the context of aspiration pneumonia is almost invariably misinterpreted.

- The granulomatous inflammation of particulate matter aspiration is quite distinctive. The most prominent feature is the presence of at least a few multinucleated, foreign-body-type giant cells (foreign-body granulomas). These may be embedded within fibroblast plugs of organizing pneumonia, or they may surround foci of dirty necrosis (Figures 2.52 to 2.55), or clusters of neutrophils, forming microabscess-like foci known as suppurative granulomas. In many cases, a single multinucleated giant cell can be seen attached to one side of a degenerating particle. In other cases, several multinucleated giant cells surround particulate matter fragments. Pink necrosis of the

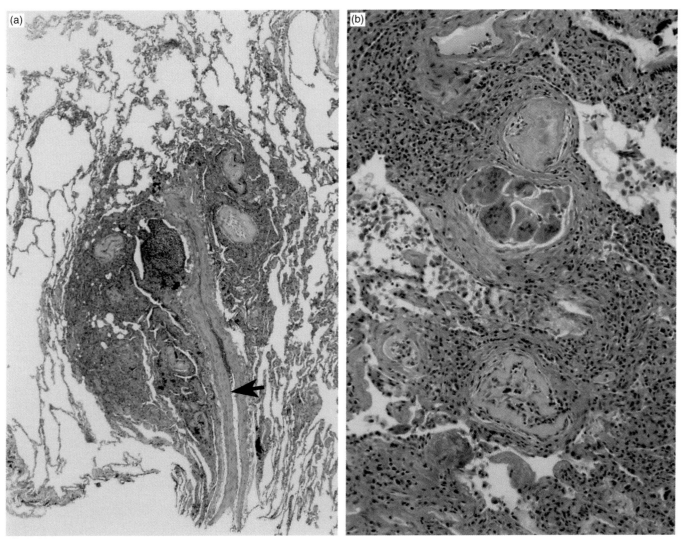

Figure 2.54. Peribronchiolar distribution of particulate matter aspiration. (a) Degenerating food particles are present in peribronchiolar lung parenchyma on both sides of a bronchovascular bundle. The pulmonary artery is unaffected and is seen here in longitudinal section (arrow). Its presence is a clue to the anatomic location of the changes. **(b)** Degenerating food particles in peribronchiolar interstitium. Note prominent multinucleated giant cells. Bronchovascular bundle is at top.

type seen in mycobacterial or fungal granulomas is uncommon, but does occasionally occur. Well-formed sarcoid-type granulomas are absent.

- Particulate matter aspiration in lung biopsies is frequently associated with organizing pneumonia. The latter is characterized by polyp-like or serpiginous plugs of fibroblasts embedded in a pale-staining matrix. These plugs are most prominent within the lumens of respiratory bronchioles, alveolar ducts and adjacent alveoli. They often contain granulomas or giant cells, which in turn contain aspirated vegetable particles (Figures 2.52 to 2.55).

Variable pathologic findings

- Acute inflammation, including acute bronchiolitis and acute bronchopneumonia, is seen in many but not all cases. Clusters of neutrophils may be found within fibroblast plugs, granulomas or multinucleated giant cells. Fragments of particulate matter are frequently present within these

clusters. Tiny microabscess-like collections of neutrophils may be surrounded by giant cells or histiocytes, forming suppurative granulomas.

- Aspirated vegetable particles are seldom birefringent. They may be pigmented.
- Chronic bronchiolitis is a common but non-specific finding in particulate matter aspiration.

Diagnostic work-up

In classic cases, no further histologic work-up is required. Special stains for microorganisms are indicated only if particulate matter is not clearly identified. The pathologist should encourage the clinician to identify risk factors that may predispose to food and particulate matter aspiration (Table 2.5). These include esophageal and gastric causes, drugs that may depress sensorium (including narcotics for chronic pain), and neurologic causes that impair swallowing. We have also seen cases occurring in the context of severe alcoholism.

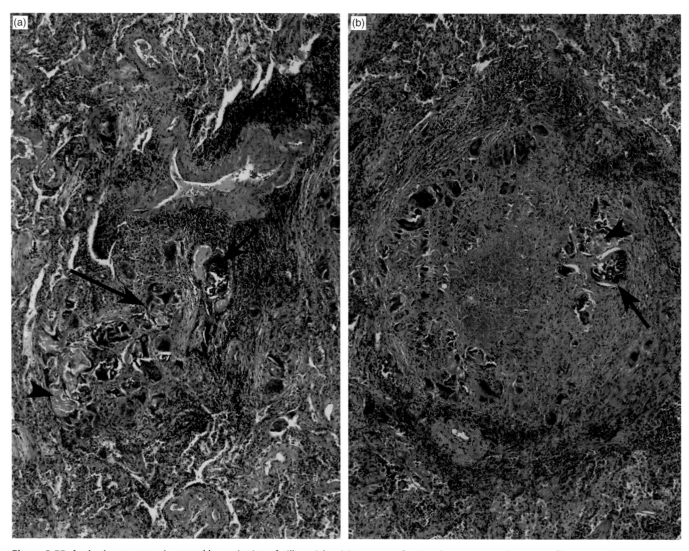

Figure 2.55. Aspiration pneumonia caused by aspiration of pill particles. (a) Low magnification, showing a granulomatous infiltrate in peribronchiolar parenchyma. A large multinucleated giant cell containing a basophilic, coral-like crospovidone particle is visible in a bronchiolar lumen (short arrow). Other giant cells contain colorless microcrystalline cellulose particles (arrowhead) or both microcrystalline cellulose and crospovidone (long arrow). **(b)** Necrotizing granuloma from the same case. Multinucleated giant cells engulfing pill excipients surround a central area of necrosis. Arrow: crospovidone. Arrowhead: microcrystalline cellulose. This tissue reaction should not be misinterpreted as IV drug abuse (talc granulomatosis).

Clinical profile

Aspiration can occur at any age. Patients with particulate matter aspiration are usually adults. The reported age range is 26 to 85, with a mean of 57. The condition occurs in both sexes. The most common symptom is dyspnea, followed by cough, fever, chest pain and hemoptysis. A history of recurrent pneumonias is typical, and should prompt the pathologist to conduct a careful search for aspirated food particles.

Radiologic findings

Particulate matter aspiration manifests as nodules or infiltrates in one or both lungs. Nodules are more common than infiltrates. Occasional lesions can manifest as a solitary PET-positive lung mass. Although conventional wisdom contends that aspiration pneumonia is a disease of the right lower lobe, it is well documented that aspirated particulate matter can be found in any lobe in either lung, including the upper lobes. The

right lung is more commonly affected. Prior studies have shown that any lobe can be affected, depending on the position of the patient during the aspiration episode.

Differential diagnosis

- The combination of granulomas and organizing pneumonia can also be seen in mycobacterial and fungal infections. Identification of either particulate matter or organisms is diagnostic.
- The differential diagnosis with GPA was addressed in that section earlier in this chapter. Identification of particulate matter or necrotizing vasculitis should resolve the issue.
- Talc granulomatosis (intravenous injection of crushed pills) can enter the differential diagnosis of pill fragment aspiration. The two entities share the presence of filler particles in the lung and multinucleated giant cells. However, organizing pneumonia and acute inflammation

Table 2.5. Conditions that predispose to particulate matter aspiration

Predisposing factors[a]	Examples
Esophageal	Esophageal carcinoma, +/− surgery Hiatal hernia, +/− surgery Esophageal dilatation for stricture Systemic sclerosis Esophageal dysmotility Achalasia
Gastric	Gastric bypass surgery Gastric surgery for peptic ulcer disease Gastric carcinoma Gastric outlet obstruction
Neurologic	Stroke Multiple sclerosis Seizures Lambert–Eaton syndrome Narcolepsy Aphasia
Drug use	Intravenous drugs Cocaine Methadone Hydromorphone Hydrocodone Drug overdose
Others	Severe alcoholism Severe reflux
Multiple causes	Gastric surgery + seizures Gastric surgery + hydrocodone Hiatal hernia repair + methadone

[a] Compiled from Mukhopadhyay and Katzenstein, *Am J Surg Pathol* 2007 (see references)

are seen only in aspiration. Further, the location of the abnormalities in peribronchiolar parenchyma, airway lumens or airspaces is diagnostic of aspiration. In contrast, the filler particles and giant cells in talc granulomatosis are restricted to alveolar septal capillaries, small blood vessels and alveolar septa. Organizing pneumonia and acute inflammation are not seen in talc granulomatosis.

Treatment and prognosis

The optimal treatment of particulate matter aspiration is unknown because the syndrome is underdiagnosed and not well described in the clinical literature.

Sample diagnosis on pathology report

Lung, left lower lobe, surgical biopsy – Organizing aspiration pneumonia (See comment).
  or
Lung, right upper lobe, surgical biopsy – Organizing particulate matter aspiration pneumonia (See comment).

Talc granulomatosis (perivascular foreign-body granulomas caused by intravenous injection of oral pills)

Talc granulomatosis is the term traditionally used to describe the formation of perivascular foreign-body-type granulomas in the lungs of individuals who inject aqueous solutions of oral pills containing stimulants or narcotics intravenously in order to obtain a more rapid or more potent "high". The oral pills most commonly abused in this way are methadone, tripelennamine (Pyribenzamine), methylphenidate (Ritalin), pentazocine (Talwin) and hydromorphone (Dilaudid). A recent report suggests that injection of acetaminophen/hydrocodone (Vicodin) can result in identical findings. While the actual psychoactive medication dissolves in the bloodstream, tiny insoluble *filler* particles in the pills persist in the circulation. From the systemic veins, they drain into the vena cava, right side of the heart and lungs, where they are trapped within tiny alveolar septal capillaries. Extrusion of these particles from capillary lumens results in the characteristic foreign-body giant cell response within alveolar septa after which the entity is named. While the condition is often associated with intravenous drug abusers, it is important to recognize that this practice differs from the "usual" intravenous injection of cocaine, heroin or methamphetamines, which may or may not be associated with insoluble contaminant substances. In talc granulomatosis, it is the *intravenous injection of oral pills* that results in the distinctive pathologic findings. Although the practice certainly qualifies as drug abuse, these individuals do not always fit the stereotypic profile of the "typical" intravenous drug abuser or drug addict. In fact, we have observed that these individuals often vigorously deny drug use, even when confronted with evidence to the contrary. Given the illicit nature of the behavior, clinical "confirmation" of the diagnosis is problematic and often impossible.

The insoluble fillers in pills, also known as *excipients*, provide bulk to the pill and function as binders, lubricants or disintegrants. The most common fillers are microcrystalline cellulose, talc and crospovidone. In past years, talc was the predominant filler, but most cases in recent years show microcrystalline cellulose. Since the filler is not always talc, the term *talc granulomatosis* is not always strictly accurate; however, the term has the twin virtues of brevity and familiarity, and has been in use for several decades.

Talc granulomatosis has traditionally been a diagnosis made at autopsy, but cases are increasingly diagnosed in surgical biopsies. The diagnostic pathologic features can also be recognized in transbronchial lung biopsies.

Major diagnostic findings

- Granulomas or multinucleated giant cells within alveolar septa (interstitium) (Figures 2.56 and 2.57, Figure 2.1d). The most florid cases feature extensive and easily visible granulomas that mimic sarcoidosis, whereas in others the findings are subtle and easily missed. Most often, the granulomatous component consists of multinucleated

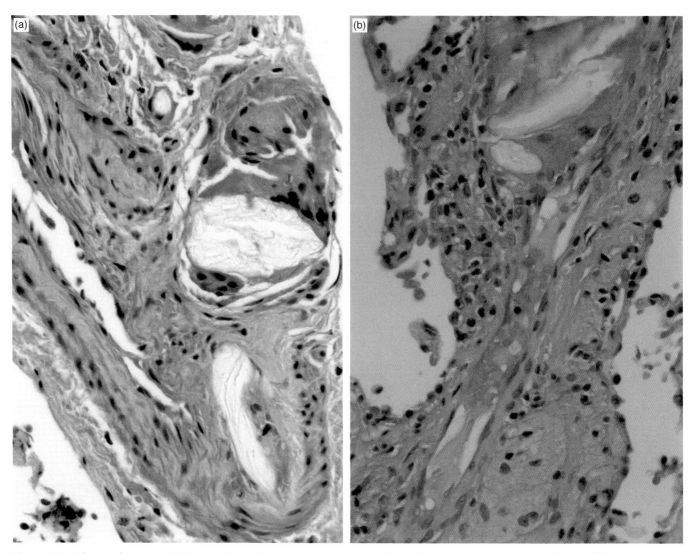

Figure 2.56. Talc granulomatosis. (a) Microcrystalline cellulose particles are surrounded by multinucleated giant cells in the wall of a small blood vessel. The material is disrupting the vessel wall and extruding into the perivascular interstitium. **(b)** Foreign-body granuloma in the interstitium adjacent to a small blood vessel. The giant cell contains foreign particles. Airspaces are uninvolved.

giant cells in the alveolar septa, engulfing birefringent foreign particles.

- Foreign (filler) material. Like the granulomas, the foreign material may be abundant and obvious, or very scant and subtle. The most common material, microcrystalline cellulose, is a colorless, fiber-like particle that is often mistaken for suture material by the novice. It is strongly birefringent and stains yellow with the Movat pentachrome stain. The material may occasionally be inside capillary lumens or the lumens or walls of other small blood vessels, but more commonly it is found in the perivascular interstitium (alveolar septa) (Figures 2.56 and 2.57, Figure 2.1d).
- "Does it polarize?" is an often-asked question when the specter of drug abuse is raised. Birefringence under polarized light is an important and diagnostically helpful feature of microcrystalline cellulose and talc, but the presence of birefringent material alone is insufficient for the diagnosis of talc granulomatosis.

- Organizing pneumonia, suppuration, fibrinous exudates in peribronchiolar parenchyma or aspirated food particles should prompt consideration of aspiration (rather than intravenous injection) of pill fragments (see previous section).

Variable pathologic findings

- Thrombi are often present within the affected blood vessels.
- Foci of necrosis in association with talc granulomatosis may be a sign of septic emboli. The necrotic foci may contain filler particles, suggesting that bacteria may "piggyback" on these particles to the lung from the skin, cardiac vegetations or other infective foci in the bloodstream.
- Pulmonary hypertension and cor pulmonale can develop in advanced cases, but these features are infrequent and are not necessary for the diagnosis. They include thickening of the media and intima, and plexiform changes in advanced cases.

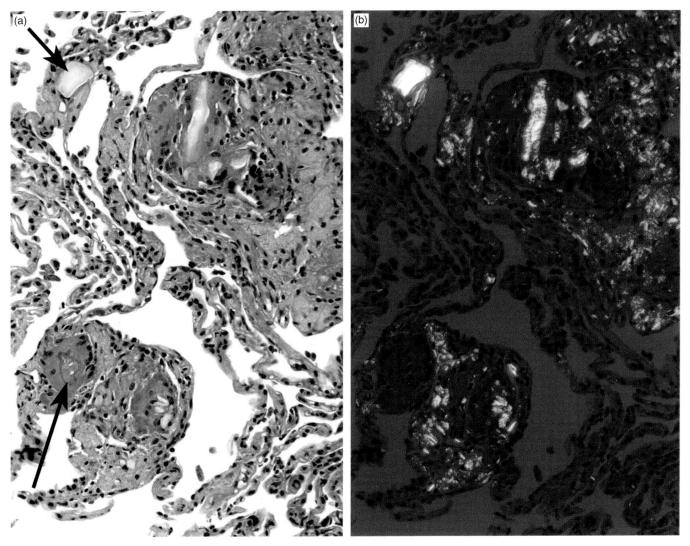

Figure 2.57. Talc granulomatosis. (a) Microcrystalline cellulose (short arrow) and crospovidone (long arrow) within multinucleated giant cells in the alveolar septa. **(b)** Same field under polarized light. Microcrystalline cellulose particles are strongly birefringent but crospovidone is not. It is clear that examination under polarized light greatly facilitates recognition of filler particles.

- Foamy macrophages are sometimes found within alveolar septa adjacent to the foreign-body granulomas.
- Size measurement of the foreign particles has been suggested as a means of differentiating inhaled and injected talc, but this is not necessary in practice since the location of the particles reliably differentiates the two. Furthermore, this method does not help to confirm or exclude aspiration of pill fragments.

Diagnostic work-up

No special stains are necessary for the diagnosis. However, the Movat pentachrome can be helpful in that it distinguishes between microcrystalline cellulose (yellow) and talc (blue), and highlights blood vessels and the associated vascular damage.

Clinical profile

Talc granulomatosis is usually encountered in young or middle-aged adults of either sex, reflecting the age of the

pill-abusing population. Patients may present with recurrent pneumonias, and may develop infective endocarditis and bacteremia. *Pseudomonas* bacteremia appears to be particularly common. More than one organism may grow in blood cultures.

A word of caution is in order regarding "clinical correlation" in this condition. Although some patients with talc granulomatosis may be known or suspected intravenous drug abusers, others may have no declared history of drug abuse. Some of these individuals go to great lengths to conceal their illegitimate drug use in order to avoid adverse consequences, which might include abrupt denial of access to their drug supply, and social stigma. Therefore, pathologists and clinicians must be prepared for vehement denials when such individuals are confronted with the pathologic findings. Clues to illicit drug use in such individuals may come from other subtle features such as a history of excessive narcotic use for chronic pain, constant demands for pain medication, and availability of easy intravenous access through an indwelling catheter or peripherally inserted central catheter (PICC) line. Other soft pointers may also be present, such as a history of homelessness, frequent changes of health care providers, visits to various hospitals, usage of multiple medications for pain control or a background of medical training.

Radiologic findings

The usual radiologic findings in talc granulomatosis are bilateral nodules or infiltrates. Multiple tiny bilateral nodules in a centrilobular or miliary pattern may be seen. Some cases show minimal or no findings on imaging studies.

Differential diagnosis

- The differential diagnosis with pill fragment aspiration has been addressed in the preceding section on particulate matter aspiration.
- Florid talc granulomatosis can mimic sarcoidosis since granulomas are interstitial in both conditions. Furthermore, sarcoidosis has been reported to occasionally contain large numbers of birefringent (endogenous) particles. However, unlike talc granulomatosis, sarcoid granulomas also occur in the pleura and bronchovascular bundles and are associated with dense hyalinized fibrosis. Sarcoidosis is excluded if birefringent particles are found *within* capillaries and other small blood vessels, or if crospovidone is present.
- Talc pneumoconiosis is a rare condition allegedly caused by excessive inhalation of talc, for example in talcum powder. The histologic features are neither well described nor well illustrated in the literature, but one would expect inhaled talc to be present in airways and/or airspaces rather than within alveolar septa.

Treatment and prognosis

There is no known cure for established talc granulomatosis. Lung transplantation has been tried in some centers for advanced cases. Pulmonary hypertension caused by occlusion of the pulmonary vasculature is a major cause of morbidity and mortality. The prognosis is poor.

Sample diagnosis on pathology report

Lung, left lower lobe and lingula, transbronchial biopsy – Talc granulomatosis (florid perivascular foreign-body giant cell reaction to particulate material) (See comment).

Berylliosis (chronic beryllium disease)

Berylliosis, also known as chronic beryllium disease, is a classic example of the discordance that can occur between textbook teaching and clinical reality. Due in large part to dogma derived from medical textbooks, generations of physicians and pathologists reflexively think of berylliosis as the main condition in the differential diagnosis of sarcoidosis when faced with non-necrotizing granulomas in the lung. In practice, pathologically well-documented cases of berylliosis are rare. The reasons for this discordance are unclear.

Berylliosis is most likely to be diagnosed in a transbronchial lung biopsy when a pathologist is provided with a clinical history of beryllium exposure.

Major diagnostic findings

- Granulomatous inflammation without necrosis. The granulomas of berylliosis are interstitial and non-necrotizing (Figure 2.58), a picture that is allegedly "indistinguishable from sarcoidosis". Since there are no recent well-illustrated pathologic studies of berylliosis, this oft-repeated statement is difficult to substantiate. The origin of this assertion can be traced back to a pathologic series from 1970 (Freiman and Hardy) and a case report from 1992 (Lewman and Kreiss). However, a critical review of the illustrations in these articles as well as textbooks of pulmonary pathology reveals histologic features that bear a closer resemblance to hypersensitivity pneumonitis than sarcoidosis. The granulomas of berylliosis vary from fairly well formed to loose but they are not as circumscribed as sarcoid granulomas, lack the dense hyalinized fibrosis that typically surrounds sarcoid granulomas, and are not distributed along lymphatic pathways.
- Significant interstitial chronic inflammation composed mainly of lymphocytes appears to be a prominent finding in berylliosis. It is fairly diffuse and extends into the interstitium beyond the granulomas.
- The main role of the pathologist in the diagnosis of berylliosis is to identify granulomas in lung biopsies and exclude infection. The finding of granulomas in a beryllium-exposed individual with a positive beryllium lymphocyte proliferation test is currently considered diagnostic of berylliosis (chronic beryllium disease). From the point of view of the surgical pathologist, it is impractical to raise the question of chronic beryllium disease every time non-necrotizing granulomas are encountered in a lung biopsy, since the vast majority of such cases represent sarcoidosis. This is especially true in cases where the pathologic findings are typical of sarcoidosis.

Variable pathologic findings

Variable findings include Langhans-type multinucleated giant cells, Schaumann bodies and peribronchiolar metaplasia.

Diagnostic work-up

As with sarcoidosis, special stains (AFB, GMS) should be performed to exclude infection. If granulomas are initially absent in a biopsy strongly suspected to represent berylliosis, deeper cuts may help to identify granulomas.

Clinical profile

Chronic beryllium disease occurs predominantly in men of all ages. Symptoms are non-specific. They include dyspnea, cough, fatigue, arthralgias and chest pain. Pulmonary function tests can show restrictive, obstructive or mixed physiology, usually with a decreased diffusing capacity.

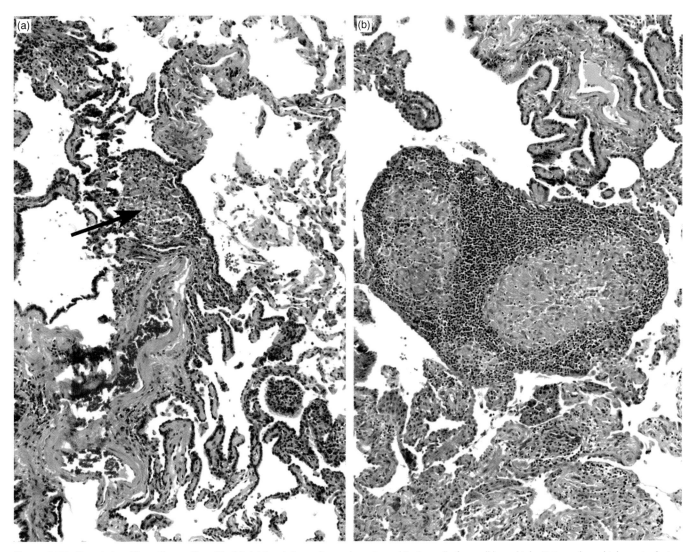

Figure 2.58. Chronic beryllium disease (berylliosis). (a) Poorly formed granuloma (arrow) in the wall of a small bronchiole. Note peribronchiolar metaplasia. **(b)** Larger, better-formed granulomas are seen in another picture from the same case. Note interstitial inflammation away from granulomas. Unlike typical granulomas of sarcoidosis, there is no hyalinized fibrosis (compare to Figures 2.43, 2.44, 2.49, 2.50).

The highest risk of exposure to beryllium occurs in individuals involved in metal production and machining. Other settings associated with beryllium exposure include dental laboratories, engine development, the automobile industry, manufacture of brass or beryllium-containing alloys, metallurgic factories, aircraft production and maintenance, production of non-sparking tools, radiation shielding, fluorescent lamps, microelectronics, engraving of gems and ore mining. Cases have also been documented in individuals with brief and trivial exposures, such as persons living near beryllium processing plants or secretaries working in offices attached to factories.

The beryllium lymphocyte proliferation test (BeLPT), which can be performed on blood samples as well as bronchoalveolar lavage (BAL) fluid, is very useful in confirming the diagnosis. The test is generally considered a good marker of beryllium sensitization, in that it is positive in 70 to 75% of beryllium-exposed individuals and negative in most unexposed healthy individuals. However, considerable inter-observer variability between laboratories has been reported, casting some doubt on the reliability of the test.

Radiologic findings

Chest radiographs may be normal early in the disease, but can progress to diffuse infiltrates, said to be indistinguishable from sarcoidosis.

Differential diagnosis

- Sarcoidosis. The combination of beryllium exposure and a positive beryllium lymphocyte proliferation test is currently the best way to separate sarcoidosis and berylliosis. However, the assumption that patients with sarcoidosis cannot also be exposed to beryllium, or have a positive beryllium lymphocyte proliferation test is questionable.
- Hypersensitivity pneumonitis. Chronic beryllium disease has many features in common with hypersensitivity pneumonitis, including interstitial inflammation, granulomas, genetic susceptibility, a known exposure source, and development of disease in some patients with

only minimal exposure. The exposure history is the key differentiating feature.

Treatment and prognosis

Standard management involves cessation of beryllium exposure combined with corticosteroid therapy. Response to corticosteroid therapy is usually good, but side effects are common, and the disease often relapses upon stopping therapy. Azathioprine therapy has been reported to be successful in one patient. The long-term prognosis is poor. Estimates of mortality range from 5.8 to 38%.

Sample diagnosis on pathology report

Lung, right middle lobe, core needle biopsy – Interstitial chronic inflammation with non-necrotizing granulomas (See comment).

Miscellaneous and rare causes of granulomas in the lung

Lung granulomas have also been described in other rare situations, both infectious and non-infectious. These are listed in Table 2.6.

Granulomas of unknown etiology

The etiology of granulomas in the lung often remains unknown, even after special stains, and pathologic features are often hopelessly non-specific. Worldwide, pulmonary granulomas are histologically unexplained in 8 to 41% of cases. Often, the failure to find an etiology can be attributed to the small size of the sample or the absence of necrosis. However, even in surgically resected necrotizing granulomas, which provide the best chance for identifying an organism and for finding specific histologic features of non-infectious granulomatous disease, a definite etiology cannot be established in approximately 25% of cases.

What should pathologists do in such situations? Are any special studies or clinical tests helpful? Should additional blocks be stained? Does it help to perform additional stains on the same block? Do molecular studies such as PCR help in difficult cases when bug stains are negative? Is it helpful to state "clinicopathologic correlation recommended" in the pathology

Table 2.6. Miscellaneous causes of lung granulomas

Cause	Examples
Infection	Pneumocystis pneumonia
	Sporotrichosis
	Candidiasis
	Echinococcosis
	Paracoccidioidomycosis
	Adiaspiromycosis
	Schistosomiasis
Non-infectious causes	Chronic granulomatous disease
	Crohn's disease
	Drug reactions (etanercept)

report? What types of clinical and radiologic information might be helpful in reaching a diagnosis?

In histoplasmosis-endemic areas, re-examining the original GMS-stained slides can detect missed fungal yeasts, and staining additional blocks may reveal fungi in a few cases.

In some cases, waiting for results of microbiologic cultures may be productive, as mycobacteria may grow in cultures even when they are undetectable in histologic sections.

A diagnosis of GPA can be made in a few cases by reviewing the histology for necrotizing vasculitis, ANCA testing, and clinical follow-up for subsequent development of overt vasculitis.

A history of rheumatoid arthritis and multiple lung nodules helps to establish a diagnosis of rheumatoid nodule.

Sarcoidosis may occasionally be diagnosed by review of the original histology, which may reveal well-formed, predominantly non-necrotizing granulomas in a lymphangitic distribution surrounded by hyalinized fibrosis in a compatible clinical setting.

A small number of resected pulmonary necrotizing granulomas remain unexplained after rigorous re-examination of the original histology and incorporation of clinical and laboratory information as described above. Patients with such lesions do well on long-term follow-up, even without medical therapy.

Sample diagnosis on pathology report

Lung, right middle lobe, surgical biopsy – Necrotizing granulomatous inflammation (See comment).

References

Tuberculosis

Attorri S, Dunbar S, Clarridge JE, III. Assessment of morphology for rapid presumptive identification of *Mycobacterium tuberculosis* and *Mycobacterium kansasii. J Clin Microbiol* 2000;**38**:1426–9.

Fukunaga H, Murakami T, Gondo T, Sugi K, Ishihara T. Sensitivity of acid-fast staining for *Mycobacterium tuberculosis* in formalin-fixed tissue. *Am J Respir Crit Care Med* 2002;**166**:994–7.

Koch ML, Cote RA. Comparison of fluorescence microscopy with Ziehl-Neelsen stain for demonstration of acid-fast bacilli in smear preparations and tissue sections. *Am Rev Respir Dis* 1965;**91**:283–4.

Medlar EM. The behavior of pulmonary tuberculous lesions; a pathological study. *Am Rev Tuberc* 1955;**71**:1–244.

Mukhopadhyay S, Farver CF, Vaszar LT, *et al.* Causes of pulmonary granulomas: a retrospective study of 500 cases from seven countries. *J Clin Pathol* 2012;**65**:51–7.

Mukhopadhyay S, Gal AA. Granulomatous lung disease: An approach to the differential diagnosis. *Arch Pathol Lab Med* 2010;**134**:667–90.

Nayak NC, Sabharwal BD, Bhathena D, Mital GS, Ramalingaswami V. The pulmonary tuberculous lesion in North India: a study in medico-legal autopsies. I. Incidence, nature, and evolution. *Am Rev Respir Dis* 1970;**101**:1–17.

Renshaw AA. The relative sensitivity of special stains and culture in open lung biopsies. *Am J Clin Pathol* 1994;**102**:736–40.

Salian NV, Rish JA, Eisenach KD, Cave MD, Bates JH. Polymerase chain reaction to detect *Mycobacterium tuberculosis* in histologic specimens. *Am J Respir Crit Care Med* 1998;**158**:1150–5.

Slavin RE, Walsh TJ, Pollack AD. Late generalized tuberculosis: a clinical pathologic analysis and comparison of 100 cases in the preantibiotic and antibiotic eras. *Medicine* 1980;**59**:352–66.

Non-tuberculous mycobacterial infection

Fujita J, Ohtsaki Y, Suemitu I, *et al.* Pathological and radiological changes in resected lung specimens in *Mycobacterium avium intracellulare* complex disease. *Eur Respir J* 1999;**13**:535–40.

González J, Tudó G, Gómez J, García A, Navarro M, Jiménez de Anta MT. Use of microscopic morphology in smears prepared from radiometric cultures for presumptive identification of *Mycobacterium tuberculosis* complex, *Mycobacterium avium* complex, *Mycobacterium kansasii*, and *Mycobacterium xenopi*. *Eur J Clin Microbiol Infect Dis* 1998;**17**:493–500.

Griffith DE, Aksamit T, Brown-Elliott BA, *et al.* An official ATS/IDSA statement: diagnosis, treatment, and prevention of nontuberculous mycobacterial diseases. *Am J Respir Crit Care Med* 2007;**175**:367–416.

Kwon KY, Myers JL, Swensen SJ, Colby TV. Middle lobe syndrome: a clinicopathological study of 21 patients. *Hum Pathol* 1995;**26**:302–7.

Marchevsky A, Damsker B, Gribetz A, Tepper S, Geller SA. The spectrum of pathology of nontuberculous mycobacterial infections in open-lung biopsy specimens. *Am J Clin Pathol* 1982;**78**:695–700.

Mukhopadhyay S, Farver CF, Vaszar LT, *et al.* Causes of pulmonary granulomas: a retrospective study of 500 cases from seven countries. *J Clin Pathol* 2012;**65**:51–7.

Mukhopadhyay S, Gal AA. Granulomatous lung disease. An approach to the differential diagnosis. *Arch Pathol Lab Med* 2010;**134**:667–90.

Mukhopadhyay S, Wilcox B, Myers JL, *et al.* Pulmonary necrotizing granulomas of unknown etiology: clinical and pathologic analysis of 131 patients with completely resected nodules. *Chest* 2013;**144**:813–24.

Schulz S, Cabras AD, Kremer M, *et al.* Species identification of mycobacteria in paraffin-embedded tissues: frequent detection of nontuberculous mycobacteria. *Mod Pathol* 2005;**18**:274–82.

Wallace JM, Hannah JB. *Mycobacterium avium* complex infection in patients with the acquired immunodeficiency syndrome. A clinicopathologic study. *Chest* 1988;**93**:926–32.

Histoplasmosis

Doxtader EE, Mukhopadhyay S, Katzenstein AL. Core needle biopsy in benign lung lesions: pathologic findings in 159 cases. *Hum Pathol* 2010;**41**:1530–5.

Goodwin RA, Jr., Shapiro JL, Thurman GH, Thurman SS, Des Prez RM. Disseminated histoplasmosis: clinical and pathologic correlations. *Medicine (Baltimore)* 1980;**59**:1–33.

Mukhopadhyay S, Aubry MC, Pulmonary granulomas: differential diagnosis, histologic features and algorithmic approach. *Diagnostic Histopathology* 2013;**19**:288–97.

Mukhopadhyay S, Doxtader EE. Visibility of *Histoplasma* within histiocytes on H&E distinguishes disseminated histoplasmosis from other forms of pulmonary histoplasmosis. *Hum Pathol* 2013;**44**:2346–52.

Mukhopadhyay S, Wilcox B, Myers JL, *et al.* Pulmonary necrotizing granulomas of unknown etiology: clinical and pathologic analysis of 131 patients with completely resected nodules. *Chest* 2013;**144**:813–24.

Peikert T, Colby TV, Midthun DE, *et al.* Fibrosing mediastinitis: clinical presentation, therapeutic outcomes, and adaptive immune response. *Medicine* 2013;**90**:412–23.

Puckett TF. Pulmonary histoplasmosis; a study of twenty-two cases with identification of *H. capsulatum* in resected lesions. *Am Rev Tuberc* 1953;**67**:453–76.

Ulbright TM, Katzenstein AL. Solitary necrotizing granulomas of the lung: differentiating features and etiology. *Am J Surg Pathol* 1980;**4**:13–28.

Weydert JA, Van Natta TL, DeYoung BR. Comparison of fungal culture versus surgical pathology examination in the detection of Histoplasma in surgically excised pulmonary granulomas. *Arch Pathol Lab Med* 2007;**131**:780–3.

Wheat LJ, Freifeld AG, Kleiman MB, *et al.* Clinical practice guidelines for the management of patients with histoplasmosis: 2007 update by the Infectious Diseases Society of America. *Clin Infect Dis* 2007;**45**:807–25.

Cryptococcosis

Baker RD, Haugen RK. Tissue changes and tissue diagnosis in cryptococcosis; a study of 26 cases. *Am J Clin Pathol* 1955;**25**:14–24.

Farmer SG, Komorowski RA. Histologic response to capsule-deficient *Cryptococcus neoformans*. *Arch Pathol* 1973;**96**:383–7.

Gal AA, Koss MN, Hawkins J, Evans S, Einstein H. The pathology of pulmonary cryptococcal infections in the acquired immunodeficiency syndrome. *Arch Pathol Lab Med* 1986;**110**:502–7.

Kent TH, Layton JM. Massive pulmonary cryptococcosis. *Am J Clin Pathol* 1962;**38**:596–604.

Kerkering TM, Duma RJ, Shadomy S. The evolution of pulmonary cryptococcosis. Clinical implications from a study of 41 patients with and without compromising host factors. *Ann Intern Med* 1981;**94**:611–6.

Lazcano O, Speights VO Jr., Strickler JG, Bilbao JE, Becker J, Diaz J. Combined histochemical stains in the differential diagnosis of *Cryptococcus neoformans*. *Mod Pathol* 1993;**6**:80–4.

McDonnell JM, Hutchins GM. Pulmonary cryptococcosis. *Hum Pathol* 1985;**16**:121–8.

Perfect JR, Dismukes WE, Dromer F, *et al.* Clinical practice guidelines for the management of cryptococcal disease: 2010 update by the Infectious Disease Society of America. *Clin Infect Dis* 2010;**50**:291–322.

Ro JY, Lee SS, Ayala AG. Advantage of Fontana-Masson stain in capsule-deficient cryptococcal infection. *Arch Pathol Lab Med* 1987;**111**:53–7.

Sarosi G. Cryptococcal lung disease in patients without HIV infection. *Chest* 1999;**115**:610–1.

Blastomycosis

Chapman SW, Dismukes WE, Proia LA, *et al.* Clinical practice guidelines for the management of blastomycosis: 2008 update by the Infectious Diseases Society of America. *Clin Infect Dis* 2008;**46**:1801–12.

Moore M. Morphologic variation in tissue of the organisms of the blastomycoses and of histoplasmosis. *Am J Pathol* 1955;**31**:1049–63.

Patel AJ, Gattuso P, Reddy VB. Diagnosis of blastomycosis in surgical pathology and cytopathology: correlation with microbiologic culture. *Am J Surg Pathol* 2010;**34**:256–61.

Pfaller MA, Diekema DJ. Epidemiology of invasive mycoses in North America. *Crit Rev Microbiol* 2010;**36**:1–53.

Sarosi GA, Davies SF. Blastomycosis. *Am Rev Respir Dis* 1979;**120**:911–38.

Schwarz J. The diagnosis of deep mycoses by morphologic methods. *Hum Pathol* 1982;**13**:519–33.

Schwarz J, Salfelder K. Blastomycosis. A review of 152 cases. *Curr Top Pathol* 1977;**65**:165–200.

Taxy JB. Blastomycosis: contributions of morphology to diagnosis. A surgical pathology, cytopathology and autopsy pathology study. *Am J Surg Pathol* 2007;**31**:615–23.

Vanek J, Schwarz J, Hakim S. North American blastomycosis: a study of ten cases. *Am J Clin Pathol* 1970;**54**:384–400.

Watts JC, Chandler FW, Mihalov ML, Kammeyer PL, Armin AR. Giant forms of *Blastomyces dermatitidis* in the pulmonary lesions of blastomycosis. Potential confusion with *Coccidioides immitis. Am J Clin Pathol* 1990;**93**:575–8.

Coccidioidomycosis

Alznauer RL, Rolle C, Pierce WF. Analysis of focalized pulmonary granulomas due to *Coccidioides immitis. AMA Arch Pathol* 1955;**59**:641–55.

Bayer AS. Fungal pneumonias: pulmonary coccidioidal syndromes (Part 2). Miliary, nodular, and cavitary pulmonary coccidioidomycosis; chemotherapeutic and surgical considerations. *Chest* 1981;**79**:686–91.

Deppisch LM, Donowho EM. Pulmonary coccidioidomycosis. *Am J Clin Pathol* 1972;**58**:489–500.

DiCaudo DJ. Coccidioidomycosis: a review and update. *J Am Acad Dermatol* 2006;**55**:929–42.

Jude CM, Nayak NB, Patel MK, Deshmukh M, Batra P. Pulmonary coccidioidomycosis: pictorial review of chest radiographic and CT findings. *Radiographics* 2014;**34**:912–25.

Mukhopadhyay S, Aubry MC. Pulmonary granulomas: differential diagnosis, histologic features and algorithmic approach. *Diagnostic Histopathology* 2013;**19**:288–97.

Mukhopadhyay S, Gal AA. Granulomatous lung disease. An approach to the differential diagnosis. *Arch Pathol Lab Med* 2010;**134**:667–90.

Shekhel TA, Ricciotti RW, Blair JE, Colby TV, Sobonya RE, Larsen BT. Surgical pathology of pleural coccidioidomycosis: a clinicopathological study of 36 cases. *Hum Pathol* 2014;**45**:961–9.

Sobonya RE, Yanes J, Klotz SA. Cavitary pulmonary coccidioidomycosis: pathologic and clinical correlates of disease. *Hum Pathol* 2014;**45**:153–9.

Zimmerman LE. Demonstration of *Histoplasma* and *Coccidioides* in so-called tuberculomas of lung. *Am Arch Intern Med* 1954;**91**:690–9.

Chronic necrotizing pulmonary aspergillosis

Binder RE, Faling LJ, Pugatch RD, Mahasaen C, Snider GL. Chronic necrotizing pulmonary aspergillosis: a discrete clinical entity. *Medicine (Baltimore)* 1982;**61**:109–24.

Caras WE, Pluss JL. Chronic necrotizing pulmonary aspergillosis: pathologic outcome after itraconazole therapy. *Mayo Clin Proc* 1996;**71**:25–30.

Franquet T, Müller NL, Giménez A, Guembe P, de la Torre J, Bagué S. Aspergillosis: histologic, clinical and radiologic findings. *Radiographics* 2001;**21**:825–37.

Gefter WB, Weingrad TR, Epstein DM, et al. "Semi-invasive" pulmonary aspergillosis: a new look at the spectrum of *Aspergillus* infections of the lung. *Radiology* 1981;**140**:313–21.

Nagata N, Sueishi K, Tanaka K, Iwata Y. Pulmonary aspergillosis with bronchocentric granulomas. *Am J Surg Pathol* 1990;**14**:485–88.

Saraceno JL, Phelps DT, Ferro TJ, Futerfas R, Schwartz DB. Chronic necrotizing pulmonary aspergillosis: approach to management. *Chest* 1997;**112**:541–8.

Soubani AO, Chandrasekar PH. The clinical spectrum of pulmonary aspergillosis. *Chest* 2002;**121**:1988–99.

Tron V, Churg A. Chronic necrotizing pulmonary aspergillosis mimicking bronchocentric granulomatosis. *Pathol Res Pract* 1986;**181**:621–4.

Walsh TJ, Anaissie EJ, Denning DW, et al. Treatment of aspergillosis: clinical practice guidelines of the Infectious Diseases Society of America. *Clin Infect Dis* 2008;**46**:327–60.

Yousem SA. The histological spectrum of chronic necrotizing forms of pulmonary aspergillosis. *Hum Pathol* 1997;**28**:650–6.

Allergic bronchopulmonary aspergillosis

Aubry MC, Fraser R. The role of bronchial biopsy and washing in the diagnosis of allergic bronchopulmonary aspergillosis. *Mod Pathol* 1998;**11**:607–11.

Bosken CH, Myers JL, Greenberger PA, Katzenstein AL. Pathologic features of allergic bronchopulmonary aspergillosis. *Am J Surg Pathol* 1988;**12**:216–22.

Franquet T, Müller NL, Giménez A, Guembe P, de la Torre J, Bagué S. Aspergillosis: histologic, clinical and radiologic findings. *Radiographics* 2001;**21**:825–37.

Greenberger PA. When to suspect and work up allergic bronchopulmonary aspergillosis. *Ann Allergy Asthma Immunol* 2013;**111**:1–4.

Hinson KFW, Moon AJ, Plummer NS. Broncho-pulmonary aspergillosis. A review and a report of eight new cases. *Thorax* 1952;**7**:317–33.

Katzenstein AL, Liebow AA, Friedman PJ. Bronchocentric granulomatosis, mucoid impaction, and hypersensitivity reactions to fungi. *Am Rev Respir Dis* 1975;**111**:497–537.

Mukhopadhyay S, Gal AA. Granulomatous lung disease. An approach to the differential diagnosis. *Arch Pathol Lab Med* 2010;**134**:667–90.

Stevens DA, Schwartz HJ, Lee JY, et al. A randomized trial of itraconazole in allergic bronchopulmonary aspergillosis. *N Engl J Med* 2000;**342**:756–62.

Travis WD, Kwon-Chung KJ, Kleiner DE, et al. Unusual aspects of allergic bronchopulmonary fungal disease: report of two cases due to *Curvularia* organisms associated with allergic fungal sinusitis. *Hum Pathol* 1991;**22**:1240–8.

Walsh TJ, Anaissie EJ, Denning DW, et al. Treatment of aspergillosis: clinical practice guidelines of the Infectious Diseases Society of America. *Clin Infect Dis* 2008;**46**:327–60.

Dirofilariasis

Asimacopoulos PJ, Katras A, Christie B. Pulmonary dirofilariasis. The largest single-hospital experience. *Chest* 1992;**102**:851–5.

Ciferri F. Human pulmonary dirofilariasis in the United States: a critical review. *Am J Trop Med Hyg* 1982;**31**:302–8.

Darrow JC, Lack EE. *Dirofilaria immitis* as an unusual cause of the peripheral coin lesion in man. *J Surg Oncol* 1981;**16**:219–24.

Flieder DB, Moran CA. Pulmonary dirofilariasis: a clinicopathologic study of 41 lesions in 39 patients. *Hum Pathol* 1999;**30**:251–6.

Gutierrez Y. Diagnostic features of zoonotic filariae in tissue sections. *Hum Pathol* 1984;**15**:514–25.

Portnoy LG. Dirofilariasis. In: Connor DH, Chandler FW, Schwartz DA, Manz HJ, Lack EE, eds. *Pathology of infectious diseases*, Volume II. Stamford, CT: Appleton and Lange, 1997. pp. 1391–6.

Risher WH, Crocker EF Jr., Beckman EN, Lacklock JB, Ochsner JL. Pulmonary dirofilariasis. *J Thorac Cardiovasc Surg* 1989;**97**:303–8.

Ro JY, Tsakalakis PJ, White VA, *et al.* Pulmonary dirofilariasis: the great imitator of primary or metastatic lung tumor. A clinicopathologic analysis of seven cases and a review of the literature. *Hum Pathol* 1989;**20**:69–76.

Schmidt LH, Dirksen U, Reiter-Owona I, *et al.* Pulmonary dirofilariasis in a Caucasian patient with metastasized osteosarcoma in a non-endemic European region. *Thorax* 2011;**66**:270.

Simón F, Siles-Lucas M, Morchón R, *et al.* Human and animal dirofilariasis. The emergence of a zoonotic mosaic. *Clin Microbiol Rev* 2012;**25**:507–44.

Paragonimiasis

Boland JM, Vaszar LT, Jones JL, *et al.* Pleuropulmonary infection by *Paragonimus westermani* infection in the United States: a rare cause of eosinophilic pneumonia after ingestion of live crabs. *Am J Surg Pathol* 2011;**35**:707–13.

Castilla EA, Jessen R, Scheck DN, Procop GW. Cavitary mass lesion and recurrent pneumothoraces due to *Paragonimus kellicotti* infection. North American Paragonimiasis. *Am J Surg Pathol* 2003;**27**:1157–60.

DeFrain M, Hooker R. North American Paragonimiasis. Case report of a severe clinical infection. *Chest* 2002;**121**:1368–72.

Diaz JH. Paragonimiasis acquired in the United States: native and non-native species. *Clin Microbiol Rev* 2013;**26**:493–504.

Griffin AT, Farghaly H, Arnold FW. Cough and hemoptysis in a Burmese immigrant. *Infect Dis Clin Pract* 2013;**21**:204–7.

Mukae H, Taniguchi H, Matsumoto N, *et al.* Clinicoradiologic features of pleuropulmonary *Paragonimus westermani* on Kyusyu Island, Japan. *Chest* 2001;**120**:514–20.

Osaki T, Takama T, Nakagawa M, Oyama T. Pulmonary *Paragonimus westermani* with false-positive fluorodeoxyglucose positron emission tomography mimicking primary lung cancer. *Gen Thorac Cardiovasc Surg* 2007;**55**:470–2.

Procop GW, Marty AM, Scheck DN, Mease DR, Maw GM. North American paragonimiasis: a case report. *Acta Cytol* 2000;**44**:75–80.

Procop GW. North American paragonimiasis (caused by *Paragonimus kellicotti*) in the context of global paragonimiasis. *Clin Microbiol Rev* 2009;**22**:415–46.

Robertson KB, Janssen WJ, Saint S, Weinberger SE. The missing piece. *N Engl J Med* 2006;**355**:1913–8.

Granulomatosis with polyangiitis (GPA, Wegener's)

Carrington CB, Liebow A. Limited forms of angiitis and granulomatosis of Wegener's type. *Am J Med* 1966;**41**:497–527.

Fienberg R, Mark EJ, Goodman M, McCluskey RT, Niles JL. Correlation of antineutrophil cytoplasmic antibodies with the extrarenal histopathology of Wegener's (pathergic) granulomatosis and related forms of vasculitis. *Hum Pathol* 1993;**24**:160–8.

Gal AA, Velasquez A. Antineutrophil cytoplasmic autoantibody in the absence of Wegener's granulomatosis or microscopic polyangiitis: implications for the surgical pathologist. *Mod Pathol* 2002;**15**:197–204.

Gaudin PB, Askin FB, Falk RJ, Jennette JC. The pathologic spectrum of pulmonary lesions in patients with anti-neutrophil cytoplasmic autoantibodies specific for anti-proteinase 3 and anti-myeloperoxidase. *Am J Clin Pathol* 1995;**104**:7–16.

Jennette JC, Falk RJ, Bacon PA, *et al.* 2012 Revised international Chapel Hill consensus conference nomenclature of vasculitides. *Arthritis Rheum* 2013;**65**:1–11.

Katzenstein AL, Locke WK. Solitary lung lesions in Wegener's granulomatosis. Pathologic findings and clinical significance in 25 cases. *Am J Surg Pathol* 1995;**19**:545–52.

Lombard CM, Duncan SR, Rizk NW, Colby TV. The diagnosis of Wegener's granulomatosis from transbronchial biopsy specimens. *Hum Pathol* 1990;**21**:838–42.

Mark EJ, Matsubara O, Tan-Liu NS, Fienberg R. The pulmonary biopsy in the early diagnosis of Wegener's (pathergic) granulomatosis: a study based on 35 open lung biopsies. *Hum Pathol* 1988;**19**:1065–71.

Travis WD, Hoffman GS, Leavitt RY, Pass HI, Fauci AS. Surgical pathology of the lung in Wegener's granulomatosis. Review of 87 open lung biopsies from 67 patients. *Am J Surg Pathol* 1991;**15**:315–33.

Yoshikawa Y, Watanabe T. Pulmonary lesions in Wegener's granulomatosis: a clinicopathologic study of 22 autopsy cases. *Hum Pathol* 1986;**17**:401–10.

Eosinophilic granulomatosis with polyangiitis (EGPA, Churg–Strauss syndrome)

Chumbley L, Harrison E Jr., DeRemee R. Allergic granulomatosis and angiitis (Churg-Strauss syndrome). Report and analysis of 30 cases. *Mayo Clin Proc* 1977;**52**:477–84.

Churg J, Strauss L. Allergic granulomatosis, allergic angiitis, and periarteritis nodosa. *Am J Pathol* 1951;**27**:277–301.

Churg A. Recent advances in the diagnosis of Churg-Strauss syndrome. *Mod Pathol* 2001;**14**:1284–93.

Comarmond C, Pagnoux C, Khellaf M, *et al.* Eosinophilic granulomatosis with polyangiitis (Churg-Strauss). Clinical characteristics and long-term followup of the 383 patients enrolled in the French Vasculitis Study Group Cohort. *Arthritis Rheum* 2013;**65**:270–81.

Finan MC, Winkelmann RK. The cutaneous extravascular necrotizing granuloma (Churg-Strauss granuloma) and systemic disease: a review of 27 cases. *Medicine (Baltimore)* 1983;**62**:142–58.

Katzenstein AL. Diagnostic features and differential diagnosis of Churg-Strauss syndrome in the lung. A review. *Am J Clin Pathol* 2000;**114**:767–72.

Koss MN, Antonovych T, Hochholzer L. Allergic granulomatosis (Churg-Strauss syndrome): pulmonary and renal morphologic findings. *Am J Surg Pathol* 1981;**5**:21–8.

Lanham JG, Elkon KB, Pusey CD, Hughes GR. Systemic vasculitis with asthma and eosinophilia: a clinical approach to the Churg-Strauss syndrome. *Medicine (Baltimore)* 1984;**63**:65–81.

Mouthon L, Dunogue B, Guillevin L. Diagnosis and classification of eosinophilic granulomatosis with polyangiitis (formerly named Churg-Strauss syndrome). *J Autoimmunity* 2014;**48–49**:99–103.

Reid AJ, Harrison BD, Watts RA, Watkin SW, McCann BG, Scott DG. Churg-Strauss syndrome in a district hospital. *QJM* 1998;**91**:219–29.

Rheumatoid nodules

Baruch AC, Steinbronn K, Sobonya R. Pulmonary adenocarcinomas associated with rheumatoid nodules: a case report and review of the literature. *Arch Pathol Lab Med* 2005;**129**:104–6.

Beumer HM, van Belle CJ. Pulmonary nodules in rheumatoid arthritis. *Respiration* 1972;**29**:556–64.

Glace B, Gottenberg J-E, Mariette X, *et al.* Efficacy of rituximab in the treatment of pulmonary rheumatoid nodules: findings in 10 patients from the French autoimmunity and Rituximab/Rheumatoid Arthritis registry (AIR/PR registry). *Ann Rheum Dis* 2012;**71**:1429–31.

Highton J, Hung N, Hessian P, Wilsher M. Pulmonary rheumatoid nodules demonstrating features usually associated with rheumatoid synovial membrane. *Rheumatology* 2007;**46**:811–4.

Jolles H, Moseley PL, Peterson MW. Nodular pulmonary opacities in patients with rheumatoid arthritis. A diagnostic dilemma. *Chest* 1989;**96**:1022–5.

Lamblin C, Bergoin C, Saelens T, Wallaert B. Interstitial lung diseases in collagen vascular diseases. *Eur Respir J* 2001;**18** (**Suppl.32**):69s–80s.

Mukhopadhyay S, Wilcox B, Myers JL, *et al.* Pulmonary necrotizing granulomas of unknown etiology: clinical and pathologic analysis of 131 patients with completely resected nodules. *Chest* 2013;**144**:813–24.

Mukhopadhyay S, Gal AA. Granulomatous lung disease. An approach to the differential diagnosis. *Arch Pathol Lab Med* 2010;**134**:667–90.

Yousem SA, Colby TV, Carrington CB. Lung biopsy in rheumatoid arthritis. *Am Rev Respir Dis* 1985;**131**:770–7.

Yue CC, Park CH, Kushner I. Apical fibrocavitary lesions of the lung in rheumatoid arthritis. Report of two cases and review of the literature. *Am J Med* 1986;**81**:741–6.

Sarcoidosis

Baughman RP, Culver DA, Judson MA. A concise review of pulmonary sarcoidosis. *Am J Respir Crit Care Med* 2011;**183**:573–81.

Baughman RP, Teirstein AS, Judson MA, *et al.* Clinical characteristics of patients in a case control study of sarcoidosis. *Am J Respir Crit Care Med* 2001;**164**:1885–9.

Gal AA, Koss MN. The pathology of sarcoidosis. *Curr Opin Pulm Med* 2002;**8**:445–51.

Hsu RM, Connors AF Jr., Tomashefski JF Jr. Histologic, microbiologic, and clinical correlates of the diagnosis of sarcoidosis by transbronchial biopsy. *Arch Pathol Lab Med* 1996;**120**:364–8.

Mukhopadhyay S, Gal AA. Granulomatous lung disease. An approach to the differential diagnosis. *Arch Pathol Lab Med* 2010;**134**:667–90.

Mukhopadhyay S, Farver CF, Vaszar LT, *et al.* Causes of pulmonary granulomas: a retrospective study of 500 cases from seven countries. *J Clin Pathol* 2012; **65**:51–7.

Reid JD, Andersen ME. Calcium oxalate in sarcoid granulomas. With particular reference to the small ovoid body and a note on the finding of dolomite. *Am J Clin Pathol* 1988;**90**:545–58.

Rosen Y, Moon S, Huang CT, Gourin A, Lyons HA. Granulomatous pulmonary angiitis in sarcoidosis. *Arch Pathol Lab Med* 1977;**101**:170–4.

Visscher D, Churg A, Katzenstein AL. Significance of crystalline inclusions in lung granulomas. *Mod Pathol* 1988;**1**:415–9.

Xu L, Kligerman S, Burke A. End-stage sarcoid lung disease is distinct from usual interstitial pneumonia. *Am J Surg Pathol* 2013;**37**:593–600.

Hot tub lung

Aksamit TR. Hot tub lung: infection, inflammation, or both? *Semin Respir Infect* 2003;**18**:33–9.

Cappelluti E, Fraire AE, Schaefer OP. A case of "hot tub lung" due to *Mycobacterium avium* complex in an immunocompetent host. *Arch Intern Med* 2003;**163**:845–8.

Donato J, Phillips CT, Gaffney AW, VanderLaan PA, Mouded M. A case of hypercalcemia secondary to hot tub lung. *Chest* 2014;**146**:e186–9.

Embil J, Warren P, Yakrus M, *et al.* Pulmonary illness associated with exposure to *Mycobacterium-avium* complex in hot tub water. Hypersensitivity pneumonitis or infection? *Chest* 1997;**111**:813–6.

Fjallbrant H, Akerstrom M, Svensson E, Andersson E. Hot tub lung: an occupational hazard. *Eur Respir Rev* 2013;**22**:88–90.

Hanak V, Kalra S, Aksamit TR, Hartman TE, Tazelaar HD, Ryu JH. Hot tub lung: presenting features and clinical course of 21 patients. *Respir Med* 2006;**100**:610–5.

Kahana LM, Kay JM, Yakrus MA, Waserman S. *Mycobacterium avium* complex infection in an immunocompetent young adult related to hot tub exposure. *Chest* 1997;**111**:242–5.

Khoor A, Leslie KO, Tazelaar HD, Helmers RA, Colby TV. Diffuse pulmonary disease caused by nontuberculous mycobacteria in immunocompetent people (hot tub lung). *Am J Clin Pathol* 2001;**115**:755–62.

Sood A, Sreedhar R, Kulkarni P, Nawoor AR. Hypersensitivity pneumonitis-like granulomatous lung disease with nontuberculous mycobacteria from exposure to hot water aerosols. *Environ Health Perspect* 2007;**115**:262–6.

Travaline JM, Kelsen SG. Hypersensitivity pneumonitis associated with hot tub use. *Arch Intern Med* 2003;**163**:2250; author reply 2250–1.

Granulomatous lung disease caused by aspiration of food and other particulate gastric contents

Barnes TW, Vassallo R, Tazelaar HD, Hartman, Ryu J. Diffuse bronchiolar disease due to chronic occult aspiration. *Mayo Clin Proc* 2006;**81**:23–34.

Bulmer SR, Lamb D, McCormack RGM, Walbaum PR. Aetiology of unresolved pneumonia. *Thorax* 1978;**33**:307–14.

Crome L, Valentine JC. Pulmonary nodular granulomatosis caused by inhaled vegetable particles. *J Clin Pathol* 1962;**15**:21–5.

Emery JL. Two cases of lentil pneumonitis. *Proc R Soc Med* 1960;**53**:952–3.

Head MA. Foreign body reaction to inhalation of lentil soup: giant cell pneumonia. *J Clin Pathol* 1956;**9**:295–9.

Knoblich R. Pulmonary granulomatosis caused by vegetable particles. So-called lentil pulse pneumonia. *Am Rev Respir Dis* 1969;**99**:380–9.

Marom EM, McAdams HP, Erasmus JJ, Goodman PC. The many faces of pulmonary aspiration. *AJR Am J Roentgenol* 1999;**172**:121–8.

Mukhopadhyay S, Katzenstein AL. Pulmonary disease due to aspiration of food and other particulate matter: a clinicopathologic study of 59 cases diagnosed on biopsy or resection specimens. *Am J Surg Pathol* 2007;**31**:752–9.

Teabeaut JR, II. Aspiration of gastric contents; an experimental study. *Am J Pathol* 1952;**28**:51–67.

Vidyarthi SC. Diffuse miliary granulomatosis of the lungs due to aspirated vegetable cells. *Arch Pathol* 1967;**83**:215–8.

Talc granulomatosis (perivascular foreign-body granulomas caused by intravenous injection of oral pills)

Ganesan S, Felo J, Saldana M, Kalasinsky VF, Lewin-Smith MR, Tomashefski JF, Jr. Embolized crospovidone (poly[N-vinyl-2-pyrrolidone]) in the lungs of intravenous drug users. *Mod Pathol* 2003;**16**:286–92.

Houck RJ, Bailey GL, Daroca PJ, Jr., Brazda F, Johnson FB, Klein RC. Pentazocine abuse. Report of a case with pulmonary arterial cellulose granulomas and pulmonary hypertension. *Chest* 1980;**77**:227–30.

Kringsholm B, Christoffersen P. The nature and the occurrence of birefringent material in different organs in fatal drug addiction. *Forensic Sci Int* 1987;**34**:53–62.

Lewman LV. Fatal pulmonary hypertension from intravenous injection of methylphenidate (Ritalin) tablets. *Hum Pathol* 1972;**3**:67–70.

Pare JA, Fraser RG, Hogg JC, Howlett JG, Murphy SB. Pulmonary 'mainline' granulomatosis: talcosis of intravenous methadone abuse. *Medicine (Baltimore)*. 1979;**58**:229–39.

Sigdel S, Gemind JT, Tomashefski JF Jr. The Movat pentachrome stain as a means of identifying microcrystalline cellulose among other particulates found in lung tissue. *Arch Pathol Lab Med* 2011;**135**:249–54.

Tomashefski JF, Jr., Felo JA. The pulmonary pathology of illicit drug and substance abuse. *Curr Diagnostic Pathol* 2004;**10**:413–26.

Tomashefski JF, Jr., Hirsch CS. The pulmonary vascular lesions of intravenous drug abuse. *Hum Pathol* 1980;**11**:133–45.

Tomashefski JF, Jr., Hirsch CS, Jolly PN. Microcrystalline cellulose pulmonary embolism and granulomatosis. A complication of illicit intravenous injections of pentazocine tablets. *Arch Pathol Lab Med* 1981;**105**:89–93.

Zeltner TB, Nussbaumer U, Rudin O, Zimmermann A. Unusual pulmonary vascular lesions after intravenous injections of microcrystalline cellulose. A complication of pentazocine tablet abuse. *Virchows Arch A Pathol Anat Histol* 1982;**395**:207–16.

Berylliosis (chronic beryllium disease)

Barna BP, Culver DA, Yen-Lieberman B, Dweik RA, Thomassen MJ. *Clin Diagn Lab Immunol* 2003;**10**:990–4.

Freiman DG, Hardy HL. Beryllium disease. The relation of pulmonary pathology to clinical course and prognosis based on a study of 130 cases from the U.S. beryllium case registry. *Hum Pathol* 1970;**1**:25–44.

Frome EL, Newman LS, Cragle DL, Colyer SP, Wambach PF. Identification of an abnormal beryllium lymphocyte proliferation test. *Toxicology* 2003;**183**:39–56.

Maier LA, Martyny JW, Liang J, Rossman MD. Recent chronic beryllium disease in residents surrounding a beryllium facility. *Am J Respir Crit Care Med* 2008;**177**:1012–17.

Mukhopadhyay S, Gal AA. Granulomatous lung disease. An approach to the differential diagnosis. *Arch Pathol Lab Med* 2010;**134**:667–90.

Müller-Quernheim J, Gaede KI, Fireman E, Zissel G. Diagnoses of chronic beryllium disease within cohorts of sarcoidosis patients. *Eur Respir J* 2006;**27**:1190–5.

Newman LS, Kreiss K. Nonoccupational beryllium disease masquerading as sarcoidosis: identification by blood lymphocyte proliferative response to beryllium. *Am Rev Respir Dis* 1992;**145**:1212–4.

Ribeiro M, Fritscher LG, Al-Musaed AM, et al. Search for chronic beryllium disease among sarcoidosis patients in Ontario, Canada. *Lung* 2011;**189**:233–41.

Salvator H, Gille T, Hervé A, Bron C, Lamberto C, Valeyre D. Chronic beryllium disease: azathioprine as a possible alternative to corticosteroid treatment. *Eur Respir J* 2013;**41**:234–6.

Williams WJ. A histological study of the lungs in 52 cases of chronic beryllium disease. *Br J Ind Med* 1958;**15**:84–91.

Miscellaneous and rare causes of granulomas in the lung

Bouvry D, Mouthon L, Brillet P-Y, et al. Granulomatosis-associated common variable immunodeficiency disorder. A case-control study versus sarcoidosis. *Eur Respir J* 2013;**41**:115–22.

Casey MB, Tazelaar HD, Myers JL, et al. Noninfectious lung pathology in patients with Crohn's disease. *Am J Surg Pathol* 2003;**27**:213–9.

England DM, Hochholzer L. Primary pulmonary sporotrichosis. Report of eight cases with clinicopathologic review. *Am J Surg Pathol* 1985;**193**:193–204.

England DM, Hochholzer L. Adiaspiromycosis: an unusual fungal infection of the lung. Report of 11 cases. *Am J Surg Pathol* 1993;**17**:876–86.

Flieder DB, Moran CA. Pulmonary dirofilariasis: a clinicopathologic study of 41 lesions in 39 patients. *Hum Pathol* 1999;**30**:251-6.

Hartel PH, Shilo K, Klassen-Fischer M, et al. Granulomatous reaction to *Pneumocystis jirovecii*. Clinicopathologic review of 20 cases. *Am J Surg Pathol* 2010;**34**:730–4.

Khemasuwan D, Farver CF, Mehta AC. Parasites of the air passages. *Chest* 2014;**145**:883–95.

Kurtin PJ, Myers JL, Adlakha H, et al. Pathologic and clinical features of primary pulmonary extranodal marginal zone B-cell lymphoma of MALT type. *Am J Surg Pathol* 2001;**25**:997–1008.

Moskaluk CA, Pogrebniak HW, Pass HI, Gallin JI, Travis WD. Surgical pathology of the lung in chronic granulomatous disease. *Am J Clin Pathol* 1994;**102**:684–91.

Granulomas of unknown etiology

Aubry MC. Necrotizing granulomatous inflammation: what does it mean if your special stains are negative? *Mod Pathol* 2012;**25**(Suppl 1):S31–8.

Doxtader EE, Mukhopadhyay S, Katzenstein AL. Core needle biopsy in benign lung lesions: pathologic findings in 159 cases. *Hum Pathol* 2010;**41**:1530–5.

Katzenstein AL, Locke WK. Solitary lung lesions in Wegener's granulomatosis. Pathologic findings and clinical significance in 25 cases. *Am J Surg Pathol* 1995;**19**:545–52.

Mukhopadhyay S, Gal AA. Granulomatous lung disease. An approach to the differential diagnosis. *Arch Pathol Lab Med* 2010;**134**:667–90.

Mukhopadhyay S, Aubry MC, Pulmonary granulomas: differential diagnosis, histologic features and algorithmic approach. *Diagnostic Histopathology* 2013;**19**:288–97.

Mukhopadhyay S, Wilcox B, Myers JL, et al. Pulmonary necrotizing granulomas of unknown etiology: clinical and pathologic analysis of 131 patients with completely resected nodules. *Chest* 2013;**144**:813–24.

Mukhopadhyay S, Farver CF, Vaszar LT, et al. Causes of pulmonary granulomas: a retrospective study of 500 cases from seven countries. *J Clin Pathol* 2012;**65**:51–7.

Schulz S, Cabras AD, Kremer M, et al. Species identification of mycobacteria in paraffin-embedded tissues: frequent detection of nontuberculous mycobacteria. *Mod Pathol* 2005;**18**:274–82.

Ulbright TM, Katzenstein AL. Solitary necrotizing granulomas of the lung: differentiating features and etiology. *Am J Surg Pathol* 1980;**4**:13–28.

Weydert JA, Van Natta TL, DeYoung BR. Comparison of fungal culture versus surgical pathology examination in the detection of *Histoplasma* in surgically excised pulmonary granulomas. *Arch Pathol Lab Med* 2007;**131**:780–3.

Chapter 3

Infections of the lung, non-granulomatous

This chapter discusses infections of the lung in which the usual tissue reaction is not granulomatous. They are separated from granulomatous infections because the identification of granulomatous inflammation changes the differential diagnosis considerably (Chapter 2). It must be noted that some of the infections discussed here may occasionally elicit a granulomatous response; this will be addressed where appropriate.

The list of causes of lung infections includes ordinary bacteria, mycobacteria, viruses, fungi and parasites, among others. However, the focus of this chapter is on organisms that often require lung biopsies for diagnosis and are therefore likely to be encountered by surgical pathologists. For example, *Pneumocystis* is included here because lung biopsies are frequently performed as part of the diagnostic work-up. In contrast, ordinary bacterial and viral infections are not discussed because pathologic examination plays little or no role in these diseases.

Figure 3.1 shows examples of a few organisms that can be diagnosed in lung biopsies and are associated with tissue reactions other than granulomatous inflammation. Figure 3.2 shows an algorithm listing common tissue reactions in infections of the lung, and the organisms most frequently associated with them. It also provides a list of organisms that should be at the top of a surgical pathologist's differential diagnosis when a history of immunosuppression is provided. The list is far from comprehensive, but provides a useful starting point for a pathologic work-up. Table 3.1 provides a few pearls and pitfalls in the diagnosis of non-granulomatous infections in lung biopsies.

Pneumocystis pneumonia

Pneumocystis jirovecii (formerly *Pneumocystis carinii*) is a fungal organism that exclusively infects immunocompromised individuals. The organism was formerly thought to be a parasite, but ribosomal RNA sequencing studies resulted in its reclassification as a fungal organism. Interestingly, despite the widespread acceptance that *Pneumocystis* is a fungus, the nomenclature used for structures that it forms in lung tissues (*cysts* and *trophozoites*) differs from standard terminology applied to most fungi (yeasts and hyphae).

Pneumocystis pneumonia (PCP) is probably the most common infection diagnosed by surgical pathologists in immunocompromised hosts, especially those with HIV/AIDS. The infection can be diagnosed in transbronchial biopsies as well as by cytologic examination of BAL fluid. Transbronchial biopsies are especially valuable when BAL fluid cytology and microbiologic tests such as direct immunofluorescence are negative.

Table 3.1. Pearls and pitfalls in non-granulomatous lung infections

Always consider performing special stains if there is a history of immunosuppression, even if the tissue reaction is nondescript

Intensify your search for organisms in biopsies from immunosuppressed patients

Pneumocystis enters the differential diagnosis of virtually any tissue reaction, including no inflammation, minimal inflammation, granulomatous inflammation and diffuse alveolar damage. It is easy to miss because organisms may be rare

Consider the possibility of *Pneumocystis* before you identify a fungus as *Histoplasma* or *Cryptococcus*

Septate hyphae with narrow-angle branching are not always *Aspergillus*; *Pseudallescheria* and *Fusarium* can appear identical

Angioinvasion is a key pathologic finding in invasive aspergillosis

If you see necrosis but no granulomatous inflammation in a small biopsy, consider the possibility that the biopsy has sampled the center of a necrotizing granuloma and obtain AFB and GMS stains

Most viruses are impossible to identify by histology: the most common exceptions are cytomegalovirus, herpes simplex virus and adenovirus

Bacteria can be detected in lung biopsies on Gram stains, but most cannot be definitively identified

Parasites are very infrequent in lung biopsies: the most common are *Dirofilaria*, *Strongyloides* and *Paragonimus*

Organisms are seldom found in non-specific chronic inflammation, unless the patient is severely immunocompromised

Cases with atypical radiologic features or non-diagnostic transbronchial biopsies may require surgical lung biopsy.

Major diagnostic findings

- The most classic histologic feature of *Pneumocystis* pneumonia is the presence of frothy intra-alveolar eosinophilic material (Figure 3.3a, Figure 3.1b). At high magnification, the frothy material contains clear spaces within which tiny dots are faintly visible. The spaces are formed by the cyst form of the organism, while the dots represent trophozoites. Cysts are not clearly seen on H&E but can be highlighted with a GMS stain (Figure 3.3b). Trophozoites are GMS-negative. The froth-with-dots appearance on H&E is pathognomonic of PCP.

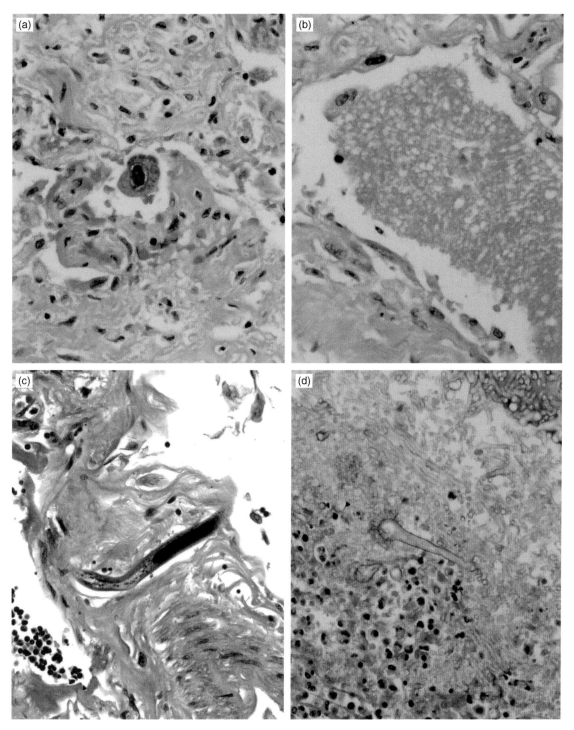

Figure 3.1. Lung infections with non-granulomatous tissue reactions. (a) Cytomegalovirus pneumonia. **(b)** *Pneumocystis* pneumonia. **(c)** Strongyloidiasis. **(d)** Fruiting bodies in an aspergilloma.

- Minimal to mild interstitial thickening. This important feature of the tissue reaction in PCP is often overlooked because it may be subtle. The alveolar septa may appear normal in places, but at least minimal interstitial thickening is usually present (Figure 3.4a). Prominent type 2 pneumocytes occasionally line the thickened alveolar septa, and a few lymphocytes may be present within the thickened interstitium. The appearance may mimic non-specific interstitial pneumonia (NSIP).

Variable pathologic findings

- Granulomatous inflammation is an uncommon and underappreciated feature of *Pneumocystis* pneumonia. It varies from small to large areas of parenchymal necrosis rimmed by epithelioid histiocytes (Figure 3.4b), to well-formed necrotizing granulomas, scattered multinucleated giant cells or non-necrotizing granulomas associated with organizing pneumonia. The necrosis may show a hint of

123

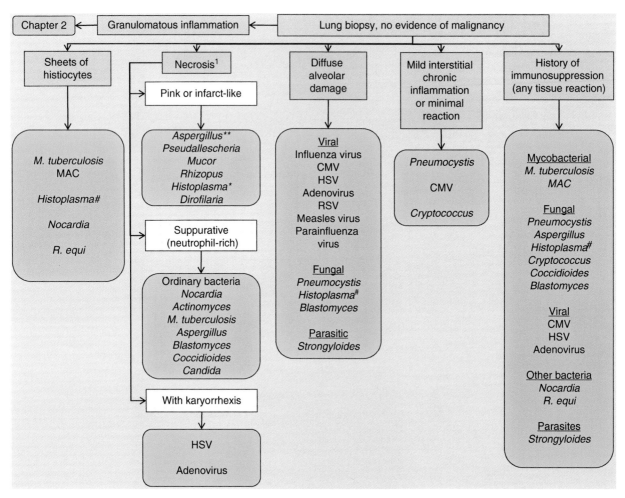

Figure 3.2. Algorithm for pathologic diagnosis of lung infections that lack a granulomatous component. This algorithm provides a starting point for pathologists to consider specific organisms based on the tissue reaction and history of immune suppression. *Histoplasmoma; #disseminated histoplasmosis; **invasive aspergillosis; [1]in small biopsies, always consider the possibility that the necrosis may represent the center of a necrotizing granuloma. CMV – cytomegalovirus; HSV – herpes simplex virus; MAC – *M. avium* complex; *R. equi* – *Rhodococcus equi* (malakoplakia); RSV – respiratory syncytial virus.

the typical frothy material, but organisms usually cannot be seen clearly without a GMS stain. The key to the diagnosis may lie in the surrounding alveoli if areas with the typical froth-with-dots appearance can be identified. Rarely, a discrete, well-formed necrotizing granuloma mimicking other fungal and mycobacterial infections may be formed, and the diagnostic frothy material may be absent.

- Diffuse alveolar damage represents another pitfall for the unwary. It can be avoided if one is cognizant of the fact that PCP in immunocompromised individuals can manifest as diffuse alveolar damage without the typical frothy material. In this form of the disease, organisms are very few in number and difficult to find. The diagnosis is easy to miss unless a GMS stain is meticulously examined with *Pneumocystis* in mind.

- A florid lymphocytic vasculitis can be seen in cases with granulomatous inflammation. It is characterized by extensive infiltration of the media and intima of arteries by large numbers of lymphocytes and occasional histiocytes. Necrotizing vasculitis is not seen. The overall appearance mimics lymphomatoid granulomatosis, and is similar to

acute pulmonary histoplasmosis or acute tuberculosis in immunocompromised patients.

Diagnostic work-up

- No special stains are required if the classic "froth-with-dots" appearance is evident on H&E. However, GMS staining does help to highlight the organisms (Figure 3.3b). *Pneumocystis* cysts are tiny, and overlap with the size range of *Histoplasma* (Table 3.2). They vary from round to helmet-shaped to crescent-like, folded or collapsed. Budding is absent. On GMS, the cysts may contain a black intra-cystic dot (Figure 3.5b). As mentioned previously, trophozoites do not stain with GMS.

- GMS staining is very helpful when the classic frothy material is absent, or in cases manifesting as minimal interstitial chronic inflammation, diffuse alveolar damage or granulomatous inflammation. In these situations, GMS will stain cysts that cannot be visualized on H&E. A GMS stain must be performed on all immunocompromised patients with mild interstitial thickening or a hint of froth within the alveoli.

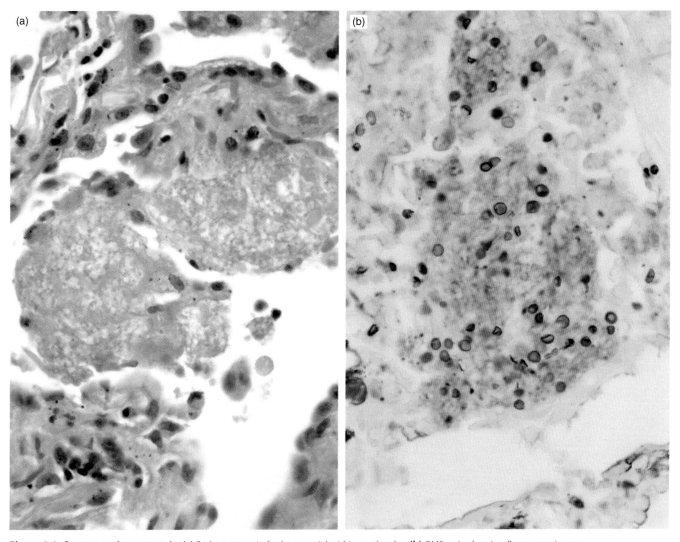

Figure 3.3. *Pneumocystis* **pneumonia. (a)** Pathognomonic frothy material within an alveolus. **(b)** GMS stain showing *Pneumocystis* cysts.

- Giemsa, Diff-Quik and other similar stains are helpful in cytologic material, since they stain trophozoites. The morphology of the organisms in well-stained cytologic preparations can be diagnostic (Figure 3.5).
- Once *Pneumocystis* organisms are identified, pathologists must look for other organisms because co-infection is common in severely immunocompromised hosts, especially those with AIDS. The most common co-infecting organisms are cytomegalovirus, non-tuberculous mycobacteria, *Histoplasma* and *Cryptococcus* (Figure 3.11 in the section on cytomegalovirus shows an example). Pathologists must also be alert to the possibility of concurrent Kaposi sarcoma.

Clinical profile

PCP invariably occurs in immunocompromised hosts. In practice, virtually all patients are adults, but children may also be infected. In fact, some of the earliest reported cases of PCP in humans occurred in malnourished European infants in the 1930s and 1940s and in infants and children in the United States in the 1960s.

HIV/AIDS is the most common setting in which PCP occurs, but other conditions are becoming increasingly common as HIV/AIDS is better managed with highly active antiretroviral therapy. The most frequent cause of PCP in HIV-negative individuals is corticosteroid therapy. The median dose of prednisone in such individuals is 30 to 40 mg per day with a median duration of exposure of 12 to 16 weeks. The lowest reported corticosteroid doses in which PCP has been reported are 16 mg per day with monotherapy and 5 mg per day in conjunction with other immunosuppressive drugs. PCP can also occur in patients with acute leukemia, lymphoma, severe combined immunodeficiency syndrome, and hematologic or solid tumors being treated with chemotherapy. It is rare in lung transplant recipients and recipients of allogenic bone marrow transplants, probably because of routine Bactrim prophylaxis.

Most patients with *Pneumocystis* pneumonia present with worsening respiratory distress and severe hypoxia. Fever, dry cough and dyspnea are common, as are non-specific constitutional symptoms. The presentation tends to be more acute in HIV-negative individuals, with rapid progression to respiratory failure.

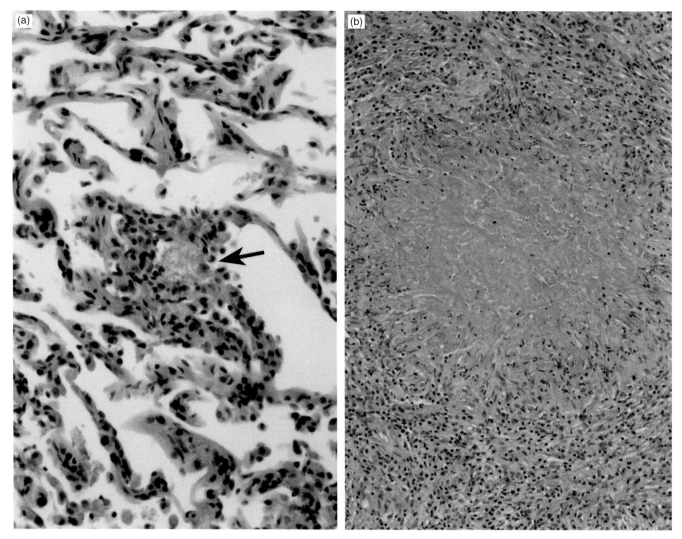

Figure 3.4. Atypical features in *Pneumocystis* pneumonia. (a) Non-descript tissue reaction with subtle, focal interstitial thickening. The diagnosis can easily be missed if the tiny focus of frothy material within an alveolus (arrow) is not recognized **(b)**. Necrotizing granuloma in *Pneumocystis* pneumonia. Organisms were present within the necrosis on GMS and diagnostic frothy material was present elsewhere in the biopsy (not shown).

Pneumocystis does not grow in cultures. However, it can be detected in the microbiology laboratory by direct immuno-fluorescence testing of induced sputum. Currently, PCR and/or immunofluorescence testing of BAL fluid are routinely used for diagnosis. PCR has been shown to be more sensitive than biopsy, although it is unclear whether this increased sensitivity detects clinically relevant infections or non-pathogenic respiratory flora. These techniques often provide a rapid diagnosis even before the corresponding transbronchial biopsy is available for histologic examination.

Radiologic findings

Chest radiographs show bilateral interstitial infiltrates but can be normal in some instances. On chest CT, the classic finding is the presence of bilateral ground-glass opacities. These opacities often spare the periphery of the lungs. Less common findings include airspace consolidation, reticular opacities, nodules, cavitary lesions and pneumothorax. Individuals with granulomatous inflammation usually present with lung nodules or

masses, which are typically multiple. *Pneumocystis* infection presenting as a solitary lung nodule is rare.

Differential diagnosis

The differential diagnosis mainly includes *Histoplasma* and *Cryptococcus* (Table 3.2). This issue arises predominantly in cases that lack a froth-with-dots appearance and show granulomatous features.

Treatment and prognosis

Trimethoprim/sulfamethoxazole (Bactrim) is the standard antimicrobial agent. Corticosteroids are added in some cases. Timely diagnosis and therapy is the most important factor in improving survival. Outcomes are worse in HIV-negative patients (48% mortality) than in HIV-positive individuals (17% mortality). The mortality rate in HIV-negative patients increases to 60% in cases where mechanical ventilation is required for respiratory failure.

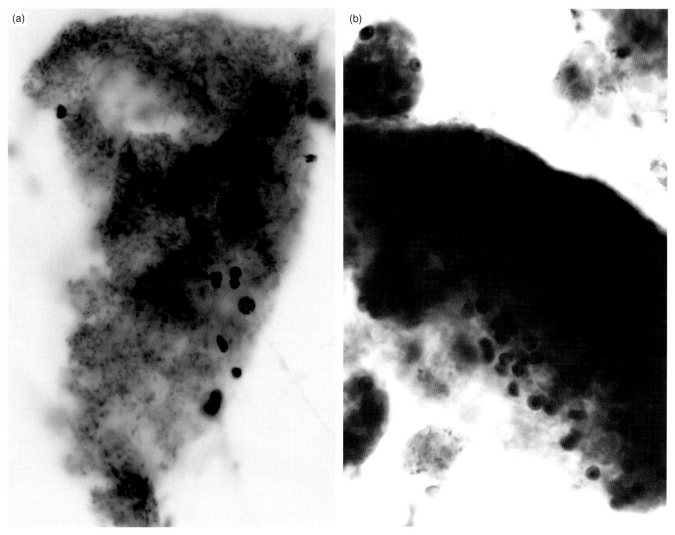

Figure 3.5. BAL fluid in *Pneumocystis* pneumonia. (a) Diff-Quik. A clump of frothy material contains multiple tiny dots (trophozoites). This should not be misinterpreted as an artifact or non-specific debris. **(b)** GMS stain highlights cysts. Note intra-cystic dots.

Sample diagnosis on pathology report

Lung, right upper lobe, transbronchial biopsy – Pneumocystis pneumonia (See comment).

Invasive aspergillosis

Aspergillus is a ubiquitous fungus; i.e., it is encountered worldwide. The most common species involved in lung disease is *A. fumigatus*, followed by *A. niger* and *A. flavus*. *Aspergillus* forms hyphae (mycelia) in tissues. Pulmonary aspergillosis has a wide clinical and pathologic spectrum depending on the immune status of the host, including invasive, semi-invasive, saprophytic and allergic disease. This section focuses on invasive aspergillosis, which is the most dreaded manifestation of aspergillosis in the lung, typically occurring in immunocompromised hosts.

Invasive aspergillosis can be diagnosed in small biopsies such as needle biopsies or transbronchial biopsies of the lung, as well as in larger specimens.

Major diagnostic findings

- Invasive aspergillosis is characterized by necrosis containing septate fungal hyphae. The necrosis is usually pink, bland and smudgy, and is often admixed with hemorrhage. It is frequently infarct-like, i.e., ghosts of necrotic alveoli are visible within the necrosis. In most cases, the necrosis is cell-poor, without a significant inflammatory infiltrate or basophilic nuclear debris. Fungal hyphae can be appreciated within the necrosis on H&E, although they are often pale-staining and can be missed at low magnification (Figure 3.6a).
- Vascular invasion is a key finding in invasive aspergillosis. It involves invasion of fungal hyphae through the walls of blood vessels into their lumens (Figure 3.6b). The involved vessels are usually found within the necrosis. Vascular lumens are often plugged with fungal hyphae, explaining the infarct-like appearance of the necrosis.

Table 3.2. How to differentiate *Pneumocystis*, *Histoplasma* and *Cryptococcus*

Feature	Pneumocystis	Histoplasma	Cryptococcus
Usual tissue reaction	Froth with dots within alveoli	Necrotizing granuloma	Non-necrotizing granulomatous inflammation with multinucleated giant cells
Granulomas	Occasionally	Yes, mostly	Yes, mostly
Necrotizing granulomatous inflammation	Possible	Usual	Occasional
Organisms visible on H&E	Cysts: no (froth visible) Trophozoites: Yes	In necrotizing granuloma: No In disseminated histoplasmosis: yes	Yes: yeasts with gray cell walls and surrounding halo
GMS	Positive	Positive	Positive
Shape of organisms on GMS	Round, crescentic, helmet-shaped, sickle-shaped, collapsed	Round, oval, tapered	Round
Collapsed forms	Characteristic	Occasional	Occasional
Size on GMS	4 to 6 µm	1 to 5 µm	4 to 10 µm
Size variation on GMS	Moderate	Minimal	Marked
Intra-cystic dot on GMS	Occasional	No	No
Budding	No	Narrow-based	Narrow-based
Mucicarmine	Negative	Negative	Often positive
Immunohistochemistry for *Pneumocystis*	Positive	Negative	Negative
Immunocompromised host	Always	Variable	Variable
Radiology	If nodules, usually multiple	Nodules may be solitary or multiple	Nodules may be solitary or multiple

- *Aspergillus* forms long, thin, uniform septate hyphae with narrow-angle branching (Figure 3.7a). The term *dichotomous branching* refers to the fact that the fungus bifurcates into two branches, each of which may give rise to two further branches, and so on. The branch angle in *Aspergillus* is usually described as 45° but in reality there is considerable variation and any angle less than 90° is acceptable. The hyphae appear round when cut in cross section. Large fusiform dilatations or varicosities are not uncommon. Other septate hyphae such as *Pseudallescheria* and *Fusarium* may show identical morphologic features in tissue and therefore cannot be reliably differentiated from *Aspergillus* (Figure 3.7b). Hence, the term *aspergillosis* should be used only after microbiologic confirmation that the organism is indeed *Aspergillus*. Cases in which microbiologic results are unavailable can be termed *invasive fungal pneumonia*. Needless to say, identification down to the species level (*A. fumigatus* vs. *A. niger*, for example) is neither possible nor expected in pathologic material.

Variable pathologic findings

- The necrosis in some cases of invasive aspergillosis may contain a prominent neutrophilic infiltrate, resembling a necrotizing bronchopneumonia.
- The fungal hyphae in invasive aspergillosis often have a "streaming" appearance in which the hyphae are arranged approximately parallel to each other. This is distinct from the tangled, haphazard arrangement of fungal hyphae in mycetomas.
- The histologic appearance of the wall of the lesion is variable. In some cases, the wall contains granulation tissue or fibrosis. In others, necrosis abuts the surrounding viable lung without a well-defined wall. Occasionally, the wall may contain granulomatous inflammation.
- Necrotizing tracheobronchitis or pseudomembranous tracheobronchitis is a variant of invasive aspergillosis. As implied by the name, this involves necrosis of the trachea and bronchi and formation of a pseudomembrane on the luminal surface.

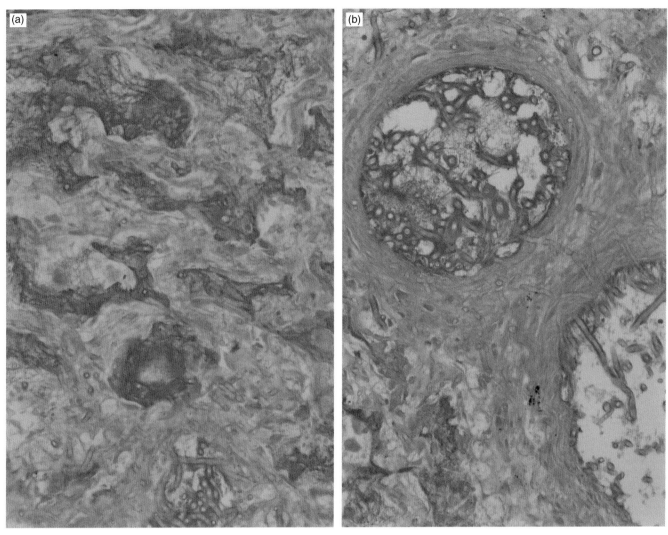

Figure 3.6. Invasive aspergillosis. (a) Fungal hyphae in a background of infarct-like hemorrhagic necrosis. There is no significant inflammation. **(b)** Vascular invasion. Fungal hyphae invade the vessel wall and plug the lumen.

- The concept of *semi-invasive aspergillosis* is discussed in detail in the chapter on granulomatous disease (Chapter 2).
- As in mycetomas, calcium oxalate crystals may be present in some cases. They are thought to result from the combination of oxalic acid derived from the fungus and calcium derived from the host.

Diagnostic work-up

GMS staining is not always required since *Aspergillus* is usually visible on H&E. However, occasionally organisms are pale staining and may be difficult to see in a necrotic background. The GMS stain can be very helpful in such situations. Also, as in other fungal infections, GMS stains help to highlight the number of organisms.

Clinical profile

Invasive aspergillosis is a disease of immunocompromised hosts. The most common settings are acute leukemia (especially patients with acute myeloid leukemia undergoing induction chemotherapy), hematopoietic stem cell transplantation, severe neutropenia, prolonged therapy with high-dose corticosteroids, and graft-versus-host disease. Recipients of lung transplants are also at increased risk, as are individuals with COPD, AIDS, chronic granulomatous disease, critically ill patients in intensive care units, and the elderly. Although invasive aspergillosis is the most common fungal pneumonia in patients with hematologic malignancies, it is infrequently seen by pathologists in the United States because of the widespread availability of non-invasive laboratory tests and increased awareness of its characteristic findings on chest CT.

Galactomannan testing in serum and BAL fluid is now widely used for the diagnosis of invasive aspergillosis. The sensitivity and specificity of serum testing is between 70 and 80%. Reported sensitivity for the BAL galactomannan assay is 85%, and the specificity is greater than 94%.

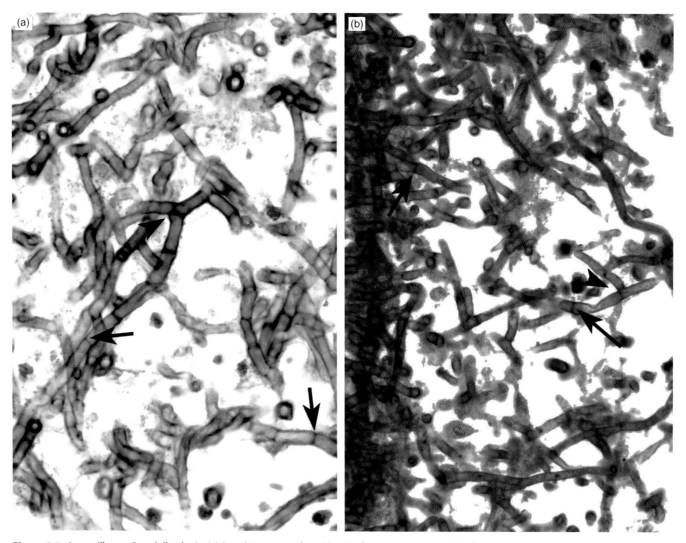

Figure 3.7. *Aspergillus* vs. *Pseudallescheria*. (a) Branching septate fungal hyphae from a patient who died of invasive pulmonary aspergillosis. Arrows: septa, arrowhead: narrow-angle branch point. Cultures grew *Aspergillus fumigatus*. **(b)** Fungal hyphae with narrow-angle branching (arrowhead) and septa (arrows), histologically indistinguishable from *Aspergillus*. These fungi were seen in a necrotic endobronchial lesion that developed after chemoradiation for lung cancer. Cultures grew *Pseudallescheria boydii*.

Radiologic findings

The classic lesion of invasive aspergillosis is a nodule surrounded by a halo of ground-glass attenuation (*halo sign*). Other findings include pleura-based wedge-shaped areas of consolidation corresponding to hemorrhagic infarction, the air crescent sign characterized by separation of necrotic lung from the adjacent viable lung, cavities, tree-in-bud opacities and the *hypodense sign*.

Differential diagnosis

- Invasive aspergillosis should be distinguished from invasive fungal pneumonia caused by other hyphal fungi such as *Mucor* and *Rhizopus*. These infections can cause necrotizing, granulomatous and/or angioinvasive lesions identical to aspergillosis. To compound the problem, *Aspergillus* often contains greatly swollen and distorted hyphae with varicosities, mimicking *Mucor*. However, in contrast to *Aspergillus, Mucor* shows wide-angle branching

(typically 90°) and forms hyphae that lack septa. If present, calcium oxalate crystals and fruiting heads favor *Aspergillus*.

- Invasive aspergillosis should also be distinguished from other forms of pulmonary aspergillosis. These are outlined in Table 3.3.

Treatment and prognosis

Voriconazole is currently the drug of choice for invasive pulmonary aspergillosis. In individuals who cannot tolerate voriconazole, liposomal amphotericin B is an alternative. Caspofungin has been used successfully in patients who fail to respond to first-line therapy. The prognosis is poor. The mortality rate for invasive pulmonary aspergillosis exceeds 50% in neutropenic patients, and may be as high as 90% in hematopoietic stem cell transplant recipients. HIV-infected individuals with invasive pulmonary aspergillosis have a median survival of 3 months.

Table 3.3. Differential diagnosis of the major forms of pulmonary aspergillosis

	Invasive aspergillosis	Chronic necrotizing aspergillosis	Mycetoma	Allergic bronchopulmonary aspergillosis
Aspergillus present in lung	Yes	Yes	Yes	Yes
Type of disease	Invasive	Semi-invasive	Saprophytic (non-invasive)	Allergic (non-invasive)
Typical immune status of patient	Severely impaired, often neutropenic	Normal or mildly compromised	Normal	Atopic (usually asthmatic)
Pre-existing lung disease	None	None, or emphysema	Pre-existing cavitary lung disease	Asthma
Radiologic features	Nodules, consolidation, halo sign	New and progressive cavity	Air–fluid levels in pre-existing cavity	Central bronchiectasis, mucoid impaction
Key clinical tests	Galactomannan testing, radiology, cultures	Radiology, cultures	Radiology, cultures	Radiology, IgE, cultures, skin testing
Morphology of fungal hyphae	Streaming	Streaming	Tangled, lamellated	Degenerated
Main histologic features	Necrosis, angioinvasion	Necrotizing granulomatous inflammation	Lamellated masses of fungal hyphae	Numerous eosinophils, allergic mucin, granulomatous inflammation
Wall of lesion	None, or granulation tissue	Granulomatous inflammation	Fibrosis and chronic inflammation	Eosinophils, granulomatous inflammation
Granulomas	Occasional	Always	No	Almost always
Necrosis	Yes	Yes	Scant debris	Often
Vascular invasion	Yes	No	No	No
Treatment	Voriconazole	Variable, often anti-fungals	None unless hemoptysis	Steroids

Sample diagnosis on pathology report

With culture confirmation that the organism is *Aspergillus*:

Lung, right middle lobe, surgical biopsy – Invasive aspergillosis (See comment).

Without culture confirmation:

Lung, left middle lobe, surgical biopsy – Invasive fungal pneumonia (See comment).

Mycetoma (fungus ball, aspergilloma)

A mycetoma is a tangled mass of fungal hyphae (fungus ball) that forms within a pre-existing cavity derived from the bronchial tree, presumably by saprophytic colonization. The term aspergilloma is used when the fungus is microbiologically proven to be *Aspergillus*. Aspergilloma is a common form of pulmonary aspergillosis. Since the fungi colonize pre-existing cavities and do not invade lung parenchyma, aspergilloma is regarded as a non-invasive form of aspergillosis. The fungus isolated from most mycetomas is *Aspergillus*, but other organisms have been rarely reported, including *Pseudallescheria*, *Cladosporium*, *Penicillium* and *Coccidioides*. Among *Aspergillus* species, *A. fumigatus* is by far the most common.

As mentioned above, aspergillomas form within pre-existing lung cavities. The common settings in which such cavities arise include sarcoidosis, lung cancer and bronchiectasis.

Major diagnostic findings

- Fungus ball. The main histologic finding is the presence of a mass of tangled fungal hyphae (mycelial mats) floating within a cavity-like space (Figure 3.8). The fungus ball typically has a lamellated appearance at low magnification caused by the alternation of densely packed and loosely packed hyphae (Figure 3.9). Since it is freely mobile and non-invasive, it often separates from the wall and may need to be submitted in a separate cassette.
- By definition, there is no evidence of tissue invasion, including granulomatous inflammation in the wall, vascular invasion or parenchymal invasion.
- Microbiologic cultures are required for definitive identification of *Aspergillus*. Fungus balls without microbiologic confirmation can be diagnosed as mycetoma. The most common specimens from which *Aspergillus* is isolated are bronchial brushings and BAL

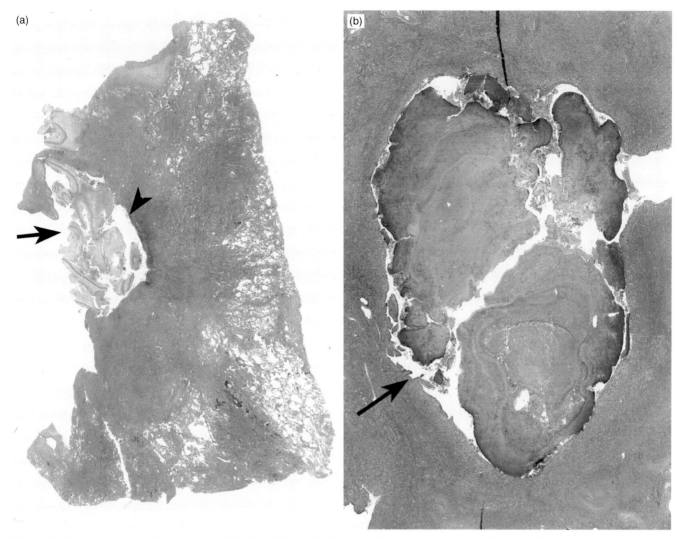

Figure 3.8. Mycetoma (aspergilloma), low magnification. (a) Fungal hyphae (arrow) float in a cavity (arrowhead). The lamellated appearance of the fungal masses is visible even at this very low magnification. **(b)** In this example from another case, the epithelial lining of the fungus-filled cavity is visible (arrow), as is the surrounding chronic inflammation and fibrosis.

fluid. *A. fumigatus* is by far the most common species, followed by *A. niger* and *A. flavus*. A few referral laboratories offer PCR testing on formalin-fixed paraffin-embedded tissues for subtyping fungal hyphae.

Variable pathologic findings

- The cavity in which a mycetoma forms is essentially a dilated and inflamed bronchus. Hence, a respiratory lining composed of ciliated columnar cells is usually present unless ulceration or denudation supervenes. The wall of the cavity shows dense chronic inflammation or fibrosis or both (Figure 3.8). The inflammatory infiltrate is usually composed of lymphocytes and plasma cells. Granulomatous inflammation is not a feature of mycetomas, and should suggest semi-invasive disease.
- The lumen of the cavity often contains small amounts of admixed mucin or inflammatory debris, especially at the periphery. However, extensive necrosis should suggest an alternative diagnosis (semi-invasive/granulomatous aspergillosis or invasive aspergillosis).

- The lining of the cavity may be extensively ulcerated. Ulceration is most likely the underlying basis of hemoptysis in patients with mycetomas.
- There may be organizing pneumonia in the lung adjacent to the mycetoma.
- Features of the underlying disease that led to the cavity may be present in the background.
- Massive numbers of oxalate crystals have been observed in some cases. They appear as irregular bright crystals that are birefringent under polarized light. These crystals may appear dumbbell-like, sheaf-like or rosette-like. They may be found in association with the fungus, or in the necrotic debris between the fungus and the wall, or in the wall of the cavity. Oxalate crystals are more common in *A. niger* infections.
- The fungal hyphae in mycetomas may produce fruiting bodies, also known as fruiting heads or conidiophores (Figure 3.9, Figure 3.1d). These spectacular flower-like fungal forms are composed of a stalk (hypha) containing a round swollen structure (vesicle) at one end. From the

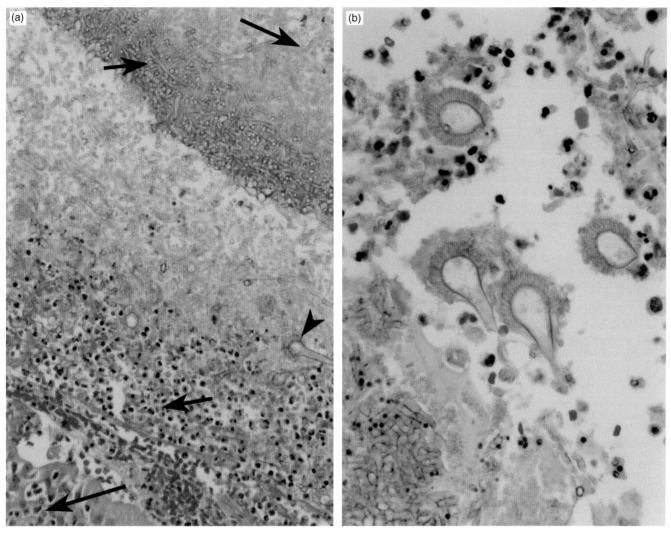

Figure 3.9. Mycetoma (aspergilloma), high magnification. (a) Layers of a resected pulmonary aspergilloma (mycetoma or fungus ball). The wall of the cavitary lesion is lined by respiratory epithelium (long arrow, bottom). Inflammatory debris is present within the lumen at the edge of the fungus ball (short arrow, bottom). Fruiting bodies are also visible (arrowhead). Densely packed and haphazardly tangled fungal hyphae (short arrow, top) alternate with loosely arranged hyphae (long arrow, top), giving rise to the characteristic lamellated appearance. **(b)** Fruiting bodies.

vesicle, radiating spokes (phialides) bearing tiny round spores (conidia) emanate like petals on a flower. The spores are often found in the background singly and in clusters, detached from their parent fruiting bodies, and are often golden yellow in color. They do not bud. Fruiting bodies are the reproductive form of the fungus. Their formation requires an oxygen supply, which in turn requires a patent communication between the fungus ball and the tracheobronchial tree. For this reason, fruiting bodies are usually seen in aspergillomas and invasive tracheobronchitis. We have also seen them in an *Aspergillus* empyema presumably caused by a bronchopleural fistula. Their presence in association with septate hyphae with narrow-angle branching suggests that the organism is *Aspergillus*, and is considered confirmatory by some. Structural differences in the fruiting bodies of the common species of *Aspergillus* (*A. fumigatus, A. flavus and A. niger*) have

been described. For example, *A. fumigatus* has a flask-shaped vesicle from which straight phialides arise directly, covering the upper two-thirds of the vesicle. In contrast, *A. niger* has a spherical vesicle covered on all sides by carrot-like structures known as metulae from which V-shaped phialides arise.

- Mycetomas are usually solitary, but multiple and bilateral examples have been reported.
- Grossly, mycetomas consist of tan or light-brown putty-like material within a lung cavity. This gross appearance is not diagnostic, since it can also be seen in chronic necrotizing aspergillosis (See Figures 2.32 and 2.33, Chapter 2).

Diagnostic work-up

The organisms are obvious on H&E, and GMS staining is not required.

Clinical profile

Mycetomas can develop in both genders and at all ages, reflecting the wide variety of conditions that can cause lung cavities. These include bronchiectasis (most commonly caused by tuberculosis, cystic fibrosis or lung carcinoma) and sarcoidosis. Other reported underlying conditions include intralobar sequestration, bronchogenic cyst and pneumatocele.

Since mycetomas develop in individuals with pre-existing cavitary lung disease, when symptoms develop it is difficult to determine whether they are related to the underlying disease or should be attributed to the mycetoma. A significant minority of patients are completely asymptomatic, the mycetoma being discovered incidentally on chest imaging performed for other reasons. Aspergillomas can be present for many years without causing symptoms. In symptomatic individuals, the most common and clinically significant symptom is hemoptysis, which can be sudden and life-threatening. Cough and dyspnea are also commonly reported, but these may be related to the underlying cavitary lung disease rather than the mycetoma. Fever is rare in the absence of superimposed bacterial infection.

Sputum cultures are negative in 50% of cases. When they are positive, *A. fumigatus* is the most common organism isolated. Serum IgG antibodies to *Aspergillus* are positive in many cases.

Radiologic findings

The diagnosis is usually made on radiologic grounds. The classic finding is a lung cavity containing a solid, round or oval mass that moves when the patient's position is changed. The upper lobes are most commonly involved. A characteristic *air-crescent* is often seen between the mycetoma and the cavity wall, but is not specific since it can be seen in hematomas, abscesses, tumors and hydatid cysts. The cavity wall or the adjacent pleura may be thickened.

Differential diagnosis

The differential diagnosis of mycetoma and other forms of pulmonary aspergillosis is addressed in Table 3.3.

Treatment and prognosis

Most patients with mycetomas can be followed without specific therapy, especially if they are asymptomatic. There is no evidence that mycetomas respond to anti-fungal agents. In cases where anti-fungals have been used, they have been shown to be ineffective. Surgery (lobectomy, segmentectomy or pneumonectomy) is indicated for uncontrollable, life-threatening hemoptysis, but is associated with high mortality (7 to 23%). Surgery may also be performed to determine the etiology of the lesion if radiologic findings are not definitive. Bronchial artery embolization is occasionally performed in patients who cannot tolerate surgery. Approximately 10% of mycetomas resolve spontaneously. Unfortunately, post-operative complications are common after surgery for mycetomas. They include bronchopleural fistula, sepsis and death.

Sample diagnosis on pathology report

In cases without a culture-proven organism:

Lung, right upper lobe, lobectomy – Mycetoma (See comment).

In cases with culture-proven *Aspergillus*:

Lung, right upper lobe, lobectomy – Aspergilloma (See comment).

Cytomegalovirus pneumonia

Cytomegalovirus (CMV) is by far the most common virus identified by surgical pathologists in lung biopsies. Lung infection (CMV pneumonia) occurs mainly in immunocompromised individuals. Some authors use the equivalent term CMV pneumonitis. CMV is recognizable in tissues by the characteristic morphologic changes that it produces in the cells it infects, known as *viral cytopathic effect*. CMV is one of the few viruses that produce a viral cytopathic effect in the lung. Although individual viruses are too tiny to be seen with a light microscope, large numbers of viral particles conglomerate to form *inclusions* that can be seen on routine H&E-stained sections. The morphology of the inclusions in CMV infection is described below.

In the lung, CMV infection can be diagnosed by pathologists in bronchoalveolar lavage fluid, transbronchial biopsies and even core needle biopsies.

Major diagnostic findings

- The viral cytopathic effect of CMV is characterized by the presence of enlarged cells with nuclear and cytoplasmic inclusions (Figure 3.10, Figure 3.1a). The infected cells may be alveolar macrophages, alveolar pneumocytes, endothelial cells or fibroblasts. They may be found within the airspaces or in the interstitium. The nucleus is enlarged and contains a central dark red or purple, round or irregular inclusion surrounded by a clear space, resulting in an "owl's-eye" appearance. However, the clear space is not always present. The cytoplasm also contains inclusions but these are smaller and often less prominent, and may be absent depending on the plane of section. Conversely, since the infected cells are greatly enlarged, the plane of section may show cytoplasmic inclusions only. When cytoplasmic inclusions are present, they appear as multiple tiny purple granules. The number of cells with inclusions varies from rare (and difficult to find) to numerous and prominent. The combination of cellular enlargement, nuclear inclusions and cytoplasmic inclusions with the morphologic features described above is pathognomonic of CMV.
- The nuclear inclusions of CMV are often described as "Cowdry type A" inclusions, which are eosinophilic intranuclear inclusions accompanied by margination of the nuclear chromatin onto the nuclear membrane. They are named after Edmund Cowdry, a cytologist and anatomist who attempted to subclassify nuclear inclusions in 1934. Interestingly, CMV was not included in Cowdry's original

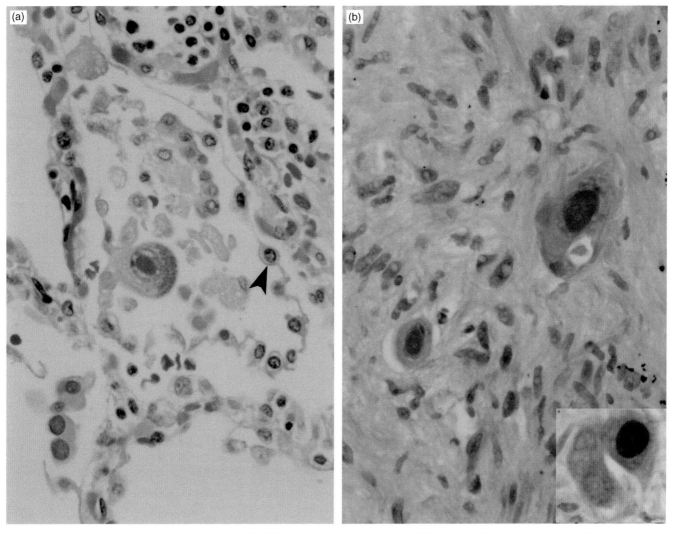

Figure 3.10. Cytomegalovirus pneumonia. (a) Enlarged cell showing cytopathic effect typical of CMV, with nuclear inclusion surrounded by a clear zone, as well as cytoplasmic inclusions. Compare size of cell to type 2 pneumocyte (arrowhead). Note minimal interstitial inflammatory infiltrate.
(b) Two CMV-infected cells in a core needle biopsy of the lung from an immunosuppressed individual with a cavitary lung mass. The cells are enlarged and contain nuclear inclusions. Cytoplasmic inclusions are harder to appreciate. Other cells in the biopsy contained nuclear and cytoplasmic inclusions (not shown), and immunohistochemistry for CMV was positive (inset).

list of viruses with type A inclusions. Similar intranuclear inclusions can also be seen in infections caused by herpes simplex virus and varicella zoster, both of which were on Cowdry's original list. Unlike CMV, however, neither of these viruses forms intracytoplasmic inclusions. Cowdry type B inclusions – eosinophilic inclusions of variable size without margination of the nuclear membrane – are poorly characterized. They are allegedly seen in polio.

Variable pathologic findings

- The tissue reaction in CMV pneumonia is extremely variable. Many cases show no tissue reaction at all. Since CMV inclusions do not occur in immunocompetent, healthy individuals, this appearance should probably be regarded as abnormal.
- Minimal or mild interstitial chronic inflammation (interstitial pneumonia/interstitial pneumonitis) is also

common in cytomegalovirus pneumonia (Figure 3.10). When a concurrent infection such as *Pneumocystis* pneumonia is present, it is difficult to ascertain which organism is responsible for the inflammatory reaction. This phenomenon complicates interpretation of unusual tissue reactions reported in CMV pneumonia.

- Diffuse alveolar damage occurs in some cases. It is characterized by the presence of hyaline membranes, fibrinous exudates within the alveoli, alveolar septal thickening by edema and fibroblasts, and reactive type 2 pneumocytes.
- Numerous histiocytes may occasionally be present within airspaces. They may have foamy or clear cytoplasm.
- A miliary pattern with necrosis has been described in some patients in surgical biopsies or autopsies from bone marrow transplant recipients with CMV pneumonia. It is characterized by multiple tiny spherical lesions with a central neutrophilic response, cellular debris within alveoli,

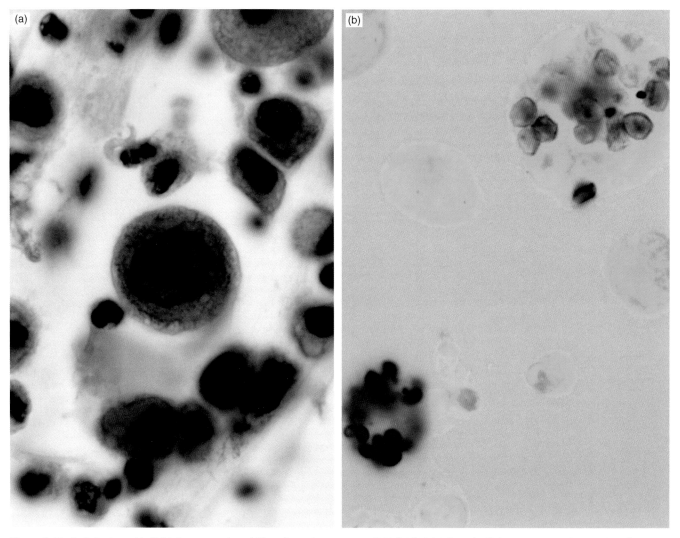

Figure 3.11. Co-infection with CMV, *Pneumocystis* and *Histoplasma* in same case (BAL fluid). (a) Enlarged cell showing CMV viral cytopathic effect (Pap stain). **(b)** Same case stained with GMS, showing co-infection with *Pneumocystis* (top right) and *Histoplasma* (bottom left). The *Histoplasma* yeasts are smaller than the *Pneumocystis* cysts. The patient had HIV/AIDS, diagnosed 15 years earlier but never treated. The CD4 count was 14 cells/mm³.

hemorrhage and numerous CMV-infected cells, but relatively little change in the intervening lung.

- Necrotizing tracheobronchitis has been reported in AIDS patients with CMV infection.
- Co-infection with other opportunistic organisms is common (Figure 3.11). These include *Pneumocystis*, *Histoplasma*, *Cryptococcus* and mycobacteria. A search for these organisms should always be performed when CMV inclusions are found. Co-existent Kaposi sarcoma is also common. Indeed, there is evidence to suggest that isolated CMV pneumonia is less common than CMV in combination with another infection or Kaposi sarcoma.

Diagnostic work-up

- Immunohistochemistry for CMV can be helpful when inclusions are equivocal or atypical on H&E (Figure 3.10). Immunostaining often highlights more inclusions than are apparent at first glance. However, the random use of immunohistochemistry in the absence of inclusions on

H&E can be problematic. Some studies of positive immunohistochemical staining in the absence of inclusions have shown some correlation of such staining with elevated CMV viral loads in BAL fluid. However, it is unclear whether such cases represent clinically significant CMV pneumonia. See "clinical profile", below, for a more detailed discussion of this issue.

- The cytoplasmic inclusions of CMV-infected cells can be PAS- and/or GMS-positive, ostensibly because they contain a mucopolysaccharide coat.
- Electron microscopy has been used for viral identification in the past, but it has been replaced by immunohistochemistry in most centers.

Clinical profile

CMV pneumonia can occur at any age, including neonates, infants and children. Most patients are immunocompromised. The infection is best known in the setting of HIV/AIDS but organ transplant recipients are also at risk. Of the latter, the highest risk is in bone marrow transplant recipients followed by recipients of combined heart–lung transplants and kidney transplants. CMV pneumonia is probably the most common infection in lung transplant recipients encountered by surgical pathologists. Cases also occur in patients treated with corticosteroids or chemotherapy. A few histologically well-documented cases of CMV pneumonia have been reported in immunocompetent individuals.

The clinical presentation is non-specific. The most common symptoms are fever and shortness of breath. Some individuals are asymptomatic. The clinical course varies from insidious to fulminant.

The diagnosis of CMV pneumonia is made in the presence of radiologic infiltrates and laboratory evidence of CMV infection, which may come from cultures of BAL fluid or biopsied tissue, or identification of inclusions in BAL fluid or transbronchial biopsies. Measurement of viral loads in the blood by quantitative PCR is commonly performed in transplant recipients.

The relative merits of inclusions (on H&E or BAL cytology), immunohistochemistry and cultures for the diagnosis of CMV infection have been examined in several studies. Most authors agree that the finding of CMV inclusions by routine morphology correlates well with clinically significant disease. Viral cultures are more sensitive than histology but do not always correlate with clinically significant disease since they are able to detect low, clinically insignificant viral burdens. The clinical significance of positive CMV immunohistochemistry in the absence of inclusions on H&E remains unclear. In some studies, identification of CMV inclusions by immunohistochemistry in BAL fluid correlated better with symptomatic CMV infection and lung infiltrates. Others have shown that atypical immunohistochemical staining, defined as positive immunohistochemistry in non-cytomegalic cells without inclusions, correlates with intermediate-level viral loads in BAL fluid, possibly representing incipient CMV pneumonia. It is unclear whether routine immunohistochemical staining for CMV is justified in the absence of inclusions, and whether the use of immunohistochemistry should differ depending on the setting (immunocompetent individuals vs. transplant recipients).

Radiologic findings

Typical findings on chest X-rays are bilateral interstitial infiltrates with lower lobe predominance. Bilateral ground-glass opacities are most common on chest CT. Other findings include mixed alveolar-interstitial opacities, poorly defined centrilobular nodules, consolidation, bronchial dilatation and thickened interlobular septa. Solitary or multiple lung nodules mimicking malignancy occur in some patients, although it is unclear whether they can be attributed solely to CMV. A histologically documented case of CMV pneumonia presenting as a solitary cavitary mass has also been reported. A specific diagnosis of CMV pneumonia cannot be made on the basis of radiologic findings, since they overlap greatly with other viral infections.

Differential diagnosis

- Reactive type 2 pneumocytes. Type 2 pneumocytes may be enlarged in a variety of interstitial lung diseases and occasionally contain intracytoplasmic Mallory hyalin, but nuclear and cytoplasmic inclusions are absent.
- Other viral inclusions. The combination of enlarged size and nuclear and cytoplasmic inclusions serves to differentiate CMV from other types of viral inclusions. Measles pneumonia can feature both intranuclear and intracytoplasmic inclusions but the infected cells are multinucleated whereas CMV-infected cells are not. *Herpes*, *Varicella* and adenovirus feature intranuclear inclusions but lack intracytoplasmic inclusions. Other common viral infections of the lung either show only intracytoplasmic inclusions (RSV, parainfluenza) or lack viral cytopathic changes (influenza, Hantavirus, severe acute respiratory syndrome (SARS) coronavirus).
- Malignant cells such as the Reed-Sternberg cell of Hodgkin lymphoma can have a similar appearance, but nuclear features of malignancy are usually obvious and the background contains a prominent mixed inflammatory infiltrate composed of small lymphocytes, histiocytes, plasma cells or eosinophils.
- Viral shedding. The frequent finding of CMV in cultures from asymptomatic patients has led to the concept of *viral shedding*, which suggests that the virus is present but clinically insignificant. The finding of inclusions on routine H&E-stained sections favors a true clinically significant infection and argues against viral shedding.

Treatment and prognosis

Intravenous ganciclovir is the drug of choice for CMV pneumonia. CMV hyperimmune globulin is added in some cases. Foscarnet is used for ganciclovir-resistant cases. The prognosis is variable. Some patients develop tachypnea and hypoxia and die rapidly with fulminant acute respiratory failure. Reported mortality rates range from 15 to 75%. In the post-ganciclovir era, the mortality of CMV infection in lung transplant recipients ranges from 2 to 12%.

Sample diagnosis on pathology report

Lung, right lower lobe, transplant transbronchial biopsy – Cytomegalovirus pneumonia (See comment).

Respiratory syncytial virus bronchiolitis and pneumonia

Respiratory syncytial virus (RSV) is the most common viral cause of respiratory tract infections in infants and children and is second only to influenza as a cause of viral lung infections overall. It is estimated that 5% of hospitalizations in children less than 5 years of age are attributable to RSV. Worldwide, it is estimated that 50% of children in the first year of life, and virtually all children by the first few years, are infected by this virus, which is easily transmitted by aerosols or direct contact. The infection is rampant in day-care centers and pre-schools in the United States. Outbreaks are common in the late autumn or winter. RSV typically causes upper respiratory tract infection but may progress down the respiratory tract, causing laryngitis, tracheobronchitis, bronchiolitis and pneumonia.

Infections in adults are uncommon, but do occur occasionally in immunocompromised hosts. Since the diagnosis is usually based on clinical features and laboratory tests, RSV is not commonly seen by surgical pathologists. Occasional cases may be encountered at autopsy or in lung biopsies from immunocompromised hosts.

Major diagnostic findings

The viral cytopathic effect of RSV consists of multinucleated giant cells that form a "syncytium" after which the virus is named. The cells may line alveoli or airways, or may be desquamated. Small round eosinophilic intracytoplasmic inclusions have been described in some cases. They may be surrounded by a thin clear halo. Necrosis of the giant cells can occur. Unfortunately, these viral cytopathic changes are not always identifiable.

Variable pathologic findings

- Interstitial chronic inflammation, or *interstitial pneumonia*, is probably the most common finding. It consists of mild alveolar septal thickening by variable numbers of inflammatory cells, mainly lymphocytes. This tissue response is similar to the reaction seen in other viral infections such as parainfluenza or influenza, and may co-exist with diffuse alveolar damage.
- Diffuse alveolar damage is a form of acute lung injury seen in severe cases of RSV infection involving the lung parenchyma. The findings include variable alveolar septal widening by edema and fibroblasts and prominent reactive type 2 pneumocytes. Hyaline membranes may be present in the acute stage. DAD is also a feature of other severe viral infections and can be seen in many other infectious and non-infectious settings.
- *Bronchiolitis* is a well-known feature of RSV, but there are no distinctive pathologic clues to indicate a specific etiology other than the cytopathic effect described above. Syncytial giant cells may be found adjacent to the intraluminal cellular debris. Reported changes include chronic inflammation in bronchiolar walls, lymphoid aggregates, ulceration and sloughing of bronchiolar epithelium, luminal debris composed of mucin, necrotic epithelial cells or inflammatory cells and reactive or regenerative changes such as hyperplasia and squamous metaplasia. Necrotizing bronchiolitis has also been described. The lymphocytes are predominantly CD3-positive T-cells.
- A particularly florid version of RSV pneumonia characterized by numerous multinucleated syncytial giant cells in the lung parenchyma associated with diffuse alveolar damage has been described in a child with severe combined immunodeficiency syndrome.
- Edema and lymphatic dilatation have been described in a few cases.

Diagnostic work-up

Monoclonal and polyclonal antibodies to RSV antigen are available for immunohistochemistry, and can be very useful for confirming the diagnosis in formalin-fixed paraffin-embedded tissue. The antibody stains the cytoplasm or membrane of the syncytial giant cells. Staining has also been described in bronchial and bronchiolar ciliated columnar cells, alveolar pneumocytes, bronchial and alveolar luminal debris and macrophages.

Clinical profile

Infants and children are most commonly affected. The typical symptoms are those of an upper respiratory tract infection. They include rhinorrhea, cough, sneezing and fever. Severe disease is associated with dyspnea, tachypnea, cyanosis, nasal flaring, wheezing and hypoxia. Physical findings include intercostal retractions, hyper-resonant chest and rales. Apneic episodes occur in 20% of hospitalized infants. In adults, half the cases involve upper respiratory tract infection characterized by cough, pharyngitis and low-grade fever. Secondary bacterial infections are common.

Most cases of RSV infection are diagnosed presumptively on clinical grounds without microbiologic confirmation. If required, the latter can be obtained by a nasopharyngeal aspirate or swab, which can be tested by cultures, enzyme immunoassays, direct or indirect immunofluorescence, or PCR-based assays. RT-PCR is currently the gold standard, and some viral panels now allow multiplex PCR testing for several common respiratory tract viruses including RSV. Cultures have traditionally been the gold standard but take 2 to 5 days to become positive and are less sensitive than PCR. Multiplex point-of-care direct antigen detection tests are practical and widely available, but are less sensitive than PCR. Serology is not helpful because 10 to 30% of patients with acute RSV infection are seronegative.

Radiologic findings

Lung infiltrates suggestive of bronchiolitis or pneumonia may be present. In children, common findings are peribronchial thickening and air trapping suggestive of bronchiolitis, or patchy consolidation suggestive of pneumonia. On chest CT, mosaic attenuation, airway-centered changes or multifocal airspace findings are common. In one study, the most common CT finding in microbiologically confirmed RSV infection was the presence of tree-in-bud opacities. Other common findings include bronchial wall thickening and multifocal consolidation, similar to other viral infections. A small proportion of cases show no abnormalities on chest CT.

Differential diagnosis

- Diffuse alveolar damage can have numerous etiologies, both infectious and non-infectious. Diagnosis of RSV as a cause requires identification of the characteristic viral cytopathic effect, RSV immunohistochemistry, or microbiologic confirmation by a nasopharyngeal aspirate or swab.

- Other viral infections can cause identical histologic findings. The absence of nuclear inclusions differentiates RSV from CMV, herpes and measles. Parainfluenza is the only other major viral lung infection that causes intracytoplasmic inclusions. Definitive differentiation from RSV requires immunohistochemistry or microbiologic confirmation.
- Hard metal lung disease can cause multinucleated giant cells and interstitial chronic inflammation. In most cases, the acute clinical picture of RSV pneumonia should be easy to differentiate from the insidious onset of hard metal lung disease. Histologically, prominent emperipolesis favors hard metal lung disease, whereas intracytoplasmic inclusions point to RSV pneumonia.
  Immunohistochemistry or microbiology can confirm the diagnosis.

Treatment and prognosis

Routine use of nebulized ribavirin in infants and children with RSV bronchiolitis is not recommended. Management in children is supportive, consisting mainly of supplemental oxygen, hydration and chest physiotherapy. Palivizumab prophylaxis is indicated for pre-term infants in the first year of life. In immunosuppressed adults, inhaled ribavirin is the drug of choice.

The prognosis is excellent in most cases, with spontaneous resolution of symptoms over days to weeks. Some children deteriorate for 2 to 3 days after onset of the disease but subsequently improve. The mortality of RSV bronchiolitis is low. Rare deaths have been reported in previously healthy, immunocompetent children. Reported long-term sequelae include persistent hypoxia and pulmonary function abnormalities.

Sample diagnosis on pathology report

In the presence of supportive microbiologic or immunohistochemical evidence:

Lung, right middle lobe, transbronchial biopsy – Diffuse alveolar damage with multinucleated giant cells, consistent with respiratory syncytial virus pneumonia (See comment).

In the absence of supportive microbiologic or immunohistochemical evidence:

Lung, right middle lobe, transbronchial biopsy – Organizing diffuse alveolar damage (See comment).

Influenza

Influenza is the most common viral infection of the lungs. It is highly infectious, has a seasonal distribution, and has been responsible for several well-known pandemics. It is caused by the influenza virus, which is classified into three main antigenic types or genera (A, B and C). Of these, influenza A is the most common and clinically significant. Together, influenza A and influenza B account for most cases of seasonal influenza. Each antigenic type is further classified into serotypes based on permutations of the surface viral proteins hemagglutinin (HA) and neuraminidase (NA). Of these serotypes, three (H1N1, H1N2 and H3N2) currently cause most human infections in the United States.

A variant of the influenza A virus came into the spotlight during the 2008/2009 influenza season. It was known variously as novel influenza A(H1N1) virus, pandemic A/H1N1 virus, new influenza virus, swine-like influenza virus, swine-origin influenza virus or colloquially as "swine flu". It contained genes derived from two types of swine influenza, one of which was a triple reassortant of human, avian and swine influenza A strains. In this way, novel influenza A(H1N1) virus was distinct from seasonal influenza A(H1N1) virus. Another serotype of influenza A that has received attention in recent years is avian influenza A virus (H5N1). This virus is endemic in poultry but has also caused disease in humans in Asian countries with high mortality.

From the point of view of the surgical pathologist, influenza is very difficult to diagnose since it does not cause a viral cytopathic effect. Further, the non-specific tissue reaction is common to many other viral infections as well as a wide range of infectious and non-infectious etiologies.

Major diagnostic findings

There is no known viral cytopathic effect and there are no pathognomonic histologic findings. The diagnosis relies on demonstration of the virus by immunohistochemistry, immunofluorescence, PCR-based tests or testing of clinical samples such as nasopharyngeal swabs or aspirates, bronchial washings, bronchoalveolar lavage specimens or biopsied lung tissue.

Variable pathologic findings

- The histologic findings can be divided into those caused by the virus and those attributable to superimposed bacterial infection. The two often co-exist. Findings attributed to viral infection include diffuse alveolar damage, intra-alveolar hemorrhage, acute necrotizing tracheobronchitis, bronchitis and bronchiolitis. A similar spectrum of findings is seen in novel influenza A(H1N1) and avian influenza (H5N1). The main finding attributable to superimposed bacterial infection is acute bronchopneumonia, characterized by a neutrophilic infiltrate within alveolar spaces accompanied by fibrin, edema and/or macrophages. The most common superinfecting bacteria are *Staphylococcus aureus*, *Streptococcus pneumoniae* and *Haemophilus influenzae*.
- Inflammatory changes of the trachea, bronchi and bronchioles occur in most cases between days 3 and 13 of the illness. Reactive and regenerative changes of the lining epithelium are also common. Squamous metaplasia may occur, and is sometimes so striking as to suggest squamous cell carcinoma.
- Diffuse alveolar damage (DAD) is the most consistent histologic manifestation of influenza pneumonia. It can be seen as early as the second day of illness and as late as day 21. It is more prominent in patients requiring mechanical ventilation and supplemental oxygen. Other viruses that cause DAD include novel influenza A(H1N1) (Figure 3.12), avian influenza (H5N1), severe acute respiratory syndrome (SARS) coronavirus, adenovirus, hantavirus, herpes virus,

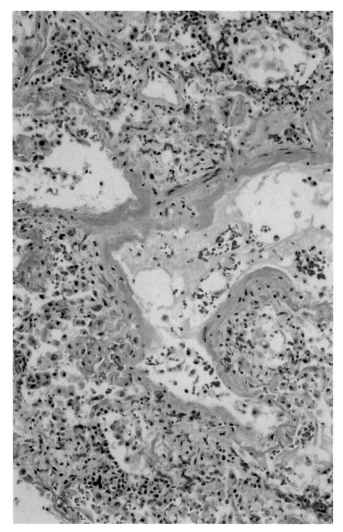

Figure 3.12. H1N1 influenza (swine flu). Diffuse alveolar damage in novel influenza A(H1N1) diagnosed at autopsy. Hyaline membranes are present. There is no viral cytopathic effect. The diagnosis was confirmed by RT-PCR testing of a pre-mortem nasal aspirate and a post-mortem nasal swab at a reference lab.

CMV, parainfluenza virus and measles virus. DAD can also be caused by chemotherapy, radiation, toxic inhalants, gastric acid aspiration and connective tissue disease. In the vast majority of cases, the histologic features of DAD are similar regardless of the underlying cause. Therefore, knowledge of the clinical setting and ancillary tests are usually required to establish a specific etiology.

Diagnostic work-up

- Immunohistochemical techniques have demonstrated viral antigens within airway epithelium. Antibodies have been used on formalin-fixed paraffin-embedded tissue, but are not widely available.
- Clinical testing of respiratory secretions with a polymerase chain reaction (PCR) based test, often in a multiplex PCR panel that includes other common respiratory viruses, is currently the most common means of confirming the diagnosis. Common panels currently in use generally test for influenza A and B, RSV, parainfluenza and adenovirus, among others.
- In fatal cases, seasonal influenza virus or novel influenza A (H1N1) virus infection can be detected by real-time polymerase chain reaction testing of autopsied tissue samples.

Clinical profile

Influenza can occur at any age but adults are most commonly affected. It involves previously healthy immunocompetent individuals as well as those with underlying medical illnesses, pre-existing lung disease or compromised immune systems.

Most patients present with fever, cough, chills, myalgia, malaise, headache or anorexia. These systemic manifestations, more common during the first few days of the illness, are referred to as "flu-like" symptoms since influenza is the prototype. However, similar symptoms are common in many other viral and non-viral infections that mimic influenza. In the latter part of the first week, common symptoms are nasal discharge, sore throat and dry cough. There may be a history of contact with other individuals exhibiting flu-like symptoms.

The clinical course can be severe, especially in elderly individuals with comorbid illnesses. Shortness of breath tends to be associated with the development of pneumonia. Severe disease occasionally occurs in previously healthy young people, or in those with underlying illnesses. Some individuals have a distinctly "non-respiratory" presentation. Rarely, influenza virus is recovered from the lungs of patients lacking premonitory symptoms of a flu-like illness.

Even with a high index of suspicion, the clinical diagnosis can be difficult because confirmatory testing can take a few days to a week. Laboratory confirmation most commonly comes from testing of nasopharyngeal aspirates, washings or swabs. Bronchoalveolar lavage fluid, bronchial washings and tissue samples can also be tested. PCR-based tests are currently the gold standard, since they are more sensitive than viral cultures. They are also highly specific, provide rapid results, and are of especially high clinical utility when used in a multiplex assay that detects other respiratory viruses. Please see the preceding section on respiratory syncytial virus for additional discussion of these tests.

Radiologic findings

The radiologic findings overlap greatly with other viral infections. Common abnormalities attributable to influenza bronchiolitis include bronchial wall thickening and tree-in-bud opacities. Severe influenza is associated with multiple foci of consolidation, interstitial/alveolar infiltrates and ground-glass opacities, changes that usually correspond pathologically to diffuse alveolar damage. Chest CTs are normal in a larger proportion of influenza infections than other common respiratory tract viral infections.

Differential diagnosis

The differential diagnosis from the pathologist's standpoint includes other causes of bronchiolitis and diffuse alveolar damage. In most cases, the etiology of these injury patterns cannot be determined on histologic grounds. However, some cases of diffuse alveolar damage may show specific pathologic findings such as viral inclusions (CMV, herpes simplex virus, adenovirus, parainfluenza virus), fungal organisms (*Histoplasma, Blastomyces, Pneumocystis*) or particulate matter aspiration.

Treatment and prognosis

Mild influenza does not require antiviral therapy. The neuraminidase inhibitors oseltamivir and zanamivir are the drugs of choice for severe influenza, including influenza pneumonia. Benefit from antiviral treatment in seasonal influenza is strongest when treatment is started within 48 hours of the onset of illness. Approximately 10% of seasonal influenza A cases are resistant to oseltamivir whereas novel influenza A(H1N1) is usually sensitive. Currently, mortality from influenza is approximately 2% overall and 29 to 71% in influenza pneumonia. The reported mortality rate of avian influenza A(H5N1) is approximately 60%.

Sample diagnosis on pathology report

Lung, right middle lobe, surgical biopsy – Diffuse alveolar damage (See comment).

Herpes tracheobronchitis and pneumonia

Herpes of the lower respiratory tract is caused by herpes simplex virus (HSV). Although HSV commonly causes ulcers in the mouth and esophagus, disease of the lower respiratory tract is rare. It includes tracheobronchitis and pneumonia. Lung infection is thought to result from downward extension of the virus from upper respiratory tract disease or by hematogenous dissemination. It appears that the virus is truly causative in some cases and an incidental finding in others. The latter is especially true when the virus is detected by cultures alone.

The diagnosis can be made by endobronchial or transbronchial biopsy if the characteristic inclusions are sampled. The inclusions can also be identified in cytologic specimens.

Major diagnostic findings

- Cowdry type A inclusions (Figure 3.13a). HSV is the only common virus included in Edmund Cowdry's original list of viruses with type A inclusions. Such inclusions were subsequently named "Cowdry type A" and the concept was extended to other viruses such as CMV and RSV. As described by Cowdry, type A inclusions are eosinophilic inclusions within the nucleus surrounded by a clear halo that marginates the remaining nuclear chromatin to the periphery of the nucleus, up against the nuclear membrane.
- The other major type of nuclear inclusion seen in HSV is the ground-glass inclusion, which causes the nucleus to appear hazy or opaque (Figure 3.13b). The name is derived from the similarity to ground-glass, a type of glass the surface of which has been ground to produce a rough (matte) finish.
- HSV does not form intracytoplasmic inclusions. Unlike CMV, the infected cells are not enlarged. The viral cytopathic effect of HSV in cytologic preparations is often summarized as **m**ultinucleation, **m**olding and **m**argination

of nuclear chromatin (the "3 Ms"). However, in the lung, multinucleated cells are uncommon, and molding is not always present.

Variable pathologic findings

- *Necrotizing bronchiolitis* with extensive *karyorrhectic nuclear debris*. The destruction of bronchioles by necrosis containing abundant karyorrhectic debris is the most helpful clue to the diagnosis (Figure 3.14). Karyorrhexis is characterized by breakdown of necrotic nuclei into numerous minute basophilic fragments. Other tissue reactions in HSV pneumonia include organizing diffuse alveolar damage with florid interstitial fibroblast proliferation and intra-arterial thrombi, secondary vasculitis adjacent to areas of necrosis, and interstitial mononuclear cell infiltrates. Florid squamous metaplasia may be seen in some cases.
- Ulcers are a common manifestation of HSV infection of the upper respiratory tract as well as the airways, including the trachea, bronchi and bronchioles (Figure 3.15). They are often accompanied by necrosis, granulation tissue, and necrotic exudates within bronchiolar lumens. Viral inclusions are commonly found in the residual epithelium or ulcer bed.
- Some cases show evidence of concurrent bacterial pneumonia.

Diagnostic work-up

A combined immunohistochemical stain for HSV type 1 (HSV-1) and HSV type 2 (HSV-2) can be very helpful in confirming the diagnosis when viral inclusions are identified or suspected on H&E. Staining is seen in the nuclei of epithelial cells as well as macrophages.

Clinical profile

Adults and children of either sex can develop HSV infection of the lower respiratory tract, but most cases are reported in young adults. Symptoms include progressive dyspnea, fever, painful cough, pleuritic chest pain, headache, myalgia and malaise. Fever may be absent in some cases.

HSV pneumonia is exceedingly rare in immunocompetent individuals, and is uncommon even in immunocompromised hosts. The disease is thought to spread mainly through the airways, consistent with the pathologic findings. However, hematogenous dissemination is thought to be the mechanism of lung infection in some immunocompromised patients, as well as in neonates. There is an increased risk of HSV infection of the lower respiratory tract in patients with ARDS, and in individuals with severe cutaneous burns. Other reported risk factors include endotracheal intubation and prior open thoracic surgery. Combinations of factors seem to be especially potent. For example, many cases have been reported in patients who previously underwent endotracheal intubation for ARDS, suggesting that intubation predisposes to lower respiratory tract infection, possibly by driving viral particles down into the lungs from the airways and upper respiratory tract foci. This hypothesis is

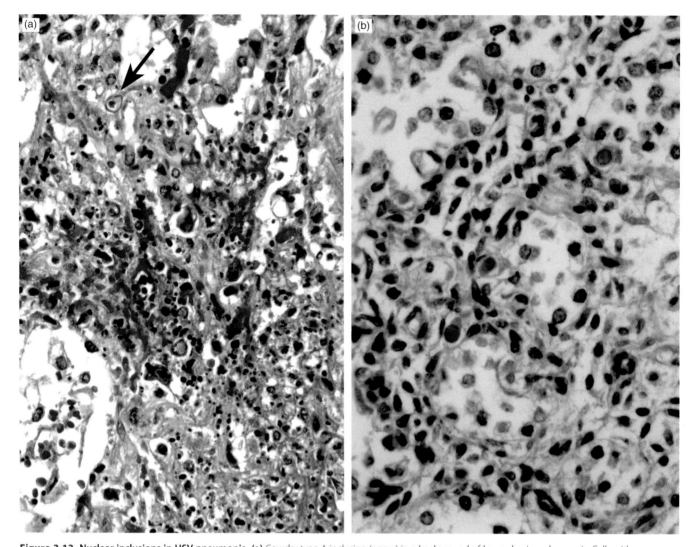

Figure 3.13. Nuclear inclusions in HSV pneumonia. (a) Cowdry type A inclusion (arrow) in a background of karyorrhexis and necrosis. Cells with ground-glass nuclear inclusions are also present. **(b)** Ground-glass intranuclear inclusion in a case of neonatal herpes pneumonia. Cases courtesy of Dr. Carol Farver.

supported by the finding of HSV in the tracheobronchial secretions (tracheal aspirates and BAL fluid) of up to 30% of critically ill patients with ARDS, rare reports of HSV tracheobronchitis and pneumonia in patients with herpes labialis, and the bronchoscopic finding of tracheal or bronchial ulcers in some patients with HSV pneumonia.

It is well documented that HSV pneumonia can occur in patients who have tested negative on commonly used respiratory panels performed on nasopharyngeal swabs. The virus can grow in cultures, but culture positivity does not necessarily indicate true infection. As with CMV, histopathologic demonstration of viral inclusions is thought to be a more robust indicator of clinically significant disease than positive cultures.

Radiologic findings

The radiologic findings – diffuse bilateral infiltrates – overlap with those of ARDS. Chest radiographs may show white-out of the affected lungs, multiple foci of airspace consolidation, or unilateral interstitial and alveolar infiltrates. On chest CT, HSV pneumonia enters the differential diagnosis of diffuse bilateral ground-glass opacities without additional findings. Bilateral foci of airspace consolidation in a peribronchovascular distribution have also been described. Overall, the radiologic features are non-specific, and do not allow a confident diagnosis in the absence of microbiologic or pathologic confirmation.

Differential diagnosis

- CMV also shows Cowdry A-type intranuclear inclusions, but is easily distinguished from HSV because the infected cells are greatly enlarged and also contain intracytoplasmic inclusions. Ground-glass inclusions, multinucleation and molding are not seen in CMV.
- Adenovirus features necrosis, karyorrhectic debris and intranuclear inclusions without cytoplasmic inclusions. In contrast to HSV, the inclusions are smudgy rather than ground-glass. Cowdry A inclusions are usually absent, as are multinucleation and nuclear molding. In difficult cases, immunohistochemistry for CMV and adenovirus helps to resolve the issue.

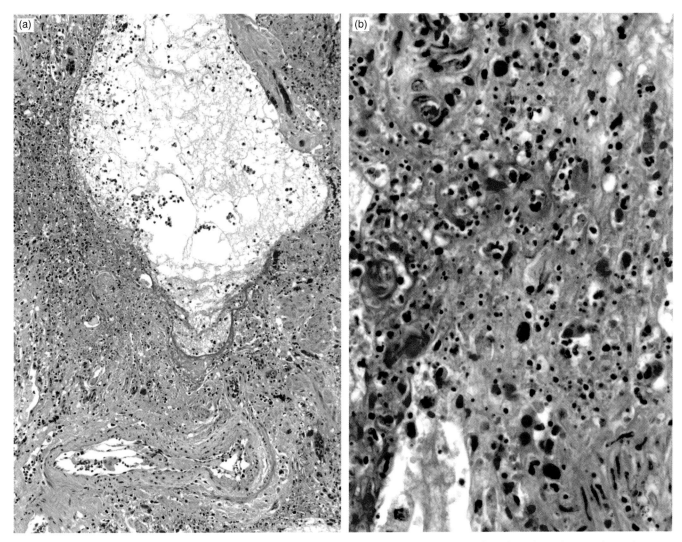

Figure 3.14. Bronchiolar necrosis and karyorrhectic debris in HSV pneumonia. (a) A bronchovascular bundle is shown here. The artery (bottom) is intact but the bronchiole (top) is completely necrotic. **(b)** Necrosis with abundant karyorrhectic debris.

Treatment and prognosis

The drug of choice for HSV pneumonia is acyclovir. Significant improvement of symptoms, clearing of infiltrates and disappearance of inclusions on repeat biopsies has been reported with prompt therapy.

Sample diagnosis on pathology report

Lung, right upper lobe, endobronchial biopsy – Ulcer with necrosis (Herpes inclusions present).

    or

Lung, left lower lobe, surgical biopsy – Necrotizing bronchiolitis (Herpes simplex inclusions present).

Adenovirus pneumonia

Adenovirus infections are not commonly encountered by surgical pathologists; the decrease in incidence of this infection in adults has been attributed to the development of a live attenuated vaccine. Adenovirus can cause pharyngitis, pharyngoconjunctivitis, laryngitis, tracheobronchitis, bronchiolitis and pneumonia. Unfortunately, because of difficulties in antemortem diagnosis, this infection is generally seen by pathologists only at autopsy.

Major diagnostic findings

Viral cytopathic effect characterized by smudgy intranuclear inclusions ("smudge cells") (Figure 3.16). These inclusions are found in bronchiolar or alveolar epithelial cells, often adjacent to necrosis and karyorrhectic debris. They may be numerous and prominent, or few in number and difficult to find. The inclusions are basophilic or amphophilic and homogeneous. They fill and enlarge the nucleus, resulting in loss of the normal chromatin pattern. In contrast to Cowdry A inclusions, there is no halo around the inclusion, and no margination of nuclear chromatin.

Variable pathologic findings

- Diffuse alveolar damage is the characteristic tissue reaction in adenovirus pneumonia. As in diffuse alveolar damage in other settings, it features hyaline membranes, thickened alveolar septa, reactive type 2 pneumocytes and fibrinous

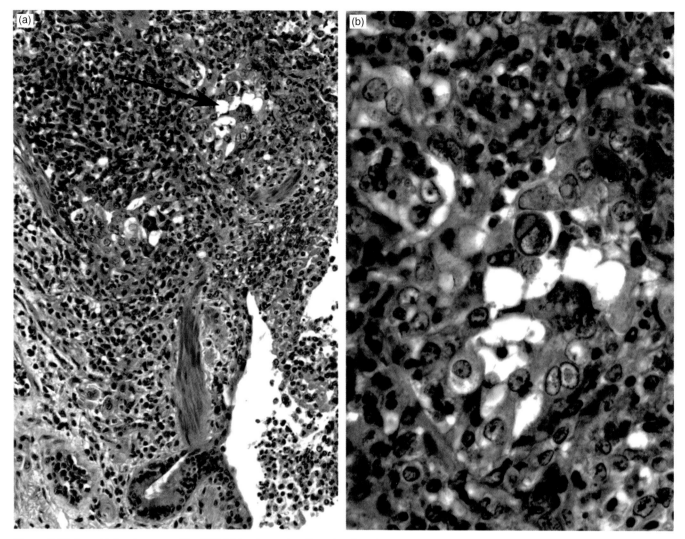

Figure 3.15. Bronchiolar ulcer caused by HSV. (a) An ulcerated and heavily inflamed bronchiole contains cells with HSV inclusions in the ulcer bed (arrow), shown at high magnification in b. **(b)** Intranuclear inclusions with margination of chromatin and nuclear molding. Immunohistochemistry for HSV was strongly positive. Case courtesy of Dr. A. V. Arrossi.

exudates within the airspaces. Viral inclusions may be found adjacent to these areas (Figure 3.16). In the organizing phase, the interstitium may be diffusely thickened. An interstitial pneumonia composed of lymphocytes may accompany the DAD, and contribute to the interstitial thickening.

- Necrosis with karyorrhectic debris. Although it may not be obvious at low magnification, necrosis is often present in adenovirus pneumonia. It almost invariably involves and destroys small bronchioles and adjacent alveoli causing necrotizing bronchiolitis and necrotizing bronchopneumonia. A valuable tip-off to the diagnosis is the presence of karyorrhectic debris, characterized by minute dot-like basophilic particles derived from necrotic disintegrating nuclei. It is found within the lumens of bronchioles and alveoli.

- Another type of inclusion described in adenovirus infection is eosinophilic and surrounded by a halo. It is less well defined than Cowdry A inclusions.

- Organizing pneumonia has been reported adjacent to the characteristic necrotic areas. Changes attributable to other concomitant infections may be present, especially in transplant recipients.

Diagnostic work-up

Immunohistochemistry for adenovirus is feasible and is the most convenient and rapid method for confirming the diagnosis. The staining pattern is nuclear and cytoplasmic. Immunofluorescence has also been used for confirming the diagnosis, but it requires specialized equipment and fresh tissue, and is not widely available. In situ hybridization can also be used to detect viral particles in formalin-fixed paraffin-embedded tissue. The viral particles can also be identified by electron microscopy, where they are arranged in hexagonal groups referred to as a *lattice-like* or *honeycomb* pattern.

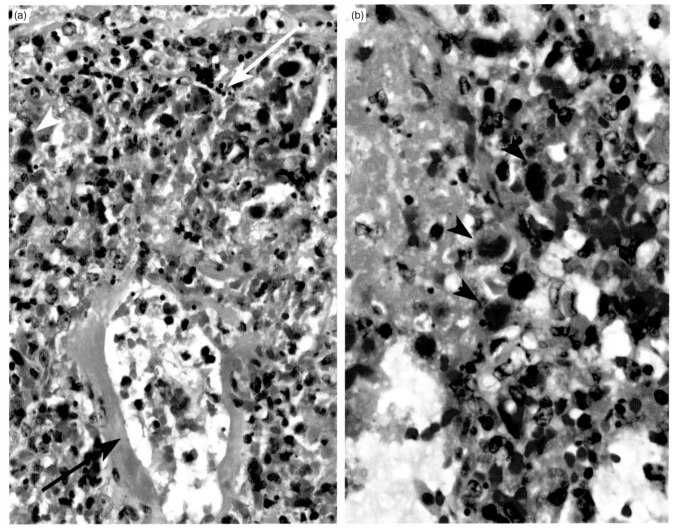

Figure 3.16. Adenovirus pneumonia. (a) Note hyaline membrane (long arrow), karyorrhectic debris (white arrow) and smudge cells (white arrowhead). **(b)** High magnification, showing smudgy texture of nuclear chromatin characteristic of adenovirus viral cytopathic effect (arrowheads). Case courtesy of Dr. Carol Farver.

Clinical profile

Adenovirus infection can occur in immunocompromised as well as immunocompetent individuals, and may affect both children and adults. Most infections occur in infants and children less than 5 years of age. Infection of the upper respiratory tract is common, but adenovirus pneumonia is rare. It is estimated that up to 2 to 5% of respiratory infections in children are caused by adenovirus.

Although rare in neonates, adenovirus pneumonia has been reported in premature and term babies with no obvious risk factors. Transplant recipients, especially infants and young children, are particularly susceptible. Recipients of bone marrow or stem cell transplants are highest risk, but infections have also been reported in recipients of lung (1 to 2%), heart, heart–lung and renal transplants.

Symptoms of adenovirus pneumonia include fever, cough, dyspnea, wheezing and acute respiratory distress. A prodrome of conjunctivitis or morbilliform rash may occur prior to development of respiratory symptoms. In pediatric lung transplant recipients, the interval between transplantation and onset of symptoms ranges from 3 to 9 days to as late as 40 days. Patients may develop acute respiratory failure and often require mechanical ventilation. It has been suggested that a normal or decreased white cell count associated with lymphocytosis and progression of disease despite antibiotic therapy should suggest the possibility of adenovirus pneumonia.

PCR-based testing of nasopharyngeal swabs for respiratory tract pathogens is currently the most common means of confirming the diagnosis. Tracheal aspirates and lung aspirates can also be tested. Adenovirus is part of many currently available multiplex PCR tests. Viral cultures of bronchoalveolar lavage fluid may also yield a diagnosis, but can take as long as 4 to 8 days to become positive.

Radiologic findings

Chest radiographs show bilateral interstitial infiltrates, or the picture can mimic bacterial pneumonia. In children, the most common radiologic findings on chest CT are diffuse bilateral infiltrates, severe overinflation due to air trapping and lobar atelectasis, especially of the right upper lobe or left lower lobe. Overinflation/air trapping is thought to be a manifestation of bronchiolar involvement. Other radiologic findings include bronchial wall thickening, lobar or segmental consolidation, bilateral consolidation and pleural effusions.

Differential diagnosis

- Other viral infections. HSV is the main viral infection in the differential diagnosis since it can cause diffuse alveolar damage accompanied by karyorrhexis, bronchiolar necrosis and small airway inflammation. Further, the ground-glass inclusions of HSV can appear similar to the smudgy inclusions of adenovirus. Cowdry type A inclusions support a diagnosis of HSV, as does multinucleation or nuclear molding. In difficult cases, immunohistochemistry for HSV and adenovirus can be very helpful.
- Other causes of necrosis with karyorrhexis such as necrotizing capillaritis may enter the differential diagnosis. This is rarely a significant diagnostic problem since capillaritis involves alveolar septa whereas adenovirus infection is a bronchiolocentric process.

Treatment and prognosis

Most adenovirus infections are indolent and self-limited, and do not require specific therapy. The drug of choice for adenovirus pneumonia is cidofovir. γ-interferon or intravenous immunoglobulin is sometimes given as adjunctive therapy. Adenovirus is thought to be the most aggressive of the viral causes of pneumonia. Although most patients recover from adenovirus lower respiratory tract infections, the prognosis of severe adenovirus pneumonia is poor, especially in neonates and transplant recipients. In the latter group, adenovirus is the most lethal viral infection, with most reported cases resulting in death, graft failure or early development of obliterative bronchiolitis. In children who survive acute episodes of adenovirus bronchiolitis and pneumonia, bronchiectasis and obliterative bronchiolitis are well-documented long-term sequelae, occurring especially in infections caused by adenovirus type 21. Mortality rates of invasive adenovirus disease following stem cell transplantation vary from 25 to 75%. This high rate seems to have decreased after the introduction of cidofovir, but the prognosis of patients with adenovirus pneumonia remains dismal.

Sample diagnosis on pathology report

Lung, right upper lobe, surgical biopsy – Diffuse alveolar damage (adenovirus inclusions present) (See comment).

Parainfluenza virus

Parainfluenza virus is a common cause of respiratory infections in infants and children. In the United States, parainfluenza virus types 1–3 have been found to be responsible for up to one-third of lower respiratory tract infections in children less than 5 years of age. This virus is perhaps best known as the etiologic agent of *croup*, a syndrome characterized by barking cough, stridor, fever and subglottic narrowing in infants and young children. The pathologic correlate of croup is *laryngotracheitis*. Lower respiratory tract infections, characterized by bronchiolitis or pneumonia, are usually caused by parainfluenza virus 3. Although most cases of parainfluenza occur in immunocompetent individuals, the infection is most severe and fatal in immunocompromised hosts.

Major diagnostic findings

Viral cytopathic effect with immunohistochemical confirmation. The characteristic viral cytopathic effect of parainfluenza virus consists of multinucleated (syncytial) giant cells with intracytoplasmic inclusions (Figure 3.17). The giant cells are most commonly derived from alveolar pneumocytes.

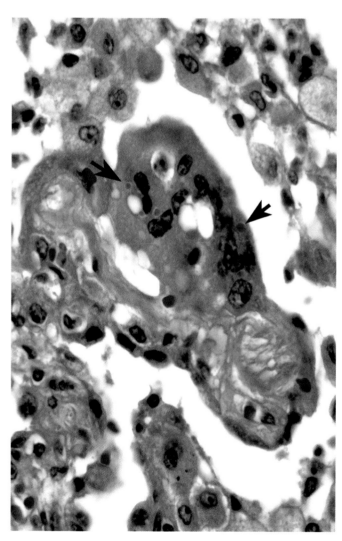

Figure 3.17. Parainfluenza viral cytopathic effect. Multinucleated syncytial cell lining an alveolar septum in a case of parainfluenza pneumonia. Note intracytoplasmic eosinophilic inclusions (arrows), some of which are surrounded by a small clear space. Case courtesy of Dr. Carol Farver.

Intranuclear inclusions are absent, although nucleoli may be prominent. The inclusions may also be found in the trachea or bronchi.

Variable pathologic findings

Viral inclusions are not always present. Some cases feature tracheobronchitis, bronchiolitis, diffuse alveolar damage or interstitial pneumonia.

Diagnostic work-up

Monoclonal antibodies against parainfluenza virus are commercially available for use in immunohistochemistry. The staining pattern is granular and cytoplasmic. Electron microscopy has also been used for confirming the diagnosis.

Clinical profile

Most parainfluenza infections occur in infants and children between the ages of 7 and 36 months, with a peak in the second and third years of life. Upper respiratory tract illnesses and croup are the best-recognized manifestations. Parainfluenza pneumonia occurs mainly in immunocompromised individuals, especially children with congenital immune deficiencies. The best known of these is *severe combined immunodeficiency* (SCID), a disorder that impairs both T- and B-cell function and presents in infancy with multiple infections. Cases of parainfluenza pneumonia have also been documented in bone marrow and stem cell transplant recipients, 5 to 15% of lung transplant recipients and children with acute leukemia who have received high-dose chemotherapy. In pediatric organ transplant recipients, most cases occur less than 3 months after transplantation. Reported symptoms in parainfluenza pneumonia include fever, cough, rhinorrhea, wheezing and tachypnea. Direct identification of the virus can be obtained by multiplex PCR-based respiratory panels or viral cultures of respiratory tract specimens, including biopsied tissues. The prognosis of parainfluenza pneumonia in immunocompromised individuals is poor. Several deaths have been reported.

Radiologic findings

There are no distinctive radiologic findings. Bibasilar infiltrates described as "interstitial" or "patchy" have been described on chest radiographs.

Differential diagnosis

- RSV. Pathologic features shared by RSV and parainfluenza include cytoplasmic inclusions, absence of nuclear inclusions, multinucleation and interstitial pneumonia. Multinucleation is more prominent in parainfluenza, but this feature cannot be relied upon for a definitive diagnosis. The best way to resolve the differential diagnosis is by immunohistochemistry.

- Measles pneumonia also features multinucleated giant cells with intracytoplasmic inclusions, but intranuclear inclusions are additionally present.
- Giant cell interstitial pneumonia (due to hard metal lung disease or other causes) also features multinucleated giant cells and an interstitial pneumonia. The clinical setting (acute in parainfluenza vs. chronic in giant cell interstitial pneumonia) and the presence of viral inclusions in parainfluenza will settle the issue in most cases.

Treatment and prognosis

There are no antiviral agents with proven efficacy against parainfluenza. Severe croup can be treated with a single dose of corticosteroids or nebulized epinephrine. Most parainfluenza virus infections are self-limited. The reported mortality of bone marrow transplant recipients with parainfluenza virus infection is 37 to 60%.

Sample diagnosis on pathology report

Lung, right upper lobe, surgical biopsy – Diffuse alveolar damage with multinucleated giant cells (intracytoplasmic inclusions present) (See comment).

Strongyloidiasis

Strongyloidiasis is caused by the nematode (roundworm) *Strongyloides stercoralis*. The disease occurs worldwide, with endemic areas in tropical or subtropical regions such as Southeast Asia. However, strongyloidiasis has also been reported in Western countries. In the United States, pockets of high prevalence have been reported in Kentucky, southern Virginia and North Carolina. The disease has been reported in aboriginal populations in Northern Australia. Immigrants to Western countries from endemic areas are also at high risk for strongyloidiasis, especially if they are receiving immunosuppressive therapy. The infection has been reported in Vietnam veterans, for example. It is thought that infection can last for many years in immunocompetent individuals with minimal or no symptoms.

Strongyloidiasis is contracted mainly by direct contact with soil contaminated with free-living larvae, for example by walking barefoot in contaminated soil. Rare cases of person-to-person transmission have also been documented. Infective (filariform) larvae of *Strongyloides* enter humans through the skin, penetrate the dermis and spread hematogenously to the lungs. There, they migrate into the airways, move upwards to the pharynx and are swallowed into the gastrointestinal tract. In the small intestine, larvae mature into adult female worms, which lay eggs that turn into rhabditiform larvae. Some of these turn into filariform larvae that can re-enter the bloodstream. This phenomenon, known as *auto-infection*, is a distinctive feature of the life cycle of *Strongyloides*. Re-entry in small numbers results in persistent, low-level disease. However, in immunocompromised

147

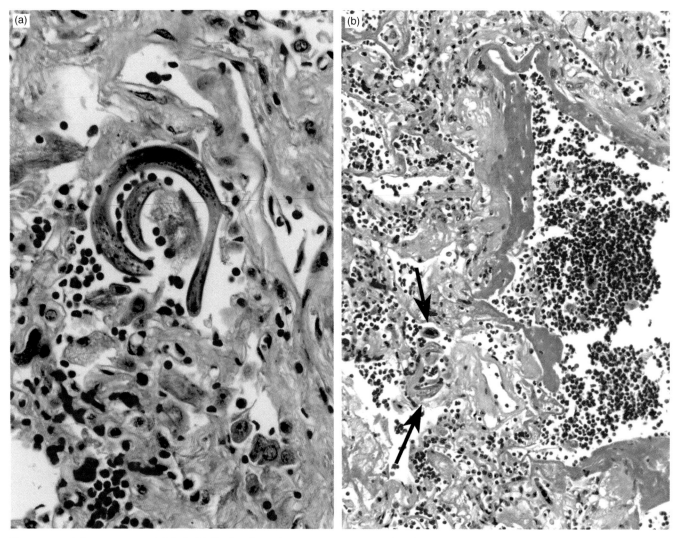

Figure 3.18. Pulmonary strongyloidiasis. (a) Filariform larva of *Strongyloides* in the lung. **(b)** Diffuse alveolar damage. Hyaline membranes are obvious, but larvae are easy to miss at this magnification (arrows). Case courtesy of Dr. Carol Farver.

hosts, large numbers of larvae re-enter the bloodstream, resulting in disseminated strongyloidiasis and the *hyperinfection syndrome*.

Major diagnostic findings

Strongyloides larvae are tiny, elongated, pink to purple structures with a tapered end and a broad end. They are often coiled, curved or S-shaped (Figure 3.18, Figure 3.1c). The blunt end lacks a prominent buccal cavity. Filariform (slender) larvae are far more common in the lung than rhabditiform (non-slender) larvae. They have a cylindrical esophagus that occupies half the body length. Dot-like structures may be present within the larvae, and help to identify the organism (Figure 3.18, Figure 3.1c). Larvae may be found within bronchiolar lumens, airspaces, lymphatics or the walls and lumens of pulmonary arteries.

Variable pathologic findings

- The tissue reaction is quite variable. There may be no inflammatory reaction, or larvae may be surrounded by neutrophils, fibrin or granulomatous inflammation.

- Diffuse alveolar damage (DAD) is a common feature of acute lung injury in severe strongyloidiasis. Larvae may be found within injured alveoli adjacent to hyaline membranes (Figure 3.18).
- Acute bronchopneumonia. The acute inflammatory exudate may contain filariform larvae surrounded by neutrophils and fibrin. It has been suggested that acute bronchopneumonia in these patients is caused by enteric bacteria *piggybacking* on larvae.
- Poorly formed granulomas or multinucleated giant cells may be found within the interstitium. Rarely, these may contain filariform larvae.
- Patchy interstitial fibrosis has been described, especially within interlobular septa.
- Infections by other opportunistic pathogens such as CMV are common.
- The parasite is well described in the cytology literature. Sputum samples may contain filariform or rhabditiform larvae. The organisms may also be found in BAL fluid.

- Adult worms are only rarely found in the lung, but may be seen in stool samples or duodenal biopsies.

Diagnostic work-up

There are no special stains or immunohistochemical markers. The larvae are empty-looking (non-staining) on Diff-Quik and positive (black) on GMS. They may stain red or blue on a Gram stain.

Clinical profile

Most infected individuals are asymptomatic or have minimal symptoms. The most common symptoms reported are cough, dyspnea, wheezing and hemoptysis. Others include choking sensation, hoarseness and chest pain. Bacteremia and sepsis also occur commonly, presumably due to piggy-backing of enteric bacteria into the bloodstream on the backs of invading larvae. Spontaneous pneumothorax is extremely rare.

Immunocompromised hosts develop a severe form of strongyloidiasis known as the *hyperinfection syndrome*, which involves hematogenous dissemination of large numbers of organisms from the intestinal tract to extra-intestinal organs. Most patients that develop this syndrome are on corticosteroids, but the condition has also been described in HIV/AIDS, organ transplant recipients and patients with malignancies. Clinically, the syndrome is characterized by exacerbation of gastrointestinal or pulmonary symptoms and detection of large numbers of larvae in gastrointestinal or respiratory tract specimens.

Strongyloidiasis is usually diagnosed on the basis of laboratory testing. Larvae may be found in the stool, sputum, bronchial brushings, bronchoalveolar lavage fluid, bronchoscopic lung biopsies, duodenal aspirates, small intestinal biopsies, tracheal aspirates or pleural fluid. Adult worms may be found in stool samples and duodenal biopsies. Surgical lung biopsies are required in some patients, and provide the best opportunity to evaluate the associated tissue reaction. Some cases are diagnosed only at autopsy. Serology (ELISA) is fairly sensitive (except in the first 4 weeks) but non-specific.

Radiologic findings

Chest X-rays most commonly show bilateral or focal interstitial infiltrates. Pleural effusions are present in 40%, and lung abscesses in 15%.

Differential diagnosis

Strongyloides is the only parasite whose larval forms are seen in the lungs with any appreciable frequency. The two other parasites that may be seen in the lung by surgical pathologists are discussed in Chapter 2. The diagnostic form in pulmonary dirofilariasis is the adult worm. In pulmonary paragonimiasis, it is generally the eggs and rarely an adult worm. In lung pathology, the presence of

larvae derived from parasites other than *Strongyloides* is vanishingly rare. If the diagnosis is in doubt, serologic testing can be confirmatory.

Treatment and prognosis

The drug of choice for uncomplicated strongyloidiasis is oral ivermectin. The hyperinfection syndrome has a high mortality rate (up to 87%).

Sample diagnosis on pathology report

Lung, right upper lobe, surgical biopsy – Diffuse alveolar damage (*Strongyloides* larvae present).

Nocardiosis

Nocardia is a filamentous gram-positive bacterium that causes lung disease in immunocompromised individuals. The nomenclature of this organism has undergone considerable change in recent years. Consequently, many *Nocardia* isolates that in the past would have been classified as *Nocardia asteroides* are now known as *Nocardia cyriacigeorgica*. In the twenty-first century, *Nocardia* is speciated by sequence analysis of its 16S rRNA gene. Details of the basis of this shift in nomenclature are outside the scope of this book, but it is worth mentioning that at present, using modern subtyping techniques, the species most frequently isolated from pulmonary nocardiosis are *N. nova*, *N. cyriacigeorgica*, *N. farcinica* and *N. abscessus*. Pulmonary disease caused by *N. carnea*, *N. grenadensis*, *N. veterana*, *N. otitidiscaviarum* and *N. brasiliensis* has also been reported. *Nocardia farcinica* is notable for ceftriaxone-resistance and a propensity for skin and deep soft tissue infections. *Nocardia* can be identified by pathologists in core needle biopsies as well as in surgical lung biopsies. Biopsies of brain lesions may also be diagnostic.

Major diagnostic findings

- The inflammatory reaction in pulmonary nocardiosis is characterized by variable combinations of *neutrophils, histiocytes* and/or *necrosis* (Figure 3.19). The neutrophilic component may manifest as acute inflammation admixed with histiocytes, acute bronchopneumonia, necrotizing acute bronchopneumonia, suppurative necrosis or abscess formation. The histiocytic component is also usually prominent. It can form nodular lesions characterized by extensive filling of airspaces by sheets of foamy or pink histiocytes admixed with a few scattered neutrophils, vaguely granulomatous areas, or occasional multinucleated giant cells. Well-formed non-necrotizing sarcoid-like granulomas and well-formed necrotizing granulomas are not features of nocardiosis.
- *Nocardia* is not visible on H&E, and it does not form sulfur granules. The latter is described further in the discussion on differential diagnosis. The role of special stains is discussed

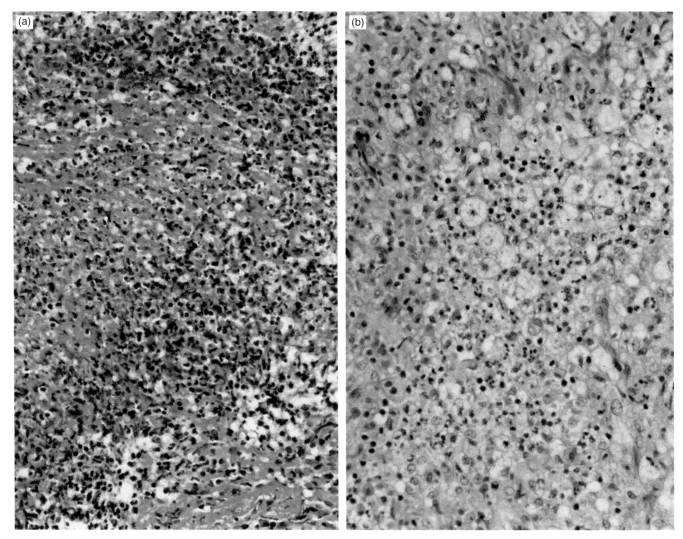

Figure 3.19. Nocardia pneumonia (H&E). (a) Suppurative necrosis resembling an abscess. **(b)** Sheets of histiocytes admixed with neutrophils. A vaguely granulomatous area is at top left.

in the section on diagnostic work-up. Briefly, on GMS or Gram stains, the organisms are slender, filamentous (thread-like), elongated, branching, gram-positive rods (Figure 3.20).

Variable pathologic findings

Occasional pathologic findings in pulmonary nocardiosis include secondary vasculitis adjacent to necrotic areas and small foci of organizing pneumonia. The pleura or bronchial tree may be involved.

Diagnostic work-up

- From the perspective of the surgical pathologist, the most useful stain for the diagnosis is GMS. *Nocardia* is invariably GMS-positive. It appears as slender, elongated, branching, thread-like structures (Figure 3.20). The organisms are much longer than ordinary bacterial rods, and far more slender and thread-like than fungal hyphae.

- A tissue Gram stain such as Brown-Hopps or Brown-Brenn is often helpful, although it is more capricious than the GMS stain. *Nocardia* is gram-positive, i.e. it stains blue. The other morphologic features mentioned above can also be appreciated in Gram-stained slides.

- *Nocardia* is famously included in the list of acid-fast organisms. This property may be attributable to the presence of tuberculostearic acids in its wall. However, *Nocardia* is *AFB-negative* on the standard AFB stain, which is the Ziehl-Neelsen. This is generally attributed to the strong acid (3% acid-alcohol) used for removing carbol fuchsin in the staining procedure. Positive acid-fast staining requires the Fite modification of the AFB stain, also known as Fite-Faraco or simply as Fite. The weak acid used in this stain (1% acid-alcohol) and the inclusion of peanut oil-xylene results in retention of acid-fast staining in weakly acid-fast organisms such as *Nocardia* and *Mycobacterium leprae*. On the Fite stain, using microbiologic smears, *Nocardia* is described as weakly and

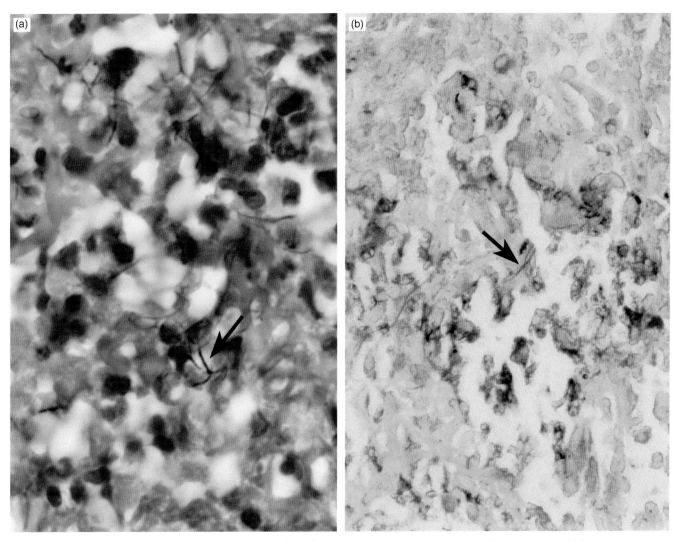

Figure 3.20. Nocardia organisms on GMS and Gram stains. (a) Slender elongated gram-positive rods (arrow, oil immersion lens). **(b)** Slender GMS-positive rods (arrow, 40x objective).

partially acid-fast. In other words, some organisms are AFB-positive while others are AFB-negative. In surgical pathology material, *Nocardia* is often AFB-negative in culture-confirmed cases, even if the Fite stain is used. Therefore, for practical purposes, negative acid-fast staining should not preclude a pathologic diagnosis of nocardiosis.

Clinical profile

The reported age range in pulmonary nocardiosis is 3 to 81 years, and it may occur in either sex. Nocardiosis almost exclusively involves immunocompromised hosts. In a recent review of the literature, only 13 cases out of 448 were identified in apparently immunocompetent individuals. The most common predisposing condition is prior treatment with corticosteroids. Other settings include solid organ transplantation, hematopoietic stem cell transplantation, HIV/AIDS, COPD (often being treated with corticosteroids), hematologic malignancies, other malignancies, chronic granulomatous disease and pulmonary alveolar proteinosis (PAP). The association

with PAP is especially notable, although the total number of reported cases is small (32 cases by 2012). Nocardiosis is the most common infection in patients with PAP. Infection may precede the diagnosis of PAP, may be diagnosed concurrently with PAP, or may occur subsequently in patients with established PAP. The cause is unknown but is thought to be related to macrophage dysfunction. Nocardiosis should be suspected in any patient with PAP that develops nodules or cavitary lesions in the lung or brain.

The symptoms of pulmonary nocardiosis are non-specific. They include fever, cough, expectoration, dyspnea, pleuritic chest pain and constitutional symptoms. Fever is absent in many cases. Hemoptysis is unusual. Patients with concurrent brain lesions may present with headache or altered sensorium. Laboratory findings are unhelpful, but may include leukocytosis. After the lungs, the brain is the most commonly involved site, followed by the skin.

Definitive identification of the organism requires microbiologic confirmation, but *Nocardia* may or may not grow in cultures. Cultures take a minimum of 48 to 72 hours to become

Table 3.4. *Nocardia* vs. *Actinomyces*

Feature	*Nocardia*	*Actinomyces*
Nature of the organisms	Bacteria	Bacteria
Organisms visible on H&E	No	Yes
Acid-fast staining	Negative on Ziehl-Neelsen Weakly positive on Fite (variable)	Negative
Gram stain	Gram-positive rods	Gram-positive rods
GMS	Positive	Positive
Filamentous (Gram, GMS)	Yes	Yes
Branching (Gram, GMS)	Yes	Yes
Suppurative necrosis and acute inflammation	Yes	Yes
Granules and Splendore-Hoeppli material in lung	No	Yes
Typical host	Immunocompromised	Immunocompetent; may have underlying lung disease
Site of infection	Lung (most common), brain, skin	Skin and soft tissues (most common), lung (rare)
Treatment	Sulfonamides	Penicillin

positive. For pathologists, the practical implication is that the organism may be seen in biopsy samples before culture confirmation. *Nocardia* can grow in cultures of sputum, BAL fluid, bronchial washings, cerebrospinal fluid, blood or biopsied tissue (lung, brain or skin).

Radiologic findings

Chest radiographs most commonly show infiltrates, nodules, cavities, consolidation or pleural effusion. Chest CTs show a similarly wide spectrum of findings, of which nodules and nodular opacities are probably the most common. They are typically multiple and bilateral but may be solitary. Cavitation is a frequent finding. A ground-glass halo may be present around the nodules in some cases. Pleural effusions, empyema and chest wall involvement have also been reported. There is no predilection for any side or lobe. None of the radiologic findings are specific for nocardiosis.

Differential diagnosis

- Clinically, *Nocardia* can be difficult to differentiate from *Actinomyces*, especially in destructive, draining skin and soft tissue infections of the feet. There are also several similarities between the two organisms (Table 3.4). However, the difficulty in distinguishing between these organisms in lung pathology is generally overstated, given that *Actinomyces* forms *sulfur granules*, which are easily visible on H&E (Figure 3.21). In contrast, *Nocardia* does not form sulfur granules in the lung, and cannot be seen on H&E. Sulfur granules, also known simply as *granules* or *grains*, are spherical aggregates of bacteria that may be large enough to be visible grossly as tiny yellow granules. Pathologists are familiar with these structures since they are common in tonsils. The center of each granule appears basophilic because it contains innumerable bacteria packed together in a compact aggregate (Figure 3.21). The periphery is usually eosinophilic. It is composed of radiating, acellular, club-like material thought to be derived from antigen–antibody complexes. This peripheral eosinophilic material is known as *Splendore-Hoeppli material* and the process involving its deposition is known as the *Splendore-Hoeppli phenomenon*. Splendore-Hoeppli material can also be seen around many other bacterial, fungal and parasitic organisms, the best known of which is *Sporothrix*, where the material forms so-called *asteroid bodies*. In skin and soft tissue infections, granules can be formed by *Actinomyces*, *Nocardia* (Madura foot), other bacteria such as *Staphylococcus* (botryomycosis), and a variety of fungi. Granules have never been documented in pulmonary nocardiosis.
- Granulomatous infections and ordinary bacteria also enter the differential diagnosis given the rather broad range of inflammatory reactions. These should be easily excluded by AFB, GMS and Gram stains. *Nocardia* is AFB-negative on standard Ziehl-Neelsen staining, and is longer than mycobacteria. On GMS, it is much more slender and thread-like than fungal hyphae.
- Pulmonary malakoplakia, a rare infection caused by *Rhodococcus equi*, enters the differential diagnosis of histiocyte-rich inflammatory infiltrates with variable acute inflammation or necrosis in immunocompromised individuals. It can be differentiated from nocardiosis by the presence of targetoid, basophilic, iron-positive/von Kossa-positive *Michaelis-Guttman bodies*, striking positivity for PAS within the histiocytes, and absence of filamentous organisms on GMS.

Treatment and prognosis

Pulmonary nocardiosis responds well to sulfonamides. The most commonly used drug is trimethoprim/sulfamethoxazole (cotrimoxazole, Bactrim). A combination of imipenem and amikacin is used in some cases. Alternatives include linezolid and ceftriaxone. Importantly, several cases of pulmonary nocardiosis have been reported in patients receiving sulfonamide prophylaxis.

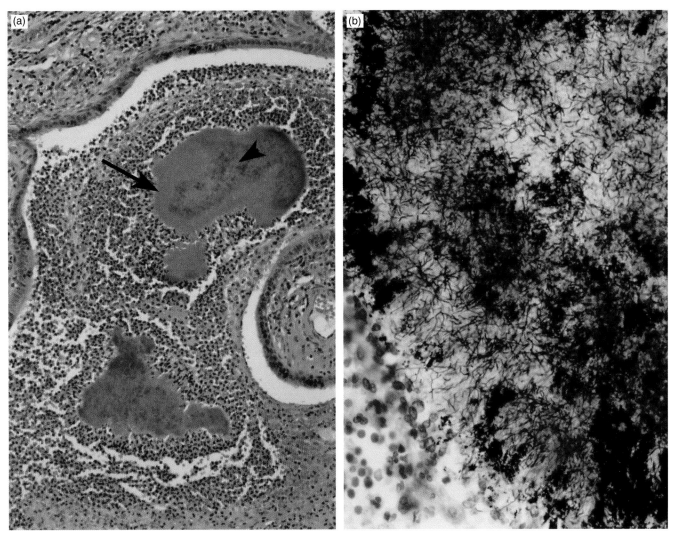

Figure 3.21. Actinomycosis of the lung. (a) Actinomycotic granules (sulfur granules) within the lumen of a bronchiole, surrounded by an acute inflammatory exudate. The basophilic center of each granule contains bacteria (arrowhead). The eosinophilic periphery is composed of Splendore-Hoeppli material (arrow). **(b)** Gram stain, showing large numbers of filamentous gram-positive rods within the granule.

The most dreaded complication is disseminated disease, especially to the brain. The overall mortality of pulmonary nocardiosis varies from 14 to 40%. Dissemination to the central nervous system increases the mortality rate to 64 to 100%.

Sample diagnosis on pathology report

Lung, right upper lobe, needle biopsy – Suppurative necrosis with histiocytic infiltrate (Gram-positive bacteria most consistent with Nocardia present) (See comment).

References

Pneumocystis pneumonia

Askin FB, Katzenstein AL. *Pneumocystis* infection masquerading as diffuse alveolar damage: a potential source of diagnostic error. *Chest* 1981;**79**:420–2.

Bleiweiss IJ, Jagirdar JS, Klein MJ, *et al.* Granulomatous *Pneumocystis carinii* pneumonia in three patients with the acquired immune deficiency syndrome. *Chest* 1988;**94**: 580–3.

El Ghoul R, Eckardt SM, Mukhopadhyay S, Ashton RW. Fever and dyspnea in a 61-year-old woman with metastatic breast cancer. *Chest* 2009;**136**:634–8.

Foley NM, Griffiths MH, Miller RF. Histologically atypical *Pneumocystis carinii* pneumonia. *Thorax* 1993;**48**:996–1001.

Gal AA, Plummer AL, Langston AA, Mansour KA. Granulomatous *Pneumocystis carinii* pneumonia complicating hematopoietic cell transplantation. *Pathol Res Pract* 2002;**198**:553–8.

Hartel PH, Shilo K, Klassen-Fischer M, *et al.* Granulomatous reaction to *Pneumocystis*

jirovecii: clinicopathologic review of 20 cases. *Am J Surg Pathol* 2010;**34**:730–4.

Krajicek BJ, Thomas CF Jr., Limper AH. *Pneumocystis* pneumonia: current concepts in pathogenesis, diagnosis and treatment. *Clin Chest Med* 2009;**30**:265–78.

Thomas CF Jr., Limper AH. *Pneumocystis* pneumonia. *N Engl J Med* 2004;**350**:2487–98.

Travis WD, Pittaluga S, Lipschik GY, *et al.* Atypical pathologic manifestations of *Pneumocystis carinii* pneumonia in the acquired immune deficiency syndrome. Review of 123 lung biopsies from 76 patients with emphasis on cysts, vascular invasion, vasculitis, and granulomas. *Am J Surg Pathol* 1990;**14**:615–25.

Weber WR, Askin FB, Dehner LP. Lung biopsy in *Pneumocystis carinii* pneumonia: a histopathologic study of typical and atypical features. *Am J Clin Pathol* 1977;**67**:11–9.

Invasive aspergillosis

Chai LY, Hsu LY. Recent advances in invasive pulmonary aspergillosis. *Curr Opin Pulm Med* 2011;**17**:160–6.

Denning DW. Invasive aspergillosis. *Clin Infect Dis* 1997;**26**:781–805.

De Pauw B, Walsh TJ, Donnelly JP, *et al.* Revised definitions of invasive fungal disease from the European Organization for Research and Treatment of Cancer/Invasive Fungal Infections Cooperative Group and the National Institute of Allergy and Infectious Diseases Mycoses Study Group (EORTC/MSG) Consensus Group. *Clin Infect Dis* 2008;**46**:1813–21.

Franquet T, Muller NL, Gimenez A, *et al.* Spectrum of pulmonary aspergillosis: histologic, clinical and radiologic findings. *Radiographics* 2001;**21**:825–37.

Fraser RS. Pulmonary aspergillosis: pathologic and pathogenetic features. *Pathol Annu* 1993;**28 Pt 1**:231–77.

Greene RE, Schlamm HT, Oestmann J-W, *et al.* Imaging findings in acute invasive pulmonary aspergillosis: clinical significance of the halo sign. *Clin Infect Dis* 2007;**44**:373–9.

Orr DP, Myerowitz RL, Dubois PJ. Patho-radiologic correlation of invasive pulmonary aspergillosis in the compromised host. *Cancer* 1978;**41**:2028–39.

Patterson TF, Kirkpatrick WR, White M, *et al.* Invasive aspergillosis: disease spectrum, treatment practices, and outcomes. *Medicine (Baltimore)* 2000;**79**:250–60.

Watts JC, Chandler FW. Morphologic identification of mycelial pathogens in tissue sections. A caveat. *Am J Clin Pathol* 1998;**109**:1–2.

Young RC, Bennett JE, Vogel CL, Carbone PP, DeVita VT. Aspergillosis. The spectrum of the disease in 98 patients. *Medicine (Baltimore)* 1970:**49**:147–73.

Mycetoma (fungus ball, aspergilloma)

Aquino SL, Lee ST, Warnock ML, Gamsu G. Pulmonary aspergillosis: imaging findings with pathologic correlation. *AJR Am J Roentgenol* 1994;**163**:811–5.

Franquet T, Muller NL, Gimenez A, *et al.* Spectrum of pulmonary aspergillosis: histologic, clinical and radiologic findings. *Radiographics* 2001;**21**:825–37.

Fraser RS. Pulmonary aspergillosis: pathologic and pathogenetic features. *Pathol Annu* 1993;**28 Pt 1**:231–77.

Kurrein F, Green GH, Rowles SL. Localized deposition of calcium oxalate around a pulmonary *Aspergillus niger* fungus ball. *Am J Clin Pathol* 1975;**64**:556–63.

McGregor DH, Papasian CJ, Pierce PD. Aspergilloma within cavitating pulmonary adenocarcinoma. *Am J Clin Pathol* 1989;**91**:100–3.

Nime FA, Hutchins GM. Oxalosis caused by *Aspergillus* infection. *Johns Hopkins Med J* 1973;**133**:183–94.

Regnard JF, Icard P, Nicolosi M, *et al.* Aspergilloma: a series of 89 surgical cases. *Ann Thorac Surg* 2000;**69**:898–903.

Smith FB, Beneck D. Localized *Aspergillus* infestation in primary lung carcinoma. Clinical and pathological contrasts with post-tuberculous intracavitary aspergilloma. *Chest* 1991;**100**:554–6.

Villar TG, Pimentel JC, Freitas E, Costa M. The tumour-like forms of aspergillosis of the lung (pulmonary aspergilloma). A report of five new cases and a review of the Portuguese literature. *Thorax* 1962;**17**:22–38.

Young RC, Bennett JE, Vogel CL, Carbone PP, DeVita VT. Aspergillosis. The spectrum of disease in 98 patients. *Medicine (Baltimore)* 1970:**49**:147–73.

Cytomegalovirus pneumonia

Beschorner WE, Hutchins GM, Burns WH, Saral R, Tutschka PJ, Santos GW. Cytomegalovirus pneumonia in bone marrow transplant recipients: miliary and diffuse patterns. *Am Rev Respir Dis* 1980;**122**:107–14.

Browning JD, More IAR, Boyd JF. Adult pulmonary cytomegalic inclusion disease. Report of a case. *J Clin Pathol* 1980;**33**:11–8.

Chemaly RF, Yen-Lieberman B, Castilla EA, *et al.* Correlation between viral loads of cytomegalovirus in blood and bronchoalveolar lavage specimens from lung transplant recipients determined by histology and immunohistochemistry. *J Clin Microbiol* 2004;**42**:2168–72.

Craighead JE. Pulmonary cytomegalovirus infection in the adult. *Am J Pathol* 1971;**63**:487–504.

Gorelkin L, Chandler FW, Ewing EP. Staining qualities of cytomegalovirus inclusions in the lungs of patients with the acquired immunodeficiency syndrome: a potential source of diagnostic

misinterpretation. *Hum Pathol* 1986;**17**:926–9.

Karakelides H, Aubry MC, Ryu JH. Cytomegalovirus pneumonia mimicking lung cancer in an immunocompetent host. *Mayo Clin Proc* 2003;**78**:488–90.

Macasaet FF, Holley KE, Smith TF, Keys TF. Cytomegalovirus studies of autopsy tissue. II. Incidence of inclusion bodies and related pathologic data. *Am J Clin Pathol* 1975;**63**:859–65.

Shibata M, Terashima M, Kimura H, *et al.* Quantitation of cytomegalovirus DNA in lung tissue of bone marrow transplant recipients. *Hum Pathol* 1982;**23**:911–5.

Strickler JG, Manivel JC, Copenhaver CM, Kubic VL. Comparison of in situ hybridization and immunohistochemistry for detection of cytomegalovirus and herpes simplex virus. *Hum Pathol* 1990;**21**:443–8.

Wallace JM, Hannah J. Cytomegalovirus pneumonitis in patients with AIDS. Findings in an autopsy series. *Chest* 1987;**92**:198–203.

Respiratory syncytial virus bronchiolitis and pneumonia

Aherne W, Bird T, Court SDM, Gardner PS, McQuillin J. Pathological changes in virus infections of the lower respiratory tract in children. *J Clin Pathol* 1970:**23**:7–18.

Delage G, Brochu P, Robillard L, Jasmin G, Joncas JH, Lapointe N. Giant cell pneumonia due to respiratory syncytial virus. Occurrence in severe combined immunodeficiency syndrome. *Arch Pathol Lab Med* 1984;**108**:623–5.

Englund JA, Sullivan CJ, Jordan C, Dehner LP, Vercellotti GM, Balfour HH Jr. Respiratory syncytial virus infection in immunocompromised adults. *Ann Intern Med* 1988;**109**:203–8.

Henrickson KJ, Hall CB. Diagnostic assays for respiratory syncytial virus disease. *Pediatr Infect Dis J* 2007;**344**:S36–40.

Johnson JE, Gonzales RA, Olson SJ, Wright PF, Graham BS. The histopathology of fatal untreated human respiratory syncytial virus infection. *Mod Pathol* 2007;**20**:108–19.

Kurlandsky LE, French G, Webb PM, Porter DD. Fatal respiratory syncytial virus pneumonitis in a previously healthy child. *Am Rev Respir Dis* 1988;**138**:468–72.

Levenson RM, Kantor OS. Fatal pneumonia in an adult due to respiratory syncytial virus. *Arch Intern Med* 1987;**147**:791–2.

Miller WT Jr., Mickus TJ, Barbosa E, Mullin C, Van Deerlin VM, Shiley KT. CT of viral lower respiratory tract infection in adults. Comparison among viral organisms and between viral and bacterial infections. *AJR Am J Roentgenol* 2011;**197**:1088–95.

Ventre K, Randolph A. Ribavirin for respiratory syncytial virus infection of the lower respiratory tract in infants and young children. *Cochrane Database Syst Rev* 2007;**1**: CD000181.

Wright C, Oliver KC, Fenwick FI, Smith NM, Toms GL. A monoclonal antibody pool for routine immunohistochemical detection of human respiratory syncytial virus antigens in formalin-fixed, paraffin-embedded tissue. *J Pathol* 1997;**182**:238–44.

Influenza

Gatherer D. The 2009 H1N1 influenza outbreak in its historical context. *J Clin Virol* 2009;**45**:174–8.

Guarner J, Shieh WJ, Paddock CD, *et al.* Histopathologic and immunohistochemical features of fatal influenza virus infection in children during the 2003–2004 season. *Clin Infect Dis* 2006;**43**:132–40.

Guarner J, Shieh WJ, Dawson J, *et al.* Immunohistochemical and in situ hybridization studies of influenza A virus infection in human lungs. *Am J Clin Pathol* 2000;**114**:227–33.

Hers JF, Masurel N, Mulder J. Bacteriology and pathology of the respiratory tract and lungs in fatal Asian influenza. *Lancet* 1958;**2**:1141–3.

Kim EA, Lee KS, Primack SL, *et al.* Viral pneumonia in adults: radiologic and pathologic findings. *Radiographics* 2002;**22**: S137–49.

Martin CM, Kunin CM, Gottlieb LS, Barnes MW, Liu C, Finland M. Asian influenza A in Boston, 1957–1958. I. Observations in thirty-two influenza-associated fatal cases. *AMA Arch Intern Med* 1959;**103**:515–31.

Mukhopadhyay S, Phillip AT, Stoppacher R. Pathologic findings in novel influenza A (H1N1) virus ("swine flu") infection. Contrasting clinical manifestations and lung pathology in two fatal cases. *Am J Clin Pathol* 2010;**133**:380–7.

Noble RL, Lillington GA, Kempson RL. Fatal diffuse influenzal pneumonia: premortem diagnosis by lung biopsy. *Chest* 1973;**63**:644–7.

Parker RGF. The pathology of uncomplicated influenza. *Postgrad Med J* 1963;**39**:564–6.

Yeldandi AV, Colby TV. Pathologic features of lung biopsy specimens from influenza pneumonia cases. *Hum Pathol* 1994;**25**:47–53.

Herpes tracheobronchitis and pneumonia

Assink-de Jong E, Groeneveld AB, Pettersson AM, *et al.* Clinical correlates of herpes simplex virus type 1 loads in the lower respiratory tract of critically ill patients. *J Clin Virol* 2013;**58**:79–83.

Boundy KE, Fraire AE, Oliveira PJ. A patient with progressive dyspnea and multiple foci of airspace consolidation. *Chest* 2014;**145**:167–72.

Byers RJ, Hasleton PS, Quigley A, *et al.* Pulmonary herpes simplex in burns patients. *Eur Respir J* 1996;**9**:2313–7.

Cowdry EV. The problem of intranuclear inclusions in virus diseases. *Arch Pathol* 1934;**18**:527–42.

Geradts J, Warnock M, Yen TS. Use of the polymerase chain reaction in the diagnosis of unsuspected herpes simplex viral pneumonia: report of a case. *Hum Pathol* 1990;**21**:118–21.

Martinez E, de Diego A, Paradis A, Perpiña M, Hernandez M. Herpes simplex pneumonia in a young immunocompetent man. *Eur Respir J* 1994;**7**:1185–8.

Nakamura Y, Yamamoto S, Tanaka S, *et al.* Herpes simplex viral infection in human neonates: an immunohistochemical and electron microscopic study. *Hum Pathol* 1985;**16**:1091–7.

Nash G. Necrotizing tracheobronchitis and bronchopneumonia consistent with herpetic infection. *Hum Pathol* 1972;**3**:283–90.

Ramsey PG, Fife KH, Hackman RC, Meyers JD, Corey L. Herpes simplex virus pneumonia. Clinical, virologic and pathologic features in 20 patients. *Ann Intern Med* 1982;**97**:813–20.

Vernon SE. Herpetic tracheobronchitis: immunohistologic demonstration of herpes simplex virus antigen. *Hum Pathol* 1982;**13**:683–6.

Adenovirus pneumonia

Abbondanzo SL, English CK, Kagan E, McPherson RA. Fatal adenovirus pneumonia in a newborn identified by electron microscopy and in situ hybridization. *Arch Pathol Lab Med* 1989;**113**:1349–53.

Becroft DM. Histopathology of fatal adenovirus infection of the respiratory tract in young children. *J Clin Pathol* 1967;**20**:561–9.

Doan ML, Mallory GB, Kaplan SL, *et al.* Treatment of adenovirus pneumonia with cidofovir in pediatric lung transplant recipients. *J Heart Lung Transplant* 2007;**26**:883–9.

Gavin PJ, Katz BZ. Intravenous ribavirin treatment for severe adenovirus disease in immunocompromised children. *Pediatrics* 2002;**110**:e9.

Kim EA, Lee KS, Primack SL, *et al.* Viral pneumonia in adults: radiologic and pathologic findings. *Radiographics* 2002;**22**: S137–49.

Ohori NP, Michaels MG, Jaffe R, Williams P, Yousem SA. Adenovirus pneumonia in lung transplant recipients. *Hum Pathol* 1995;**26**:1073–9.

Pham TTL, Burchette JL, Jr., Hale LP. Fatal adenovirus infections in immunocompromised patients. *Am J Clin Pathol* 2003;**120**:575–83.

Pinto A, Beck R, Jadavji T. Fatal neonatal pneumonia caused by adenovirus type 35: report of one case and review of the literature. *Arch Pathol Lab Med* 1992;**116**:95–9.

Rocholl C, Gerber K, Daly J, Pavia AT, Byington CL. Adenoviral infections in children: the impact of rapid diagnosis. *Pediatrics* 2004;**113**:e51–6.

Schonland M, Strong ML, Wesley A. Fatal adenovirus pneumonia: clinical and pathological features. *S Afr Med J* 1976;**50**:1748–51.

Parainfluenza virus

Akizuki S, Nasu N, Setoguchi M, Yoshida S, Higuchi Y, Yamamoto S. Parainfluenza virus pneumonitis in an adult. *Arch Pathol Lab Med* 1991;**115**:824–6.

Apalsch AM, Green M, Ledesma-Medina J, Nour B, Wald ER. Parainfluenza and influenza virus infections in pediatric organ transplant recipients. *Clin Infect Dis* 1995;**20**:394–9.

Butnor KJ, Sporn TA. Human parainfluenza virus giant cell pneumonia following cord blood transplant associated with pulmonary alveolar proteinosis. *Arch Pathol Lab Med* 2003;**127**:235–8.

Cherry JD. Croup. *N Engl J Med* 2008;**358**:384–91.

Delage G, Brochu P, Pelletier M, Jasmin G, Lapointe N. Giant-cell pneumonia caused by parainfluenza virus. *J Pediatr* 1979;**94**:426–9.

Henrickson KJ. Parainfluenza viruses. *Clin Microbiol Rev* 2003;**16**:242–64.

Lewis VA, Champlin R, Englund J, *et al.* Respiratory disease due to parainfluenza virus in adult bone marrow transplant recipients. *Clin Infect Dis* 1996;**23**:1033–7.

Little BW, Tihen WS, Dickerman JD, Craighead JE. Giant cell pneumonia associated with parainfluenza type 3 infection. *Hum Pathol* 1981;**12**:478–81.

Madden JF, Burchette JL, Jr., Hale LP. Pathology of parainfluenza virus infection in patients with congenital immunodeficiency syndromes. *Hum Pathol* 2004;**35**:594–603.

Weintrub PS, Sullender WM, Lombard C, Link MP, Arvin A. Giant cell pneumonia caused by parainfluenza type 3 in a patient with acute myelomonocytic leukemia. *Arch Pathol Lab Med* 1987;**111**:569–70.

Strongyloidiasis

Apewokin S, Steciuk M, Griffin S, Jhala D. *Strongyloides* hyperinfection diagnosed by bronchoalveolar lavage in an immunocompromised host. *Cytopathology* 2010;**21**:342–51.

Haque AK, Schnadig V, Rubin SA, Smith JH. Pathogenesis of human strongyloidiasis: autopsy and quantitative parasitological analysis. *Mod Pathol* 1994;**7**:276–88.

Higenbottam TW, Heard BE. Opportunistic pulmonary strongyloidiasis complicating asthma treated with steroids. *Thorax* 1976;**31**:226–33.

Keiser PB, Nutman TB. *Strongyloides stercoralis* in the immunocompromised population. *Clin Microbiol Rev* 2004;**17**:208–17.

Khemasuwan D, Farver CF, Mehta AC. Parasites of the air passages. *Chest* 2014;**145**:883–95.

Lin AL, Kessimian N, Benditt JO. Restrictive pulmonary disease due to interlobular septal fibrosis associated with disseminated infection by *Strongyloides stercoralis*. *Am J Respir Crit Care Med* 1995;**151**:205–9.

Maayan S, Wormser GP, Widerhorn J, Sy ER, Kim YH, Ernst JA. *Strongyloides stercoralis* hyperinfection in a patient with the acquired immune deficiency syndrome. *Am J Med* 1987;**83**:945–8.

Purtilo DT, Meyers WM, Connor DH. Fatal strongyloidiasis in immunosuppressed patients. *Am J Med* 1974;**56**:488–93.

Smith B, Verghese A, Guiterrez C, Dralle W, Berk SL. Pulmonary strongyloidiasis. Diagnosis by sputum Gram stain. *Am J Med* 1985;**79**:663–6.

Williams J, Nunley D, Dralle W, Berk SL, Verghese A. Diagnosis of pulmonary strongyloidiasis by bronchoalveolar lavage. *Chest* 1988;**94**:643–4.

Nocardiosis

Brown-Elliott BA, Brown JM, Conville PS, Wallace RJ Jr. Clinical and laboratory features of the *Nocardia* spp. based on current molecular taxonomy. *Clin Microbiol Rev* 2006;**19**:259–82.

Carbonelli C, Prati F, Carretto E, Cavazza A, Spaggiari L, Magnani G. Cavitating pulmonary nodules growing in a favourable medium. *Thorax* 2013;**68**:1078.

Feigin DS. Nocardiosis of the lung: chest radiographic findings in 21 cases. *Radiology* 1986;**159**:9–14.

Kanne JP, Yandow DR, Mohammed TL, Meyer CA. CT findings of pulmonary nocardiosis. *AJR Am J Roentgenol* 2011;**197**: W266–72.

Minero MV, Marín M, Cercenado E, Rabadán PM, Bouza E, Muñoz P. Nocardiosis at the turn of the century. *Medicine (Baltimore)* 2009;**88**:250–61.

Oddó D, González S. Actinomycosis and nocardiosis. A morphologic study of 17 cases. *Pathol Res Pract* 1986;**181**:320–6.

Peleg AY, Husain S, Qureshi ZA, *et al.* Risk factors, clinical characteristics and outcome of *Nocardia* infection in organ transplant recipients: a matched case-control study. *Clin Infect Dis* 2007;**44**:1307–14.

Punatar AD, Kusne S, Blair JE, Seville MT, Vikram HR. Opportunistic infections in patients with pulmonary alveolar proteinosis. *J Infect* 2012;**65**:173–9.

Robboy SJ, Vickery AL Jr. Tinctorial and morphologic properties distinguishing actinomycosis and nocardiosis. *N Engl J Med* 1970;**282**:593–6.

Wang HL, Seo YH, LaSala PR, Tarrand JJ, Han XY. Nocardiosis in 132 patients with cancer. *Am J Clin Pathol* 2014;**142**:513–23.

Predominantly airspace abnormalities

This chapter addresses the differential diagnosis of pathologic abnormalities found mainly within the airspaces, i.e., the lumens of the alveoli. These include pulmonary alveolar proteinosis, pulmonary edema, acute bronchopneumonia, eosinophilic pneumonia, respiratory bronchiolitis (smokers' macrophages), and hemosiderin-laden macrophages. Figure 4.1 shows some of these conditions side-by-side at the same magnification. Figure 4.2 provides an algorithm with a differential diagnosis based on histologic findings. Table 4.1 lists some pearls and pitfalls, and Table 4.2 lists the differential diagnosis of abnormalities found within airspaces.

Pulmonary alveolar proteinosis

Pulmonary alveolar proteinosis (PAP) is characterized by the abnormal accumulation of granular eosinophilic material within the airspaces. The most common type of PAP seen by pathologists is autoimmune PAP, formerly known as idiopathic PAP. It accounts for 90% of all cases and is a disease of adults. It is caused by the abnormal accumulation of surfactant within alveoli. Surfactant is a phospholipid with a small proteinaceous component whose normal function is to reduce alveolar surface tension. In normal lungs, surplus surfactant is catabolized or cleared from the lungs by alveolar macrophages. In PAP, surfactant accumulates within alveoli because of defective macrophage function caused, in most cases (85 to 90%), by a neutralizing autoantibody to granulocyte-macrophage colony-stimulating factor (GM-CSF). The involvement of GM-CSF in this process may seem surprising since it is best known as a growth factor for hematopoietic cells. However, it is now well established that GM-CSF is also required by macrophages for normal clearance of surfactant from the lungs.

Less commonly, eosinophilic granular material accumulates within alveoli in other settings, and the finding in such cases is termed secondary PAP. These settings include acute silicosis (silicoproteinosis), inhalation of minerals such as talc, aluminum, cement and kaolin, hematologic malignancies such as myelodysplastic syndrome and acute myeloid leukemia, and miscellaneous conditions such as immunodeficiency, organ transplantation and lysinuric protein intolerance. An uncommon form of PAP also occurs in children, and is referred to as hereditary PAP. It is caused by mutations in genes involved in surfactant metabolism. These genes include surfactant protein B (SFTPB), surfactant protein C (SFTPC), ATP-binding cassette, sub-family A (ABCA3), and genes coding receptors for GM-CSF

(CSF2RA and CSF2RB). Some of these mutations can also manifest as non-specific tissue reactions other than PAP, such as chronic pneumonitis of infancy and increased intra-alveolar macrophages (a so-called "DIP-like" reaction).

PAP is most commonly seen by surgical pathologists in transbronchial lung biopsies, but surgical lung biopsies are occasionally required. The characteristic turbid milky fluid can also be recognized by cytopathologists in bronchoalveolar lavage specimens.

Major diagnostic findings

- The main finding in PAP is the filling of airspaces by eosinophilic, coarsely granular material (Figure 4.3). The material is present mainly within alveoli but often extends into alveolar ducts and bronchioles. Tiny cleft-like or needle-like empty spaces resembling cholesterol clefts are commonly present within the intra-alveolar material (Figure 4.3). These were termed *acicular spaces* by Rosen, Castleman and Liebow in their original description of PAP in 1958 and have been referred to as such ever since. Eosinophilic globules of varying sizes are also usually present and are a clue to the diagnosis. In some cases, the globules may be concentrically laminated.

- Since numerous contiguous alveoli are filled with the material, the findings may appear diffuse, particularly in transbronchial biopsies. However, in surgical lung biopsies, it becomes apparent that the distribution of PAP is actually quite patchy, and that the granular material fills many alveoli in some areas of the lung but spares others (Figure 4.4). In fact, relatively large pieces of lung parenchyma are usually completely uninvolved. Occasionally, the line of demarcation between involved and spared lung is an interlobular septum.

- The alveolar septa in PAP are normal in most cases, without significant inflammation or fibrosis. This feature is noteworthy because PAP is considered a form of interstitial lung disease clinically and radiologically. It is thus the best example of a process that appears interstitial clinically but is a pure airspace process pathologically. The reason for this discordance remains unclear. It has been suggested that widening of interlobular septa by edema and dilated lymphatics might explain the characteristic septal lines of the "crazy-paving" pattern on chest CT (Figure 4.4). In practice, interlobular septa are not always abnormal in PAP, and the abrupt transition between affected and spared

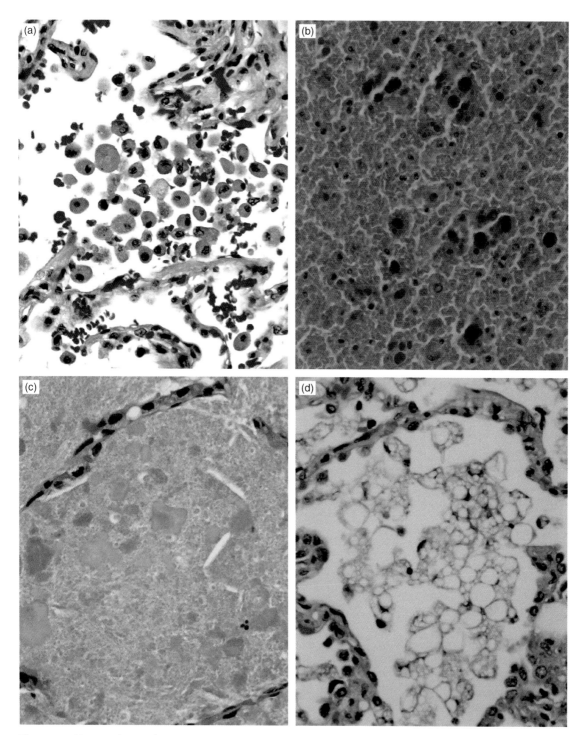

Figure 4.1. Airspace abnormalities. (a) Respiratory bronchiolitis (smoker's macrophages). **(b)** Hemosiderin-laden macrophages. **(c)** Pulmonary alveolar proteinosis. **(d)** Exogenous lipoid pneumonia.

lung does not always correspond to interlobular septa (Figure 4.4).

Variable pathologic findings

- A few scattered foamy macrophages may be present focally within the granular material in the airspaces (Figure 4.5). The macrophages are usually large and vacuolated; they may contain cholesterol clefts, and multinucleation is common. We have seen a case in which this type of multinucleated cell in a cytologic preparation also contained an asteroid body, and was incorrectly interpreted as consistent with sarcoidosis.

- Although the alveolar septa in PAP are usually pristine, a few cases have been described in which the interstitium contains a bronchiolocentric chronic inflammatory

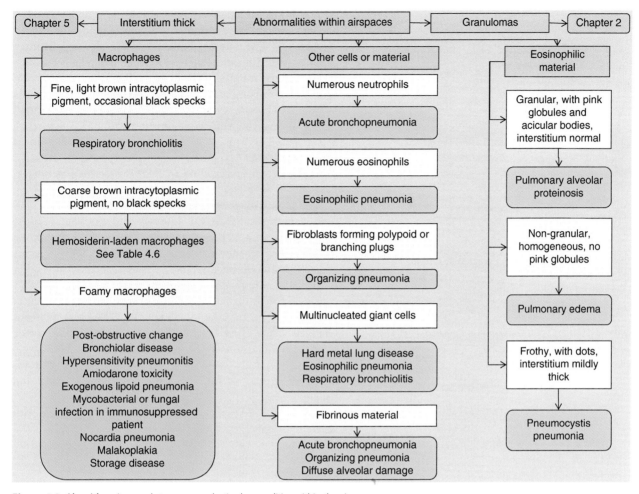

Figure 4.2. Algorithm. Approach to non-neoplastic abnormalities within the airspaces.

infiltrate with poorly formed granulomas similar to hypersensitivity pneumonitis. Clinical and radiologic findings in these cases also showed some features of both conditions. It is unclear whether these cases represent PAP with an unusual inflammatory response, hypersensitivity pneumonitis with granular intra-alveolar material, or a coincidental combination of the two.

- Mild alveolar septal fibrosis has been described but is uncommon in autoimmune PAP in adults. Type 2 pneumocytes may occasionally be prominent. However, they are inconspicuous in most cases.

- Basophilic staining has been reported in frozen section preparations stained with a rapid version of the H&E stain. In the reported cases, the expected eosinophilic staining was restored when H&E staining was performed on formalin-fixed paraffin-embedded sections.

- In most cases of PAP in adults, the microscopic appearance is remarkably constant. However, PAP in other settings such as secondary PAP (post-chemotherapy or in acute silicosis) or hereditary PAP (in children) frequently shows considerably different morphologic features, including alveolar septal thickening and interstitial chronic inflammation.

Diagnostic work-up

The granular intra-alveolar material in PAP stains weakly positive (pink) with the periodic acid-Schiff (PAS) stain (Figure 4.5). Given the pathognomonic H&E appearance and the absence of a PAS-negative entity in the differential diagnosis, the need for PAS staining is questionable. Some authors claim that the granular nature of the material is better appreciated on this stain. However, in our experience, if the H&E findings are typical, PAS staining is not essential and may in fact be misleading if it is weak or negative. We have seen occasional cases of this type that were clinically and radiologically characteristic of PAP. In autoimmune PAP, the intra-alveolar material stains positive with an antibody to surfactant apoprotein.

Clinical profile

PAP usually occurs in young adults, but it has been reported at all ages, including in neonates and the elderly (80s and 90s). The mean age in large series varies from 39 to 51 years, and the median age is 39 years. Both sexes may be affected but there is a predilection for men. A majority are smokers. Most patients present with dyspnea, cough or both. A characteristic clinical feature is that the striking radiologic findings are out of

Table 4.1. Pearls and pitfalls in airspace diseases

Pulmonary alveolar proteinosis is defined by the presence of granular eosinophilic material within the airspaces. The appearance of the material on H&E is distinctive. PAS is not always positive

Eosinophilic pneumonia is defined by the presence of intra-alveolar eosinophils, but interstitial eosinophils are also increased

It is common to find numerous macrophages within the airspaces in a wide variety of lung diseases. Avoid the use of the misnomer "DIP" to describe this non-specific finding

Most lightly pigmented macrophages within airspaces are smoker's macrophages, not "anthracotic pigment"

"Respiratory bronchiolitis" is simply the presence of smoker's macrophages within airspaces. Inflammation is not required, and the macrophages do not need to be confined to respiratory bronchioles

In the vast majority of cases, smoker's macrophages within airspaces are an incidental finding in cigarette smokers

Smoker's macrophages in patients with fibrotic interstitial lung disease are also incidental; this is not respiratory bronchiolitis-interstitial lung disease (RBILD)

Significant interstitial fibrosis excludes RBILD

RBILD is a rare diagnosis in surgical pathology and requires strict exclusion of alternative possibilities

proportion to the relatively mild clinical symptoms. Fever is uncommon. Some individuals are asymptomatic (5 to 30%).

Anti-GM-CSF autoantibody levels are elevated in most patients with autoimmune PAP. Other abnormalities such as telomerase mutations have been found in some cases. Serum LDH is commonly elevated. Physical findings include inspiratory crackles, cyanosis and clubbing. Pulmonary function tests may be restrictive (most common), obstructive or normal. There may be a disproportionate reduction in DL_{CO} relative to a modest impairment in vital capacity. Bronchoalveolar lavage fluid in PAP is described as opalescent, turbid or milky.

The clinical diagnosis in many cases is based on a combination of high-resolution CT findings and the characteristic milky appearance of bronchoalveolar lavage fluid. Therefore, lung biopsies are not required in all patients. Serology for GM-CSF antibodies is available in reference laboratories, but is not mandatory for the diagnosis.

Silicoproteinosis occurs mainly in sandblasters exposed to silica for several months to a few years. The presentation is relatively acute compared to the insidious onset of classic silicosis. Bilateral consolidation and hilar lymph node enlargement are typically seen on chest radiographs. Symptoms include shortness of breath, fever, fatigue, weight loss and cough.

Congenital PAP manifests in the neonatal period with severe hypoxia.

Table 4.2. Differential diagnosis of airspace abnormalities

Pathologic finding within airspaces	Additional clues	Pathologic diagnosis
Granular eosinophilic material	Alveolar septa normal Cholesterol clefts (acicular spaces) Eosinophilic globules "Crazy-paving" on CT	Pulmonary alveolar proteinosis
Homogeneous eosinophilic fluid	Alveolar septa normal	Pulmonary edema
Neutrophils	Fibrin, necrotic debris, involvement of respiratory bronchioles and alveolar ducts	Acute bronchopneumonia
Eosinophils	Histiocytes, fibrin in the airspaces, admixed with eosinophils Variable eosinophils, lymphocytes, plasma cells in interstitium	Eosinophilic pneumonia
Pigmented macrophages	Incidental finding	Respiratory bronchiolitis
Pigmented macrophages	Surgical lung biopsy No significant interstitial fibrosis No other pathologic explanation for ground-glass infiltrates Clinical/radiologic ILD Radiology: bilateral ground-glass infiltrates	Respiratory bronchiolitis-interstitial lung disease (RBILD)
Numerous macrophages	See next column	Desquamative interstitial pneumonia (DIP). The use of this outmoded misnomer is discouraged. See text for details
Pigmented macrophages	Hyalinized "ropy" pink interstitial fibrosis associated with emphysema	Smoking-related interstitial fibrosis (SRIF)

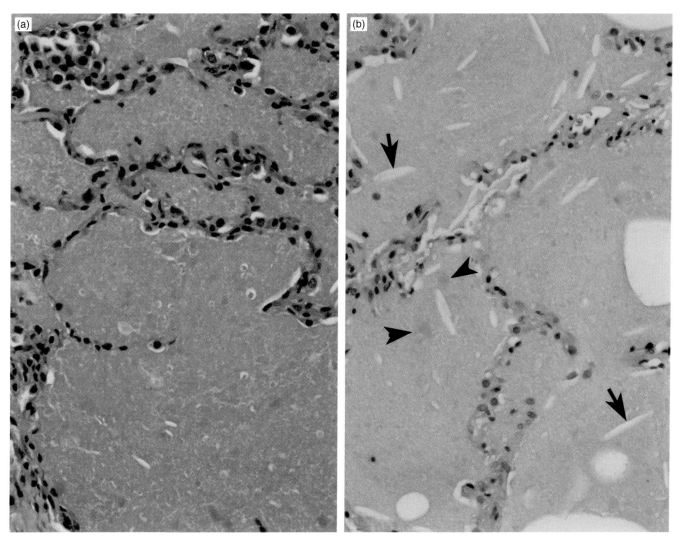

Figure 4.3. Pulmonary alveolar proteinosis. (a) Granular eosinophilic material fills the airspaces. **(b)** The material within the alveoli contains acicular spaces (arrows) and eosinophilic globules (arrowheads).

Radiologic findings

Chest X-rays show bilateral symmetric lung opacities, multifocal opacities, or consolidation, without pleural effusions or cardiomegaly. The opacities are most often perihilar (64%). On chest CT, bilateral patchy lung infiltrates in a *crazy-paving* pattern are the hallmark of PAP. This pattern is characterized by the presence of widespread bilateral ground-glass infiltrates superimposed on a background of thickened interlobular septa and intralobular lines, resembling crazy-paving. The term refers to the appearance of paving tiles of irregular shapes laid in a haphazard manner, usually in gardens. The infiltrates are often sharply demarcated from adjacent normal lung, a phenomenon known as *parenchymal sparing*; there are many variations on the precise areas of lung that are spared. The crazy-paving pattern is neither perfectly sensitive nor specific for PAP. It has also been reported in exogenous lipoid pneumonia, pulmonary edema, diffuse alveolar damage and pulmonary hemorrhage. A review of 98 cases of PAP from the Armed Forces Institute of Pathology found that the crazy-paving pattern was present in 75% of PAP, the other 25% showing ground-glass opacities

without prominent septal lines. The distribution of opacities was diffuse in 71%, chiefly central in 14%, multifocal-patchy in 11% and chiefly peripheral in 4%.

Differential diagnosis

- From the point of view of the surgical pathologist, the only condition with a similar microscopic appearance is pulmonary edema. It is characterized by the presence of eosinophilic, homogeneous fluid within the alveoli. Edema fluid lacks the coarse granularity that is characteristic of PAP (Figure 4.6). Acicular spaces, eosinophilic globules and foam cells are also absent. In difficult cases, the clinical setting can be helpful in excluding pulmonary edema, since these patients usually have clinical and radiologic features of congestive heart failure.
- *Pneumocystis* pneumonia (PCP) also enters the differential diagnosis because the typical frothy material seen in this infection is eosinophilic and intra-alveolar (Figure 4.7). However, in most instances, the froth-with-dots appearance of PCP is easily distinguished from the granular

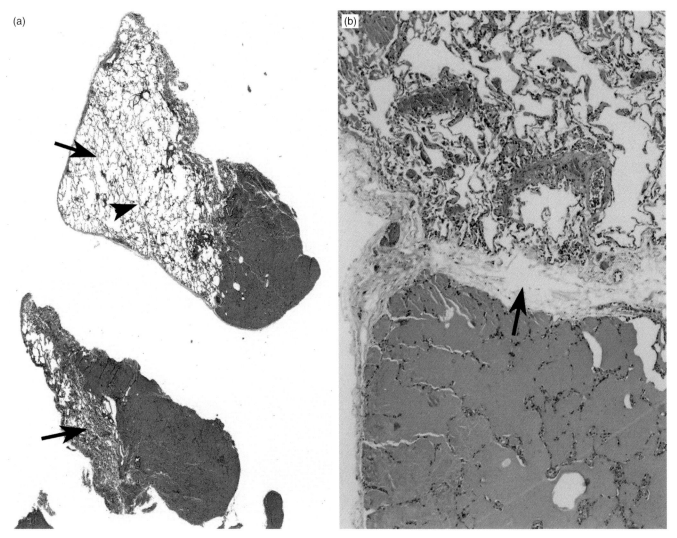

Figure 4.4. Pulmonary alveolar proteinosis. (a) At low magnification, the patchy distribution is obvious. Note spared lung (arrows) and a normal interlobular septum (arrowhead). In this example, the junction between involved and spared lung does not correspond to an interlobular septum. **(b)** In this example, the junction between involved and spared lung does correspond to an interlobular septum (arrow), which is considerably widened.

appearance of PAP on H&E-stained sections. PCP does not feature cholesterol clefts, and is usually associated with at least minimal interstitial thickening, whereas alveolar septa are usually normal in PAP. GMS staining can help in difficult cases but is not mandatory.

- Changes resembling PAP have been described secondary to bronchial obstruction by tumors. In the reported cases, there were large numbers of foamy macrophages within airspaces as well as amorphous PAS-positive eosinophilic material. The correct diagnosis was obvious because of the presence of an airway-obstructing mass, the large numbers of foamy macrophages and the prominence of an inflammatory component in the interstitium.

- Silicoproteinosis can show areas in which alveoli are filled with an eosinophilic material with acicular spaces identical to PAP (Chapter 6, Figure 6.13b). Obtaining an occupational history is the easiest way to exclude this possibility. The histologic picture is characterized by fibrotic silicotic nodules, silica particles and

interstitial pneumonia, all of which are absent in autoimmune PAP.

Treatment and prognosis

Asymptomatic individuals with PAP or those with mild symptoms do not require specific therapy, since most of these individuals remain stable or show improvement on follow-up with observation alone. For those with moderate to severe symptoms, a form of bronchoalveolar lavage (BAL) known as whole lung lavage has traditionally been the mainstay of therapy and remains the standard of care despite the availability of newer therapeutic options. The goal of whole lung lavage is to physically wash accumulated surfactant out of the lungs. In two-thirds of patients, a single whole lung lavage procedure is sufficient to induce long-term stable improvement in lung function. Unfortunately, the material re-accumulates in some cases after a median duration of 15 months, requiring periodic re-lavage.

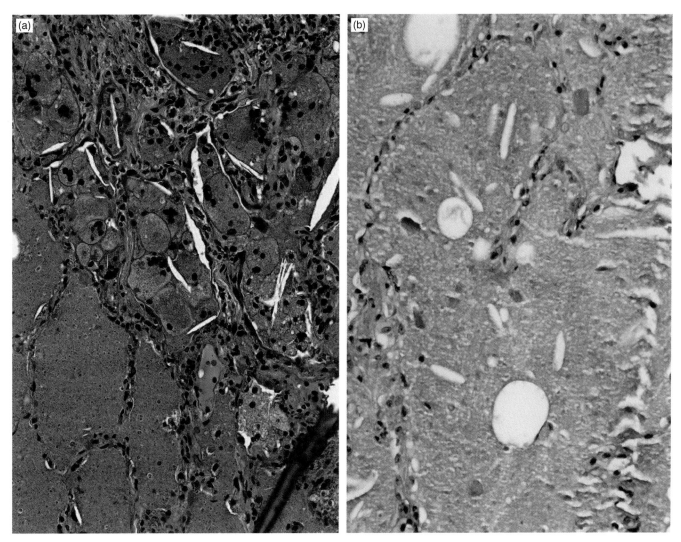

Figure 4.5. Pulmonary alveolar proteinosis. (a) Foamy macrophages. **(b)** PAS stain.

Other approaches to therapy include supplementing GM-CSF by inhaled aerosol or subcutaneous injection. Two-thirds of patients have a durable response to inhaled GM-CSF, which may last as long as 30 months. Response rates of 43 to 48% have been reported with injected GM-CSF. Those patients who do not respond to inhaled GM-CSF may require whole lung lavage. The anti-CD20 antibody rituximab has been used successfully to reduce anti-GM-CSF antibody levels. Children with PAP are also usually treated with whole lung lavage, but may eventually require lung transplantation. Pulmonary macrophage transplantation has been recently tried successfully in mice.

Patients with PAP are susceptible to several unusual infections, the most common being nocardiosis, non-tuberculous mycobacterial infections and aspergillosis. This phenomenon has been attributed to defective neutrophil function due to anti-GM-CSF antibodies.

There is a 5 to 7% rate of spontaneous remission. Data on long-term survival are lacking, but one study with 8.5 years of follow-up reported 6 deaths out of 24 patients, none of which was related to PAP. More than half of the survivors reported persistent symptoms, mainly dyspnea and cough. Overall survival currently approaches 100%.

Sample diagnosis on pathology report

Lung, right middle lobe, transbronchial biopsy – Pulmonary alveolar proteinosis. (See comment).

Eosinophilic pneumonia

Eosinophilic pneumonia is defined by the presence of eosinophils within airspaces. This finding may be associated with classic clinical and radiologic findings of eosinophilic pneumonia, or may be seen in atypical settings. There is a long list of possible etiologies, most of which need clinical investigation (Table 4.3). Notable within these are conditions like eosinophilic granulomatosis with polyangiitis (Churg–Strauss), allergic bronchopulmonary fungal disease and mucoid impaction of bronchi, which develop predominantly in patients with pre-existing asthma. In many cases of eosinophilic pneumonia where lung biopsy is performed for diagnosis, the etiology remains elusive even after a careful clinical work-up. Such cases are considered idiopathic.

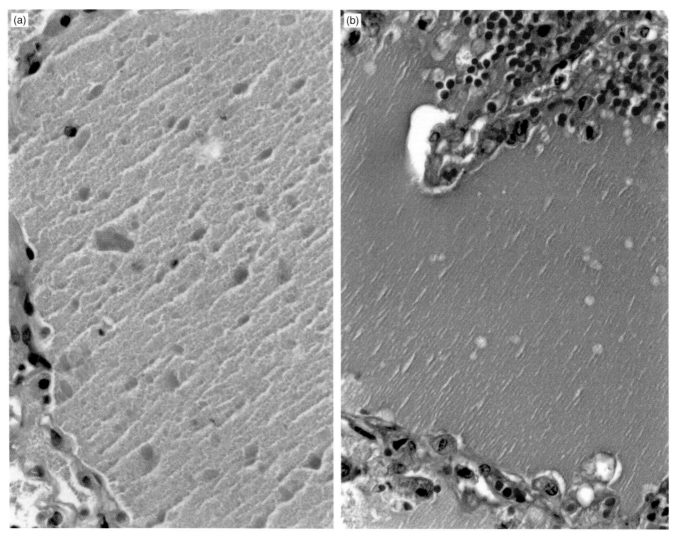

Figure 4.6. Pulmonary alveolar proteinosis vs. pulmonary edema. (a) PAP. **(b)** Pulmonary edema.

Major diagnostic findings

- Eosinophils within airspaces. The presence of eosinophils within alveoli is the cardinal feature of eosinophilic pneumonia (Figure 4.8). The eosinophils are admixed with variable numbers of histiocytes, fibrin, edema or an eosinophilic "proteinaceous exudate". The number of eosinophils varies greatly from case to case. Classic cases feature innumerable eosinophils whereas atypical cases show only a few. The latter situation is thought to occur when corticosteroid therapy is initiated prior to lung biopsy.

Variable pathologic findings

- Although it is the airspace abnormalities that define eosinophilic pneumonia, interstitial expansion may be more striking at first glance. The alveolar septa are often widened by a cellular inflammatory infiltrate composed of eosinophils, lymphocytes and plasma cells (Figure 4.9). The widened interstitium is usually lined by prominent type 2 pneumocytes. The interstitial

infiltrate may extend into the interlobular septa and pleura.
- Eosinophils may be present in and around small arteries and arterioles/venules in a perivascular, transmural or intimal distribution (Figure 4.10). This type of eosinophil-rich vasculitis is considered a secondary phenomenon. Necrotizing vasculitis is not a feature of uncomplicated eosinophilic pneumonia.
- The inflammatory and fibrinous exudate within the airspaces may show evidence of organization in the form of serpiginous fibroblast plugs (Masson bodies).
- Multinucleated giant cells may be scattered within the airspace inflammatory infiltrate (Figure 4.10). Well-formed granulomas are usually absent.
- Foamy macrophages may be present within airspaces in some cases.
- Findings indicative of an underlying etiology may be present and should always be sought. These include fungi, parasites, allergic mucin within airways, granulomas centered on bronchioles, necrotizing granulomas and necrotizing vasculitis.

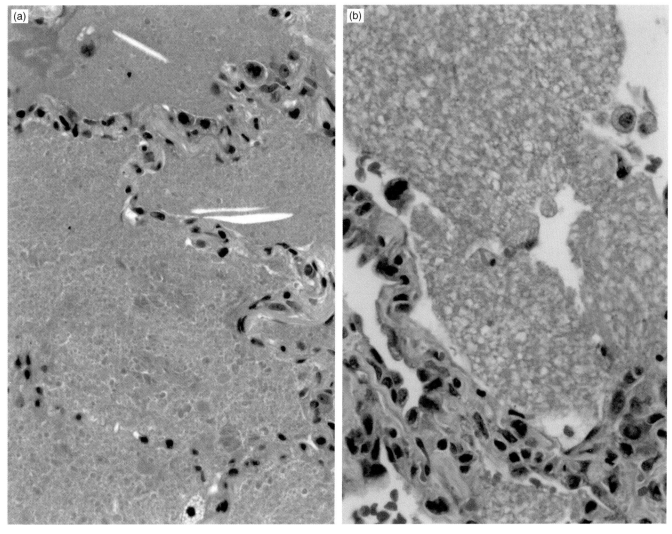

Figure 4.7. Pulmonary alveolar proteinosis vs. *Pneumocystis* pneumonia. (a) PAP. Eosinophilic material within the airspaces is coarsely granular. Note acicular spaces. **(b)** *Pneumocystis* pneumonia. Eosinophilic material within airspaces has a foamy, froth-with-dots appearance.

- Necrosis of eosinophils may occur within the airspaces, but parenchymal (interstitial) necrosis should suggest an alternative diagnosis.
- Eosinophil granules and Charcot-Leyden crystals may be found.
- The bronchi and bronchioles may show histologic features of bronchial asthma, including basement membrane thickening, goblet cell hyperplasia, smooth muscle hypertrophy and increased eosinophils.
- Eosinophils may be found in paratracheal or hilar lymph nodes.

Clinical profile

Eosinophilic pneumonia can occur in a wide variety of clinical settings, including acute and chronic diseases. These are distinguished by their clinical features, and usually do not show distinctive pathologic findings. The common factor in these entities (other than the presence of eosinophils within the alveoli) is the presence of peripheral opacities or infiltrates that appear "interstitial" radiologically. Eosinophilia in the peripheral blood (peripheral eosinophilia) may or may not be present.

Acute eosinophilic pneumonia presents as a febrile illness with hypoxemic respiratory failure. The diagnosis can be made by identifying eosinophils in BAL fluid, or by lung biopsy. There should be no evidence of infection or other specific etiologies. Cases usually have a dramatic and complete response to corticosteroids.

Chronic eosinophilic pneumonia is defined clinically by the presence of symptoms for greater than 2 weeks. Patients vary from 18 to 80 years of age; there is a 2:1 predilection for women. Clinical features include cough, dyspnea, high fever, malaise, weight loss and night sweats. Most patients have a history of asthma or other atopic diseases at presentation. However, a small but significant minority of patients have no history of asthma. Peripheral eosinophilia occurs in most patients but is not invariable. Pulmonary function tests may be obstructive or restrictive. Eosinophilia in BAL fluid is commonly used as a surrogate indicator for the presence of eosinophils within the alveoli, especially in cases that are not biopsied. In practice, lung biopsies are only performed

Table 4.3. Differential diagnosis of eosinophilic pneumonia

Etiology	How to make the diagnosis
Drug toxicity: amoxicillin, penicillin, bleomycin, daptomycin, hydrochlorothiazide, amiodarone	Careful history-taking focusing on drugs that have been associated with eosinophilic pneumonia; temporal association; exclusion of alternative causes
DRESS syndrome (**D**rug **R**ash with **E**osinophilia, **S**ystemic **S**ymptoms)	Variation on theme of drug toxicity, see above; requires presence of rash and systemic symptoms
Inhalants: cocaine, nickel carbonyl fumes	Careful social and occupational history
Parasites: *Toxocara, Trichinella, Fasciola, Strongyloides, Brugia, Wuchereria*	Careful travel history, stool examination for ova and parasites, serology for parasites Parasites on lung cytology or biopsy (*Strongyloides, Paragonimus*)
Allergic bronchopulmonary fungal disease (allergic bronchopulmonary aspergillosis)	History of asthma, peripheral eosinophilia, raised IgE level, raised *Aspergillus* IgE, radiologic findings Lung biopsy findings (allergic mucin, necrotizing granulomas, fungi)
Churg–Strauss syndrome	History of asthma, peripheral eosinophilia, multi-system disease (pericarditis, GI involvement, neuropathy), positive ANCA serology Lung biopsy findings (necrotizing granulomas, necrotizing vasculitis)
Idiopathic	No cause after appropriate clinical investigation

in a small minority of patients, generally in those in whom radiologic findings are atypical. The clinical diagnosis in most cases is based on the presence of blood or BAL eosinophilia, and predominantly peripheral lung infiltrates on radiographs.

Löffler syndrome refers to fleeting infiltrates in asymptomatic or mildly symptomatic individuals with peripheral eosinophilia. Such cases rarely come to lung biopsy.

Radiologic findings

The classic radiologic findings are bilateral infiltrates/opacities that are more prominent in the periphery of the lungs ("photographic negative of pulmonary edema"). Since some studies have used peripheral infiltrates as an inclusion criterion, it is

unclear what proportion of cases may have central or mixed infiltrates. The infiltrates are bilateral in most cases, especially on chest CT. They may exclusively involve the upper or lower lobes, or multiple lobes may be involved. Both ground-glass and dense infiltrates have been reported.

Differential diagnosis

A pathologic diagnosis of eosinophilic pneumonia should prompt a search for a specific etiology. The work-up should include stool examination for ova and parasites, and a careful history-taking, focusing on drugs that may cause eosinophilic pneumonia (Table 4.3). Other aspects of the work-up will depend on the presence of specific clinical and radiologic features.

The idiopathic form of organizing pneumonia (cryptogenic organizing pneumonia) shares many clinical and radiologic findings with eosinophilic pneumonia. The distinction between the two hinges on the demonstration of tissue eosinophilia. In cases where fibroblast plugs and eosinophils are both prominent, it may be impossible to determine whether the case represents organizing eosinophilic pneumonia or organizing pneumonia with prominent eosinophils. Differentiating between the two may not be critical, because both processes are steroid-responsive.

Diffuse alveolar damage (DAD) may enter the differential diagnosis in cases of acute eosinophilic pneumonia where DAD is part of the histologic picture. The presence of eosinophils within the interstitium and airspaces establishes the diagnosis of acute eosinophilic pneumonia in such cases.

Langerhans cell histiocytosis also features numerous eosinophils, but these are located entirely within the interstitium. Stellate interstitial nodules are a feature of Langerhans cell histiocytosis, but are not seen in eosinophilic pneumonia.

Eosinophilic granulomatosis with polyangiitis (Churg–Strauss) is always part of the differential diagnosis when eosinophilic pneumonia is seen in lung biopsies. Features that suggest a diagnosis of eosinophilic granulomatosis with polyangiitis include necrotizing granulomas and necrotizing vasculitis. Even in the absence of these findings, eosinophilic granulomatosis with polyangiitis remains a possibility because of sampling error, especially in a small biopsy.

In cases of eosinophilic pneumonia, the presence of allergic mucin should raise the possibility of allergic bronchopulmonary aspergillosis or mucoid impaction of bronchi. Diagnosis of these conditions is discussed in Chapters 2 and 9.

Hard metal lung disease occasionally enters the differential diagnosis of eosinophilic pneumonia. A few multinucleated giant cells can be seen in eosinophilic pneumonia, and occasional eosinophils can be seen in hard metal lung disease. However, the predominant finding in hard metal lung disease is interstitial chronic inflammation, and eosinophils are relatively few in number. In contrast, eosinophils dominate the histologic picture in eosinophilic pneumonia. In addition, the presence of emperipolesis of histiocytes or neutrophils within giant cells supports the diagnosis of hard metal lung disease.

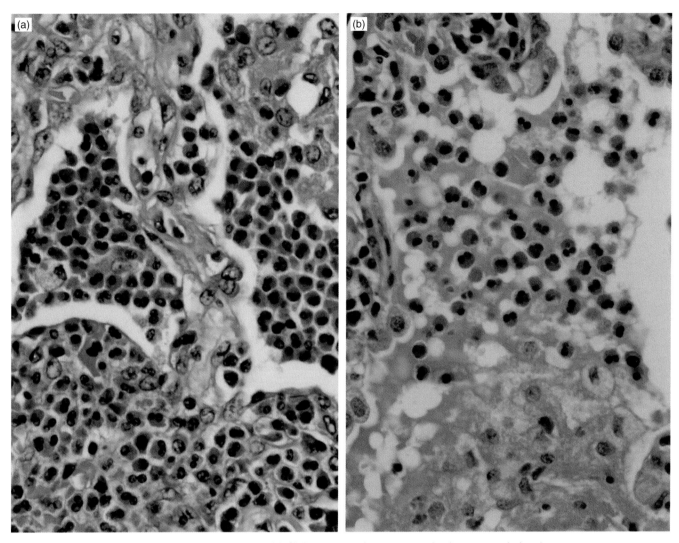

Figure 4.8. Eosinophilic pneumonia. (a) Numerous eosinophils fill the airspaces. The intervening alveolar septum is thick and type 2 pneumocytes are prominent. **(b)** Eosinophils are present in a background of edema. A few macrophages are also seen at the bottom.

Treatment and prognosis

Eosinophilic pneumonia is exquisitely sensitive to corticosteroid therapy, and the response is generally rapid (within a few days). Chest X-rays can show complete resolution of radiologic abnormalities. The prognosis is good. Symptoms, infiltrates and eosinophilia (in the peripheral blood or bronchoalveolar lavage fluid) may recur while steroids are tapered, or after cessation of steroid therapy. Relapses are steroid-responsive. On long-term follow-up, asthma develops in some patients who were non-asthmatic at presentation.

Sample diagnosis on pathology report

Lung, right middle lobe, transbronchial biopsy – Eosinophilic pneumonia (See comment).

Acute bronchopneumonia

Acute bronchopneumonia is characterized by the presence of a neutrophil-rich acute inflammatory exudate within airspaces. Differentiation between lobar pneumonia and bronchopneumonia was of some relevance in the pre-antibiotic era but is currently of little significance. The term acute bronchopneumonia can be used by pathologists regardless of whether an infectious organism is identified. The diagnosis is equally valid whether the inflammatory infiltrate is limited to peribronchiolar parenchyma or extends further into distal alveoli. The term provides a convenient way for pathologists to indicate microscopic involvement of the lung parenchyma – as opposed to bronchi and bronchioles – by an acute inflammatory exudate. Acute bronchopneumonia is most commonly caused by bacterial infection, but non-infectious causes such as aspiration and inflammatory bowel disease also exist.

Surgical pathologists may see acute bronchopneumonia in transbronchial biopsies, needle biopsies and surgical lung biopsies. It is a common finding at autopsy.

Major diagnostic findings

The defining pathologic feature of acute bronchopneumonia is the presence of an acute inflammatory exudate within

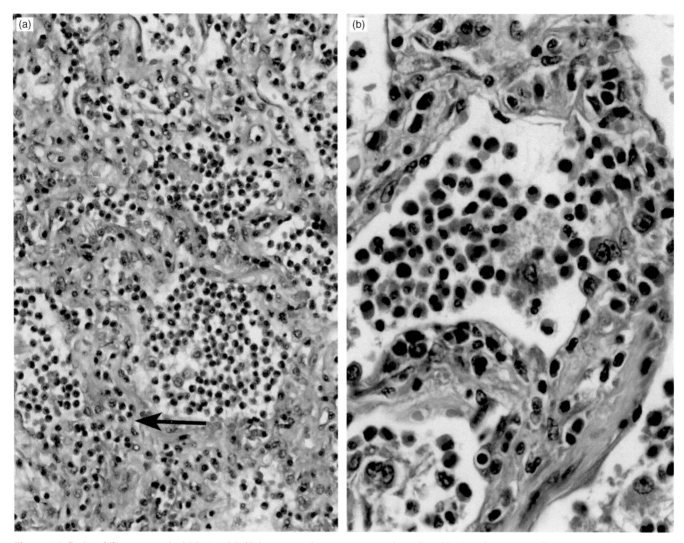

Figure 4.9. Eosinophilic pneumonia. (a) Eosinophils fill the airspaces but interstitium is also widened by the inflammatory infiltrate (arrow). **(b)** Airspace and interstitium at high magnification.

airspaces (Figures 4.11 and 4.12). Neutrophils are the predominant cell type, although macrophages are also commonly present. As mentioned above, the term is valid as long as the inflammatory infiltrate is located within alveoli. The extent of alveolar involvement does not change the pathologic diagnosis.

Variable pathologic findings

- Other common findings in acute bronchopneumonia include fibrinous exudates, edema, necrotic debris, red blood cells and macrophages within the airspaces.
- The acute inflammatory exudate may be accompanied by necrosis and destruction of alveolar septa. When a necrotic acute inflammatory lesion destroys lung parenchyma in this manner and becomes confluent, the resultant lesion is known as an *abscess*. Lung parenchyma at the periphery of abscesses frequently shows areas of organizing pneumonia, characterized by the presence of polypoid fibroblast plugs within airspaces.

- Features indicative of the etiology may be identifiable within the airspace exudate. The most common are aspirated food particles and bacterial organisms (Figures 4.11 and 4.12).
- Some histologic features are said to be associated with particular organisms. For example, amphophilic edema has been described in cases of fatal bronchopneumonia caused by *Bordetella pertussis* (Figure 4.13), and karyorrhexis is thought to be a characteristic feature of *Legionella* pneumonia. Although such findings are useful pointers, they are not specific, and require confirmation by immunohistochemistry, cultures or PCR.
- Concurrent acute bronchiolitis is common in bronchopneumonia. The demarcation between bronchiolitis and bronchopneumonia is arbitrary in some cases since the point where bronchioles turn into alveoli is not sharply defined.
- Concurrent diffuse alveolar damage is common, especially in autopsy specimens. It may reflect severe acute lung injury or concomitant viral infection.

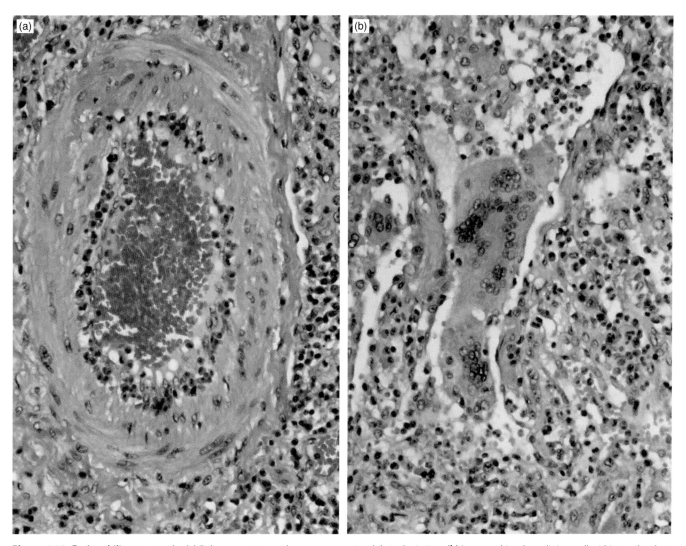

Figure 4.10. Eosinophilic pneumonia. (a) Pulmonary artery with numerous eosinophils in the intima. **(b)** Large multinucleated giant cell within an alveolus.

Diagnostic work-up

Whether a diagnostic work-up in cases of acute bronchopneumonia should be performed depends on the clinical setting, culture results and pathologic findings. One approach is to perform a tissue Gram stain (such as Brown-Brenn or Brown-Hopps) and other stains such as GMS, Dieterle or Warthin-Starry in all cases. Our experience is that the results of such stains are seldom productive and almost never change clinical management. Since most of these lesions are caused by bacterial infection, precise identification of the organism requires cultures. Furthermore, pathologic examination does not allow precise identification of the usual bacteria that cause acute bronchopneumonia. Even the seemingly simple task of distinguishing gram-positive from gram-negative bacteria is fraught with technical problems. Therefore, our approach is to use special stains when pathologic findings are unusual. Such findings include extensive necrosis, numerous admixed histiocytes and granulomas of any type. We also have a very low threshold to perform stains in immunocompromised patients, and are open to requests from clinicians to perform special stains in selected patients if the clinical picture is suspicious for infection.

Clinical profile

Patients with acute bacterial pneumonia may present with typical clinical features such as cough, fever, rusty sputum, pleuritic chest pain and hemoptysis. However, more often than not, patients who undergo lung biopsy do so because the clinical findings are atypical, or the radiologic features are unusual. Mass-like lesions are particularly likely to be biopsied since they are considered suspicious for malignancy.

Radiologic findings

Acute bronchopneumonia usually manifests as ill-defined infiltrates or consolidation. The more confluent and dense the alveolar filling, the more mass-like the lesion becomes. If organization supervenes, the infiltrates can become more nodular or mass-like. Destruction of lung parenchyma by abscess formation manifests radiologically as cavitation.

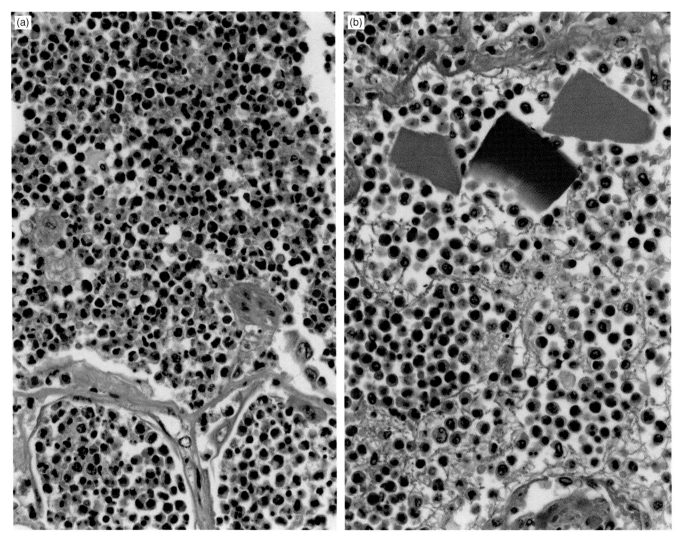

Figure 4.11. Acute bronchopneumonia. (a) Acute bronchopneumonia. The airspaces are filled with an acute inflammatory exudate containing neutrophils, macrophages and necrotic debris. **(b)** Aspirated food (skeletal muscle/meat) particles are present within the inflammatory infiltrate. This type of acute aspiration pneumonia is common in autopsy specimens. Its morphology differs considerably from particulate matter aspiration in lung biopsies (Figures 2.52–2.55, Chapter 2).

Differential diagnosis

- Diffuse alveolar damage (DAD) enters the differential diagnosis when hyaline membranes are identified in lungs that also show acute inflammation. Whether the findings should be considered as one diagnosis or as two separate entities depends on the extent of the abnormalities. For example, minimal acute inflammation in association with typical findings of DAD can be considered part of the primary process, while extensive involvement of airspaces by acute inflammatory exudates should be diagnosed separately as acute bronchopneumonia. The combination of acute bronchopneumonia and DAD should raise the possibility of viral infection with a superimposed bacterial pneumonia.
- Abscess. As mentioned above, abscesses destroy lung parenchyma (alveolar septa) and form confluent lesions, whereas the alveolar septa remain intact in uncomplicated acute bronchopneumonia.

- Bronchiolitis. Whether to label an acute inflammatory exudate as bronchiolitis or bronchopneumonia depends on the location of the inflammatory exudate. An acute inflammatory exudate within bronchiolar lumens constitutes acute bronchiolitis, whereas a similar exudate within alveoli should be termed acute bronchopneumonia. If both anatomic compartments are involved, they can both be diagnosed.

Treatment and prognosis

Treatment depends on the underlying etiology. Antibiotics are the mainstay of treatment in most patients. Prognosis depends on the virulence of the causative organism, the immune status of the host and the development of complications.

Sample diagnosis on pathology report

Lung, left lower lobe, transbronchial biopsy – Acute bronchopneumonia (See comment).

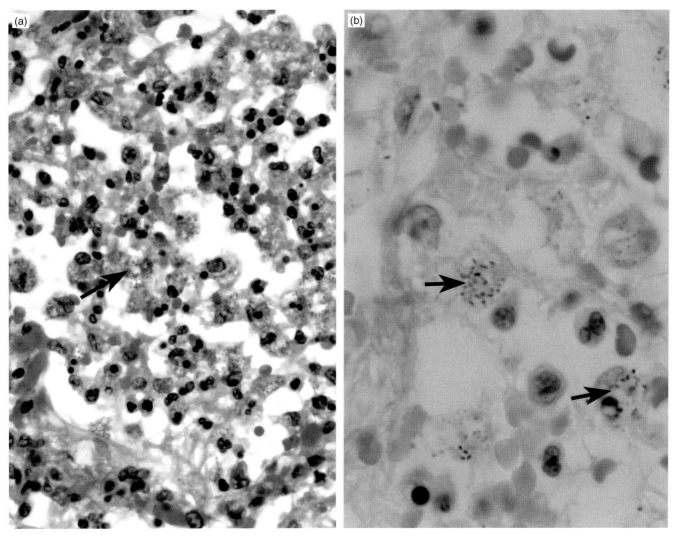

Figure 4.12. Acute bronchopneumonia. (a) Bacterial organisms are visible within macrophages on H&E in a case of acute bronchopneumonia (arrow, 40x objective lens). **(b)** A Gram stain shows that the bacteria are gram-positive cocci (arrows, oil immersion objective lens). The patient died of novel influenza A (H1N1) infection and superimposed pneumococcal pneumonia.

Smoker's macrophages (respiratory bronchiolitis, respiratory bronchiolitis–interstitial lung disease, desquamative interstitial pneumonia)

It is well known that the lungs of cigarette smokers contain pigmented macrophages within the lumens of respiratory bronchioles, alveolar ducts and alveoli. These macrophages contain a light-brown intracytoplasmic pigment derived from particles contained in cigarette smoke. By energy-dispersive X-ray spectrometry, this pigment has been shown to contain *aluminum silicates*, which are also present in tobacco and cigarette smoke.

While the presence of smoker's macrophages in the lung is easy to understand and widely accepted, the terminology associated with this finding is extremely complex, widely debated and frequently misunderstood. The confusion starts with the term *respiratory bronchiolitis*, which was first used in Niewoehner *et al*'s classic paper published in 1974. In that

study, which looked for subtle histologic changes in the lungs of young adult cigarette smokers to explain the pathologic underpinnings of emphysema, the investigators found brown-pigmented macrophages predominantly within respiratory bronchioles, which they termed respiratory bronchiolitis. The suffix "-itis" was used since the authors considered macrophages to be inflammatory cells. This awkward term has persisted to the current day. Unfortunately, it conjures up images of inflamed bronchioles, and does not adequately describe either the main pathologic finding (pigment-laden macrophages) or its clinical significance (marker of cigarette smoking).

Further confusion was added in 1987 by the description of respiratory bronchiolitis as the sole pathologic finding in six patients with clinical and radiologic evidence of interstitial lung disease. The condition was notable because the clinical and radiologic features suggested an interstitial process, whereas the pathologic findings did not. Instead, surgical lung biopsies showed a complete absence of significant fibrosis or alveolar septal pathology. The only pathologic abnormality

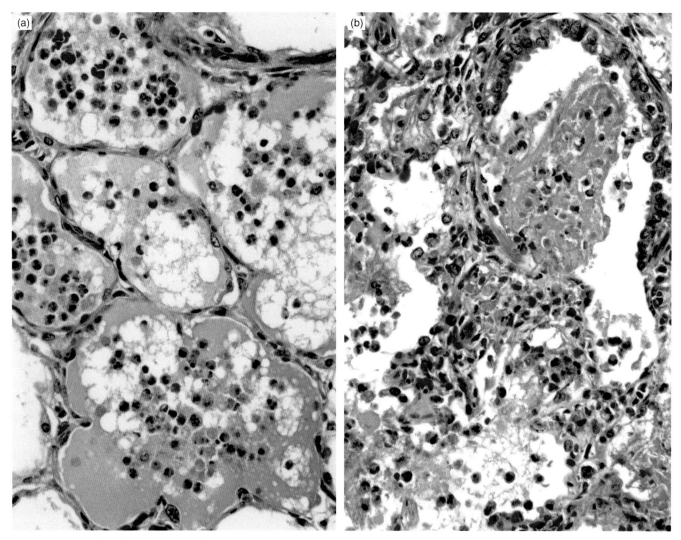

Figure 4.13. Acute bronchopneumonia in fatal *Bordetella pertussis* infection. (a) The amphophilic or basophilic appearance of the edema in the background is a clue to the diagnosis. Large numbers of *Bordetella* bacteria can be demonstrated in these areas by immunohistochemistry. **(b)** The acute inflammatory exudate spills out from a bronchiolar lumen into the adjacent airspaces. These pictures are from an autopsy of a 4-month-old child who died of pertussis. Case courtesy of Dr. Sherif Zaki.

was the presence of smoker's macrophages within airspaces. This condition is currently known as *respiratory bronchiolitis-interstitial lung disease* (RBILD). It is frequently misinterpreted and misdiagnosed by clinicians, radiologists and pathologists alike. Some clinicians incorrectly assume that a pathologic diagnosis of respiratory bronchiolitis in a patient with interstitial abnormalities on imaging is equivalent to RBILD. Radiologists make the mistake of assuming that ground-glass opacities in the upper lobes of cigarette smokers represent RBILD. From the perspective of pathologists, the most common mistake is to assume that RBILD is a combination of interstitial fibrosis and smoker's macrophages. In fact, as mentioned above, the diagnosis of RBILD requires that there should be *no pathologic evidence of interstitial abnormalities*. The radiologic interstitial abnormalities – specifically, bilateral ground-glass opacities – in RBILD are likely caused by macrophages within airspaces rather than true interstitial disease. Why radiologic interstitial abnormalities develop in some smokers but not others is unknown.

The final source of confusion in smoking-related interstitial lung disease is the entity known as *desquamative interstitial pneumonia* (DIP). This term, coined by Dr. Averill Liebow in 1965, was first used to refer to filling of the majority of alveoli in lung biopsies by "massed desquamated and proliferating cells". In the absence of immunohistochemistry, it was assumed that the cells were desquamated alveolar pneumocytes. This assumption subsequently proved to be incorrect, as the cells were shown to be macrophages. The term DIP is therefore an antiquated misnomer. It is a relic of a bygone era in which classification of interstitial lung disease was in its infancy. Over the years, the pathologic features of usual interstitial pneumonia were better defined (1986), and newer entities such as RBILD (1987), nonspecific interstitial pneumonia (1994) and smoking-related interstitial fibrosis (2010) were described. The description of these entities has removed much of the rationale for the existence of DIP. At the time of this writing (2015), DIP is rarely used by lung pathologists as a diagnostic term. In some of the instances where it is used, a more suitable diagnosis – such as RBILD, SRIF, UIP,

Table 4.4. Reasons why DIP is an unsatisfactory term

DIP is a misnomer: the cells in the alveoli are macrophages, not desquamated epithelial cells

The term does not convey the etiology of the process

The entity lumps together smoking-related interstitial lung diseases with many other unrelated etiologies

It is not clearly or exclusively a smoking-related disease – some patients are smokers, many are not

DIP was described in 1965, decades before current concepts of interstitial lung disease were defined

Many cases of DIP without fibrosis would be currently diagnosed as RBILD

Many cases that would previously be called DIP with fibrosis would currently be diagnosed as SRIF

Diagnostic criteria of DIP have never been clearly defined. The term has been used for cases without interstitial fibrosis as well as those with significant interstitial fibrosis

Its existence leads to misdiagnosis of other well-defined entities if there are numerous macrophages within airspaces

DIP is a waste-basket of several unrelated conditions of differing etiologies

DIP is classified as an "idiopathic interstitial pneumonia" even though the etiology is smoking-related in many cases

"DIP-like" changes are common, but DIP is vanishingly rare

NSIP or pulmonary Langerhans cell histiocytosis – has probably been missed. More commonly, there are dozens of entities, neoplastic and non-neoplastic, where the term "DIP-like" is used to describe filling of airspaces by cells of various types. Therefore, DIP has become a mixed bag of various unrelated conditions and the term should probably be discarded (Table 4.4).

In contrast, respiratory bronchiolitis is an extremely common finding. Surgical pathologists see smoker's macrophages in almost every type of lung specimen, including transbronchial biopsies, needle biopsies, surgical lung biopsies, lobectomies, pneumonectomies and bullectomies for pneumothorax. The diagnosis of RBILD should only be made or suggested on a surgical lung biopsy.

Major diagnostic findings

The hallmark of respiratory bronchiolitis is the presence of lightly pigmented macrophages within airspaces ("smoker's macrophages"), including alveoli, alveolar ducts and respiratory bronchioles. The pigment is light brown and finely granular, and contains a few black specks (Figure 4.14; also see Chapter 1, Figures 1.28 and 1.29, and Chapter 5, Figure 5.58). Importantly, the macrophages do not need to be confined to respiratory bronchioles.

Variable pathologic findings

- Other than the macrophages themselves, there is no significant inflammation in most cases of respiratory bronchiolitis. Specifically, lymphocytes and plasma cells are usually absent. When present, lymphocytes are few in number and limited to the walls of occasional bronchioles.
- Fibrosis is not a feature of respiratory bronchiolitis. Therefore, the presence of significant interstitial fibrosis of any type should suggest an alternative diagnosis. In such cases, respiratory bronchiolitis is either part of another pathologic process, or is simply an incidental finding.
- Respiratory bronchiolitis does not cause scarring, honeycomb change, fibroblast foci or fibroblast plugs.

Diagnostic work-up

An iron stain may be helpful when there is uncertainty whether the pigment is related to cigarette smoking or represents hemosiderin. However, the results can be difficult to interpret since smoker's macrophages are also weakly positive.

Clinical profile

Most individuals with respiratory bronchiolitis are current smokers or ex-smokers. In most cases, it is an incidental finding, and there are no associated symptoms. It can be found in smokers of all ages, and may persist for up to 32 years after cessation of cigarette smoking. In ex-smokers, the average duration between cessation of smoking and detection of respiratory bronchiolitis in lung specimens is 9 years.

Multiple clinicopathologic studies, including a detailed study by Fraig et al., have confirmed that respiratory bronchiolitis is absent in the vast majority of never-smokers. Rare exceptions have been reported, however. Potential explanations for the finding of smoker's macrophages in a never-smoker include unreliable history (the claim of being a never-smoker may be false), exposure to environmental dust or exposure to second-hand smoke from cigarette smokers.

Only rarely is respiratory bronchiolitis clinically significant. It is never an adequate explanation for a lung mass, nodule or unilateral radiologic abnormality. Therefore, in most cases where this finding is seen, one must look elsewhere to explain abnormal radiologic findings. Because respiratory bronchiolitis is such a common incidental finding, its presence in patients with interstitial lung disease often reflects sampling error, especially in transbronchial biopsies. Contrary to common misconception, the pathologic finding of respiratory bronchiolitis is *not* necessarily equivalent to a clinical diagnosis of RBILD.

Rarely, respiratory bronchiolitis is the only pathologic finding in surgical lung biopsies from individuals with clinical and radiologic features of interstitial lung disease. As mentioned previously, this situation has been termed RBILD. The most common symptoms in RBILD are mild cough and dyspnea. Patients tend to be heavy smokers, and many are in the 30- to 40-year-old age group. Pulmonary function tests may show restrictive changes or reduced diffusing capacity. The condition is occasionally detected on chest imaging performed for other reasons in asymptomatic smokers.

Radiologic findings

Radiologic abnormalities are common in cigarette smokers, especially on high-resolution CT. Some of these – especially bilateral ground-glass opacities in an upper lobe distribution – are thought to be attributable to respiratory bronchiolitis. The same findings are seen in RBILD. The findings may be upper predominant or diffuse. Other findings that have been described in RBILD include non-specific thickening of bronchial walls and centrilobular nodules.

Differential diagnosis

- Hemosiderin-laden macrophages can be misinterpreted as smoker's macrophages and vice versa. Features helpful in the differential diagnosis are shown in Table 4.5 and Figure 4.15.

Table 4.5. Smoker's macrophages vs. hemosiderin-laden macrophages

	Smoker's macrophages (respiratory bronchiolitis)	Hemosiderin-laden macrophages
Color of pigment	Brown	Brown
Coarseness of pigment	Fine granules	Coarse granules, with occasional large blobs
Occasional black specks	Present	Absent
Iron stain	Weakly positive (light blue)	Strongly positive (deep blue)
Significance	Derived from cigarette smoke	Indicative of prior hemorrhage

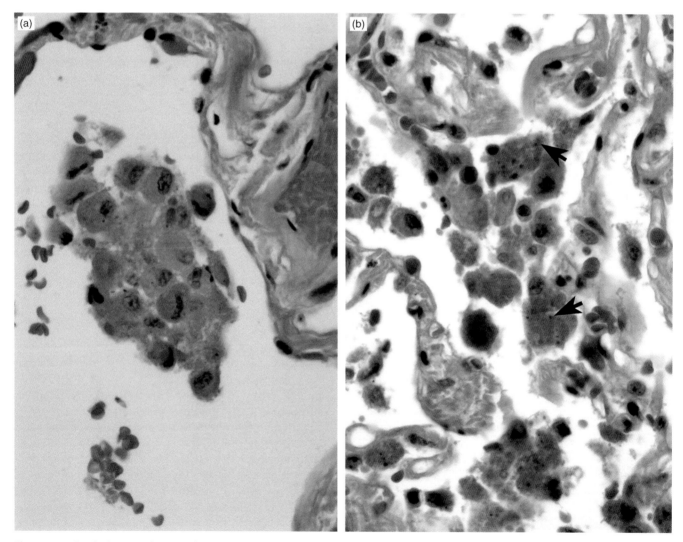

Figure 4.14. Smoker's macrophages within airspaces (respiratory bronchiolitis). (a) Lightly pigmented macrophages within an alveolus. **(b)** The pigment within the macrophages is light brown and granular. The presence of a few tiny black specks (arrows) is an important feature that helps to differentiate smoker's macrophages from hemosiderin-laden macrophages.

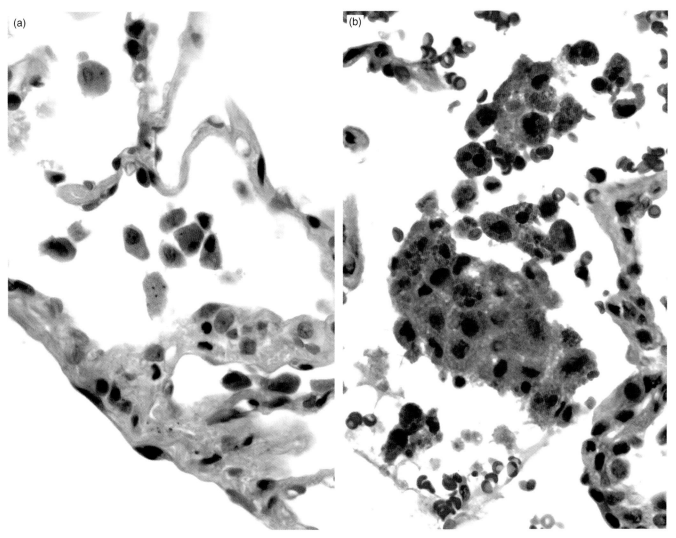

Figure 4.15. Respiratory bronchiolitis vs. hemosiderin-laden macrophages. (a) Respiratory bronchiolitis (smoker's macrophages). The intracytoplasmic pigment in these macrophages is finely granular and contains a few tiny black specks. **(b)** Hemosiderin-laden macrophages. The pigment is coarsely granular and lacks black specks. The granules are considerably larger than those of respiratory bronchiolitis.

- The possibility of RBILD should be considered if respiratory bronchiolitis is the only abnormality in a surgical (wedge) biopsy. However, pathologic findings do not distinguish between respiratory bronchiolitis and RBILD, and pathologists should never make this diagnosis in the absence of clinical information. By definition, the diagnosis of RBILD requires clinical or radiologic evidence of interstitial lung disease. The radiologic findings are typically bilateral patchy ground-glass opacities. There should be no evidence of significant fibrosis on CT scans or in biopsy specimens. Finally, the pathologist should meticulously exclude alternative explanations for ground-glass opacities such as infection, hypersensitivity pneumonitis, organizing pneumonia or diffuse alveolar damage. If these strict criteria are not met, the finding of respiratory bronchiolitis in a lung biopsy should be considered an incidental finding.
- DIP. For the reasons described above, the term DIP should be avoided altogether. In cases where numerous non-pigmented alveolar macrophages are present within airspaces, and the etiology is unknown, a descriptive diagnosis should suffice.
- *Bong lung.* Lung tissue in marijuana smokers can contain numerous intra-alveolar pigmented macrophages similar to smoker's macrophages. As with smoker's macrophages (respiratory bronchiolitis), these cells can be present within alveoli, alveolar ducts and respiratory bronchioles. Although the pigment in such cases tends to be a bit coarser than smoker's pigment, the appearance is not specific enough to make a definitive pathologic diagnosis and rests on a clinical history of marijuana smoking.

Treatment and prognosis

Cessation of cigarette smoking should be recommended in RBILD. There is no conclusive evidence that corticosteroids are beneficial. The prognosis is excellent. Most patients remain stable or improve.

Sample diagnosis on pathology report

Whether or not to mention respiratory bronchiolitis in the main diagnosis is a matter of judgement and context. In most cases, respiratory bronchiolitis is an incidental finding that can be relegated to a comment, microscopic description or "other findings" in a lung cancer template.

In a surgical biopsy where respiratory bronchiolitis is the only finding:

Lung, right upper lobe, surgical biopsy – Respiratory bronchiolitis (See comment).

In a surgical biopsy where respiratory bronchiolitis is the only finding, and detailed clinical and radiologic information consistent with RBILD is available to the pathologist:

Lung, right upper lobe, surgical biopsy – Respiratory bronchiolitis, consistent with respiratory bronchiolitis-interstitial lung disease (See comment).

Hemosiderin-laden macrophages and/or blood within the airspaces

Hemosiderin-laden macrophages and red blood cells are common findings within alveoli in lung biopsies and resections. Pathologists should be aware of the diagnostic approach to these findings. The first step is to determine whether blood in the airspaces is artifactual or "real". This issue was previously discussed in Chapter 1 and illustrated in Figure 1.20 of that chapter. Briefly, the presence of hemosiderin, fibrin or capillaritis in association with red blood cells suggests that bleeding occurred in vivo and is not an artifact of the biopsy procedure. Rarely, intra-alveolar red blood cells without hemosiderin may represent true in vivo hemorrhage in patients with acute active hemoptysis, since it takes approximately 2 days for hemoglobin to be converted to hemosiderin.

Once it is determined that alveolar hemorrhage is not an artifact, the main role of the surgical pathologist is to identify an etiology. This is especially important in patients who present with hemoptysis and are found to have diffuse bilateral infiltrates on imaging, a situation referred to by clinicians as *diffuse alveolar hemorrhage*. The most important etiology of diffuse alveolar hemorrhage that requires pathologic interpretation for diagnosis is *capillaritis*, which is discussed in detail in Chapter 10. Rarely, other specific etiologies associated with alveolar hemorrhage or hemosiderin deposition may also be identifiable in lung biopsies. These include granulomatosis with polyangiitis (Wegener's), vascular malformations, pulmonary veno-occlusive disease (PVOD) and pulmonary capillary hemangiomatosis (PCH). Although this book deals exclusively with non-neoplastic diseases, the reader is reminded that lung metastases from epithelioid angiosarcoma can closely mimic diffuse alveolar hemorrhage clinically and pathologically. Beyond the lesions discussed above, most other causes of pulmonary hemorrhage and hemosiderin-laden macrophages require clinical input for diagnosis. Of these, the most common is congestive heart failure, which causes passive congestion in the lungs and intra-alveolar hemosiderin deposition, presumably secondary to rupture of congested capillaries. Hemosiderin-laden macrophages in heart failure are sometimes referred to as "heart failure cells". Table 4.6 lists the common causes of intra-alveolar hemosiderin-laden macrophages and blood along with the main pathologic and clinical findings helpful in diagnosis.

Major diagnostic findings

Blood and/or hemosiderin-laden macrophages within the airspaces. Hemosiderin is a granular coarse brown pigment found within the cytoplasm of macrophages (Figure 4.15; Chapter 1, Figure 1.20; Chapter 10, Figures 10.10 and 10.15). The granules vary in size and often fuse into large blobs. Unlike smoker's macrophages, small black specks are absent.

Variable pathologic findings

- The main pathologic findings helpful in the differential diagnosis are listed in Table 4.6.
- In most cases, Goodpasture syndrome is characterized by *bland hemorrhage*, which consists of red blood cells and hemosiderin-laden macrophages within the airspaces without inflammation, vasculitis, capillaritis or necrosis (Figure 4.16). Presumably vascular damage mediated by anti-GBM antibodies results in leakage of blood out of damaged capillaries without significant inflammation.
- *Capillaritis*, also known as acute necrotizing capillaritis, is a form of vasculitis involving capillaries. It is discussed in detail in Chapter 10 and illustrated in Figures 10.13 to 10.15 of that chapter. Capillaritis is the single most important cause of alveolar hemorrhage identifiable by surgical pathologists in lung biopsies. It is characterized by destruction of alveolar septal capillaries by an inflammatory infiltrate composed of neutrophils, histiocytes and karyorrhectic debris. The inflammatory changes are usually accompanied by red blood cells and numerous hemosiderin-laden macrophages within the airspaces. Capillaritis is often a difficult diagnosis because the vasculitic changes are patchy and subtle and are frequently overshadowed by blood and hemosiderin. Also, the involved capillaries and alveolar septa are often completely destroyed, leaving behind an inflammatory infiltrate that closely mimics acute bronchopneumonia. The key to the correct diagnosis is recognizing the alveolar septal-centered nature of the inflammatory infiltrate, the karyorrhectic debris and the characteristic mix of neutrophils and histiocytes.
- Diagnostic features of PVOD and PCH are discussed in Chapter 10.
- The key to the identification of metastatic angiosarcoma is the recognition of large atypical cells exceeding the size and atypia permissible in reactive pneumocytes.

Table 4.6. Diagnoses to consider when hemosiderin and/or red blood cells are found within the airspaces in a lung biopsy or resection specimen

Cause of hemosiderin-laden macrophages and/or blood within the airspaces	Key pathologic findings	Key clinical or radiologic findings
Chronic congestion (congestive heart failure)	Alveolar septa may be thickened by congested capillaries	Clinical or radiologic evidence of congestive heart failure
Granulomatosis with polyangiitis (Wegener's)	Capillaritis or medium-vessel vasculitis and necrotizing granulomas or both	Often, capillaritis or vasculitis is not identifiable after treatment ANCA serologies can be very helpful if positive
Other causes of capillaritis	Capillaritis	See Chapter 10
Goodpasture syndrome	In most cases, no capillaritis or inflammation ("bland hemorrhage") If hemoptysis is very recent, fresh hemorrhage (red blood cells) may the only pathologic finding Immunofluorescence on a fresh (unfixed) sample of lung or kidney is required for pathologic diagnosis (linear IgG staining)	Concurrent acute renal failure, or crescentic glomerulonephritis on renal biopsy; < 10% of patients have lung-limited disease Adults (bimodal, 20 to 30 years, and 60 to 70 years) Serology for anti-glomerular basement membrane (anti-GBM) antibodies
Compression of pulmonary vein by a mediastinal mass (fibrosing mediastinitis or bronchogenic cyst)	Marked alveolar septal congestion Venous infarcts Thick pulmonary arteries Lymphatic dilatation	Requires radiologic evidence of a mediastinal mass
Pulmonary vein stenosis due to radiofrequency ablation for atrial fibrillation	Changes similar to PVOD	Requires clinical history of a prior ablation procedure for atrial fibrillation
Thrombocytopenia	None	In the absence of another cause, the platelet count is usually very low (< 5000) before spontaneous pulmonary hemorrhage occurs
Pulmonary veno-occlusive disease (PVOD)	Occlusion of small veins within the lung Giant cell reaction to calcified hemosiderin in small blood vessels Elastic stain can be helpful in detecting occluded vessels	Clinical or radiologic evidence of pulmonary hypertension Absence of extrapulmonary venous obstruction
Metastatic angiosarcoma	Can be a close mimic of diffuse alveolar damage; hemorrhage and acute lung injury may overshadow tumor cells Atypical or malignant epithelioid cells mimicking type 2 pneumocytes Immunohistochemical evidence of angiosarcoma (CD34, CD31, ERG)	Multiple bilateral nodules or infiltrates Wide age range (22 to 73 years, often young men in 30s or 40s) History of an extrapulmonary mass (right atrium, penis, other soft tissue)
Lung transplantation (transplant transbronchial biopsies)	Hemosiderin is very common; possibly a consequence of multiple biopsies	Prior transbronchial biopsies
Idiopathic pulmonary hemosiderosis	No vasculitis, inflammation or necrosis No immunoglobulin deposition	Rare, usually presents in young children with anemia and/or recurrent bronchopneumonia. Hemoptysis is variable Most cases occur under the age of 10 years (8 months to 15 years, usually 3 to 5 years) No extrapulmonary involvement
Obvious causes (trauma, tumor, vascular anomaly, aspergilloma)	Histologic features of the main disease predominate Hemorrhage is found in or around the site of the obvious lesion	None of these entities causes diffuse bilateral infiltrates

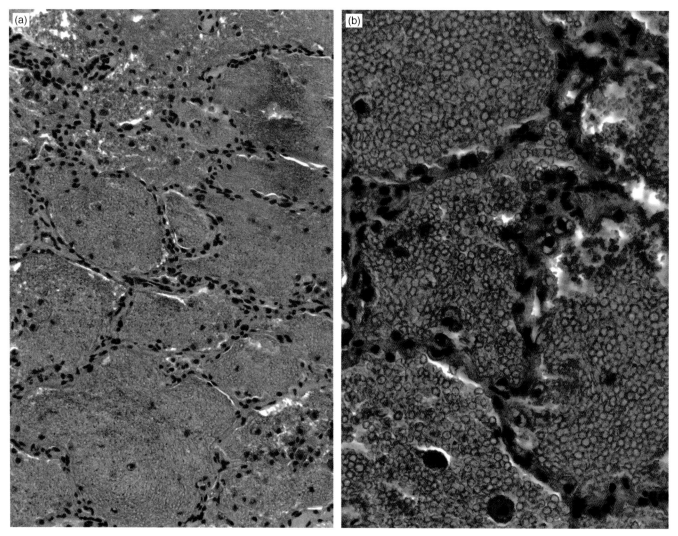

Figure 4.16. Goodpasture syndrome. (a) The airspaces are filled with red blood cells. A few scattered hemosiderin-laden macrophages are also present. **(b)** Despite the extensive hemorrhage, the alveolar septa are pristine, with no evidence of capillaritis ("bland hemorrhage"). These pictures are from a surgical lung biopsy of a 22-year-old woman. Immunofluorescence testing performed on an accompanying fresh lung sample showed linear staining for IgG along alveolar septa (not shown).

Diagnostic work-up

- An iron stain can be helpful to confirm the presence of hemosiderin.
- Immunofluorescence testing can be performed on fresh lung tissue and is very helpful in the diagnosis of Goodpasture syndrome. It can be performed on transbronchial biopsies. The classic finding in Goodpasture syndrome is the presence of diffuse linear IgG deposits along the alveolar septa (basement membranes).

Clinical profile

See Table 4.6.

Radiologic findings

See Table 4.6.

Differential diagnosis

Smoker's macrophages (respiratory bronchiolitis) are the most important entity in the differential diagnosis (see Table 4.5).

Treatment and prognosis

Treatment depends on the underlying etiology. Goodpasture syndrome requires prompt and aggressive therapy with plasmapheresis, corticosteroids and immunosuppressive agents. Idiopathic pulmonary hemosiderosis is treated with corticosteroids or other second-line immunosuppressants.

The prognosis of Goodpasture syndrome is variable. The 5-year survival currently exceeds 80%, and fewer than 30% of patients require long-term dialysis. Some patients die of massive hemoptysis or progress to end-stage renal failure.

Table 4.7. Diagnoses to consider when foamy macrophages are found within the airspaces in a lung biopsy or resection specimen

Cause of foamy macrophages within airspaces	Key pathologic findings	Key clinical or radiologic findings
Post-obstructive (endogenous lipoid pneumonia)	Foamy macrophages with fine vacuoles Airway obstruction by mass, or bronchial/bronchiolar disease (bronchiectasis, bronchiolitis, hypersensitivity pneumonitis)	Evidence of airway disease or obstruction (airway-obstructing mass, bronchiectasis, small airway disease)
Exogenous lipoid pneumonia	Foamy macrophages with large, coarse vacuoles Similar macrophages within interstitium Interstitial fibrosis See Figures 4.18, 4.19 and 4.20	Asymptomatic, or fever, weight loss, dyspnea, cough Often reflux or other factors predisposing to aspiration Ground-glass opacities, consolidation, crazy-paving pattern or mass mimicking cancer Bilateral disease more common (79%) Predilection for lower lobes, but any lobe may be involved May contain fat May be PET-positive History of using liquid paraffin (for constipation), mineral oil, oily nose drops, petroleum jelly (Vaseline), laxatives, spray lubricant, Vicks Vaporub, lip balm, lip gloss, hand lotion
Storage disorders	Finely vacuolated macrophages (Niemann–Pick) Large macrophages with striated cytoplasm, "crumpled tissue paper" appearance, cohesive groups (Gaucher) Macrophages within interstitium (Niemann–Pick and Gaucher) or capillaries (Gaucher) Admixture with eosinophilic macrophages (Gaucher) Ciliated cells with foamy cytoplasm (Niemann–Pick type B)	Usually diagnosed on the basis of extrapulmonary disease and enzyme studies Clinical evidence of sphingomyelinase (Niemann–Pick disease) or glucocerebrosidase (Gaucher disease) deficiency Adults, 23 to 53 years (Niemann–Pick), infants, children or young adults (Gaucher) Diffuse bilateral ground-glass opacities (Niemann–Pick)
Amiodarone exposure or toxicity	No specific pathologic findings Type 2 pneumocytes may be vacuolated There may be acute lung injury, lymphoid hyperplasia or increased eosinophils	History of amiodarone intake See Chapter 5 for general principles in diagnosis of drug toxicity

Idiopathic pulmonary hemosiderosis is traditionally associated with a poor outcome (median survival 2.5 years), but a recent study with a mean follow-up period of 17 years found that 80% of children who survive have a normal life in the long term.

Sample diagnosis on pathology report

Hemosiderin-filled macrophages combined with alveolar septal thickening by capillaries in a patient with congestive heart failure:

Lung, left upper lobe, surgical biopsy – Chronic congestive changes.

Blood and hemosiderin-filled macrophages without an obvious cause such as capillaritis:

Lung, right upper lobe, surgical biopsy – Numerous intra-alveolar hemosiderin-laden macrophages (See comment).

Blood and hemosiderin-filled macrophages with capillaritis:

Lung, left lower lobe, surgical biopsy – Alveolar hemorrhage with necrotizing capillaritis (See comment).

Foamy macrophages within airspaces

Foamy macrophages are very common within airspaces. Unfortunately, in most cases they are quite non-specific. In a few situations, their identification is characteristic or helpful, and may be a clue to the correct diagnosis. The main causes of intra-alveolar foamy macrophages are listed in Table 4.7.

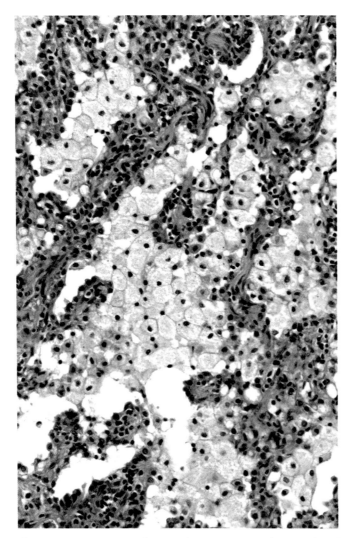

Figure 4.17. Foamy macrophages within airspaces in endogenous lipoid pneumonia. Numerous macrophages with fine cytoplasmic vacuoles fill the airspaces. This focus was adjacent to an area of bronchiectasis.

Endogenous lipoid pneumonia is not a single clinico-pathologic entity. It is simply a pathologic finding that occurs in lung parenchyma distal to obstructed or narrowed airways. It is thought that airway narrowing impedes the normal egress of macrophages from the airways, predisposing to cellular stasis and subsequent degeneration. Other macrophages then phagocytose the lipid-rich cellular debris, resulting in the characteristic appearance. The cells from which the lipid is derived are endogenous, hence the term endogenous lipoid pneumonia. The same principle is thought to underlie the presence of foamy macrophages in a wide variety of small airway disorders. The other main lesion in the differential diagnosis is *exogenous lipoid pneumonia*, which is a consequence of chronic aspiration of oily, lipid-rich substances into the lung. The word "exogenous" refers to the fact that these substances are foreign to the body.

Major diagnostic findings
See Table 4.7, and Figures 4.17 to 4.20.

Variable pathologic findings
See Table 4.7.

Diagnostic work-up
No special stains are required for the differential diagnosis. If the macrophages appear epithelioid or vaguely granulomatous, or if the patient is immunocompromised, special stains for microorganisms (AFB and GMS) should be performed.

Clinical profile
See Table 4.7.

Radiologic findings
See Table 4.7.

Differential diagnosis
See Table 4.7.

Treatment and prognosis
Treatment of exogenous lipoid pneumonia consists of cessation of exposure. In one recent large study, 46% improved, 25% were stable and 21% deteriorated. Potential complications include fibrosis, repeated episodes of infection and superinfection with atypical mycobacteria or *Aspergillus*.

Sample diagnosis on pathology report
In exogenous lipoid pneumonia:
    Lung, right upper lobe, surgical biopsy – Exogenous lipoid pneumonia (See comment).
    In post-obstructive pneumonia:
    Lung, right upper lobe, transbronchial biopsy – Chronic bronchiolitis and intra-alveolar foamy macrophages (See comment).
    If the patient is taking amiodarone:
    Lung, right middle lobe, transbronchial biopsy – Acute lung injury with numerous intra-alveolar foamy macrophages (See comment).

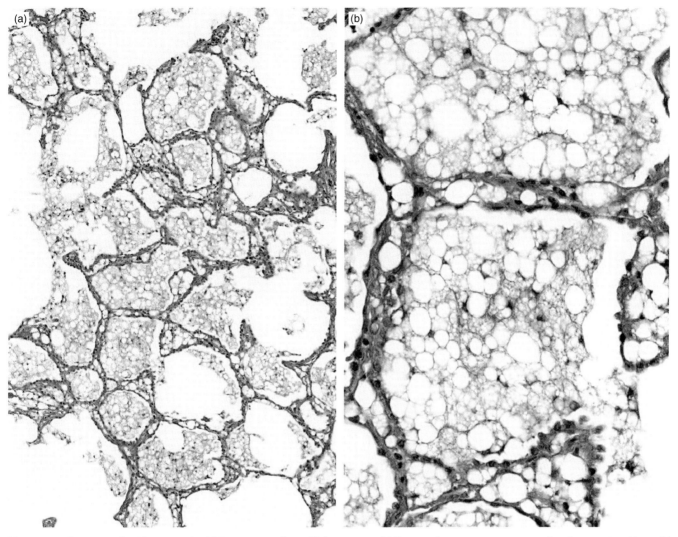

Figure 4.18. Exogenous lipoid pneumonia. (a) Foamy macrophages fill the airspaces. **(b)** The cytoplasm contains coarse vacuoles of varying sizes. Many of the vacuoles are quite large. This woman was taking mineral oil for chronic constipation. She stopped using the oil and received prednisone. Two years later, *Mycobacterium abscessus* was isolated in a sputum culture. Case courtesy of Dr. AV Arrossi.

References

Pulmonary alveolar proteinosis

Buechner HA, Ansari A. Acute silico-proteinosis. A new pathologic variant of acute silicosis in sandblasters, characterized by histologic features resembling alveolar proteinosis. *Chest* 1969;**55**:274–84.

Campo I, Mariani F, Rodi G, *et al.* Assessment and management of pulmonary alveolar proteinosis in a reference center. *Orphanet J Rare Dis* 2013;**8**:40.

Corsello BF, Choi H. Basophilic staining in pulmonary alveolar proteinosis. Report of three cases. *Arch Pathol Lab Med* 1984;**108**:68–70.

Frazier AA, Franks TJ, Cooke EO, Mohammed T-LH, Pugatch RD, Galvin JR.

From the archives of the AFIP. Pulmonary alveolar proteinosis. *RadioGraphics* 2008;**28**:883–899.

Goldstein MS, Kavuru MS, Curtis-McCarthy P, Christie HA, Farver C, Stoller JK. Pulmonary alveolar proteinosis. Clinical features and outcomes. *Chest* 1998;**114**:1357–62.

Murch CR, Carr DH. Computed tomography appearances of pulmonary alveolar proteinosis. *Clin Radiol* 1989;**40**:240–3.

Rosen SH, Castleman B, Liebow AA. Pulmonary alveolar proteinosis. *N Engl J Med* 1958;**258**:1123–42.

Seymour JF, Presneill JJ. Pulmonary alveolar proteinosis. Progress in the first 44 years. *Am J Respir Crit Care Med* 2002;**166**:215–35.

Tazawa R, Inoue Y, Arai T, *et al.* Duration of benefit in patients with autoimmune

pulmonary alveolar proteinosis after inhaled granulocyte-macrophage colony-stimulating factor therapy. *Chest* 2014;**145**:729–37.

Verma H, Nicholson AG, Kerr KM, *et al.* Alveolar proteinosis with hypersensitivity pneumonitis: a new clinical phenotype. *Respirology* 2010;**15**:1197–202.

Eosinophilic pneumonia

Allen JN, Pacht ER, Gadek JE, Davis WB. Acute eosinophilic pneumonia as a reversible cause of noninfectious respiratory failure. *N Engl J Med* 1989;**321**:569–74.

Carrington CB, Addington WW, Goff AM, *et al.* Chronic eosinophilic pneumonia. *N Engl J Med* 1969;**280**:787–98.

Cottin V, Cordier J-F. Eosinophilic lung diseases. *Immunol Allergy Clin N Am* 2012;**32**:557–86.

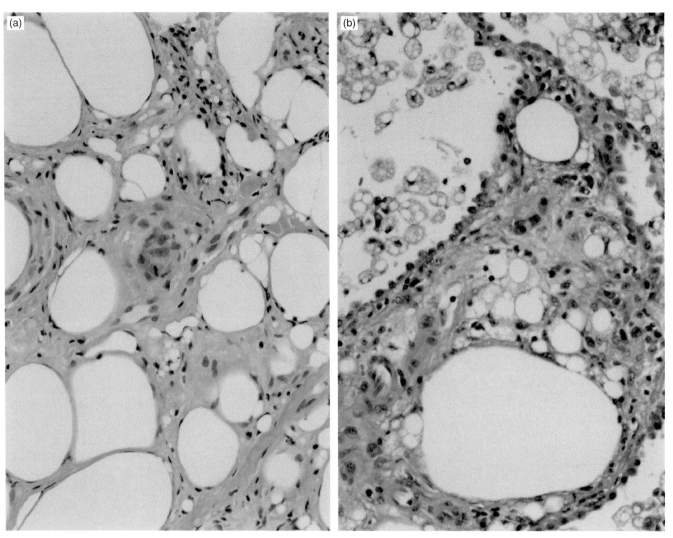

Figure 4.19. Exogenous lipoid pneumonia. (a) This needle biopsy shows fibrosis and large vacuoles within the interstitium. This woman had bilateral PET-positive masses. She was forced to take mineral oil for weight loss when she was a child. **(b)** This image from a different case shows foamy macrophages within airspaces (top) as well as the interstitium. Two large vacuoles are additionally seen in the interstitium.

Fox B, Seed WA. Chronic eosinophilic pneumonia. *Thorax* 1980;**35**:570–80.

Grantham JG, Meadows JA III, Gleich GJ. Chronic eosinophilic pneumonia. Evidence for eosinophil degranulation and release of major basic protein. *Am J Med* 1986;**80**:89–94.

Jederlinic PJ, Sicilian L, Gaensler EA. Chronic eosinophilic pneumonia. A report of 19 cases and a review of the literature. *Medicine (Baltimore)* 1988;**67**:154–62.

Liebow AA, Carrington CB. The eosinophilic pneumonias. *Medicine* 1969;**48**:251–85.

Marchand E, Reynaud-Gaubert M, Lauque D, *et al.* Idiopathic chronic eosinophilic pneumonia. A clinical and follow-up study of 62 cases. *Medicine* 1998;**77**:299–312.

Olopade CO, Crotty TB, Douglas WW, Colby TV, Sur S. Chronic eosinophilic pneumonia and idiopathic bronchiolitis obliterans organizing pneumonia:

comparison of eosinophil number and degranulation by immunofluorescence staining for eosinophil-derived major basic protein. *Mayo Clin Proc* 1990;**70**:137–45.

Tazelaar HD, Linz LJ, Colby TV, Myers JL, Limper AH. Acute eosinophilic pneumonia: histopathologic findings in nine patients. *Am J Respir Crit Care Med* 1997;**155**:296–302.

Acute bronchopneumonia

Blackmon JA, Chandler FW, Cherry WB, *et al.* Legionellosis. *Am J Pathol* 1981;**103**:429–64.

Bonifacio SL, Kitterman JA, Ursell PC. Pseudomonas pneumonia in infants: an autopsy study. *Hum Pathol* 2003;**34**:929–38.

Casey MB, Tazelaar HD, Myers JL, *et al.* Noninfectious lung pathology in patients

with Crohn's disease. *Am J Surg Pathol* 2003;**27**:213–9.

Hayden RT, Uhl JR, Qian X, *et al.* Direct detection of *Legionella* species from bronchoalveolar lavage and open lung biopsy specimens: comparison of LightCycler PCR, in situ hybridization, direct fluorescence antigen detection, and culture. *J Clin Microbiol* 2001;**39**:2618–26.

Hernandez FJ, Kirby BD, Stanley TM, Edelstein PH. Legionnaires' disease. Postmortem pathologic findings of 20 cases. *Am J Clin Pathol* 1980;**73**:488–95.

Mukhopadhyay S, Katzenstein AL. Pulmonary disease due to aspiration of food and other particulate matter: a clinicopathologic study of 59 cases diagnosed on biopsy or resection specimens. *Am J Surg Pathol* 2007;**31**:752–9.

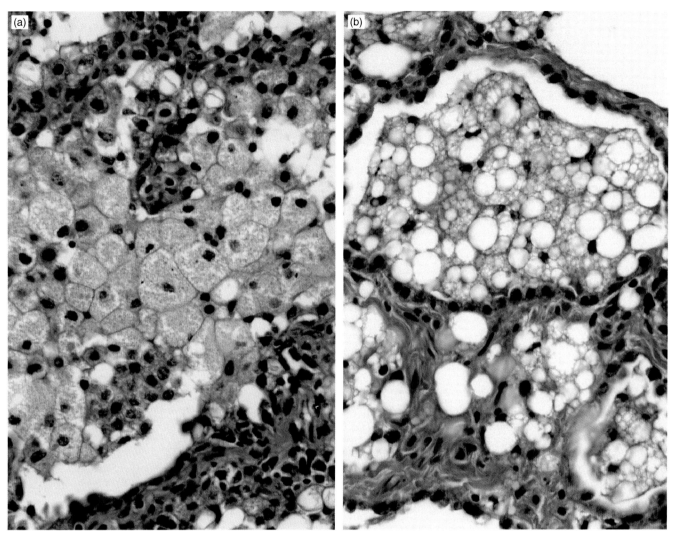

Figure 4.20. Endogenous lipoid pneumonia vs. exogenous lipoid pneumonia (identical magnification). (a) Foamy macrophages with finely vacuolated cytoplasm. **(b)** Foamy macrophages with coarsely vacuolated cytoplasm. Note presence of vacuolated cells within the interstitium, and interstitial fibrosis.

Mukhopadhyay S, Phillip AT, Stoppacher R. Pathologic findings in novel influenza A (H1N1) virus ("swine flu") infection. Contrasting clinical manifestations and lung pathology in two fatal cases. *Am J Clin Pathol* 2010;**133**:380–7.

Paddock CD, Sanden GN, Cherry JD, *et al.* Pathology and pathogenesis of fatal *Bordetella pertussis* infection in infants. *Clin Infect Dis* 2008;**47**:328–38.

Theaker JM, Tobin JOH, Jones SEC, *et al.* Immunohistological detection of *Legionella pneumophila* in lung sections. *J Clin Pathol* 1987;**40**:143–6.

Winn WC Jr, Myerowitz RL. The pathology of the *Legionella* pneumonias. A review of 74 cases and the literature. *Hum Pathol* 1981;**12**:401–22.

Smoker's macrophages (respiratory bronchiolitis, respiratory bronchiolitis–interstitial lung disease, desquamative interstitial pneumonia)

Agius RM, Rutman A, Knight RK, Cole PJ. Human pulmonary alveolar macrophages with smokers' inclusions. *Br J Exp Pathol* 1986;**67**:407–13.

Brody AR, Craighead JE. Cytoplasmic inclusions in pulmonary macrophages of cigarette smokers. *Lab Invest* 1975;**32**:125–32.

Fraig M, Shreesha U, Savici D, Katzenstein AL. Respiratory bronchiolitis: a clinicopathologic study in current smokers, ex-smokers and never-smokers. *Am J Surg Pathol* 2002;**26**:647–53.

Gill A. Bong lung: regular smokers of cannabis show relatively distinctive histologic changes that predispose to pneumothorax. *Am J Surg Pathol* 2005;**29**:980–1.

Katzenstein A-LA, Mukhopadhyay S, Zanardi C, Dexter EE. Clinically occult interstitial fibrosis in smokers: classification and significance of a surprisingly common finding in lobectomy specimens. *Hum Pathol* 2010;**41**:316–25.

Katzenstein AL. Smoking-related interstitial fibrosis (SRIF): pathologic findings and distinction from other chronic fibrosing lung diseases. *J Clin Pathol* 2013;**66**:882–7.

Myers JL, Veal CF Jr, Shin MS, Katzenstein AL. Respiratory bronchiolitis causing interstitial lung disease. A clinicopathologic study of six cases. *Am Rev Respir Dis* 1987;**135**:880–4.

Niewoehner DE, Kleinerman J, Rice DB. Pathologic changes in the peripheral airways of young cigarette smokers. *N Engl J Med* 1974;**291**:755–8.

Yousem SA, Colby TV, Gaensler EA. Respiratory bronchiolitis-associated interstitial lung disease and its relationship to desquamative interstitial pneumonia. *Mayo Clin Proc* 1989;**64**:1373–80.

Yousem SA. Respiratory bronchiolitis-associated interstitial lung disease with fibrosis is a lesion distinct from fibrotic non-specific interstitial pneumonia: a proposal. *Mod Pathol* 2006;**19**:1474–9.

Hemosiderin-laden macrophages and/or blood within the airspaces

Adem C, Aubry MC, Tazelaar HD, Myers JL. Metastatic angiosarcoma masquerading as diffuse pulmonary hemorrhage: clinicopathologic analysis of 7 new patients. *Arch Pathol Lab Med* 2001;**125**:1562–5.

Clainche LL, Bourgeois ML, Fauroux B, *et al.* Long-term outcome of idiopathic pulmonary hemosiderosis in children. *Medicine* 2000;**79**:318–26.

Colby TV, Fukuoka J, Ewaskow SP, Helmers R, Leslie KO. Pathologic approach to pulmonary hemorrhage. *Ann Diagn Pathol* 2001;**5**:309–19.

Greco A, Rizzo MI, De Virgilio A, *et al.* Goodpasture's syndrome: a clinical update. *Autoimmun Rev* 2015;**14**:246–53.

Iaochimescu OC, Stoller JK. Diffuse alveolar hemorrhage: diagnosing it and finding the cause. *Clev Clin J Med* 2008;**75**:258–80.

Lombard CM, Colby TV, Elliott CG. Surgical pathology of the lung in anti-basement antibody-associated Goodpasture's syndrome. *Hum Pathol* 1989;**20**:445–51.

Myers JL, Katzenstein AL. Wegener's granulomatosis presenting with massive pulmonary hemorrhage and capillaritis. *Am J Surg Pathol* 1987;**11**:895–8.

Travis WD, Carpenter HA, Lie JT. Diffuse pulmonary hemorrhage. An uncommon manifestation of Wegener's granulomatosis. *Am J Surg Pathol* 1987;**11**:702–8.

Travis WD, Colby TV, Lombard C, Carpenter HA. A clinicopathologic study of 34 cases of diffuse pulmonary hemorrhage with lung biopsy confirmation. *Am J Surg Pathol* 1990;**14**:1112–5.

Yang HM, Lai CK, Patel J, *et al.* Irreversible intrapulmonary vascular changes after pulmonary vein stenosis complicating catheter ablation for atrial fibrillation. *Cardiovasc Pathol* 2007;**16**:51–5.

Foamy macrophages within airspaces

Amir G, Ron N. Pulmonary pathology in Gaucher's disease. *Hum Pathol* 1999;**30**:666–70.

Burke M, Fraser R. Obstructive pneumonitis: a pathologic and pathogenetic reappraisal. *Radiology* 1988;**166**:699–704.

Garlassi E, Rossi G, Bedini A, Richeldi L. Unexpected identification of bilateral masses in an asymptomatic heavy smoker. *Thorax* 2010;**65**:846.

Gondouin A, Manzoni P, Ranfaing E, *et al.* Exogenous lipoid pneumonia: a retrospective multicentre study of 44 cases in France. *Eur Respir J* 1996;**9**:1463–9.

Kennedy JD, Costello P, Balikian JP, Herman PG. Exogenous lipoid pneumonia. *AJR Am J Roentgenol* 1981;**136**:1145–9.

Larsen BT, Vaszar LT, Colby TV, Tazelaar HD. Lymphoid hyperplasia and eosinophilic pneumonia as histologic manifestations of amiodarone-induced lung toxicity. *Am J Surg Pathol* 2012;**36**:509–16.

Marchiori E, Zanetti G, Mano CM, Irion KL, Daltro PA, Hochhegger B. Lipoid pneumonia in 53 patients after aspiration of mineral oil: comparison of high-resolution computed tomography findings in adults and children. *J Comput Assist Tomogr* 2010;**34**:9–12.

Nicholson AG, Florio R, Hansell DM, *et al.* Pulmonary involvement by Niemann-Pick disease. A report of six cases. *Histopathology* 2006;**38**:596–603.

Spickard A 3rd, Hirschmann JV. Exogenous lipoid pneumonia. *Arch Intern Med* 1994;**154**:686–92.

Verbeken EK, Demedts M, Vanwing J, Deneffe G, Lauweryns JM. Pulmonary phospholipid accumulation distal to an obstructed bronchus. A morphologic study. *Arch Pathol Lab Med* 1989;**113**:886–90.

Chapter 5

Predominantly interstitial lung disease

Diagnosis and classification of interstitial lung disease is a common indication for lung biopsies, both transbronchial and surgical. The unifying feature of these diseases is pathologic evidence of interstitial involvement, usually manifesting as widening of the alveolar septa. This chapter addresses the differential diagnosis of interstitial abnormalities. Some diseases – such as pulmonary alveolar proteinosis and respiratory bronchiolitis-interstitial lung disease – are classified as interstitial lung diseases based on clinical and radiologic features. However, they are actually airspace diseases with minimal or no pathologic involvement of the interstitium. These are discussed in Chapter 4. Figure 5.1 shows side-by-side comparisons at identical magnification of a few common types of interstitial lung disease.

The classic clinical findings of interstitial lung disease include dyspnea, cough, bilateral lung infiltrates on chest imaging and restrictive changes on pulmonary function tests. However, in practice, the complete spectrum of symptoms, signs, radiologic findings and pulmonary function abnormalities in interstitial lung disease is exceedingly wide, and frequently deviates from this stereotype. In general, the clinical features of interstitial lung disease are non-specific and do not provide a definitive diagnosis. Therefore, the diagnosis and classification of interstitial lung disease is based primarily on radiologic and pathologic findings.

The ever-expanding alphabet soup of acronyms in interstitial lung disease is arcane and difficult to master, especially for trainees, clinicians, radiologists and pathologists who only occasionally encounter these uncommon diseases. There are few conditions where so much angst and controversy surrounds nomenclature and classification of diseases that mostly lack effective therapies and are of unknown etiology. Traditional classifications of interstitial lung disease separate the "idiopathic interstitial pneumonias" from diseases of "known etiology" such as sarcoidosis or pulmonary Langerhans cell histiocytosis. However, the label "idiopathic" is applied arbitrarily. For example, UIP and NSIP are classified as *idiopathic interstitial pneumonias* because their etiology is usually unknown, but they also occur in the setting of connective tissue disease and other underlying conditions. Current classification schemes do not specify whether clinicians, radiologists or pathologists should decide if a given case of interstitial lung disease should be considered idiopathic or connective tissue disease-related. They also fail to define the precise requirements to "prove" an underlying etiology. The reason for this ambiguity is that assignment of etiology in most cases of interstitial lung disease is an arbitrary and subjective exercise.

In practice, the clinical work-up performed to unearth an etiology varies greatly from clinician to clinician. For example, many clinicians believe that patients who do not have clinical features of connective tissue disease at presentation should not undergo unnecessary "shotgun" serologic testing, whereas others perform extensive serologic testing even in the absence of clinical findings. The optimal approach remains unclear and is a matter of personal preference.

Multidisciplinary discussion (MDD) has been trumpeted in recent years as a solution for cases in which radiologic and pathologic diagnoses are discrepant, but in practice discrepancies often persist even after detailed face-to-face multidisciplinary discussion in which subspecialized expert radiologists and fellowship-trained pulmonary pathologists are shown each other's findings and presented with details of the clinical history. When multiple pulmonologists are present, clinical opinions often vary greatly from physician to physician. In these difficult cases, the so-called "consensus clinico-radiologic-pathologic (CRP) diagnosis" is an arbitrary judgement call made by the treating physician. The diagnostic accuracy of this process is questionable.

In practice, pathologists often interpret biopsies with little or no clinical information, and must be prepared to stand by their diagnosis, which should be rooted in well-defined pathologic criteria. The treating clinician can and must incorporate all available information to base treatment decisions on, but clinical features should not change the pathologic diagnosis. Useful practical tips for making a pathologic diagnosis in lung biopsies for interstitial lung disease can be found in a recent review (Katzenstein *et al, Hum Pathol* 2008).

Another problem with current classification systems is that clinicians and pathologists peruse the associated tables and expect to fit their case into one of the entities listed. However, the reality is that many cases do not fit into any of these groups and require descriptive diagnoses. Pathologists who turn to existing classifications for practical guidance on making a diagnosis do not get a sense of the entities that account for the majority of cases in practice (UIP, DAD, organizing pneumonia, pulmonary Langerhans cell histiocytosis, unclassifiable interstitial fibrosis) versus those that are rare (NSIP, acute interstitial pneumonia (AIP), RBILD) or virtually non-existent (LIP, DIP).

This chapter aims to address these problem areas. Algorithms for surgical pathologists faced with lung biopsies with interstitial abnormalities are provided in Figures 5.2, 5.3 and 5.4. Table 5.1 lists the most common entities that pathologists will encounter when evaluating lung biopsies for interstitial lung disease. Table 5.2 lists uncommon or rare

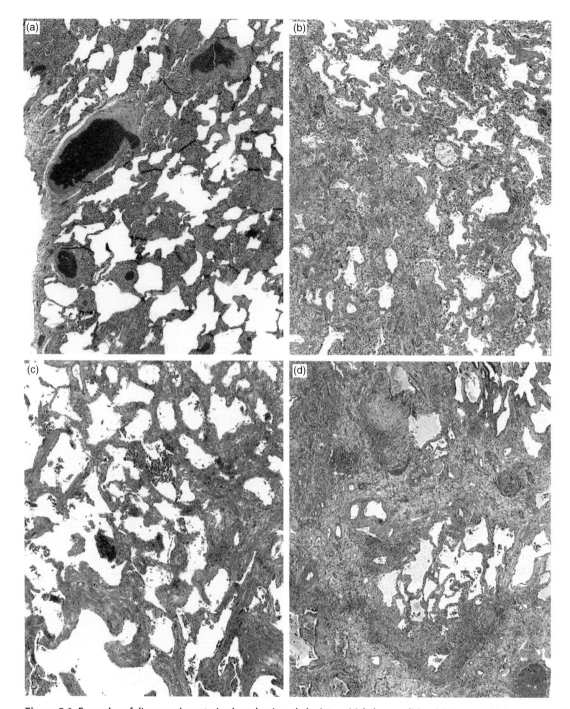

Figure 5.1. Examples of diseases characterized predominantly by interstitial abnormalities. (a) Hypersensitivity pneumonitis. **(b)** Diffuse alveolar damage. **(c)** Smoking-related interstitial fibrosis. **(d)** Usual interstitial pneumonia.

entities, some of which, such as desquamative interstitial pneumonia (DIP) and lymphoid interstitial pneumonia (LIP), are conceptually incorrect artifacts of a bygone era that have been largely replaced by other, better defined entities. Pearls and pitfalls related to interstitial lung disease are summarized in Table 5.3.

Usual interstitial pneumonia

Usual interstitial pneumonia (UIP) is a chronic fibrosing interstitial lung disease that represents the pathologic correlate of idiopathic pulmonary fibrosis (IPF). It is one of the most common forms of interstitial lung disease diagnosed by pathologists, rivalled only by sarcoidosis, organizing pneumonia and diffuse alveolar damage. UIP is a pathologic diagnosis, whereas IPF is a clinical term. According to current criteria, a radiologic or pathologic diagnosis of UIP is required for a clinical diagnosis of IPF. The history and evolution of the concepts of UIP and IPF – a fascinating topic – are outside the scope of this book.

The term UIP appears odd to those encountering it for the first time, since it neither mentions the main pathologic

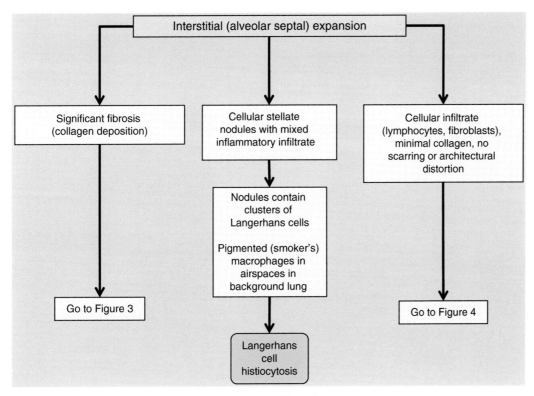

Figure 5.2. Algorithm for pathologic approach to interstitial lung disease.

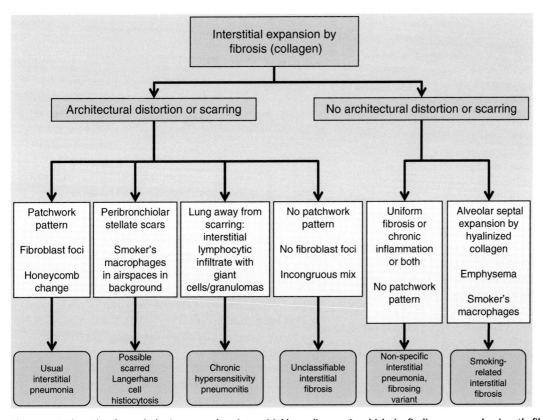

Figure 5.3. Algorithm for pathologic approach to interstitial lung diseases in which the findings are predominantly fibrotic.

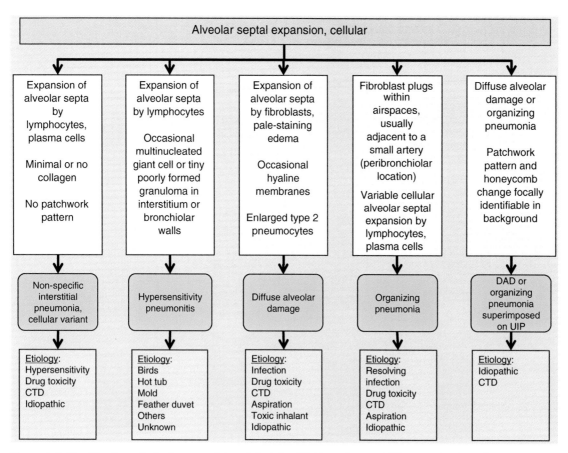

Figure 5.4. Algorithm for pathologic approach to cellular interstitial lung diseases. CTD, connective tissue disease.

feature of the disease (fibrosis) nor its etiology (unknown/idiopathic). The term dates back to histologic observations made by Dr. Averill Liebow in 1965. The word "usual" refers to the fact that UIP is the "usual" pathologic finding in patients with pulmonary fibrosis of unknown cause. The word "pneumonia" also causes confusion, since it is often interpreted as implying an infectious etiology. However, in the context of interstitial lung disease, "pneumonia" is used in a broader sense to denote "abnormality", which may include inflammation or fibrosis or both. This explains why the term "*idiopathic interstitial pneumonias*" has been used to lump together non-infectious fibrosing and inflammatory interstitial lung diseases of unknown etiology. The term "pneumonitis" as an alternative to "pneumonia" has not found much traction. The European equivalent – "cryptogenic fibrosing alveolitis" – conveyed the fibrosing nature of the process as well as the unknown etiology. However, it has fallen out of favor since the American Thoracic Society/European Respiratory Society (ATS/ERS) consensus statement in 2002, because the word "alveolitis" was felt to incorrectly focus on inflammation rather than fibrosis.

UIP is typically diagnosed in surgical lung biopsies obtained by open procedures or video-assisted thoracoscopic surgery (VATS). UIP is also encountered in lungs that have been removed at the time of lung transplantation for IPF. Transbronchial lung biopsies only rarely sample the full range of findings.

Major diagnostic findings

- Interstitial fibrosis in a "patchwork pattern" is the hallmark of UIP and is the most consistent histologic finding. It is also referred to as "spatial heterogeneity". It is characterized by abrupt juxtaposition of scarred lung with normal lung, or abrupt juxtaposition of different types of abnormalities (scarring and honeycomb change, for example) without a transition zone (Figure 5.1d and Figure 5.5). The term "patchwork" refers to the similarity of this low-magnification appearance to a quilt stitched together from a patchwork of smaller pieces.

- Parenchymal scarring (architectural distortion). The fibrosis in UIP may expand alveolar septa without distorting or obliterating lung architecture. More commonly, however, confluent fibrosis forms scars that distort lung architecture (Figure 5.6). These areas are essentially unrecognizable as lung tissue. Scarring is considered a form of architectural distortion, and is a key component in the diagnosis of UIP (Figure 5.7). At high magnification, the scarred areas contain collagen, hyperplastic smooth muscle fibers, small blood vessels and a few scattered lymphocytes (Figure 5.8). Although one expects fibrosis to be eosinophilic, the fibrosis in UIP scars is often light-staining, with a loose arrangement of collagen fibers.

Table 5.1. Common causes of interstitial lung disease

Pathologic diagnosis	Acronym	Key pathologic findings	Most common clinical setting
Usual interstitial pneumonia	UIP	Interstitial fibrosis in patchwork pattern Fibroblast foci Scarring Honeycomb change	Idiopathic pulmonary fibrosis (IPF)
Organizing pneumonia	OP or BOOP	Plugs of fibroblasts within airspaces in a pale-staining background	Abnormal residuum of prior pneumonia
Diffuse alveolar damage	DAD	Hyaline membranes (acute stage) Diffuse interstitial widening by edema and fibroblast proliferation (organizing stage)	Sick patient on ventilator with bilateral ground-glass opacities
Pulmonary Langerhans cell histiocytosis	PLCH	Irregular or stellate interstitial nodules containing sheets of Langerhans cells Smoker's macrophages in background lung	Multiple bilateral tiny (millimeter-sized) lung nodules
Smoking-related interstitial fibrosis	SRIF	Hyalinized interstitial fibrosis with glassy appearance Emphysema and smoker's macrophages	Incidental finding in lobectomy specimens with cancer and emphysema (clinically occult)
Hypersensitivity pneumonitis	HP or HSP	Mild expansion of alveolar septa by lymphocytes, more prominent around respiratory bronchioles and alveolar ducts Variable findings: foamy macrophages in peribronchiolar airspaces, occasional multinucleated giant cells or tiny, poorly formed granulomas, rare foci of organizing pneumonia	Bilateral ground-glass opacities in a never-smoker with birds in the home
Usual interstitial pneumonia with superimposed diffuse alveolar damage/ organizing pneumonia/ mixed acute lung injury	N/A	Features of UIP in background lung Hyaline membranes or diffuse interstitial edema and fibroblast proliferation or organizing pneumonia or mix of acute changes	Acute respiratory failure Acute exacerbation of idiopathic pulmonary fibrosis
Unclassifiable interstitial fibrosis (descriptive diagnosis)	None	Interstitial fibrosis that does not meet criteria for UIP, NSIP or other known forms of interstitial lung disease	Interstitial lung disease Connective tissue disease
Combined pulmonary fibrosis and emphysema	CPFE	UIP with unusually enlarged airspaces caused by emphysema	Interstitial lung disease in patients with emphysema
Non-specific interstitial pneumonia	NSIP	Uniform fibrosis and/or chronic inflammation without "patchwork pattern" No scarring or honeycomb change	Interstitial lung disease
Connective tissue disease-related interstitial lung disease	CTD-ILD	NSIP, UIP or unclassifiable interstitial fibrosis	Interstitial lung disease in individual with known connective tissue disease
Drug-related interstitial lung disease	None	Cellular chronic interstitial pneumonia (cellular NSIP), mild diffuse interstitial expansion by fibroblasts or edema (acute lung injury), diffuse alveolar damage, foamy macrophages in airspaces, UIP or unclassifiable fibrosis No pathologic evidence of infection or alternative specific diagnosis	Interstitial lung disease in individual taking drug known to be associated with lung toxicity Exclusion of alternative etiologies such as infection Regression of interstitial changes after cessation of therapy

Table 5.2. Rare causes of interstitial lung disease

Pathologic diagnosis	Acronym	Key pathologic findings	Most common clinical setting
Alveolar septal amyloidosis	None	Diffuse expansion of alveolar septa by glassy, acellular amorphous eosinophilic material Amyloid deposition in blood vessels Congo red positive	Known systemic amyloidosis
Pleuroparenchymal fibroelastosis	PPFE	Elastotic fibrosis, mainly subpleural	Interstitial lung disease
Lymphoid interstitial pneumonia	LIP	Striking interstitial expansion by lymphocytes and plasma cells	Interstitial lung disease in Sjögren syndrome or HIV
Hard metal lung disease	HMLD, GIP	Chronic inflammation or fibrosis in interstitium Multinucleated giant cells in airspaces Emperipolesis	Metal grinder
Hermansky–Pudlak syndrome	None	UIP or unclassifiable fibrosis Rarely NSIP Vacuolated type 2 pneumocytes	Interstitial fibrosis in Puerto Rican individual with oculocutaneous albinism
Desquamative interstitial pneumonia[a]	DIP	Diffuse filling of alveolar spaces by macrophages[b]	Interstitial lung disease in smoker

[a] Avoid this diagnosis unless all alternative possibilities can be excluded. Consider classifying as respiratory bronchiolitis (RB), RBILD or SRIF. A descriptive diagnosis is preferable. See Chapter 4 for details.
[b] A non-specific finding that can be seen in virtually any type of interstitial lung disease.

DIP – desquamative interstitial pneumonia; GIP – giant cell interstitial pneumonia; HMLD – hard metal lung disease; IPF – idiopathic pulmonary fibrosis; NSIP – non-specific interstitial pneumonia; RBILD – respiratory bronchiolitis-interstitial lung disease; SRIF – smoking-related interstitial fibrosis; UIP – usual interstitial pneumonia.

Table 5.3. Pearls and pitfalls in interstitial lung disease

UIP is the most common pathologic diagnosis in surgical lung biopsies performed for interstitial lung disease

IPF is a clinical diagnosis. UIP is a pathologic diagnosis

Most cases of UIP correspond to IPF

Radiologists can diagnose UIP when honeycomb change is present, but the diagnosis is usually missed when honeycomb change is microscopic (present on biopsy but not appreciable on CT)

An acute clinical presentation does not exclude underlying UIP

Granulomas and inflammation do not necessarily exclude UIP

If strict criteria are followed, true NSIP is very uncommon

Many cases of UIP show NSIP-like changes in some lobes. Corollaries: (1) many cases of NSIP represent poorly sampled UIP; (2) when there is UIP in one lobe and NSIP in another, the diagnosis is UIP

Do not diagnose NSIP if there is evidence of honeycomb change radiologically

Do not allow a radiologic "diagnosis" of NSIP to deter you from making a diagnosis of UIP if the pathologic findings are classic. A radiologic diagnosis of NSIP is notoriously inaccurate

Some cases of interstitial lung disease cannot be classified even after surgical lung biopsy

Hypersensitivity pneumonitis is a disease of lymphocytes, not eosinophils

In hypersensitivity pneumonitis, "bronchiolitis" refers to involvement of the smallest, most distal and most subtle bronchioles (respiratory bronchioles and alveolar ducts)

Do not diagnose RBILD, NSIP, DIP or LIP in transbronchial lung biopsies

Table 5.3. (cont.)

Large numbers of intra-alveolar macrophages can be found in a wide variety of unrelated lung diseases. Desquamative interstitial pneumonia (DIP) is an outdated, conceptually incorrect misnomer. In 2015, most cases that appear to be "DIP-like" can and should be classified as other specific forms of interstitial lung disease

RBILD is not a pure pathologic diagnosis, i.e., it cannot be diagnosed by pathologists in the absence of clinical and radiologic information

By definition, interstitial fibrosis is not a feature of emphysema. If you see significant interstitial fibrosis along with emphysema, consider smoking-related interstitial fibrosis (SRIF) or combined pulmonary fibrosis and emphysema (UIP + emphysema)

Do not diagnose lymphoid interstitial pneumonia (LIP) unless MALT lymphoma has been conclusively ruled out, and there is diffuse and striking alveolar septal expansion in a surgical lung biopsy

Outside the setting of Sjögren syndrome or HIV/AIDS, LIP is vanishingly rare

DIP – desquamative interstitial pneumonia; IPF – idiopathic pulmonary fibrosis; LIP – lymphoid interstitial pneumonia; NSIP – non-specific interstitial pneumonia; RBILD – respiratory bronchiolitis-interstitial lung disease; SRIF – smoking-related interstitial fibrosis; UIP – usual interstitial pneumonia.

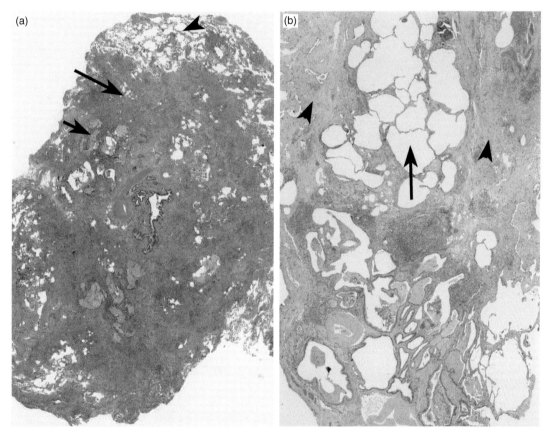

Figure 5.5. Patchwork pattern in UIP. (a) Low magnification, showing juxtaposition of normal lung (arrowhead) and scarred lung (long arrow). The latter is in turn juxtaposed to an area of microscopic honeycomb change (small arrow). **(b)** Another case, with an island of normal lung (arrow) abruptly juxtaposed to scarred lung (arrowheads). Note microscopic honeycomb change at bottom of field.

- Fibroblast foci (singular: fibroblast focus) are present in nearly all cases of UIP and are thought to be central to its pathogenesis. In contrast to the common type of fibrosis (collagen deposition), they are characterized by fibroblast proliferation. A fibroblast focus is a tiny interstitial aggregate of spindle-shaped fibroblasts and myofibroblasts in a pale-staining, myxoid background (Figure 5.9). Fibroblast foci are located exclusively within the interstitium. The side of the fibroblast focus facing the airspace is often dome-shaped, and is separated from the airspace by type 2 pneumocytes; the opposite side may be flat or curved, and blends with the interstitium. The overlying epithelium may occasionally show squamous metaplasia. Inflammatory cells are often present adjacent to fibroblast foci, but are not prominent within them. Fibroblast foci tend to be most numerous in areas of fibrosis, severe architectural distortion and honeycomb change, but they are also found in areas of minimal

191

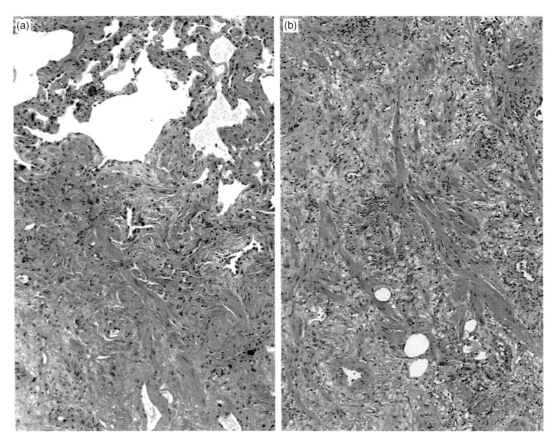

Figure 5.6. Interstitial fibrosis and parenchymal scarring in UIP. (a) Compare interstitial fibrosis without architectural distortion (top) to parenchymal scarring with architectural distortion (bottom). **(b)** Scarred parenchyma from another case of UIP. Note absence of normal lung architecture. Hyperplastic smooth muscle fibers are visible within the scarred areas in both pictures.

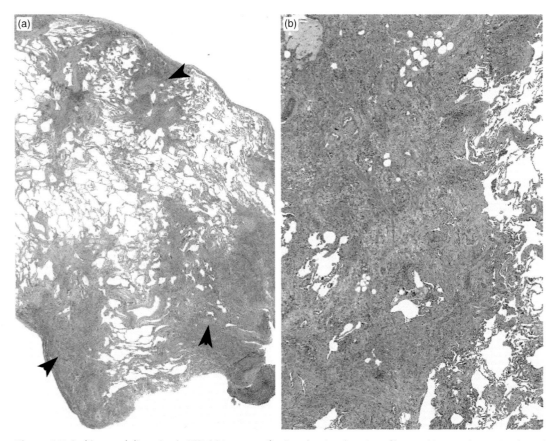

Figure 5.7. Architectural distortion in UIP. (a) Low magnification, showing distortion of lung architecture by scarring (arrowheads). **(b)** Large area of scarring unrecognizable as lung is at left. Contrast to relatively preserved lung, at right.

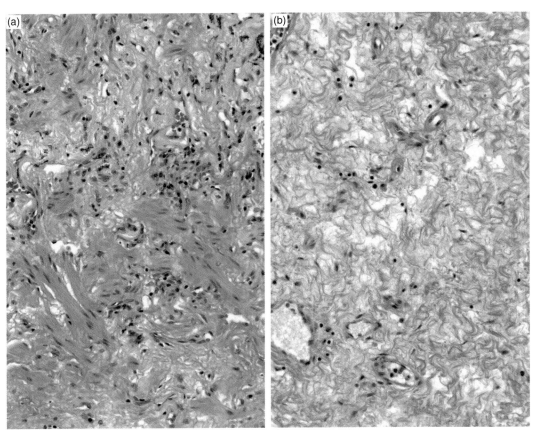

Figure 5.8. Scarred areas in UIP at high magnification. (a) Hyperplastic smooth muscle fibers. **(b)** Pale appearance, with loose arrangement of collagen bundles.

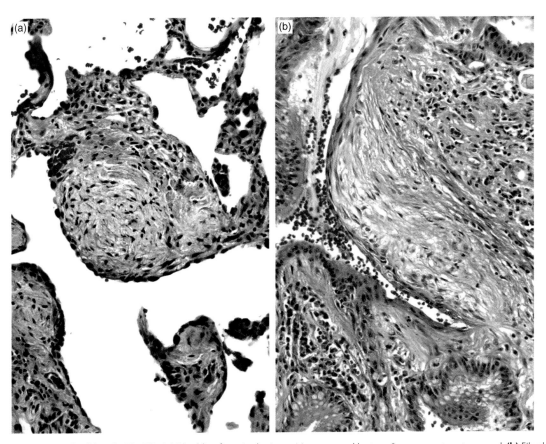

Figure 5.9. Fibroblast foci in UIP. (a) Fibroblast focus in the interstitium, covered by type 2 pneumocytes at one end. **(b)** Fibroblast focus in fibrotic lung.

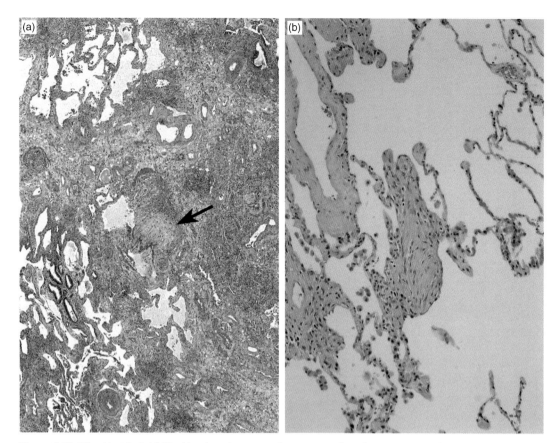

Figure 5.10. Fibroblast foci. (a) Fibroblast focus in an area of severe parenchymal scarring (arrow). **(b)** Fibroblast focus in less affected lung.

fibrosis and inflammation (Figure 5.10). Fibroblast foci are thought to represent microscopic foci of acute lung injury (a mini-version of organizing DAD), responsible for initiating and propagating fibrosis in UIP. Some studies claim that large numbers of fibroblast foci correlate with a more aggressive disease course and worse prognosis but this has been disputed by others. Fibroblast foci can also be found in other fibrosing interstitial lung diseases such as NSIP, chronic hypersensitivity pneumonitis and SRIF, but are usually few in number in these settings.

- Honeycomb change is a form of architectural distortion seen in most cases of UIP and some cases of other interstitial lung diseases with advanced fibrosis. However, it is most common and most extensive in UIP. The earliest forms of honeycomb change can only be appreciated microscopically (microscopic honeycomb change), while more advanced forms can be seen grossly as well as on high-resolution CT scans. Microscopically, it is characterized by the presence of clusters of enlarged, irregular airspaces lined at least partially by bronchiolar (ciliated columnar) epithelium, and usually filled with mucin (Figure 5.11). The enlarged airspaces may also contain neutrophils, macrophages and cell debris. Squamous metaplasia may occur in the lining epithelium. Honeycomb change often develops in the vicinity of bronchioles, and can be misinterpreted as adenocarcinoma

or bronchiectasis. The ciliated lining helps to separate the lesion from adenocarcinoma. In contrast to bronchiectasis, which is a single dilated and inflamed bronchus, the airspaces of honeycomb change are multiple and clustered. They are also significantly less inflamed, and their lumens contain mucin rather than inflammatory debris (Figure 5.12). Although the presence of a respiratory lining causes a superficial resemblance to dilated bronchioles, the dilated spaces in honeycomb change are clustered and haphazardly arranged, lack a partner artery, and are not surrounded by well-organized smooth muscle bundles (Figure 5.13). Clearance of mucin and other debris from areas of honeycomb change is poor, resulting in increasing accumulation of mucin and progressive dilatation of the spaces. Eventually, the spaces become large enough to be visible grossly or on high-resolution CT scans, this being a key feature in the radiologic diagnosis of UIP. Honeycomb change is a difficult concept to grasp since logic dictates that end-stage fibrosis should manifest as increasing amounts of collagen. It seems counterintuitive that end-stage fibrosis would be associated with dilated, mucin-filled, respiratory epithelium-lined airspaces. Despite the fact that this phenomenon is difficult to explain, the practical reality is that honeycomb change is a common and diagnostically important feature in UIP. When visible grossly, it is most prominent in subpleural lung parenchyma, where it appears as

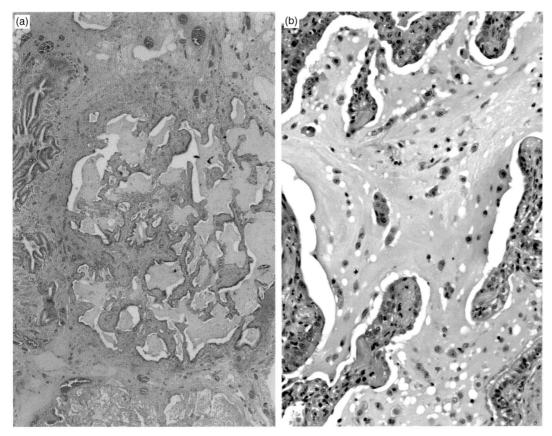

Figure 5.11. Honeycomb change in UIP. (a) Low magnification, showing cluster of dilated airspaces filled with mucin. The process has completely replaced the alveolated lung. Note fibrosis in the background and a bronchiole at the left edge of the picture. **(b)** Higher magnification of honeycomb change from a different case, showing mucin containing a few macrophages and neutrophils. Ciliated columnar epithelium is visible at the top left and bottom right.

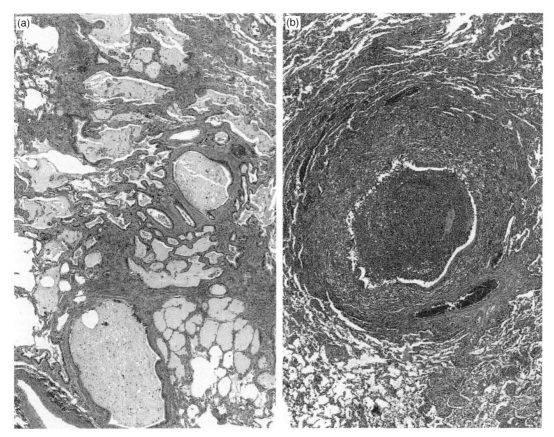

Figure 5.12. Honeycomb change vs. bronchiectasis. (a) Honeycomb change. Clustered, mucin-filled, ciliated-epithelium-lined, dilated spaces are present in a fibrotic background. **(b)** Bronchiectasis. Single dilated and severely inflamed bronchus. The lumen contains an acute inflammatory exudate rather than mucin. There is no significant fibrosis.

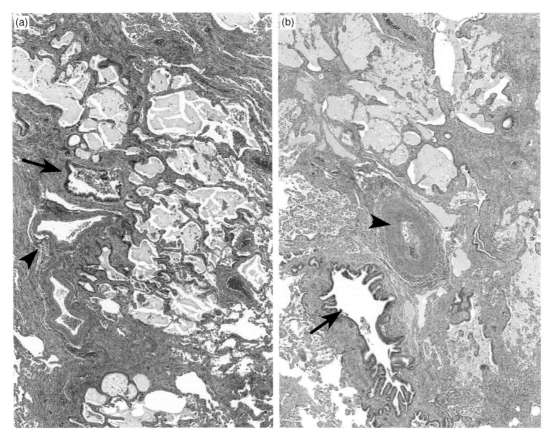

Figure 5.13. Honeycomb change vs. bronchioles. (a) In this image, a bronchiole (arrow) is accompanied by its partner artery (arrowhead). The remaining clustered, distorted and mucin-filled spaces represent honeycomb change. **(b)** Dilated bronchiole (arrow) and thick partner artery (arrowhead) with extensive honeycomb change at top and right. Note the fibrosis in the background.

multiple, variably sized, closely packed cystic spaces. When honeycombing is advanced, the gross appearance can be striking, and explains the origin of the term (Figure 5.14).

Variable pathologic findings

- Grossly, fibrosis and honeycomb change in UIP is usually more advanced and prominent in the lower lobes and less so in the upper lobes (Figure 5.15). In any lobe, peripheral lung is generally more severely affected. However, fibrosis can occur in any lobe, and may occasionally predominate in the upper lobes. The central areas of the lungs (close to the hilum, and away from the pleura) also show fibrosis microscopically, but this is less evident grossly.

- Some publications state that the distribution of fibrosis in UIP is often peripheral, subpleural or paraseptal, whereas others dispute this contention. A landmark histologic study of explant lungs with UIP showed that a peripheral distribution was absent in most cases (Katzenstein *et al*, 2002). In practice, scarring and inflammation around bronchovascular bundles is common in UIP. Additionally, as illustrated in Figures 5.11 and 5.13, honeycomb change often occurs in peribronchiolar parenchyma. The absence of a subpleural or paraseptal distribution, or the presence of

peribronchiolar fibrosis does not exclude a diagnosis of UIP.

- Areas resembling non-specific interstitial pneumonia (NSIP) are common in UIP. They are characterized by uniform expansion of alveolar septa by collagen or chronic inflammation or both (Figure 5.16). In one study, NSIP-like areas were present in 12 of 15 surgical lung biopsies and 16 of 20 explant specimens with UIP. The histologic appearance in these areas is identical to NSIP except that they occur only focally in a background otherwise diagnostic of UIP. Cases in which NSIP-like areas are prominent and extensive pose the greatest difficulty in differentiating UIP from NSIP.

- Interstitial chronic inflammation is usually minimal in UIP and is overshadowed by fibrosis. However, some cases show extensive and severe inflammation, especially in areas of scarring and honeycomb change (Figure 5.17). The inflammatory infiltrate usually consists of lymphocytes and plasma cells. Lymphoid aggregates may be present in scarred areas, even in UIP occurring in an idiopathic setting. Acute inflammation is seen in a few cases. Eosinophilic pneumonia-like foci containing large numbers of eosinophils have been described. Cases with such foci have a clinical behavior identical to more typical cases.

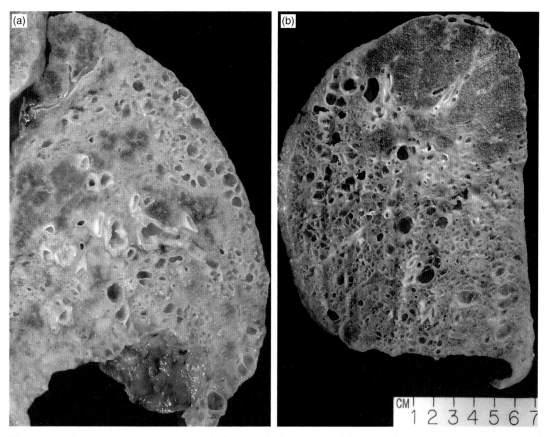

Figure 5.14. Gross appearance of honeycomb change. (a) Fibrotic lung with honeycomb change, most prominent in peripheral lung parenchyma. **(b)** Striking honeycomb change sparing only the apex of the upper lobe.

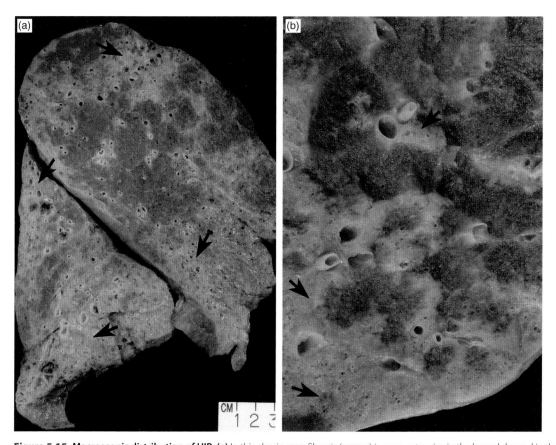

Figure 5.15. Macroscopic distribution of UIP. (a) In this classic case, fibrosis (arrows) is more extensive in the lower lobe and in the periphery of the lung. Areas of the upper lobe are grossly spared, but such areas may show microscopic evidence of fibrosis. **(b)** In this lung, fibrosis is obvious grossly (arrows) but honeycomb change is not. Honeycomb change was present microscopically.

197

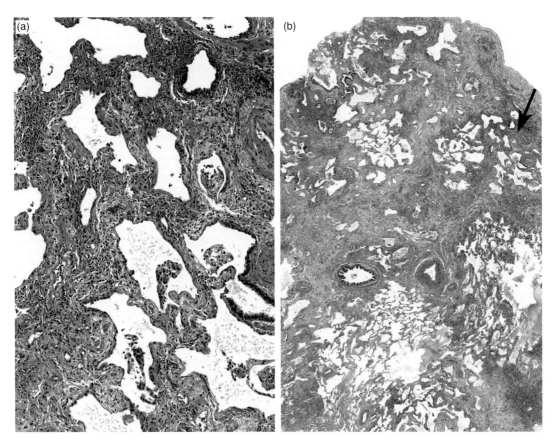

Figure 5.16. NSIP-like area in UIP. (a) Uniform expansion of alveolar septa by collagen and chronic inflammation, resembling NSIP. **(b)** Low magnification shows that the NSIP-like area is only focally present (arrow) in a patchwork pattern that is otherwise typical of UIP.

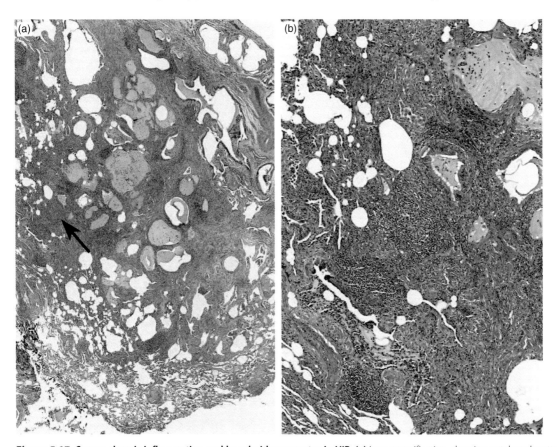

Figure 5.17. Severe chronic inflammation and lymphoid aggregates in UIP. (a) Low magnification, showing patchwork pattern with scarring and honeycomb change (top) and normal lung (bottom). The area indicated by the arrow is shown at high magnification in b. **(b)** Chronic inflammation with lymphoid aggregates.

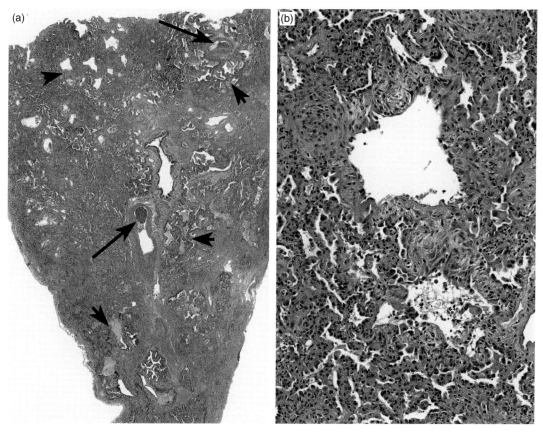

Figure 5.18. UIP with superimposed DAD. (a) Low magnification, showing areas of microscopic honeycomb change consistent with UIP (small arrows). The absence of intervening patches of normal lung is a clue to the presence of a superimposed abnormality. Thrombi in small arteries are also a tip-off (long arrows). The area indicated by the arrowhead is shown at high magnification in b. **(b)** Diffuse alveolar septal expansion by fibroblasts, typical of organizing DAD.

- Traction bronchiolectasis and traction bronchiectasis are common findings in UIP. They are characterized by the presence of dilated bronchioles and bronchi within fibrotic lung. Dilated bronchioles can be differentiated from honeycomb change by the presence of a partner artery and orderly smooth muscle bundles surrounding normal, well-oriented, often infolded bronchiolar epithelium. Dilatation of airways is thought to be a consequence of fibrosis pulling on airway walls.

- Superimposed foci of diffuse alveolar damage and organizing pneumonia are not uncommon in UIP. They should be suspected in cases with areas of uniform alveolar septal expansion or with unusually prominent pale-staining areas indicating the presence of numerous fibroblasts. These superimposed acute changes form the pathologic basis of episodic acute clinical deterioration in patients with known UIP or cases of UIP diagnosed only after the patient presents with acute respiratory failure, a phenomenon known as "accelerated UIP" or "acute exacerbation of IPF". When extensive, superimposed acute changes can obscure the underlying patchwork pattern of fibrosis and complicate the diagnosis (Figure 5.18). On the other hand, if areas of fibrotic lung without superimposed acute changes remain, underlying UIP may be readily appreciated (Figure 5.19).

- Alveolar macrophages are quite common in UIP. They may occasionally be prominent and numerous. The term "DIP-like reaction" has been used in such cases.

- Peribronchiolar metaplasia is a common finding in UIP. It is likely a precursor to microscopic honeycomb change. It is characterized by the extension of bronchiolar epithelium out of the bronchioles into areas of alveolated lung, forming clusters of gland-like spaces lined by bronchiolar epithelium in the peribronchiolar parenchyma (Figure 5.20). This appearance can mimic adenocarcinoma, but the presence of cilia indicates the benign nature of the lesion. The overall appearance is similar to microscopic honeycomb change, differing only in the degree of dilatation and filling of the lumens by mucin, both of which are greater in honeycomb change.

- Small foci of adipose tissue are often seen in the pleura or in subpleural lung parenchyma in UIP (Figure 5.21). This is thought to be a metaplastic phenomenon.

- Metaplastic bone. Scattered tiny foci of metaplastic bone are often present in UIP, usually in scarred lung parenchyma.

- Granulomas and multinucleated giant cells are often said to militate against a diagnosis of UIP and favor hypersensitivity pneumonitis. However, in practice, granulomas or giant cells may be seen in UIP. Their

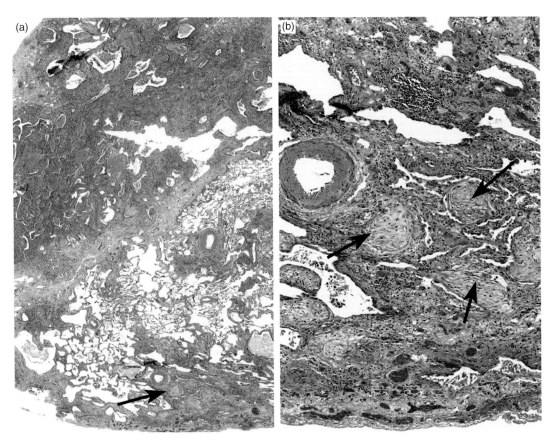

Figure 5.19. UIP with superimposed BOOP. (a) Low magnification, showing patchwork pattern with scarring and honeycomb change at top, and areas of normal lung below. The area indicated by the arrow is shown at higher magnification in b. **(b)** Organizing pneumonia, characterized by fibroblast plugs within peribronchiolar airspaces. Note small artery at left, a clue to the peribronchiolar location of the findings.

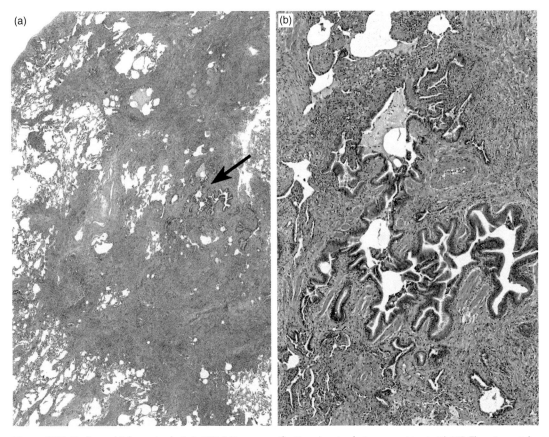

Figure 5.20. Peribronchiolar metaplasia in UIP. (a) Low magnification, showing features consistent with UIP. There is a patchwork pattern with extensive scarring juxtaposed to small areas of normal lung. The area indicated by the arrow is shown at higher magnification in b. **(b)** Bronchiolar epithelium extends out into peribronchiolar alveoli. Note fibroblast focus at top left.

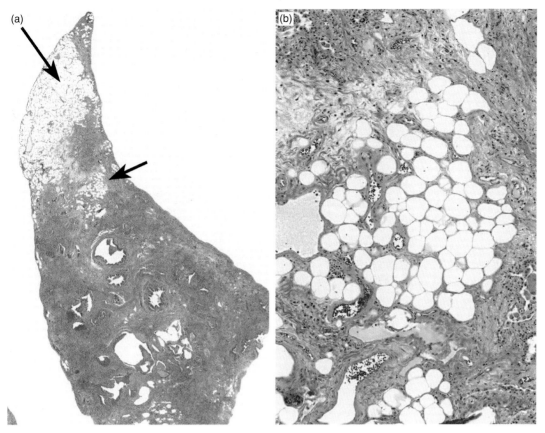

Figure 5.21. Adipose tissue in UIP. (a) Low magnification, showing extensive fibrosis and scarring. Adipose tissue is present not only in pleura (long arrow) but also within lung parenchyma (short arrow). The area indicated by the short arrow is shown at higher magnification in b. **(b)** Adipose tissue.

significance depends on the location, morphology and background of the granulomas. Scattered multinucleated giant cells are often present in the airspaces or interstitium in areas of scarring and honeycomb change, and often contain cholesterol clefts (Figure 5.22). They reflect poor clearance of cell debris from scarred lung. Granulomas and giant cells may also reflect infection or particulate matter aspiration.

- Arterial thickening may accompany interstitial fibrosis of any type, but the findings are especially striking in UIP (Figure 5.23). The arteries usually show severe medial hypertrophy, but intimal fibrosis may also be present. The changes mimic pulmonary hypertension, but the key point to remember is that pulmonary artery changes in UIP and other fibrosing lung diseases do not correlate with clinical evidence of pulmonary hypertension.
- Superimposed changes related to cigarette smoking may be present. These include pigmented macrophages within the airspaces (respiratory bronchiolitis) and emphysema. Superimposed emphysema can also modify the morphology and complicate interpretation.

Diagnostic work-up

- No special stains are required for pathologic diagnosis in classic cases of UIP. The diagnosis can be readily made on H&E-stained sections.

- Although stains for collagen such as trichome stains or the Movat pentachrome can highlight collagen and fibroblasts, they are unnecessary since significant fibrosis can be easily appreciated on H&E.
- Special stains for microorganisms are occasionally performed, prompted by the presence of neutrophils within areas of honeycomb change. However, these neutrophils are a consequence of stasis, not infection, and special stains are generally unnecessary.
- As mentioned previously, UIP is a pathologic diagnosis. When honeycomb change is seen on chest CT, a reasonably accurate diagnosis of UIP can also be made radiologically, although such classic cases are seldom biopsied. In cases where all the diagnostic features are present, there is little or no need for clinical information.
- Although UIP is a pathologic diagnosis, IPF is a clinical diagnosis, which is used by clinicians in cases with a pathologic or radiologic diagnosis of UIP for which no etiology is apparent on clinical grounds. Once the pathologist or radiologist has made a diagnosis of UIP, the clinician must make a subjective judgement regarding whether the disease is idiopathic (i.e., IPF) or should be attributed to an underlying condition such as connective tissue disease. Attributing an etiology to fibrotic lung diseases is a highly subjective exercise based primarily on personal preference. The clinical work-up performed to

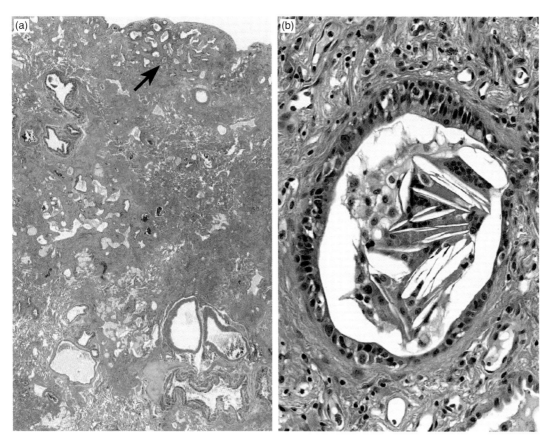

Figure 5.22. Granulomas and giant cells in UIP. (a) Low magnification, showing patchwork pattern typical of UIP. The area indicated by the arrow is shown at higher magnification in b. **(b)** Multinucleated giant cells containing cholesterol clefts are present within an airspace in an area of honeycomb change.

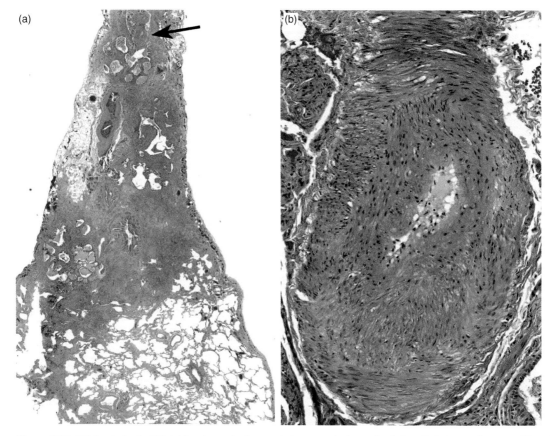

Figure 5.23. Thick arteries in UIP. (a) Scarring and microscopic honeycomb change (top) abruptly juxtaposed to normal lung (bottom). The area indicated by the arrow is shown at higher magnification in b. **(b)** This artery shows striking medial hypertrophy. In UIP, such arterial changes do not reliably correlate with pulmonary artery pressures.

discover an etiology varies widely from institution to institution and clinician to clinician. Many clinicians attribute UIP that develops in patients with known underlying connective tissue disease or some occupational exposures to these "etiologies", but the validity of this assumption is unclear. Specifically, it is impossible to be certain that UIP in such patients is caused by the underlying disease or exposure and is not an unrelated, idiopathic process. This problem is compounded by the fact that there is extensive overlap in the histologic features of UIP that occurs in an idiopathic setting and UIP that occurs in other settings such as connective tissue disease or asbestos exposure. Notably, the prognosis of pathologically confirmed UIP is poor, regardless of the presumed underlying etiology.

- Some cases with pathologic features of UIP do not have classic clinical or radiologic features of IPF. Clinicians often attribute such cases to "chronic hypersensitivity pneumonitis", "non-specific interstitial pneumonia" or "connective tissue disease-related interstitial lung disease". Whether UIP in such cases represents IPF with atypical clinical features or other, distinct forms of interstitial lung disease remains a subjective and unanswerable question, even after extensive clinical, radiologic and pathologic correlation.

- Multi-disciplinary discussion between clinicians, radiologists and pathologists has been touted as a magic bullet for diagnosing difficult cases of interstitial lung disease. The key role of radiologists and pathologists in the diagnosis is not surprising, since the recognition, diagnosis and classification of interstitial lung disease is based almost entirely on radiologic and pathologic findings. However, in some cases, the radiologic interpretation differs from the pathologic diagnosis. In such cases, multi-disciplinary discussion can be helpful in showing each specialist the findings and viewpoint of the others, assessing the possibility of sampling error, and providing an opportunity to ask questions and determine the degree of confidence of each specialist. The process can be productive when either the radiology or the pathology is classic and is compatible with the opposing viewpoint, or when a key piece of clinical information emerges. In practice, consensus is often elusive in cases that stray from the norm. In some cases, consensus is not possible even after extensive multi-disciplinary discussion between clinicians experienced in interstitial lung disease, dedicated thoracic radiologists with expertise in interpreting high-resolution CTs, and experienced, fellowship-trained pulmonary pathologists. Ultimately, the onus of making a pathologic diagnosis falls squarely on the shoulders of the pathologist, while the responsibility for using or over-riding this information and making treatment decisions falls on the treating physician.

Clinical profile

UIP is usually encountered in older adults of either gender. Most cases occur in individuals greater than 50 years of age,

and the mean age hovers around 60 to 65 years. However, histologically confirmed cases of UIP have been reported in patients ranging from 24 to 90 years. Currently, approximately half of patients enrolled in clinical trials undergo confirmatory lung biopsy. In the remainder, UIP is diagnosed on radiologic grounds.

The classic clinical presentation of UIP is that of an elderly adult who presents with slowly progressive cough and dyspnea for several months. However, many cases diverge from this stereotypical presentation, and are diagnosed in atypical settings. The best known of these is acute exacerbation of IPF, in which acute respiratory symptoms or the sudden development of acute respiratory failure brings the patient to clinical attention. Such individuals may have a known pre-existing diagnosis of IPF, but more commonly the diagnosis is made after pathologic examination when the patient presents with acute symptoms. Another atypical setting in which UIP is occasionally diagnosed is in lobectomies for lung cancer. Such patients are either asymptomatic, or have minimal symptoms that are attributed to the lung tumor.

Radiologic findings

UIP manifests radiologically as bilateral interstitial infiltrates with an apicobasal gradient. That is, the radiologic abnormalities tend to be greater at the bases of the lungs than at the apices. Interestingly, although lower lobe involvement is emphasized in most reviews, upper lobe involvement is also common. Indeed, it has been shown that some degree of upper lobe involvement is characteristic of UIP.

High-resolution CT scans of the chest (section thickness of 1 or 1.5 mm at 5- or 10-mm intervals) usually show minimal ground-glass attenuation superimposed on a background of patchy reticulation, lobular distortion, intralobular lines, traction bronchiolectasis and traction bronchiectasis. The infiltrates have a peripheral and basilar predominance. Honeycombing is most prominent at the lung bases, especially in the posterior lung zones. This classic pattern – honeycombing with lower lobe predominance – is recognized by most experienced radiologists as typical of UIP. However, it is also well documented that UIP can manifest radiologically as fibrosis without honeycombing or as minimal fibrosis. Pathologists should be familiar with these atypical radiologic presentations because classic cases with honeycombing are increasingly diagnosed by radiologists, and surgical lung biopsies are increasingly reserved for atypical cases. UIP with atypical features is commonly misinterpreted by radiologists as NSIP or chronic hypersensitivity pneumonitis. The main reason for this discrepancy – underappreciated in the radiology literature – is that early (microscopic) honeycomb change is identifiable by microscopic examination but not by radiology, since the cysts are too small to be seen even on high-resolution CT scans.

It is well documented that some cases of histologically confirmed UIP manifest radiologically as ground-glass opacities. ATS/ERS guidelines on this issue have been inconsistent. Past versions have stated that ground-glass opacities are inconsistent with UIP, whereas more recent versions have illustrated

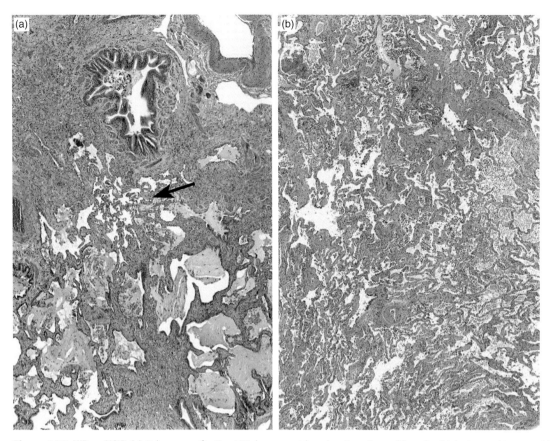

Figure 5.24. UIP vs. NSIP. (a) At low magnification, UIP shows a patchwork pattern. Scarred lung (top) is juxtaposed to normal lung (arrow), which in turn is juxtaposed to honeycomb change (bottom). **(b)** NSIP. Uniform expansion of alveolar septa without patchwork pattern, scarring, normal lung or honeycomb change.

cases with exactly this scenario. Ground-glass opacities are often interpreted by radiologists as evidence of hypersensitivity pneumonitis. In practice, ground-glass opacities are quite common in UIP, and correspond to a wide range of super-imposed abnormalities including diffuse alveolar damage, organizing pneumonia, smoking-related changes (macro-phages, fibrosis), foamy macrophages and bronchiolitis. The presence of these superimposed processes does not exclude UIP, and there is no reason why they should exclude a clinical diagnosis of IPF or exclude patients from trials of anti-fibrotic therapies.

Differential diagnosis

- Non-specific interstitial pneumonia (NSIP) can be difficult to differentiate from UIP, especially in cases with extensive fibrosis (fibrosing variant). In addition to varying degrees of fibrosis and chronic inflammation, honeycomb change and fibroblast foci can occur in both, complicating the assessment. Clinical features are similar, and radiologic findings overlap greatly, especially in cases without honeycomb change. Therefore, in the absence of honeycomb change on high-resolution CT scans, histologic examination is the only way to reliably differentiate between UIP and NSIP. The key feature is the presence of a "patchwork pattern" in UIP but not in NSIP (Figure 5.24). The presence of numerous fibroblast foci or extensive

honeycomb change and scarring also argues against NSIP. Practising pathologists should realize that UIP – the "usual" form of interstitial pneumonia – is far more common than NSIP. The rarity of NSIP is demonstrated by the fact that in the original report, only 64 cases of this condition were found in a busy lung pathology consultation practice over a period of 10 years, amounting to 6 to 7 cases a year (Katzenstein and Fiorelli, 1994). By comparison, in the same practice, cases of UIP were seen daily, easily amounting to a few hundred cases a year. Another point to remember before diagnosing NSIP is that NSIP-like areas are common in UIP. It is well documented in several studies that cases with UIP in one lobe and NSIP in another behave as UIP and should be diagnosed as such. In patients who undergo biopsies of multiple lobes, the risk of mortality is 16 times greater if one lobe shows UIP and the other shows NSIP than if both lobes show NSIP, and 24 times greater if both lobes show UIP. Therefore, UIP trumps NSIP, and what appears to be NSIP in one or more lobes may represent poorly sampled UIP. For these reasons, a pathologic diagnosis of NSIP should not be made in cases with radiologic evidence of UIP or honeycomb change in any lobe, and should be avoided in cases with a biopsy of a single lobe.

- Chronic hypersensitivity pneumonitis. Many experts currently believe that the chronic form of hypersensitivity pneumonitis can develop extensive

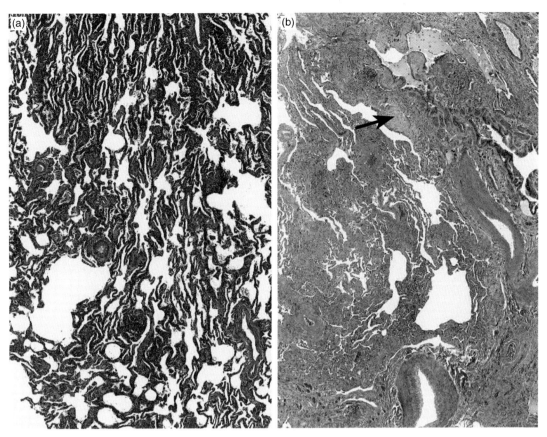

Figure 5.25. Hypersensitivity pneumonitis vs. UIP. (a) Hypersensitivity pneumonitis is characterized by mild, uniform and cellular expansion of alveolar septa. **(b)** In UIP, some areas are fibrotic (top right) while others are normal (bottom left). Note fibroblast focus (arrow).

fibrosis and may be histologically indistinguishable from UIP. This dogma has been taken to such an extreme that histologically classic cases of UIP are labeled as chronic hypersensitivity pneumonitis based on such radiologic features as upper lobe predominance, peribronchial disease, ground-glass opacities or air trapping. The belief that these cases represent end-stage hypersensitivity pneumonitis remains unchanged even though these cases behave in a fashion identical to UIP, have a dismal prognosis and are unresponsive to therapy. The practical consequence of this dogma is that these patients are not given a clinical label of IPF and are thus not candidates for trials of anti-fibrotic therapy. Although it is true that chronic hypersensitivity pneumonitis can be associated with fibrosis and honeycomb change, we believe that this diagnosis should only be made if lung parenchyma away from the scarred areas shows classic histologic features associated with subacute hypersensitivity pneumonitis, including a cellular chronic interstitial pneumonia, peribronchiolar accentuation and scattered multinucleated giant cells (Figure 5.25 illustrates the differences between subacute hypersensitivity pneumonitis and UIP). Peribronchial fibrosis occurs commonly in UIP and is not a specific indicator of hypersensitivity pneumonitis. Similarly, granulomas and multinucleated giant cells can occur in UIP, and do not necessarily indicate hypersensitivity

pneumonitis. It is likely that many cases currently classified as chronic hypersensitivity pneumonitis actually represent UIP with atypical radiologic features.
- Unclassifiable interstitial fibrosis. Cases that show significant interstitial fibrosis but cannot be readily classified into UIP or NSIP are common in practice. The usual reason for diagnostic difficulty is that the fibrosis is fairly diffuse but the honeycomb change is relatively focal. Another common finding that leads to difficulties in classification is patchy fibrosis in which the degree of inflammation seems excessive for UIP (Figure 5.26).
- Organizing pneumonia. It can be difficult to determine if an individual aggregate of fibroblasts represents a fibroblast focus or a fibroblast plug of organizing pneumonia, but the differentiation is not difficult if the whole picture is examined. The fibroblast plugs of organizing pneumonia occur within lumens, tend to be clustered, are located in peribronchiolar airspaces, and have shapes varying from round to elongated and branching (Figures 5.27 to 5.29). In contrast, fibroblast foci occur in the interstitium (not airspaces), are single (not clustered), randomly located (not peribronchiolar), and uniform in size and shape. Another helpful feature is that fibroblast plugs occasionally constrict as they pass from one alveolus to another, forming a dumbbell like structure, while fibroblast foci do not.

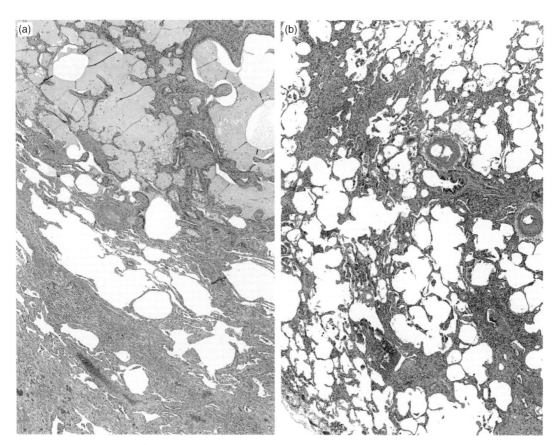

Figure 5.26. UIP vs. unclassifiable interstitial fibrosis. (a) UIP. Note transition from honeycomb change (top) to normal lung (center) to scarred lung (bottom). **(b)** This case shows interstitial fibrosis but was considered unclassifiable. The patchy nature of the fibrosis with areas of spared lung excludes NSIP. UIP is certainly a consideration, and a fibroblast focus is seen towards the bottom of the picture. However, there is too much inflammation for UIP, no honeycomb change, and the inflammation extends into lung away from the fibrotic areas. The possibility of chronic hypersensitivity pneumonitis or underlying connective tissue disease should be considered in such cases.

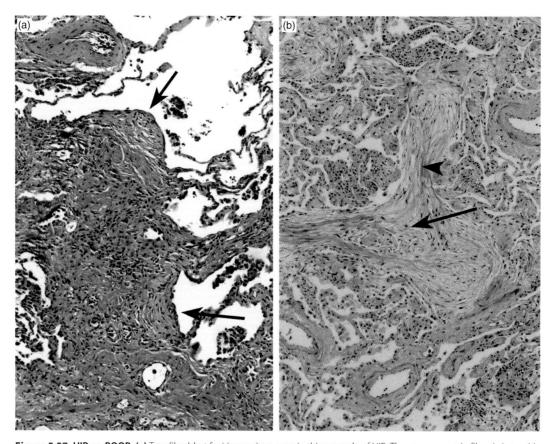

Figure 5.27. UIP vs. BOOP. (a) Two fibroblast foci (arrows) are seen in this example of UIP. They are present in fibrotic interstitium, which is juxtaposed abruptly to normal lung. They are dome-shaped rather than polyp-like. **(b)** Organizing pneumonia. This fibroblast plug (arrow) is characterized by a polyp-like shape and branching configuration. It is present within airspaces, and constricts as it passes from one airspace to another (arrowhead). A small artery is present nearby. There is mild interstitial inflammation but no collagen-type fibrosis.

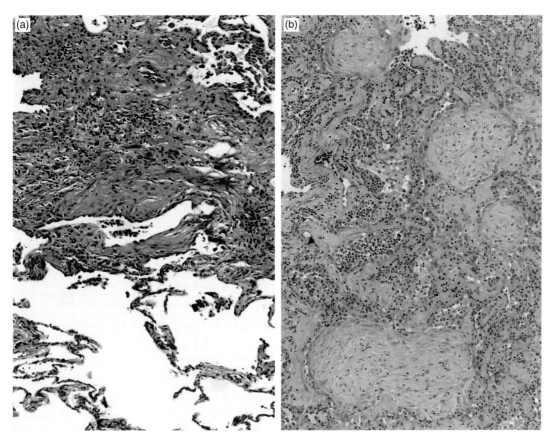

Figure 5.28. Fibroblast foci (UIP) vs. fibroblast plugs (organizing pneumonia). (a) Fibroblast foci tend to occur singly. **(b)** Fibroblast plugs are usually found in clusters.

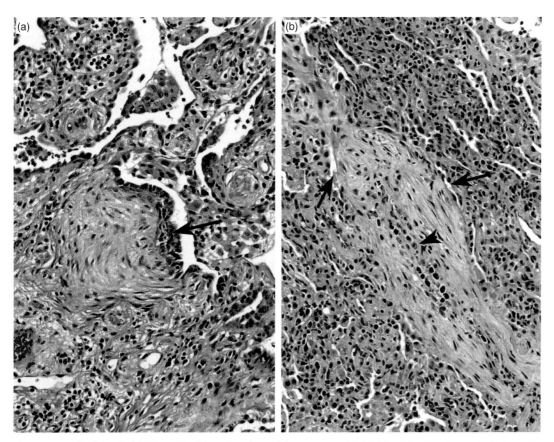

Figure 5.29. Fibroblast foci (UIP) vs. fibroblast plugs (organizing pneumonia). (a) A fibroblast focus is seen in the interstitium. It is separated from the airspace by respiratory epithelium (arrow). There is no cleft on the opposite surface, which blends into the fibrotic interstitium. No inflammatory cells are seen within the fibroblast focus. **(b)** Fibroblast plug from a case of organizing pneumonia fills and is separated from the adjacent interstitium on both sides by clefts (arrows). Inflammatory cells – including plasma cells – are present within the fibroblast plug (arrowhead).

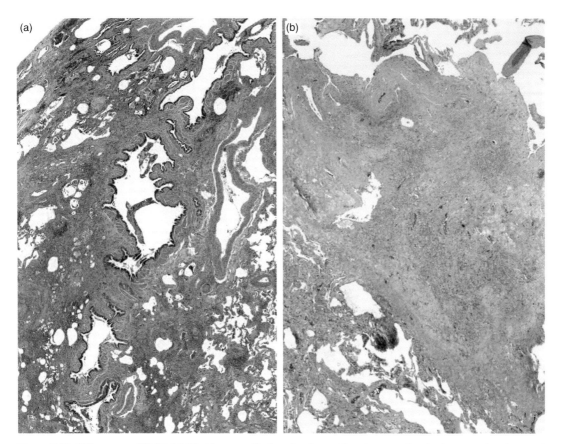

Figure 5.30. UIP vs. scarred PLCH. (a) UIP at low magnification, showing patchwork pattern. Scarring is present, but does not have a peribronchiolar predilection. **(b)** Scarred pulmonary Langerhans cell histiocytosis. This scar is peribronchiolar (note adjacent artery), and is vaguely similar to the stellate lesions seen in the cellular phase of the disease. Without concurrent cellular lesions, scarred pulmonary Langerhans cell histiocytosis can be very difficult to distinguish from UIP.

- Scarred pulmonary Langerhans cell histiocytosis can show a patchwork pattern and fibroblast foci. In the absence of diagnostic cellular areas, the presence of stellate scars in a peribronchiolar distribution is the most helpful finding (Figure 5.30).
- End-stage sarcoidosis can cause extensive fibrosis, which is caused by progressive replacement of granulomas by eosinophilic masses of hyalinized collagen (Figure 5.31). These fibrotic areas typically contain "cracks". Whether sarcoidosis can progress to form fibroblast foci and honeycomb change is controversial. Our view is that such changes represent UIP/IPF in patients who also happen to have sarcoidosis, rather than fibrosis related to sarcoidosis per se.
- Smoking-related interstitial fibrosis is usually easy to separate from UIP because the fibrosis is uniform and hyalinized, in contrast to the patchwork pattern of UIP (Figure 5.32). Emphysema and respiratory bronchiolitis are almost invariably present. Fibroblast foci and honeycomb change are rare.
- Combined pulmonary fibrosis and emphysema (CPFE) is an entity in which UIP and severe emphysema are both present. Clinically and pathologically, this entity can present diagnostic challenges because the presence of emphysema modifies the pathologic and the clinical features of the fibrotic lung (Figure 5.33).

Treatment and prognosis

Currently, there is no effective therapy for UIP. Treatment with conventional anti-inflammatory agents such as prednisone fails to reverse the fibrosis, and may actually be harmful. An anti-fibrotic agent (pirfenidone) and a tyrosine kinase inhibitor (nintedanib) have been recently shown to slow the rate of decline of lung function over the course of 1 year, but neither has been shown to cure the disease, reverse fibrosis or improve survival.

The clinical course of UIP is variable. However, most patients progress or die of progressive respiratory failure or acute exacerbations within 3 to 5 years after diagnosis. Development of ground-glass opacities in such patients often heralds the development of superimposed diffuse alveolar damage. Some patients develop acute respiratory failure and diffuse alveolar damage immediately after surgical lung biopsy. This complication may be caused by high positive end-expiratory pressure (PEEP) to the non-biopsied lung. Other patients progress slowly over the years, with declining FEV1 and a gradual increase in fibrosis and size of the honeycomb cysts on follow-up chest CTs. Others remain clinically stable for as long as 63 months after diagnosis. Rarely, patients with biopsy-proven UIP in the setting of IPF survive beyond 10 years. In the largest study of biopsy-proven UIP in the setting of IPF to date (203

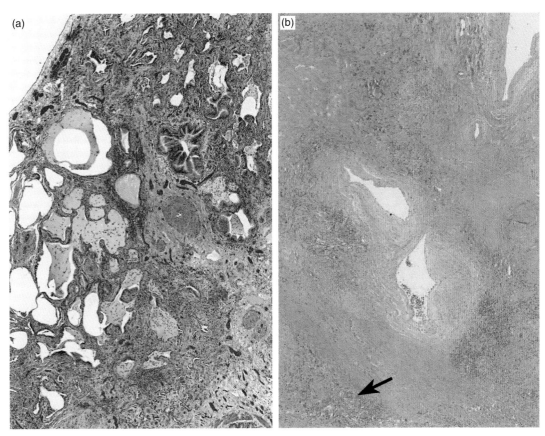

Figure 5.31. UIP vs. end-stage sarcoidosis. (a) UIP: Honeycomb change and peribronchiolar metaplasia. **(b)** Dense hyalinized fibrosis with few burnt-out non-necrotizing granulomas (arrow).

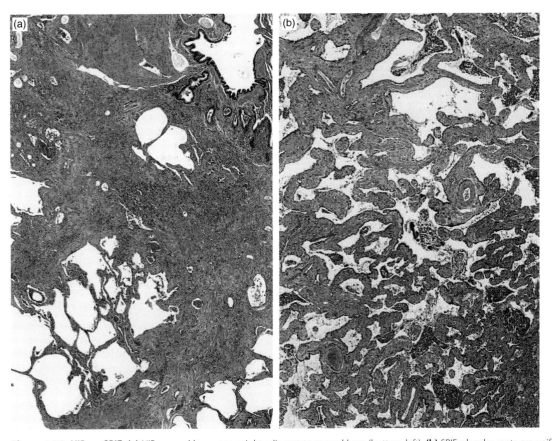

Figure 5.32. UIP vs. SRIF. (a) UIP: scarred lung at top right adjacent to normal lung (bottom left). **(b)** SRIF: alveolar septa are uniformly expanded by dense hyalinized fibrosis. The lung is emphysematous, and numerous smoker's macrophages are present within airspaces.

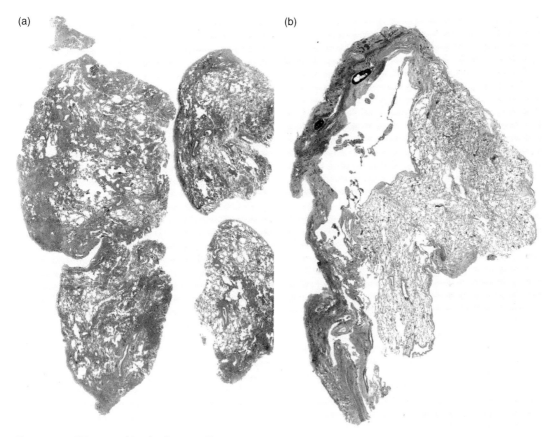

(a)

(b)

Figure 5.33. UIP vs. combined pulmonary fibrosis and emphysema (CPFE). (a) UIP: fibrosis in a patchwork pattern, including subpleural fibrosis. **(b)** Combined pulmonary fibrosis and emphysema: considerable subpleural fibrosis is present (left), but concurrent severe emphysema greatly distorts the architecture and masks the extent of the fibrosis.

patients, Park *et al*), there were five survivors beyond 10 years and one who survived 15 years. Gruden *et al* recently reported a case where the patient was alive 102 months after a pathologic diagnosis of UIP.

The prognosis of UIP is very poor, with a median survival of only 2 to 3 years from the time of diagnosis. It has been suggested that the outcome is worse in the idiopathic setting than in the setting of underlying connective tissue disease. In recent large studies, the survival for UIP in the setting of IPF was 4.4 (median) to 5 years (mean), versus 7.1 (median) to 10 years (mean) for UIP in the setting of connective tissue disease. Interestingly, some studies have documented a 5-year survival in UIP in the setting of IPF of as high as 44% and a 5-year transplant-free survival of as high as 24%. It has been suggested that the likelihood of long-term survival is higher in patients who survive beyond the 5-year period. The median survival of IPF post-lung transplantation is 4.5 years.

Sample diagnosis on pathology report

Lung, right lower lobe and right middle lobe, surgical biopsies – Usual interstitial pneumonia (See comment).

The concept of acute lung injury

Before we discuss the next two entities, it is important to introduce the concept of *acute lung injury*, a term that is used differently by clinicians and pathologists. Clinically, acute lung injury is considered a slightly less severe form of the acute respiratory distress syndrome (ARDS). Clinical criteria for ARDS include: (1) acute onset, (2) PaO_2/FIO_2 ratio ≤ 200 mmHg, (3) bilateral pulmonary infiltrates on chest radiographs, and (4) the absence of congestive heart failure, defined as pulmonary artery wedge pressure ≤ 18 mmHg (when measured) or no clinical evidence of left atrial hypertension. The clinical criteria for acute lung injury are identical to those for ARDS, with the exception of the PaO_2/FIO_2 ratio, which is ≤ 300 mmHg. Thus defined, the diagnosis of ARDS and acute lung injury does not require histologic input and is a mixed bag in terms of etiology and underlying pathology. The causes of ARDS and acute lung injury include infection/sepsis, shock, trauma, aspiration and oxygen toxicity, among many others. Some cases occur without an apparent cause. The underlying pathology in ARDS and acute lung injury is most commonly diffuse alveolar damage (DAD), but infectious pneumonias, culture-negative acute bronchopneumonia, organizing pneumonia, capillaritis with alveolar hemorrhage and eosinophilic pneumonia are found in a high proportion of cases. Clinicians managing patients with ARDS and acute lung injury may occasionally perform lung biopsies in order to identify cases with a treatable or potentially reversible cause such as infection.

From a pathologic standpoint, *acute lung injury* describes the spectrum of pathologic changes in the lung

Table 5.4. Causes of organizing pneumonia

Cause	Notes
Idiopathic	The cause of organizing pneumonia remains unknown in the majority of cases seen by pathologists. In the appropriate clinical and radiologic setting, this can be termed cryptogenic organizing pneumonia (COP)
Localized finding at the edge of another histologically obvious process	Fungal or mycobacterial granulomas, granulomatosis with polyangiitis (Wegener's), abscess, infarct, malignant tumors
Minor part of the pathologic findings of another process	Hypersensitivity pneumonitis, non-specific interstitial pneumonia, cryptococcal pneumonia, eosinophilic pneumonia, aspiration of particulate matter (important cause for pathologists to recognize, see Chapter 2)
Abnormal residuum of prior infection	Resolving pneumococcal pneumonia, resolving viral infection (influenza)
Acute exacerbation of idiopathic pulmonary fibrosis	Organizing pneumonia in these cases is a manifestation of superimposed acute lung injury. Diagnosis requires radiologic or pathologic evidence of underlying UIP
Inhalation of toxic substances	Needs clinical history for diagnosis. Examples include crack cocaine, silo-filler's lung, spray printing
Connective tissue disease	Usually obvious at presentation. Rheumatoid arthritis and dermatomyositis-polymyositis are the most common. Also reported in systemic lupus erythematosus, CREST and Sjögren syndrome
Drug-related	Ever-expanding list. *Amiodarone, nitrofurantoin* and *bleomycin* are the most common. Others include sulfasalazine, gold, minocycline and rituximab. Needs history of drug intake, exclusion of alternative etiologies and evidence of clinical response to cessation of drug therapy
Radiation	For breast cancer. Organizing pneumonia can occur outside the radiation field
Bronchial obstruction	The cause (tumor or aspirated foreign-body) is usually obvious
Lung transplantation	Fairly common, but of unclear pathogenesis; important to distinguish organizing pneumonia from constrictive bronchiolitis (bronchiolitis obliterans syndrome, see Chapter 11)
Miscellaneous causes	CLIPPER syndrome

resulting from acute injury, regardless of the exact cause. The term encompasses *diffuse alveolar damage (DAD)* and *organizing pneumonia*. DAD is typically associated with more severe clinical disease and widespread acute lung injury, whereas organizing pneumonia tends to be more indolent and subacute, reflecting a limited form of acute lung injury.

The concept that these two entities are related is supported by autopsy findings in patients who die of acute lung injury, which often show a mix of DAD and organizing pneumonia. The presence of proliferating fibroblasts in a pale-staining background in both entities also supports their relatedness. The term *acute lung injury pattern* is sometimes used by pathologists when both DAD and organizing pneumonia are present in the same biopsy, or if the findings cannot be easily pigeonholed into either category.

Organizing pneumonia

Organizing pneumonia, previously known as *bronchiolitis obliterans-organizing pneumonia* (BOOP), is one of two major histologic manifestations of acute lung injury, the other being diffuse alveolar damage (DAD). Organizing pneumonia is a common pathologic finding in lung specimens, characterized by the presence of polyp-like collections of fibroblasts within airspaces, variously referred to as *fibroblast plugs*, Masson bodies or granulation tissue polyps. Since fibroblast plugs are located predominantly within airspaces, organizing pneumonia is, strictly speaking, an airspace process. However, there are several reasons to discuss it with other interstitial lung diseases. First, fibroblast plugs originate in the interstitium and only secondarily fill airspaces. Second, the interstitium adjacent to fibroblast plugs is often inflamed and mildly thickened. Third, organizing pneumonia is often admixed with or superimposed on true interstitial processes such as organizing diffuse alveolar damage and usual interstitial pneumonia. Fourth, the lesion may present clinically as bilateral lung infiltrates, mimicking interstitial lung disease.

The major causes of organizing pneumonia are listed in Table 5.4. Pathologists will encounter histologic findings of organizing pneumonia in several distinct clinical and radiologic settings:

1. As an incidental finding at the periphery of localized mass lesions such as lung carcinoma, necrotizing granulomas, infections and abscesses, or as part of the histologic picture of well-defined entities such as

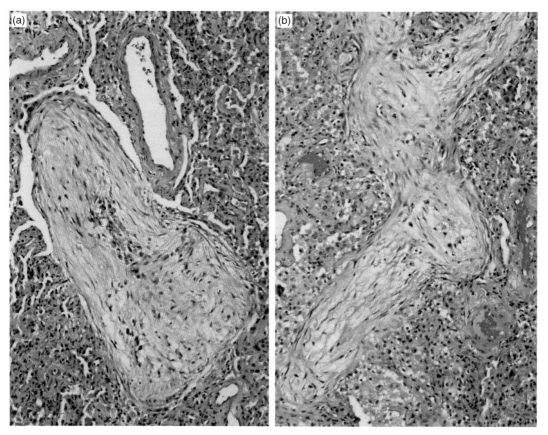

Figure 5.34. Organizing pneumonia. (a) A polyp-like fibroblast plug fills an airspace adjacent to a small artery. Note the pale, myxoid-appearing stroma. **(b)** This serpiginous, branching fibroblast plug mimics the contours of the airspaces it occupies.

cryptococcal pneumonia or organizing particulate matter aspiration pneumonia.

2. As the abnormal residuum of a prior acute bronchopneumonia. Acute bronchopneumonia and organizing pneumonia are occasionally seen together in the same biopsy, supporting the contention that the two are related.

3. As solitary or multiple lung nodules or masses, with no other associated lesion, and no definite evidence of prior infection. This form of organizing pneumonia is seen in core needle biopsies or surgical resections of lung nodules.

4. As a subacute form of interstitial lung disease presenting with cough, shortness of breath, fever and bilateral lung infiltrates. Clinical work-up for infection is typically negative. Lung biopsies show organizing pneumonia but no other specific findings. This idiopathic condition is known as *cryptogenic organizing pneumonia* (COP), and is important to recognize because it is steroid-responsive and has a better prognosis than other forms of chronic interstitial lung disease.

Organizing pneumonia can be diagnosed in any type of lung specimen, including surgical lung biopsies, transbronchial biopsies (Chapter 1, Figure 1.35) and core needle biopsies (Chapter 1, Figure 1.48).

Major diagnostic findings

The histologic hallmark of organizing pneumonia is the *fibroblast plug* (Masson body). The appearance of this structure has been variously described as "intra-alveolar buds of granulation tissue", "fibromyxoid connective tissue plugs", "granulation tissue plugs", and "fibrillated connective tissue". Fibroblast plugs are polyp-like collections of proliferating fibroblasts in a pale-staining, myxoid-appearing background (Figure 5.34). They are found predominantly within airspaces, especially peribronchiolar alveoli adjacent to small respiratory bronchioles and alveolar ducts. The characteristic clusters of round, oval, branching or serpiginous plugs are quite characteristic, even at low magnification (Figure 5.35). The branching and serpiginous shapes reflect the fact that fibroblast plugs follow the contours of airspaces, including alveoli, alveolar ducts and respiratory bronchioles. Using high magnification to determine whether fibroblastic lesions are located within the interstitium or airspaces can be treacherous. At this magnification, is it easy to misinterpret fibroblast plugs as interstitial, because they are often epithelialized on one or both sides by type 2 pneumocytes (Figure 5.36). Points of attachment are almost always identifiable between fibroblast plugs and the adjacent interstitium, causing fibroblast plugs to be misinterpreted as fibroblast foci. Stepping back to a lower magnification to assess the big picture is the best way to avoid

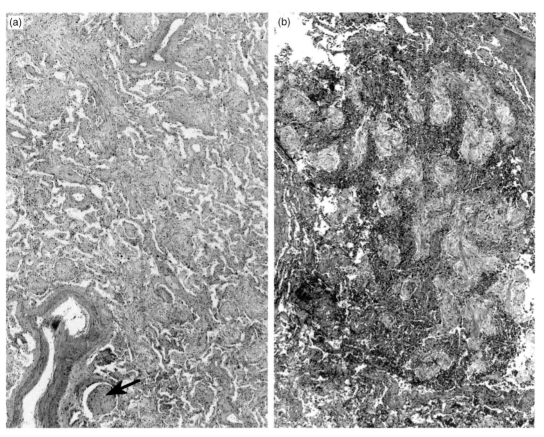

Figure 5.35. Organizing pneumonia – low magnification. (a) Cluster of pale fibroblast plugs. A bronchovascular bundle is seen at bottom left, including a respiratory bronchiole containing a fibroblast plug (arrow), indicating that the majority of fibroblast plugs in this image are within peribronchiolar alveoli. **(b)** The pale, myxoid appearance of fibroblast plugs can be appreciated even at low magnification.

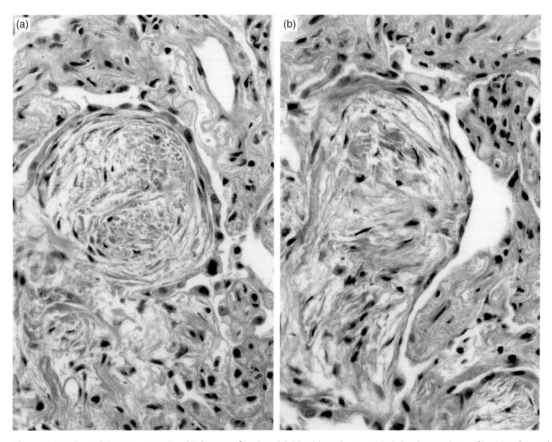

Figure 5.36. Organizing pneumonia – high magnification. (a) Fibroblast plug is epithelialized, mimicking a fibroblast focus. **(b)** The epithelial lining causes this fibroblast plug to appear interstitial.

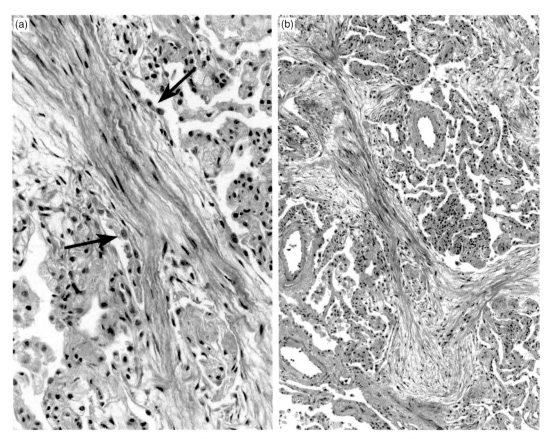

Figure 5.37. Avoiding misinterpretation of fibroblast plugs. (a) At high magnification, this fibroblast plug is lined by epithelial cells (arrows) and appears interstitial, mimicking fibroblast foci of UIP. **(b)** Stepping back to a lower magnification reveals the branching shape of the fibroblast plug and its location adjacent to small arteries, neither of which is a feature of fibroblast foci.

misinterpretation, because the branching shape of the plugs and the presence of a nearby small artery usually becomes apparent (Figure 5.37).

Variable pathologic findings

- Organizing pneumonia involves the lung parenchyma in and around the very smallest and most peripheral bronchioles. Pathologists expecting to see plugs within classic bronchioles with a ciliated lining will be disappointed since these structures are usually uninvolved. The affected airways (respiratory bronchioles and alveolar ducts) are smaller and more distal, lack a ciliated lining and merge almost imperceptibly into alveoli, giving the impression that the plugs are present randomly within alveoli. However, careful examination will often reveal the presence of small arteries adjacent to the fibroblast plugs. These arteries are the partner vessels of respiratory bronchioles and alveolar ducts, and thus serve as a clue to the peribronchiolar location of the changes (Figure 5.34a, and Figure 1.35, Chapter 1).
- Lymphocytes, histiocytes and plasma cells are frequently, but not invariably, admixed with fibroblast plugs. Plasma cells are particularly common (Figure 5.38). In contrast, inflammatory cells are generally absent in fibroblast foci of UIP.

- The adjacent interstitium may be thickened by mild chronic inflammation or may be normal (Figure 5.39). If alveolar septal thickening is diffuse and persists in the interstitium away from the fibroblast plugs, the possibility of a synchronous underlying chronic interstitial process should be considered.
- Ball-like masses of fibrin are often present within the alveoli in organizing pneumonia. This is an early form of the condition, occurring before the appearance of fibroblasts and the pale-staining matrix. Fibrinous and myxoid plugs can sometimes be seen in the same biopsy, supporting the interpretation that they represent different stages of the same process (Figure 5.40). When the plugs are purely fibrinous, the process has been termed acute fibrinous and organizing pneumonia (AFOP).
- Macrophages are frequently present with the alveoli in organizing pneumonia, and depending on their morphologic features there may be several explanations for their presence (Figure 5.41). Foamy macrophages are thought to be a consequence of airway narrowing or obstruction. Their accumulation is thought to be caused by impairment of the usual egress of macrophages from the alveoli through the airways. Since macrophages normally ingest cell debris from damaged cells, any form of airway

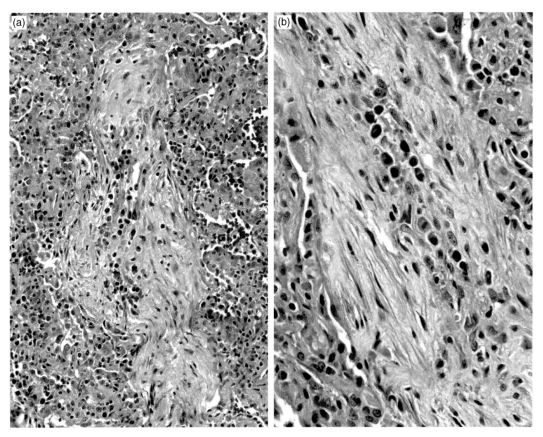

Figure 5.38. Organizing pneumonia: inflammatory cells in fibroblast plugs. (a) Inflammatory cells are visible within this fibroblast plug, even at low magnification. **(b)** Most of the inflammatory cells in this example are plasma cells.

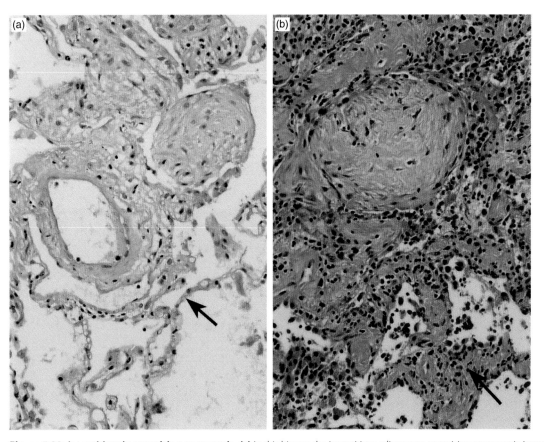

Figure 5.39. Interstitium in organizing pneumonia. (a) In this biopsy, the interstitium adjacent to organizing pneumonia is normal (arrow). **(b)** In this example, the interstitium is mildly thickened (arrow).

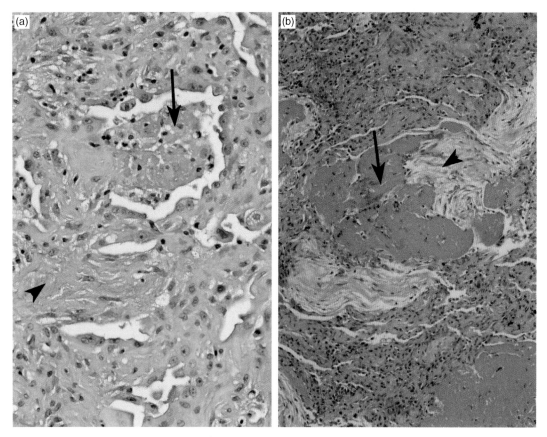

Figure 5.40. Organizing pneumonia: intra-alveolar fibrin. (a) Intra-alveolar fibrin (arrow) merges into a conventional fibroblast plug (arrowhead). **(b)** Another example illustrating the continuum between ball-like clusters of fibrin (arrow) and fibroblast plugs (arrowhead).

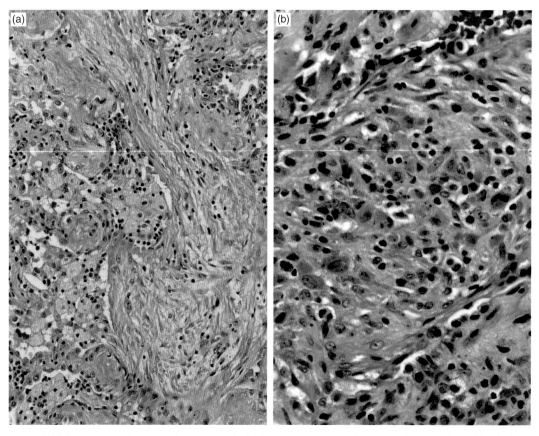

Figure 5.41. Macrophages in organizing pneumonia. (a) Foamy macrophages adjacent to a fibroblast plug. **(b)** Smoker's macrophages within a fibroblast plug.

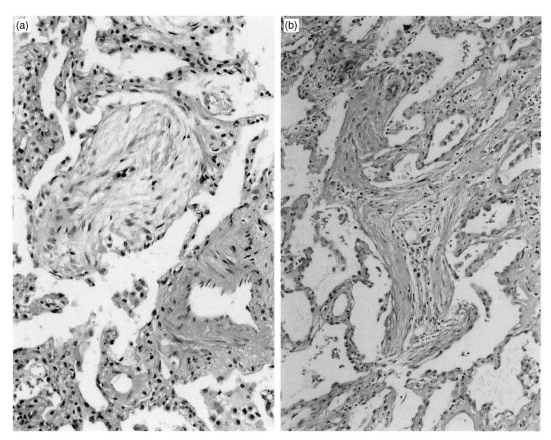

Figure 5.42. Shapes of fibroblast plugs in organizing pneumonia. (a) Oval fibroblast plug. **(b)** Branching fibroblast plug.

obstruction can result in build-up of lipid-containing substances presumably derived from cell membranes. When macrophages ingest these lipids, their cytoplasm appears foamy. Foamy macrophages are of no additional significance, and do not merit a separate diagnostic term, although this finding has been referred to in the older literature as "endogenous lipoid pneumonia". Smoker's macrophages (respiratory bronchiolitis) can also be present as an incidental finding in cigarette smokers with organizing pneumonia (Figure 5.41). These macrophages are often embedded within fibroblast plugs in respiratory bronchioles, alveolar ducts or alveoli, and contain a light-brown pigment with black specks. Finally, hemosiderin-laden macrophages may be embedded in fibroblast plugs within the alveoli. The differential diagnosis for hemosiderin-laden macrophages is wide (discussed in Chapter 4), but the most common cause is underlying congestive heart failure. Lung biopsies from individuals with treated granulomatosis with polyangiitis (Wegener's) but no active vasculitis or granulomas occasionally show organizing pneumonia with numerous hemosiderin-laden macrophages, located within fibroblast plugs or in the adjacent airspaces. A rare entity known as the "BOOP-like" variant of granulomatosis with polyangiitis (Wegener's) has also been described. It is characterized by a predominant picture of organizing pneumonia, with at least focal areas of necrotizing vasculitis, suppurative granulomas, tiny necrotic zones, microabscesses, or multinucleated giant cells.

- Fibroblast plugs may be of various shapes, including round, oval, branching or dumbbell-shaped (Figures 5.42 and 5.43). Dumbbell-shaped plugs are formed by constriction of fibroblast plugs as they pass from one alveolus to the next, presumably through pores of Kohn (Figure 5.43). A portion of the alveolar septum being transgressed is occasionally seen running over the dumbbell, similar to the appearance of an overpass or bridge over a highway.

- It is important to re-emphasize that the pathologic findings in organizing pneumonia mainly involve *respiratory bronchioles*, alveolar ducts and peribronchiolar alveoli. Unfortunately, most pathologists recognize bronchioles only if they have a round lumen and are lined by ciliated columnar cells. Such bronchioles, known as non-respiratory (membranous) bronchioles, are seldom involved in organizing pneumonia (Figure 5.44).

Diagnostic work-up

No special stains are required for the diagnosis in most cases. However, Movat or trichrome stains can help to highlight the pale-staining stroma, and cytokeratin stains may highlight the airspace localization of the process (Figure 5.45).

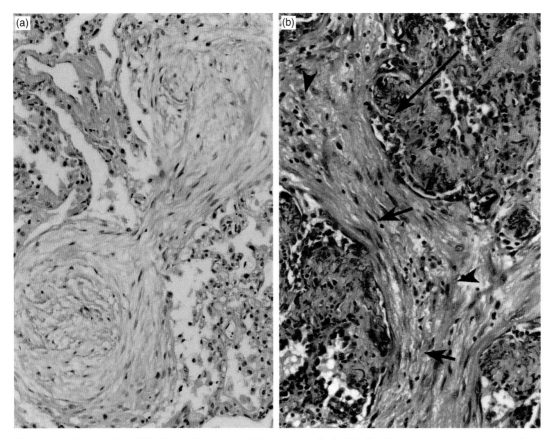

Figure 5.43. Constriction of fibroblast plugs in organizing pneumonia. (a) This fibroblast plug constricts as it passes from one alveolus to another, giving it a dumbbell-like shape. **(b)** Constricted (short arrow) and expanded (arrowhead) areas in a serpiginous fibroblast plug. Movat pentachrome stain highlights elastic tissue in the alveolar septa (long arrow), helping to confirm that the plug is intraluminal.

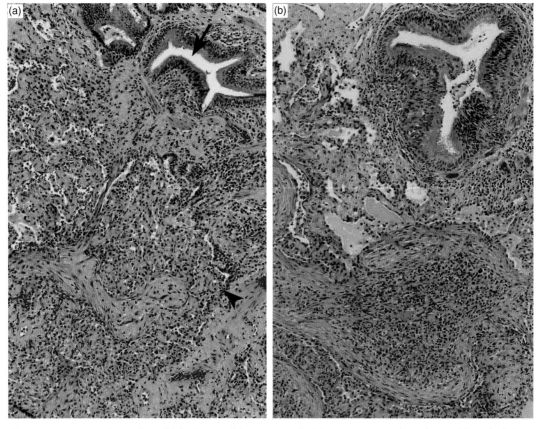

Figure 5.44. Non-respiratory bronchioles in organizing pneumonia. (a) A non-respiratory (membranous) bronchiole (top right) is uninvolved by organizing pneumonia, which fills a respiratory bronchiole (arrow: non-respiratory bronchiole; arrowhead: respiratory bronchiole) **(b)** Organizing pneumonia is seen at bottom, adjacent to an uninvolved non-respiratory (membranous) bronchiole (top right).

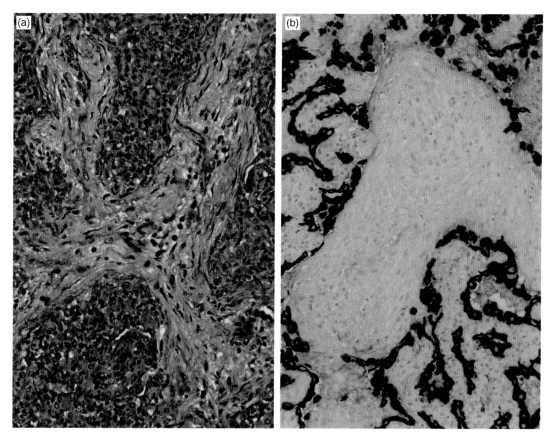

Figure 5.45. Special stains in organizing pneumonia. (a) A Movat pentachrome stain highlights the matrix in a fibroblast plug (immature matrix stains green; collagen stains yellow). Note the branching shape of the plug. **(b)** CK7 helps to show that the plug is within an airspace. Adjacent alveolar septa are lined by CK7-positive pneumocytes.

Clinical profile

Organizing pneumonia of the idiopathic type can occur at any age in persons of either sex. However, most cases have been reported in adults with a mean age in the 50s and 60s. Children are rarely affected. Common symptoms include persistent non-productive cough and shortness of breath. Dyspnea is common and may occasionally be severe. A preceding flu-like illness characterized by fever, sore throat and malaise occurs in a subset of patients. Hemoptysis is uncommon and seldom severe. Physical findings include focal sparse crackles. Wheezes are rare. There is no clubbing. Many patients have no abnormal physical findings. A wide variety of non-specific symptoms may be present, including chest pain, night sweats and mild arthralgia. Symptoms are usually present from 2 to 10 weeks prior to presentation, but some individuals have symptoms for more than 3 months. Almost all patients are treated for presumed infectious pneumonia, without a significant response. Clinical concern for interstitial lung disease is typically prompted by non-resolving infiltrates on imaging studies.

There are no specific findings on pulmonary function tests. A mild or moderate restrictive ventilatory defect is most common. Other reported findings include reduced vital capacity, impaired gas exchange and reduced single breath diffusing capacity. An obstructive pattern is uncommon.

Radiologic findings

Organizing pneumonia can result in a wide range of radiologic manifestations depending on the number and proximity of fibroblast plugs, and the presence of associated interstitial abnormalities. They include unilateral or bilateral opacities (infiltrates), and solitary, multiple or bilateral lung nodules (masses). The changes may involve any lobe.

On chest radiographs, the infiltrates of cryptogenic organizing pneumonia are usually bilateral and patchy. Any lobe may be affected. On chest CT, airspace consolidation and ground-glass opacities are the most common findings. The opacities are often peripheral and wedge-shaped. Approximately half of all cases are lower zone-predominant. The most classic finding is the *reversed halo sign* or *atoll sign*, characterized by a focal rounded area of ground-glass opacity surrounded by a ring of consolidation. It is seen in 19% of cases of cryptogenic organizing pneumonia. However, it has also been described in pulmonary zygomycosis, invasive pulmonary aspergillosis, paracoccidioidomycosis, tuberculosis, sarcoidosis, pulmonary infarction, lung adenocarcinoma and metastatic renal cell carcinoma.

It is important to remember that no single radiologic finding, including the reversed halo sign, is completely sensitive or specific. In one radiologic study, organizing pneumonia was diagnosed on the basis of patchy subpleural and/or peribronchovascular consolidation often associated with areas of ground-glass attenuation, centrilobular nodules or bronchial

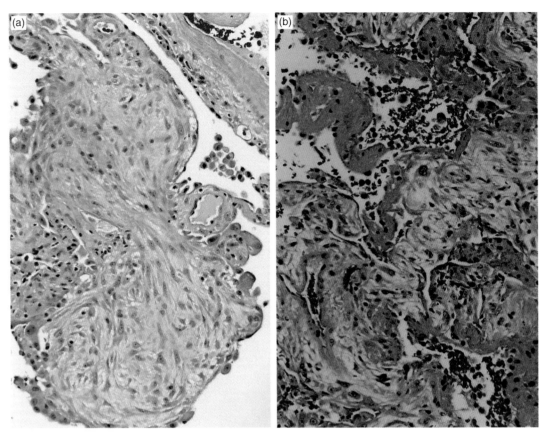

Figure 5.46. Overlap between organizing pneumonia and organizing diffuse alveolar damage. (a) Organizing pneumonia with a dumbbell-shaped fibroblast plug. **(b)** Another area from the same case, showing organizing diffuse alveolar damage, characterized by hyaline membranes and diffuse thickening of alveolar septa by fibroblasts. The case was diagnosed as mixed acute lung injury (organizing diffuse alveolar damage and organizing pneumonia). The patient was taking amiodarone.

wall thickening. Using these criteria, only 19 of 24 (79%) cases of pathologically confirmed organizing pneumonia were correctly diagnosed.

Differential diagnosis

- Usual interstitial pneumonia (UIP) is perhaps the most important entity to differentiate from organizing pneumonia because of distinct differences in therapy and prognosis. Histologically, fibroblast foci of UIP and fibroblast plugs of organizing pneumonia are both characterized by proliferating fibroblasts in a pale stroma. Historically, organizing pneumonia has been commonly misinterpreted as UIP, and we still occasionally see examples of this in consultation. Differences between fibroblast foci (of UIP) and fibroblast plugs (of organizing pneumonia) are discussed in detail in the section on UIP. Briefly, fibroblast plugs occur predominantly within airspaces, tend to be clustered, are located in peribronchiolar alveoli, and have shapes varying from polypoid to round, elongated, branched or serpiginous. In contrast, fibroblast foci are located in the interstitium, are single, randomly distributed, and fairly uniform in size and shape. A dumbbell-like shape is helpful when identified, since it is not seen in fibroblast foci. Large numbers of plasma cells are commonly found within fibroblast plugs but not in fibroblast foci.

- Diffuse alveolar damage (DAD), organizing stage. Organizing DAD and organizing pneumonia can be difficult to differentiate since fibroblast proliferation is a feature of both. The most helpful distinguishing feature is that fibroblasts are present *within alveolar septa* in organizing DAD, while they form plugs *within airspaces* in organizing pneumonia. Furthermore, in organizing pneumonia the proliferating fibroblasts are polypoid, whereas in organizing DAD alveolar septa are thickened but not in a polyp-like fashion. Classic hyaline membranes, when present, are diagnostic of DAD. Organizing pneumonia is frequently seen along with diffuse alveolar damage, especially in surgical lung biopsies and autopsies (Figure 5.46). The term *organizing acute lung injury* or *mixed acute lung injury pattern* can be used if both findings are prominent. If one finding predominates and the other is very focal, we prefer to diagnose the predominant component in order to guide therapy and provide an indication regarding severity of lung injury (more severe in DAD) and likely behavior (worse in DAD).

- Infection. Clinicians are often anxious to know whether organizing pneumonia may be infectious in etiology and are understandably reluctant to start high-dose steroids if there is a possibility of ongoing, active infection. There is no simple answer to this question, since biopsies may not always sample areas of active infection, and it is possible

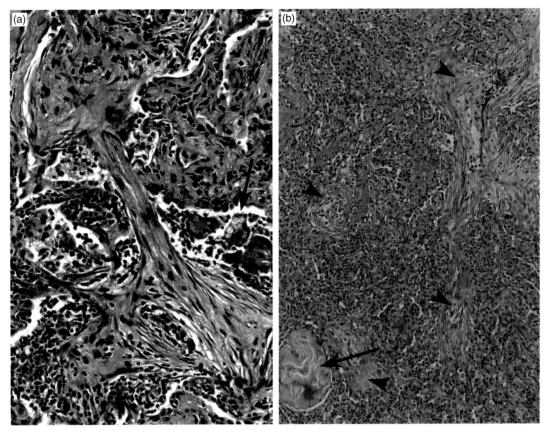

Figure 5.47. Pathologic findings that indicate the etiology of organizing pneumonia. (a) Fibroblast plug. The key to the etiology is the presence of multinucleated giant cells containing *Cryptococcus* yeasts (arrow). **(b)** Organizing pneumonia (arrowheads). The tip-off to the correct diagnosis is a degenerated vegetable particle (arrow). This is an example of organizing particulate matter aspiration.

that organizing pneumonia represents only a portion of the lesion. It is important to remember that in many cases that come to biopsy, attempts to identify an infectious process by standard clinical methods have already failed. Histologic features that may indicate an active infection or aspiration include granulomatous inflammation with or without organisms (Figure 5.47), multinucleated giant cells, necrosis and widespread acute inflammation. However, if organizing pneumonia is the only pathologic finding and cultures are negative, it is reasonable to assume that there is no ongoing active infection.

- Aspiration of particulate matter – mostly food or vegetable fragments from gastric contents – is one of the few etiologies of organizing pneumonia that can be definitively identified by pathologic examination. Tip-offs to the diagnosis are an exquisitely peribronchiolar distribution, foreign-body type granulomas rich in multinucleated giant cells, and suppurative granulomas containing neutrophils. The diagnosis is established by finding degenerating vegetable particles, other food fragments, or filler particles derived from pills (Figure 5.47). Degenerated vegetable fragments are particularly easy to overlook since they lack the typical morphology of intact plant particles. They may be few in number and difficult to find. The reader will benefit from becoming familiar with the range of histologic

appearances of aspirated particulate matter, illustrated in the section on aspiration pneumonia in Chapter 2.

Treatment and prognosis

Cryptogenic organizing pneumonia presenting as bilateral lung infiltrates of unknown cause is a steroid-responsive process with an excellent prognosis. Response to corticosteroid therapy is usually rapid. Relapses are common on cessation of therapy, but are not associated with mortality or long-term morbidity. Organizing pneumonia that presents as ARDS with severe hypoxemia has a dismal prognosis. When organizing pneumonia manifests as a focal lesion or a lung nodule, it does not relapse and no treatment is required.

Sample diagnosis on pathology report

Lung, right upper lobe, transbronchial biopsy – Organizing pneumonia (See comment).

Diffuse alveolar damage

Diffuse alveolar damage (DAD) is one of the most common forms of interstitial lung disease seen by surgical pathologists. It is the chief histologic manifestation of severe acute lung injury. Although the list of potential etiologies is long

Table 5.5. Causes of DAD

Causes of DAD	Examples
Infection	Viruses Influenza, seasonal and pandemic Herpes simplex virus type 1 Cytomegalovirus Adenovirus Respiratory syncytial virus Fungal infections Disseminated histoplasmosis Cryptococcal pneumonia Blastomycosis Non-tuberculous mycobacterial infection
Connective tissue diseases	Rheumatoid arthritis Polymyositis/dermatomyositis Systemic lupus erythematosus Systemic sclerosis (scleroderma) Mixed connective tissue disease Sjögren syndrome Anti-Jo-1 tRNA synthetase syndrome
Drugs	Amiodarone Bleomycin Busulfan Carmustine (BCNU) Cocaine Cyclophosphamide Cytosine-arabinoside (Ara-C) Gemcitabine Nitrofurantoin
Aspiration	Especially aspiration of gastric acid
Non-infectious complications of organ transplantation	Common finding, but pathogenesis is unclear
Oxygen toxicity	

Adapted from Mukhopadhyay and Parambil, *Semin Respir Crit Care Med* 2012.

(Table 5.5), the pathogenesis and tissue reaction are similar. The process is triggered by severe damage by the injurious agent to alveolar epithelium and alveolar septal capillary endothelium. Necrotic debris from the injured cells mixes with serum proteins that have exuded from injured capillaries to form linear eosinophilic structures along alveolar walls known as *hyaline membranes*. This phase of the disease is known as *acute* (or exudative) DAD. If the patient survives, fibroblasts and myofibroblasts enter the alveolar septa as part of a repair response. This phase is known as *organizing* (proliferative/fibroproliferative) DAD, and is characterized by gradual disappearance of hyaline membranes accompanied by marked proliferation of fibroblasts within the interstitium, resulting in diffuse alveolar septal thickening. It is at this stage that the interstitial nature of the process is most obvious. The interstitial fibroblasts in organizing DAD have been shown to have a high proliferative index by Ki-67 immunostaining. The presence of histologically diffuse interstitial fibroblast proliferation distinguishes organizing DAD from UIP, in which most of the fibrosis is caused by collagen deposition, with only tiny foci of fibroblast proliferation (*fibroblast foci*).

The word "diffuse" causes much confusion for pathologists, as it leads to the expectation that the abnormalities on biopsy will be diffusely distributed. However, the term DAD refers to diffuseness of injury within an individual alveolus, not the entire lung. In fact, patchy involvement of lung parenchyma is quite common in DAD, both pathologically and radiologically.

DAD is encountered in several distinct clinical settings. First, it is the usual histologic correlate of ARDS. Second, it can be the histologic manifestation of severe acute lung injury caused by a wide range of infections, gastric acid aspiration, toxic drugs, connective tissue diseases, ingestants and inhaled toxic substances. Finally, it may present as acute respiratory failure of unknown etiology in a rare condition that has been termed *acute interstitial pneumonia* (AIP).

The fact that interstitial lung disease can present as a fulminating acute illness of unknown etiology characterized by respiratory failure and bilateral lung infiltrates has been known since 1935, when Louis Hamman and Arnold Rich described four patients with exactly this presentation and diffuse interstitial fibroblast proliferation in their lungs at autopsy (*Hamman–Rich syndrome*). Over the years, the term Hamman–Rich syndrome was used incorrectly as an umbrella term for all forms of lung fibrosis of unknown cause, including the chronic interstitial lung disease that we currently recognize as UIP/IPF. One goal of the term AIP was to clarify that acute idiopathic interstitial lung disease is clinically and histologically distinct from chronic idiopathic interstitial lung disease. The diagnostic criteria for AIP are as follows:

1. Acute onset of respiratory symptoms resulting in severe hypoxia and, in most cases, acute fulminant respiratory failure.
2. Bilateral lung infiltrates on imaging.
3. No known etiology despite adequate clinical and pathologic investigation.
4. Histologic documentation of DAD.

In practice, cases fulfilling all four criteria are quite rare. The condition is misunderstood by some clinicians who apply the term to any patient with acute respiratory failure and bilateral infiltrates that are assumed to be "interstitial". If an underlying cause is identified, or there is no histologic documentation of DAD, such cases should not be labeled as AIP.

While the term AIP emphasizes the acute presentation of the disease and the prominent involvement of the interstitium, it does not mention the underlying pathology (DAD), or the requirement that known causes of DAD be excluded before making the diagnosis. Current terminology is also confusing in that DAD due to known causes is simply referred to as DAD (stating the cause), while DAD of unknown cause is termed

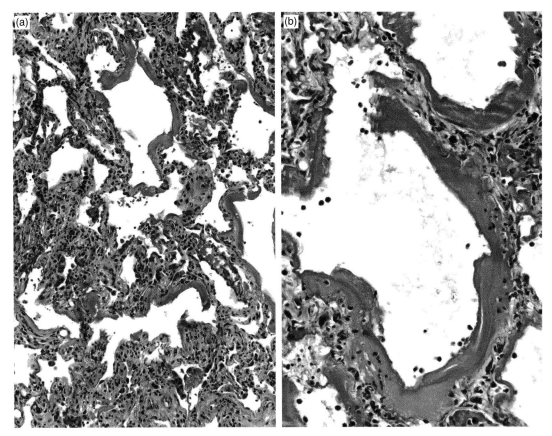

Figure 5.48. Diffuse alveolar damage, acute stage. (a) Linear eosinophilic hyaline membranes line the alveolar septa. Alveolar septa are thick, but not markedly so. **(b)** Hyaline membranes appear to be tightly adherent to the alveolar walls in this example, but they often detach into the airspaces.

AIP, implying that the failure to identify an etiology defines a discrete entity. The reader will recall that a similar situation applies to UIP, which is termed UIP (stating the cause) when it occurs in the context of a known etiology such as rheumatoid arthritis, whereas the term IPF is used when the etiology is unknown.

Major diagnostic findings

- *Hyaline membranes* are the hallmark of the acute stage of DAD. They are thick, densely eosinophilic linear structures that line the walls of alveolar septa (Figure 5.48). They are found in the acute stage of DAD and gradually disappear as the lung injury "organizes".
- *Alveolar septal thickening.* The interstitial component of DAD is less well recognized, leading to occasional misdiagnosis. The alveolar septa are abnormal at all stages of the process, but this is most obvious in the organizing stage (Figure 5.49). The interstitial thickening is caused by edema, proliferating fibroblasts, and the presence of prominent type 2 pneumocytes. Interstitial edema lends a pale, myxoid, lightly basophilic hue to the alveolar septa that resembles the pale background matrix of organizing pneumonia. In later stages of organizing DAD, hyaline membranes may be only focally present or completely absent. In summary, the pathology of DAD evolves from an early

stage where interstitial involvement is subtle and hyaline membranes are prominent (acute DAD) to a late stage where interstitial involvement is prominent and hyaline membranes are variable (organizing DAD).

Variable pathologic findings

- In addition to hyaline membranes and proliferating interstitial fibroblasts, several other histologic findings may be variably present in DAD, many of which may distract pathologists from the correct diagnosis. These include alveolar collapse/atelectasis, hyperplasia of type 2 pneumocytes (Figure 5.50), thrombi within small pulmonary arteries (Figure 5.51), squamous metaplasia (Figure 5.51) and mild interstitial chronic inflammation. Inflammatory cells – especially neutrophils – are usually scant, differentiating DAD from acute bronchopneumonia and capillaritis.
- Scarring and honeycomb change are not features of DAD. If they are present, underlying UIP should be suspected. The old paradigm that DAD can lead to honeycomb change has become outdated since the recognition that DAD can be the initial manifestation of clinically occult UIP (acute exacerbation of IPF).
- The possibility of infection should always be considered when DAD is seen in a lung biopsy. Pathologic

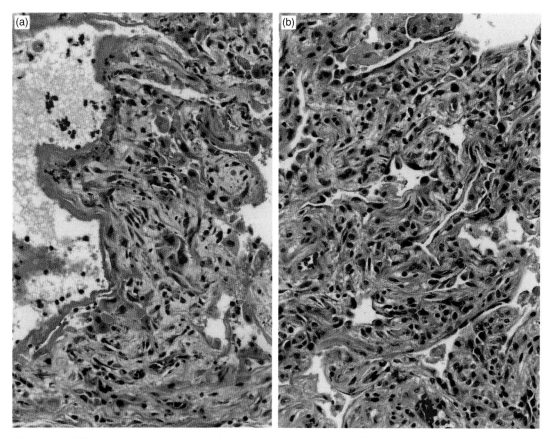

Figure 5.49. Diffuse alveolar damage, organizing stage. (a) Alveolar septum is diffusely expanded by proliferating fibroblasts and lined by a hyaline membrane. **(b)** In this example, no hyaline membranes are seen. The only finding is diffuse alveolar septal fibroblast proliferation. This picture is typical of later stages of organizing DAD.

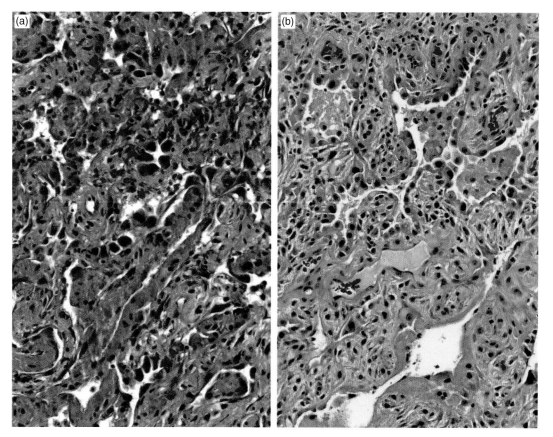

Figure 5.50. Prominent type 2 pneumocytes in diffuse alveolar damage. (a) Type 2 pneumocytes are enlarged and prominent in this example of acute DAD, but the background of hyaline membranes should prevent misinterpretation. **(b)** Organizing DAD. The even spacing of these enlarged type 2 pneumocytes is another clue to their reactive nature.

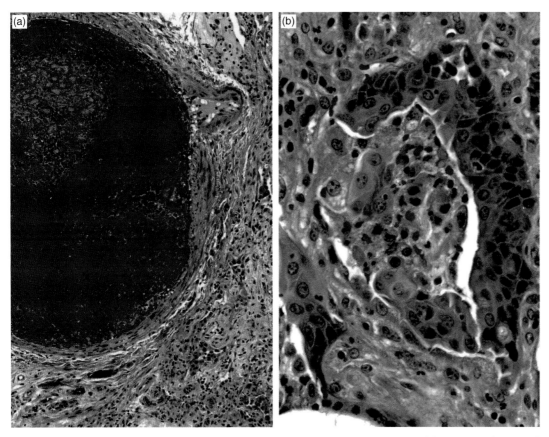

Figure 5.51. Diffuse alveolar damage. (a) Fresh thrombus in a small pulmonary artery. Interstitial changes are at bottom right. Thrombi are very common in DAD and serve as a clue to the diagnosis. **(b)** A focus of squamous metaplasia. This is another common secondary finding in DAD. Occasionally, it can be quite extensive and alarming. This finding can be misdiagnosed as squamous cell carcinoma.

examination can be invaluable for detecting organisms that are impossible to culture (e.g., *Pneumocystis*), or detected late in cultures (such as many mycobacteria, *Blastomyces* and *Histoplasma*). *Pneumocystis* pneumonia, in particular, should always be considered in the differential diagnosis of DAD, especially in immunocompromised patients, since the pathognomonic frothy exudate may be absent. CMV can also be identified in DAD by histologic examination, either by finding the pathognomonic inclusions on H&E, or by immunohistochemistry.

Diagnostic work-up

The role of lung biopsy is not just limited to identifying DAD, but also extends to identification of an underlying etiology. In a study of 58 cases of DAD diagnosed on surgical lung biopsies, histologic examination pinpointed an etiology in 6 (10%). The etiology was found mainly by identifying underlying UIP (hence establishing a diagnosis of acute exacerbation of IPF) or an infection such as CMV. In immunocompromised patients who at first glance appear to have DAD of unknown cause on histologic examination, performing a GMS stain for fungal organisms can be very helpful for diagnosing *Pneumocystis* pneumonia.

Clinical profile

DAD can occur at any age, and may involve immunocompetent as well as immunosuppressed individuals. Most patients present acutely with cough or shortness of breath over a period of days to weeks. Empiric antibiotics are often administered for presumed pneumonia. Most patients are severely hypoxic and go on to develop acute respiratory failure requiring mechanical ventilation.

The clinical work-up of patients with histologically confirmed DAD depends on the context. In some cases, the cause – such as severe burns or sepsis – may be obvious. However, in most cases, a lung biopsy is performed because the etiology of the process is unclear. Therefore, pathologists must be prepared to provide clinicians with some guidance regarding likely etiologies. The most important etiology to exclude is infection. A clinical and microbiologic work-up for viral infection should always be performed since these infections are particularly likely to cause DAD and (in most cases) cannot be identified in histologic specimens. Connective tissue diseases can also manifest pathologically as DAD. A serologic work-up for underlying connective tissue disease should therefore be considered. However, which serologic tests should be performed, and how they should be interpreted in patients who lack extrapulmonary signs of a well-defined connective tissue disease is unclear. The classic drugs that cause DAD are chemotherapeutic agents such as bleomycin and busulfan. However, these rarely cause diagnostic problems. It is the less well-known causes of drug toxicity that need to be excluded when DAD is diagnosed. Pathologists

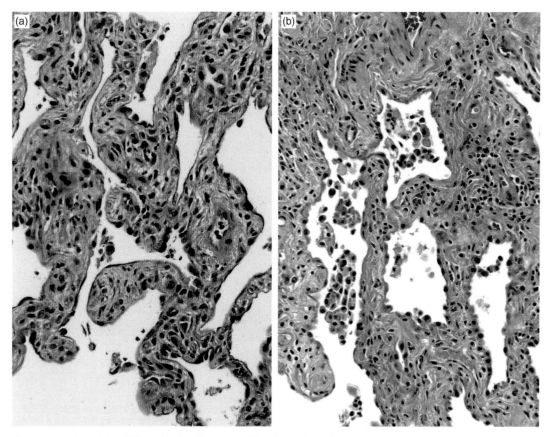

Figure 5.52. Organizing diffuse alveolar damage vs. fibrosing variant of non-specific interstitial pneumonia. (a) The alveolar septal expansion in organizing diffuse alveolar damage is caused by fibroblasts. The pale stroma gives the interstitium a "juicy" look. **(b)** In fibrosing NSIP, alveolar septal expansion is caused by a mix of collagen and lymphocytes. The fibrosis is more eosinophilic than in organizing DAD.

play a role in the diagnosis by raising this possibility, which is often overlooked by clinicians. The best examples of drug toxicities that are discovered on the basis of pathologic findings are amiodarone and nitrofurantoin. Drug-related lung disease is always difficult if not impossible to prove. In most cases, a presumptive diagnosis is based on onset of lung disease after commencement of drug therapy, exclusion of other causes such as infection, and improvement of symptoms upon cessation of the offending drug. The role of lung biopsies is to exclude infection and specify the underlying pathologic manifestation (including DAD). However, it is important to emphasize that no specific pathologic findings are unique to drug-related lung disease, or pathognomonic of any specific drug.

Differential diagnosis

Problems in diagnosis mainly arise with the organizing stage of DAD (Figures 5.52 and 5.53). Features helpful in the differential diagnosis are shown in Table 5.6.

Radiologic findings

DAD most often manifests as bilateral ground-glass opacities, "alveolar" infiltrates or opacities, or consolidation. These findings can be seen in other diseases, and are therefore nonspecific. They are often misinterpreted as "pneumonia" or "edema". The apparent presence of edema in the absence of underlying heart failure accounts for the well-known description of this condition as *non-cardiogenic pulmonary edema*. The term is not entirely accurate since true intra-alveolar pulmonary edema does not occur in DAD. Traction bronchiectasis and honeycombing have been observed in some patients with DAD, but it is likely that these features indicate underlying UIP.

Treatment and prognosis

There is no effective therapy for DAD, although high-dose intravenous corticosteroids are often tried. Many patients require mechanical ventilation and supportive care. The mortality rate of DAD due to known causes is approximately 50%, and similar rates have been reported in AIP and ARDS. Many patients with AIP die of acute respiratory failure or its complications despite mechanical ventilation and high-dose corticosteroid therapy. Overall, approximately half die within 2 months. Variable numbers of survivors have been reported in most series. Some patients with AIP survive the initial hospitalization but die of recurrent AIP, pneumonia or congestive heart failure (CHF) within a few months after discharge. No consistent clinical or pathologic features identify those patients with DAD who are likely to have a better outcome.

Table 5.6. Differential diagnosis of organizing diffuse alveolar damage

Histologic feature	Organizing DAD	Organizing pneumonia	NSIP, fibrosing variant	UIP
Significant alveolar septal thickening	Yes (fibroblast proliferation)	Variable (chronic inflammation)	Yes (collagen and lymphocytes)	Yes (collagen)
Fibroblast proliferation	Yes	Yes	No	Yes
Location of fibroblast proliferation	Alveolar septa	Airspaces (plugs)	Not applicable	Alveolar septa
Distribution of proliferating fibroblasts	Diffuse, in alveolar septa	In fibroblast plugs	Not applicable	Focal, in fibroblast foci
Hyaline membranes	Variable (may be absent)	No	No	No (unless there is superimposed DAD)
Chronic inflammation	Absent or scant	Often present	Common, diffuse	Usually minimal, focal
Patchwork pattern, scarring, honeycomb change	No (presence of these features should suggest underlying UIP)	No	No	Yes
Fibroblast foci	Absent	Absent	Occasional, few	Usually present, often several

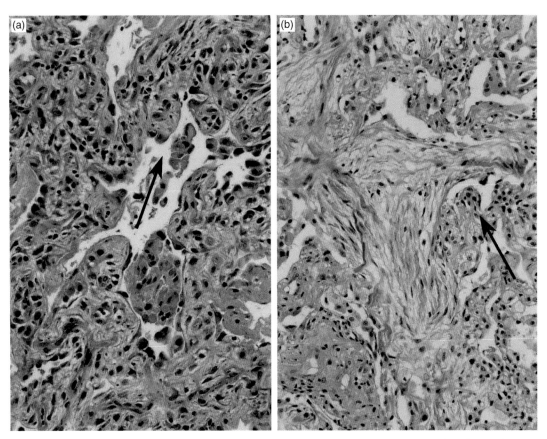

Figure 5.53. Organizing diffuse alveolar damage vs. organizing pneumonia. (a) Organizing DAD: fibroblast proliferation is in the alveolar septa. Airspaces (arrow) are open. **(b)** Organizing pneumonia: fibroblast proliferation fills the airspaces. Alveolar septa (arrow) are uninvolved. The polypoid, branching shape is also characteristic.

Table 5.7. Similarities and differences between pulmonary and extrapulmonary Langerhans cell histiocytosis

Feature	Pulmonary Langerhans cell histiocytosis	Extrapulmonary Langerhans cell histiocytosis
Langerhans cells	Present in clusters	Present in clusters
Eosinophils	Variable, often numerous	Variable, often numerous
BRAF V600E mutation	28 to 40%	37 to 57%
Age at presentation	Adults	Infants, children, young adults
Cigarette smoking	Always	Variable
Organs or tissues involved	Lung	Bone-limited, skin-limited, lymph nodes, liver, spleen, multi-organ (45%). Lung involvement is variable (10%)
Involvement of extrapulmonary tissues	Rare	Yes
Natural history and prognosis	Spontaneous resolution of nodules, or stable nodules, or progression to fibrosis	Spontaneous resolution common. ~10% mortality with disseminated disease
Treatment	Smoking cessation	Variable: observation only (skin-limited), curettage (bone-limited), chemotherapy (multi-organ disease)

Sample diagnosis on pathology report

Lung, right middle lobe, transbronchial biopsy – Diffuse alveolar damage (See comment).

Pulmonary Langerhans cell histiocytosis

Pulmonary Langerhans cell histiocytosis is a distinctive and well-characterized form of smoking-related interstitial lung disease that occurs almost exclusively in adult cigarette smokers. The disease is characterized by clusters of Langerhans cells variably admixed with other inflammatory cells in the interstitium of the lung. The terms *eosinophilic granuloma* and *histiocytosis X* – coined in the mid twentieth century and widely used for this condition prior to the recognition of Langerhans cells – are now outdated. Eponymous clinical syndromes (*Hand–Schüller–Christian disease* and *Letterer–Siwe disease*) drilled into the minds of generations of medical students have likewise fallen by the wayside, partly because they were defined clinically with little or no evidence that they represented a well-defined pathologic entity. Indeed, from a modern standpoint, it is unclear whether these syndromes were manifestations of Langerhans cell histiocytosis or other forms of histiocytic proliferation. Another term used for this condition in the past – *Langerhans cell granulomatosis* – is conceptually incorrect because collections of Langerhans cells are not granulomas (for the definition of a true granuloma, see Chapter 2).

Langerhans cells are *dendritic cells* derived from hematopoietic stem cells. It is controversial whether dendritic cells should be placed within the *mononuclear phagocyte system* or belong in a separate category. Small numbers of Langerhans cells are normally present in the skin (epidermis) and lung (airway and interstitium). They increase in number in cigarette smokers but do not form clusters. Unlike ordinary macrophages, Langerhans cells are antigen presenting cells rather than phagocytes. They have unique morphologic features (highly convoluted nuclei, Birbeck granules) and immunohistochemical characteristics (positivity for S-100, CD1a and CD207/Langerin) that help to differentiate them from ordinary macrophages.

Pulmonary Langerhans cell histiocytosis differs in several ways from extrapulmonary forms of Langerhans cell histiocytosis that occur mainly in infants, children and young adults, including age of onset, relationship to cigarette smoking, involvement of extrapulmonary tissues, natural history and treatment (Table 5.7). Features common to pulmonary Langerhans cell histiocytosis and extrapulmonary forms of Langerhans cell histiocytosis include Langerhans cell proliferation, frequent and often striking admixture with eosinophils, and the presence of *BRAF V600E* mutations in a subset of cases. Although lung involvement may occur in extrapulmonary Langerhans cell histiocytosis, this seldom causes diagnostic problems for pathologists in practice, since virtually all lung biopsies performed in this condition are from adult cigarette smokers with bilateral lung nodules, and represent pulmonary Langerhans cell histiocytosis. In contrast, the typical clinical presentation of extrapulmonary Langerhans cell histiocytosis is substantially different (skin rash in an infant, or a lytic bone lesion in the skull of a child, for example), and it is usually obvious that lung involvement, if present, is a secondary feature.

The pathologic diagnosis of pulmonary Langerhans cell histiocytosis is typically made in surgical lung biopsies, but

Table 5.8. Diagnostic modality used for tissue diagnosis of PLCH in 5 large studies

	Basset 1978	Friedman 1981	Travis 1993	Delobbe 1996	Vassallo 2002
Total number of pathologically confirmed PLCH cases	78	100	48	25	102
Surgical lung biopsy	62	100	42	24	94
Lobectomy	0	0	2	0	0
Transbronchial biopsy	1	0	4[a]	1	6[b]
CT-guided core biopsy	0	0	0	0	0
Langerhans cells (CD1a-positive) in BAL	0	0	0	0	0
Biopsies of other organs	21	0	3	0	2

Reproduced from Mukhopadhyay S *et al, Thorax* 2010.
[a] 4 of 10 transbronchial biopsies were diagnostic.
[b] 6 of 29 transbronchial biopsies were diagnostic.
PLCH = Pulmonary Langerhans cell histiocytosis; BAL = bronchoalveolar lavage.

transbronchial biopsies may also be diagnostic (Table 5.8, and Figures 1.41 and 1.42 in Chapter 1). Occasionally, the diagnosis can be made at frozen section in surgical lung biopsies. Skilled interventional radiologists can sample nodules as small as 5 mm with a CT-guided core needle biopsy, and a definitive diagnosis can be made in such cases if diagnostic areas are sampled, obviating a surgical biopsy (see Figure 1.49 in Chapter 1, and the 2010 report by Mukhopadhyay *et al* in the references). Diagnosis of pulmonary Langerhans cell histiocytosis by CD1a staining of BAL fluid receives inordinate attention in the clinical literature but is rare in practice.

Major diagnostic findings

- "Stellate" nodules with irregular edges, formed by expansion of the interstitium by a mixed inflammatory infiltrate including clusters of Langerhans cells (Figure 5.54). Some lesions are clearly interstitial but have a less solid appearance; in such cases their nodular nature is difficult to appreciate (Figure 5.55). The interstitial nature of the infiltrate is best appreciated at the edges of the nodules, where the cellular component can be clearly seen extending into alveolar septa (Figure 5.55). At low magnification, a pale, myxoid-appearing stroma is a clue to the presence of Langerhans cells (Figure 5.54 and 5.55). In contrast, pink-staining areas are usually fibrotic and lack inflammatory cells. An important feature that can be inferred at low magnification is the bronchiolocentric nature of the process. This may not be obvious at first glance since the lesions often destroy the affected bronchioles. However, the partner artery of the involved bronchiole is usually spared, providing a clue to the location of the infiltrate (Figure 5.55). The low magnification appearance of pulmonary Langerhans cell histiocytosis is virtually pathognomonic.

- The most important feature at high magnification, and one that is mandatory for a definitive diagnosis, is the presence of *clusters or sheets of Langerhans cells within the interstitium* (Figure 5.56). Langerhans cells resemble ordinary macrophages at first glance, but can be distinguished by their highly convoluted nuclei, the twisted contours of which appear walnut-like or cerebriform. Langerhans cells are numerous in the cellular phase of the disease and decrease in number as fibrosis supervenes. When fibrosis completely replaces the cellular infiltrate, a definitive pathologic diagnosis cannot be made.

- In addition to Langerhans cells, the inflammatory infiltrate in the interstitium often contains smoker's macrophages, lymphocytes, eosinophils, neutrophils and plasma cells (Figure 5.57). Since smoker's macrophages are usually found within airspaces, their presence within the interstitium is a helpful tip-off to the diagnosis. Eosinophils vary in number from case to case, and may be entirely absent in some cases. More often, they are numerous and form microabscess-like foci (Figure 5.57), explaining why many observers in prior years were prompted to name this lesion *eosinophilic granuloma*. However, as mentioned earlier, Langerhans cell histiocytosis is not a granulomatous disease since it does not contain epithelioid histiocytes.

- The alveoli in the remainder of the lung adjacent to and away from the nodules almost always contain smoker's macrophages (respiratory bronchiolitis), which is not surprising considering that nearly all patients are smokers (Figure 5.58). Since many patients are active current smokers, macrophages may be numerous in some cases, filling many alveoli and drawing attention away from the primary lesion (nodules). This type of extensive alveolar filling by macrophages is often described as "DIP-like" since it resembles

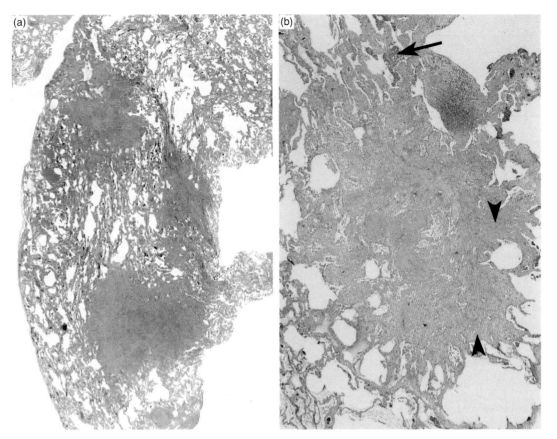

Figure 5.54. Pulmonary Langerhans cell histiocytosis, low magnification. (a) Two tiny nodules with irregular edges. **(b)** The stellate (star-shaped) configuration of this nodule is characteristic. Other typical features visible even at this magnification include the presence of macrophages within airspaces adjacent to the nodule (arrow), pale-staining areas in the nodule (arrowhead pointing up) and fibrotic areas (arrowhead pointing down).

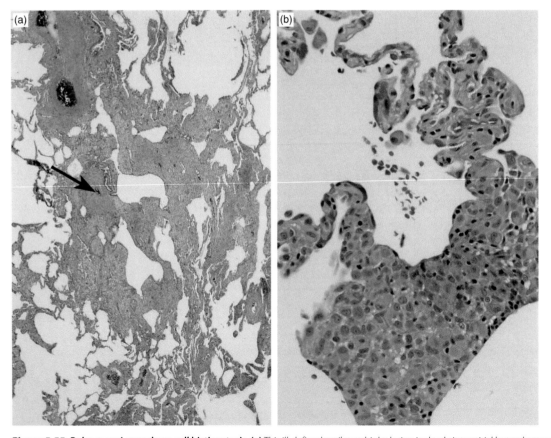

Figure 5.55. Pulmonary Langerhans cell histiocytosis. (a) This ill-defined peribronchiolar lesion is clearly interstitial but only vaguely nodular. The peribronchiolar location can be inferred from the presence of a nearby pulmonary artery (arrow). **(b)** The interstitial location of the Langerhans cell proliferation is clearly seen in this high-magnification view from another case. Airspaces are uninvolved.

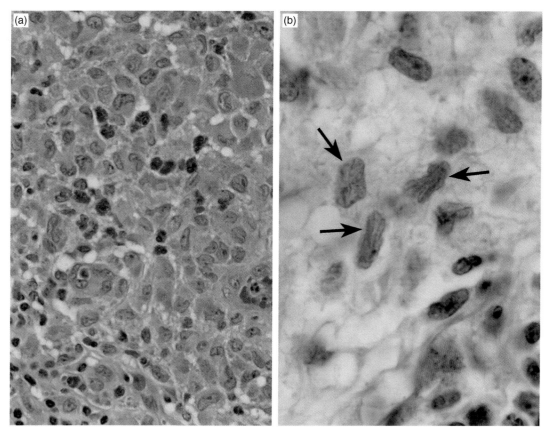

Figure 5.56. Pulmonary Langerhans cell histiocytosis, high magnification. (a) Characteristic mix of Langerhans cells and eosinophils. **(b)** Under oil immersion, the convoluted nuclei of Langerhans cells are clearly appreciated (arrows). A pigmented smoker's macrophage and an eosinophil are seen at the bottom of the picture.

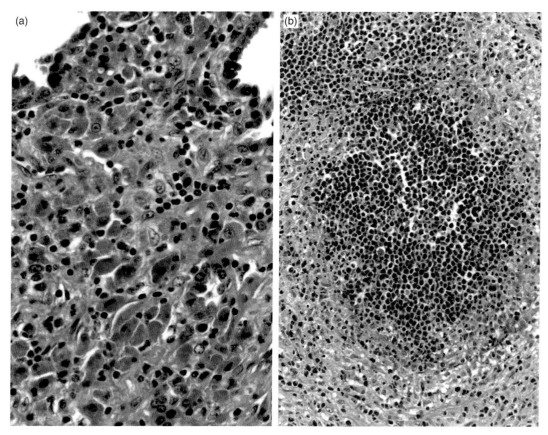

Figure 5.57. Pulmonary Langerhans cell histiocytosis. (a) Mixed inflammatory infiltrate in the interstitium containing pigmented (smoker's) macrophages, lymphocytes and occasional eosinophils. Langerhans cells are difficult to find, but the presence of smoker's macrophages within the interstitium is a clue to the diagnosis. Note prominent and slightly atypical type 2 pneumocytes at the top of the picture. **(b)** Eosinophil microabscess.

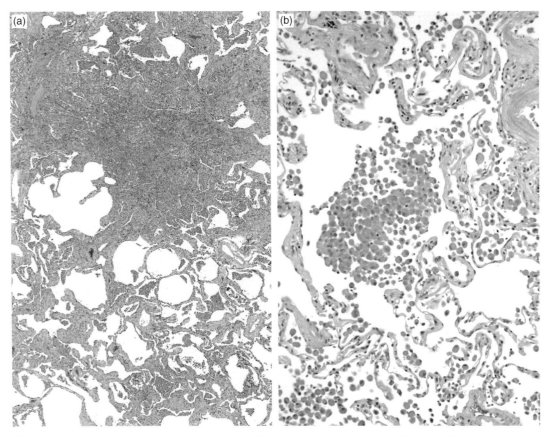

Figure 5.58. Pulmonary Langerhans cell histiocytosis. (a) Large numbers of macrophages fill the alveoli adjacent to a scarred nodule. **(b)** Higher magnification, showing numerous lightly pigmented (smoker's) macrophages. This finding should not be termed DIP.

"desquamative" interstitial pneumonia (DIP). It is one of many examples of conditions in which this conceptually incorrect term continues to be used.

Variable pathologic findings

- Interstitial fibrosis is often present in pulmonary Langerhans cell histiocytosis (Figure 5.59). It may co-exist with cellular lesions, or may gradually replace the cellular component, forming stellate peribronchiolar scars. Fibroblast foci and microscopic honeycomb change accompany the fibrosis, mimicking usual interstitial pneumonia (UIP). Another form of interstitial fibrosis that can occur in pulmonary Langerhans cell histiocytosis is SRIF. Unlike the stellate scars described above, this lesion is characterized by expansion of the alveolar septa by eosinophilic, hyalinized, ropy collagen bundles, often in association with smoker's macrophages and emphysema. For further details on SRIF, please see the next section.
- Cysts are a prominent radiologic feature of pulmonary Langerhans cell histiocytosis but are infrequently seen in surgical lung biopsies, perhaps because cases with cysts are more readily recognized by radiologists. When cysts are present, they may contain sheets of Langerhans cells in their wall (Figure 5.60). The lumen is usually empty. In many cases, they appear to represent a dilated and destroyed small bronchiole. It is unclear whether cyst

formation is related to prior necrosis or occurs via other mechanisms.
- Vasculitis is common (70%) but is usually not conspicuous. It is thought to be a secondary phenomenon. It most commonly consists of a few lymphocytes within vessel walls. Occasionally, the vascular inflammatory infiltrate is rich in eosinophils, mimicking a true primary eosinophilic vasculitis (Figure 5.61).
- Necrosis is uncommon, reported in 4% of cases. Its presence can complicate the differential diagnosis. When present, it is usually basophilic and dirty-appearing due to the presence of nuclear debris (Figure 5.62).
- As a rule, Langerhans cells are present within the interstitium. However, exceptionally they may extend into airspaces, explaining why Langerhans cells may appear in BAL fluid specimens.
- Reactive eosinophilic pleuritis has been reported in 5% of cases of pulmonary Langerhans cell histiocytosis after pneumothorax. This phenomenon is a common tissue reaction to the presence of air within the pleura. It consists of mixtures of macrophages, mesothelial cells and fibrin on the pleural surface, and has the potential to be confused with pulmonary Langerhans cell histiocytosis.
- The lung epithelium at the edges of the nodules in pulmonary Langerhans cell histiocytosis may show

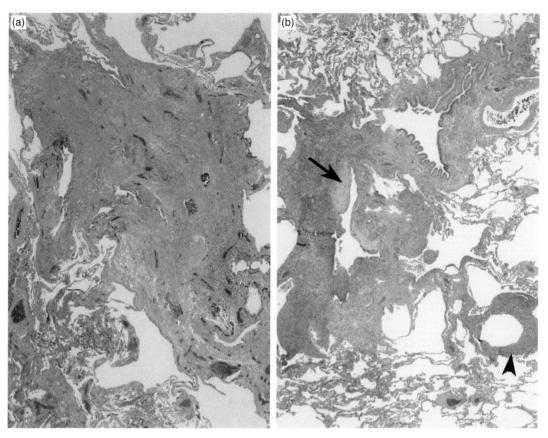

Figure 5.59. Fibrosis and scarring in pulmonary Langerhans cell histiocytosis. (a) This lesion is completely scarred and does not contain Langerhans cells, but its stellate shape and peribronchiolar location are clues to the correct diagnosis. **(b)** Another lesion from the same biopsy, showing peribronchiolar fibrosis, a fibroblast focus (arrow) and a cellular diagnostic lesion (arrowhead).

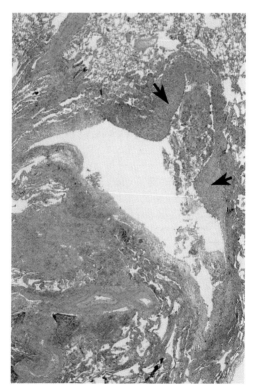

Figure 5.60. Cyst in pulmonary Langerhans cell histiocytosis. The wall of this cyst contains sheets of Langerhans cells (arrows).

prominent reactive changes, including nuclear enlargement and hyperplasia. Particularly striking examples can be difficult to distinguish from adenocarcinoma.

Diagnostic work-up

- In classic cases of pulmonary Langerhans cell histiocytosis in which clusters of Langerhans cells are easily recognizable on H&E, no immunohistochemical stains are required. If confirmation is desired, standard markers of Langerhans cells are S-100 and CD1a (Figure 5.63). S-100 marks the nucleus and cytoplasm. CD1a predominantly stains the cell membrane but may also show cytoplasmic staining. Depending on the laboratory, either marker may be more reliable in practice. Langerin (CD207) is another marker of Langerhans cells (membrane staining).

- In most surgical pathology departments, electron microscopy is no longer used for confirming the diagnosis of Langerhans cell histiocytosis, since it has been supplanted by immunohistochemistry. The most characteristic feature of Langerhans cells on electron microscopy is the intracytoplasmic *Birbeck granule*, a thin rod-like structure with longitudinal pentalaminar stripes described as zipper-like. Birbeck granules often contain a bulbous dilatation at one end, resulting in a racquet-like

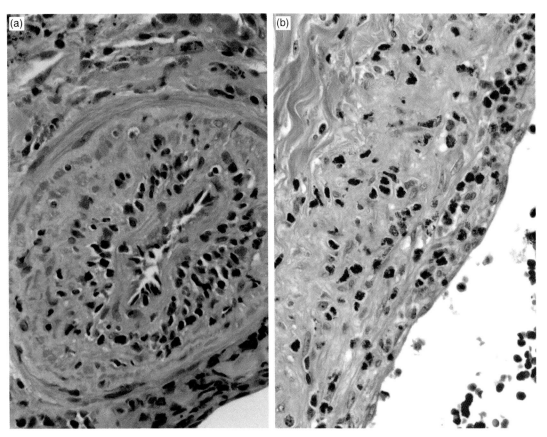

Figure 5.61. Secondary vasculitis in pulmonary Langerhans cell histiocytosis. (a) Small pulmonary artery with striking mural inflammatory infiltrate composed of lymphocytes and eosinophils. **(b)** The infiltrate in this blood vessel consists almost entirely of eosinophils. The media and intima are both involved. Case courtesy of Dr. AV Arrossi (part b).

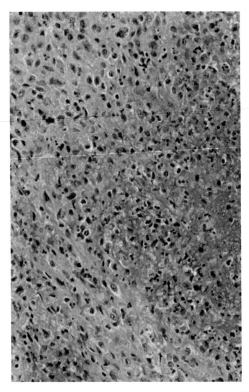

Figure 5.62. Necrosis in pulmonary Langerhans cell histiocytosis. Langerhans cells (top left) and "dirty" necrosis (right).

appearance. The deeply indented and irregular nuclear contours of Langerhans cell nuclei are also seen by electron microscopy.

Clinical profile

The age at diagnosis in pathologically confirmed cases of pulmonary Langerhans cell histiocytosis ranges from 19 to 68 years. Most patients are between 20 and 40 years of age. Both men and women are affected. Common symptoms include dyspnea, non-productive cough, wheezing and chest pain. Constitutional symptoms such as fever and weight loss occur in 15%. Hemoptysis is very unusual. Some patients present with spontaneous or recurrent pneumothoraces. Many individuals are asymptomatic at presentation. Surgical pathologists are disproportionately likely to see lung biopsies from individuals in whom multiple tiny lung nodules are discovered incidentally on chest imaging performed for unrelated reasons.

Pulmonary Langerhans cell histiocytosis is almost exclusively a disease of cigarette smokers. In most well-documented series, most or all patients are current or ex-smokers. Although a handful of cases are reported in non-smokers, some studies have included children, and the accuracy of the clinical history in such cases is unclear. In practice, the diagnosis of pulmonary Langerhans cell histiocytosis should be seriously questioned in a never-smoker.

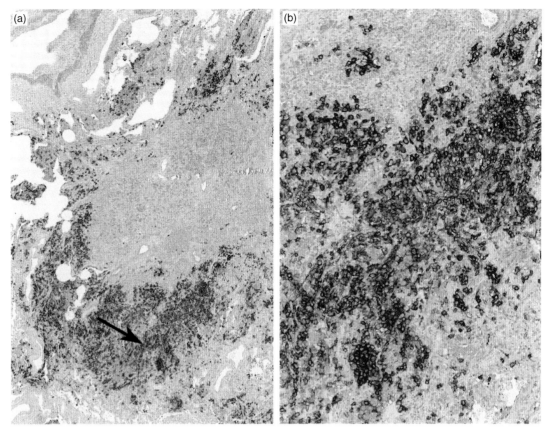

Figure 5.63. Immunohistochemistry in pulmonary Langerhans cell histiocytosis. (a) A cellular nodule, stained with CD1a. Large numbers of Langerhans cells are present in the bottom of the nodule. The area indicated by the arrow is shown at high magnification in part b. **(b)** CD1a-positive Langerhans cells.

There is no evidence of extrapulmonary involvement in the vast majority of adult smokers with pulmonary Langerhans cell histiocytosis. Pathologically confirmed extrapulmonary involvement is almost non-existent in our experience, and is uncommon in the published literature. Reported evidence of extrapulmonary involvement includes lymph node involvement at diagnosis, skin lesions, subsequent development of bone lesions and symptoms of diabetes insipidus at presentation (polyuria and polydipsia). Pathologic confirmation is seldom documented in such cases, and it remains unclear whether the findings are truly attributable to Langerhans cell histiocytosis.

Laboratory findings are non-contributory. There is no evidence of eosinophilia in the peripheral blood. Pulmonary function tests most often show evidence of airflow/airway obstruction and reduced diffusing capacity to carbon monoxide (DL_{CO}), although restrictive and mixed abnormalities also occur. In up to 20% of patients, pulmonary function tests are normal.

Radiologic findings

On chest radiographs, the most common findings are bilateral interstitial infiltrates with a reticulonodular appearance. Characteristic chest CT findings include nodules, cysts or a combination of the two. The nodules are multiple, tiny and bilateral and are almost always less than 1 cm in size. They are often described as "cavitating". In almost two-thirds of cases, nodules and cysts predominate in the upper and mid lung zones. The combination of cysts and bilateral tiny cavitating nodules in the upper lobes of a smoker is so characteristic that it is recognized with reasonable accuracy by experienced radiologists. In one study from 2003, two expert radiologists were able to correctly identify 13 of 18 cases of biopsy-proven pulmonary Langerhans cell histiocytosis with cystic change. The missed cases were misdiagnosed as RBILD/DIP or lymphoid interstitial pneumonia. Conversely, some cases of lymphoid interstitial pneumonia, emphysema and lymphangioleiomyomatosis were misinterpreted as pulmonary Langerhans cell histiocytosis.

However, the corollary of the preceding discussion is that multiple bilateral tiny nodules *without* cysts are not pathognomonic of pulmonary Langerhans cell histiocytosis. This picture is often indistinguishable from metastases to the lung or disseminated fungal/mycobacterial infections, and is most likely to prompt a lung biopsy. In our experience, many cases are detected when individuals with a known extrapulmonary malignancy undergo follow-up imaging and are found to have multiple lung nodules. Metastatic malignancy is usually the primary clinical concern in such cases.

The nodules of pulmonary Langerhans cell histiocytosis can slowly increase in number or remain stable for many years. They may be accompanied by ground-glass opacities. Scarred pulmonary Langerhans cell histiocytosis is associated with radiologic features of fibrosis, including traction bronchiectasis and honeycomb change.

Differential diagnosis

- Usual interstitial pneumonia (UIP) is easily distinguished from the cellular stage of pulmonary Langerhans cell histiocytosis, but can be very difficult to distinguish when scarring supervenes and replaces Langerhans cells. Immunohistochemical staining seldom reveals diagnostic clusters of Langerhans cells when they are not visible on routine H&E-stained sections. In such cases, the presence of peribronchiolar stellate scars, traction emphysema, severe respiratory bronchiolitis, SRIF, smoker's macrophages *within* the interstitium, and prominent type 2 pneumocytes along the edges of the scars points to Langerhans cell histiocytosis, whereas random scarring, extensive honeycomb change and numerous fibroblast foci are features of UIP (Figure 5.30).
- As mentioned in preceding paragraphs, the presence of numerous pigmented alveolar macrophages within the alveoli often prompts a knee-jerk diagnosis of "DIP" and diverts attention from the primary abnormality, which is the presence of nodular lesions. The stellate nodules of pulmonary Langerhans cell histiocytosis are usually visible at low magnification, and if correctly recognized, exclude DIP. Similarly, pulmonary Langerhans cell histiocytosis is unlikely to be mistaken for other smoking-related interstitial lung diseases such as respiratory bronchiolitis, RBILD and SRIF, since none of them forms stellate nodules or scars.
- Adenocarcinoma can enter the differential diagnosis of the florid reactive pneumocyte hyperplasia that accompanies Langerhans cell histiocytosis. The presence of Langerhans cell clusters does not exclude the possibility of a concurrent malignancy. Although this situation can be quite challenging, epithelial proliferation limited to the alveolar septa adjacent to the nodules is likely to be reactive, whereas true adenocarcinoma would be expected to extend further out into the lung parenchyma. Features such as architectural complexity, stromal invasion and degree of nuclear atypia must also be taken into account.

Treatment and prognosis

Although there are no prospective clinical trials on the treatment of pulmonary Langerhans cell histiocytosis, smoking cessation is advocated in most patients, and often results in complete resolution of nodules on chest CT. Rarely, radiologic abnormalities may disappear completely even while the patient continues to smoke. Other approaches that have been tried include corticosteroids (without success) and cladribine (with anecdotal success). Rarely, advanced fibrosis or severe pulmonary hypertension necessitates lung transplantation. The MAP kinase inhibitor vemurafenib is currently being used for other *BRAF*-driven neoplasms, and may be tried for refractory cases of Langerhans cell histiocytosis in the future.

The prognosis is good, although the disease does shorten survival compared to members of the general population. Overall, 15% of patients die from respiratory failure. The median survival is 12 to 13 years, with a 5-year survival of 74%, and a 10-year survival of 64%. Potential complications include recurrent pneumothoraces, decline in lung function and pulmonary hypertension. A recent prospective study reported that 40% of patients show at least 15% decline in lung function (FEV1, FVC or DL_{CO}) within a median of 1 year after diagnosis. Clinical features associated with poor prognosis include old age, low FEV1, FEV1/FVC or DLCO at presentation, and corticosteroid therapy. Some patients develop and die of smoking-related lung cancer, hematologic malignancies, or other pre-existing malignant tumors. There are no convincing reports of progression from isolated pulmonary Langerhans cell histiocytosis to multi-system or disseminated disease.

Sample diagnosis on pathology report

Lung, right upper lobe and right middle lobe, surgical biopsies – Pulmonary Langerhans cell histiocytosis (See comment).

Smoking-related interstitial fibrosis

Smoking-related interstitial fibrosis (SRIF) is a histologically distinctive form of interstitial fibrosis that occurs exclusively in cigarette smokers. Its unique histologic features – and the potential for misinterpretation as fibrosing NSIP – were first described in surgical lung biopsies by Yousem in 2006. The gross features were first described as "airspace enlargement with fibrosis" by Kawabata *et al* in 2008. The term SRIF was coined in 2010 by Katzenstein *et al* when histologic features similar to those described by Yousem were recognized in lung cancer lobectomies from cigarette smokers. We have used SRIF as a diagnostic term in pathology reports since 2011. There are several reasons to introduce SRIF as a clinicopathologic entity into the already confusing terminology of smoking-related interstitial lung diseases (Table 5.9).

SRIF is most commonly encountered in lobectomy specimens from cigarette smokers. Less commonly, it is seen in surgical lung biopsies for interstitial lung disease, either as the main finding, or as a minor, focal or incidental finding in the background of other types of interstitial lung disease. Prior to the introduction of SRIF, many of these cases were undoubtedly misdiagnosed as DIP or fibrosing NSIP. We have also seen SRIF in explant lungs with emphysema (where SRIF was misdiagnosed as chronic hypersensitivity pneumonitis) and in autopsies of cigarette smokers dying of other causes. Rarely, the characteristic fibrosis of SRIF can be recognized in transbronchial lung biopsies.

Major diagnostic findings

The main finding is uniform or patchy expansion of alveolar septa by eosinophilic hyalinized fibrosis, with minimal or no inflammation (Figure 5.64, Figure 5.1c, and book cover, middle image). The hyalinized appearance of the fibrosis is characteristic. It is caused by the presence of densely eosinophilic "ropy" collagen bundles within the interstitium. Emphysema and respiratory bronchiolitis (smoker's macrophages) are nearly always present in the background.

Variable pathologic findings

- Diffuse interstitial inflammation is absent in SRIF. Scattered lymphoid aggregates may occasionally be present.
- The pattern of alveolar septal expansion varies slightly from case to case. In most cases, the fibrosis is most prominent in subpleural lung parenchyma (Figure 5.65). It may also be seen in deeper lung parenchyma, either in a centrilobular or random distribution (Figure 5.66).
- Smooth muscle bundles are often scattered among the thickened alveolar septa, especially in centrilobular parenchyma around alveolar ducts (Figure 5.67).
- Emphysema is seen in nearly all cases. The interstitial fibrosis usually involves the emphysematous areas, but can also involve non-emphysematous lung parenchyma. In some cases of SRIF, scattered areas of classic emphysema without fibrosis may also be present, but they are usually focal.
- Respiratory bronchiolitis is nearly universal in SRIF. It may be very extensive, with large numbers of pigmented macrophages in nearly every respiratory

Table 5.9. Rationale for the term smoking-related interstitial fibrosis (SRIF)

Clearly definable and recognizable by pathologists in lung specimens

Readily distinguishable on pathologic grounds from other fibrosing interstitial lung diseases

Clearly conveys the etiology

Requires the presence of interstitial fibrosis, and acknowledges this succinctly

Separates smoking-related fibrosis from fibrosing NSIP in smokers

Avoids the conceptually awkward term respiratory bronchiolitis

Further reduces the need for the term DIP

Gives pathologists a diagnostic term to use when smoker's macrophages are associated with significant alveolar septal fibrosis (and emphysema)

Unlike RBILD, the diagnosis is not dependent on clinical or radiologic features

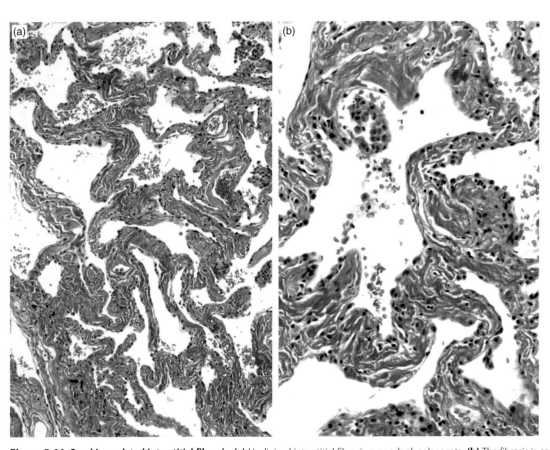

Figure 5.64. Smoking-related interstitial fibrosis. (a) Hyalinized interstitial fibrosis expands alveolar septa. **(b)** The fibrosis is composed of densely eosinophilic ropy collagen bundles. There is almost no inflammation.

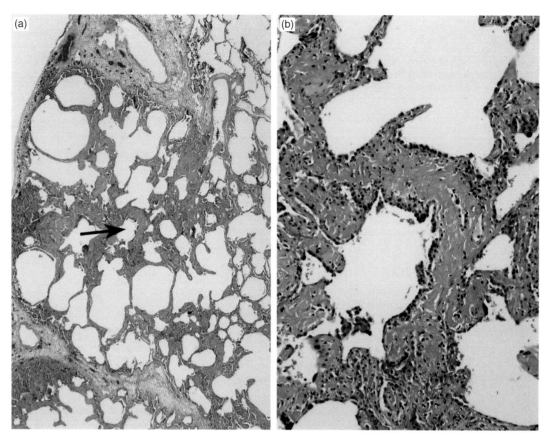

Figure 5.65. Smoking-related interstitial fibrosis. (a) Fibrosis is present mainly in subpleural parenchyma. The area indicated by the arrow is shown at high magnification in part b. **(b)** Hyalinized collagen bundles expand the alveolar septa.

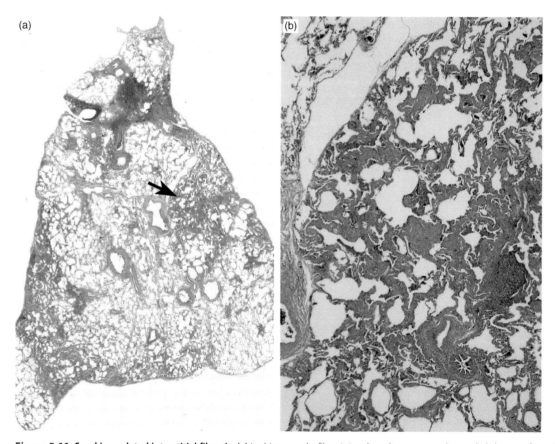

Figure 5.66. Smoking-related interstitial fibrosis. (a) In this example, fibrosis involves deeper parenchyma slightly away from the pleura. Note patchy involvement of the rest of the lung. The area indicated by the arrow is shown at high magnification in b. **(b)** Alveolar septa are thickened by patchy hyalinized fibrosis. A lymphoid aggregate is seen to the right.

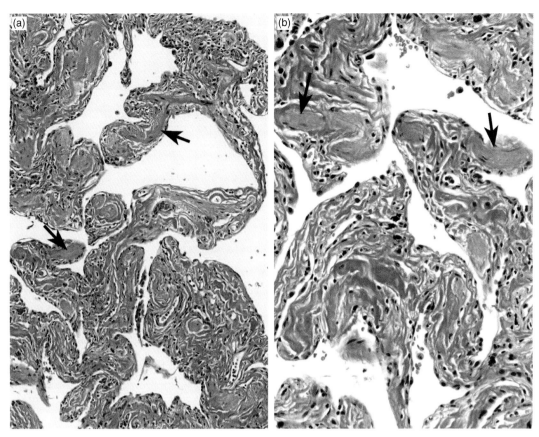

Figure 5.67. Smoking-related interstitial fibrosis. (a) Smooth muscle fibers (arrows) are often admixed with ropy collagen bundles in SRIF. **(b)** Another example of smooth muscle fibers in SRIF (arrows). Their presence probably indicates fibrosis involving alveolar ducts.

bronchiole and alveolar duct, extending into adjacent airspaces as well as airspaces adjacent to interstitial fibrosis. The overall appearance can be "DIP-like" (Figure 5.68).

- In some cases, the interstitial fibrosis stops abruptly at the interlobular septa, and is absent in the adjacent lobule.
- A few fibroblast foci can be identified in some cases, mainly within areas of fibrosis.

Diagnostic work-up

No special stains are required for the diagnosis.

Clinical profile

SRIF is usually an incidental finding in lobectomies from cigarette smokers with lung cancer. The extent to which clinical features are attributable to concurrent lung cancer or emphysema is unclear. In Yousem's series the most common symptoms were cough and dyspnea. The age range in cases reported thus far is 32 to 77 years. Both genders are affected. Patients are invariably current or ex-smokers (15 to 80 pack years).

Pulmonary function tests may show mild to moderate obstructive defects but normal results have also been reported. Mild to moderate reduction in diffusion capacity has been noted in some patients, including some with normal spirometry. In Yousem's series, mixed obstructive and restrictive patterns were common.

Radiologic findings

The radiologic findings of SRIF on high-resolution CT scans have not been adequately described. In Yousem's study, the main findings were bilateral micronodular or linear infiltrates. Ground-glass opacities were seen in 44% of cases.

Differential diagnosis

SRIF needs to be distinguished from other forms of fibrosing interstitial lung disease, including fibrosing NSIP (Figure 5.69) and UIP (Figure 5.32). Features helpful in the differential diagnosis are shown in Table 5.10.

Treatment and prognosis

It is unknown whether SRIF requires therapy, or what measures may be beneficial. In Katzenstein's study, no patient progressed to clinically significant interstitial lung disease, but follow-up was short. In Yousem's series, all patients were alive with stable or slowly progressive disease after 0.5 to 5.2 years of follow-up. Our anecdotal experience suggests that patients with SRIF who progress or die do so because of concomitant lung cancer or emphysema.

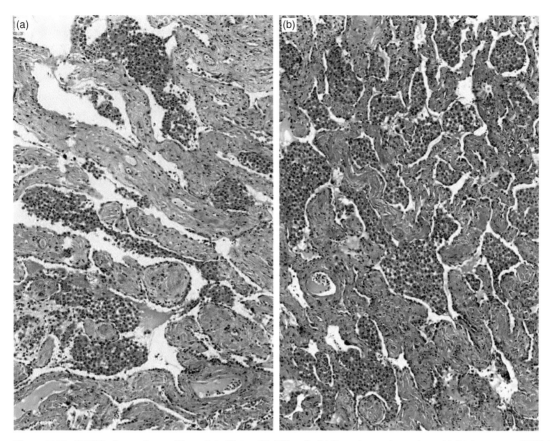

Figure 5.68. "DIP-like" areas in smoking-related interstitial fibrosis. (a) Extensive respiratory bronchiolitis in an area of SRIF. **(b)** Large clusters of smoker's macrophages fill nearly all airspaces. The presence of hyalinized interstitial fibrosis indicates the correct interpretation.

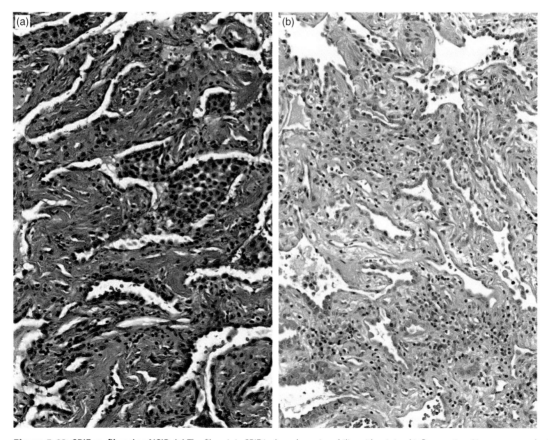

Figure 5.69. SRIF vs. fibrosing NSIP. (a) The fibrosis in SRIF is densely eosinophilic, with minimal inflammation. Numerous smoker's macrophages fill the airspaces. **(b)** The collagen in fibrosing NSIP is not hyalinized, and is admixed with chronic inflammation.

Table 5.10. Differential diagnosis of SRIF

Histologic feature	SRIF	RBILD	NSIP, fibrosing variant	UIP
Significant alveolar septal fibrosis	Yes	No	Yes	Yes
Alveolar septal expansion by ropy hyalinized collagen	Yes	No	No	No
Chronic inflammation	Absent or scant, focal	Absent or scant, focal	Common, diffuse	Usually minimal, focal
Patchwork pattern, scarring, honeycomb change	No	No	No	Yes
Fibroblast foci	Usually absent; occasionally a few	No	Occasional, few	Usually present, often several
Emphysema	Nearly all cases	Uncommon	Uncommon	Variable
Respiratory bronchiolitis	Nearly all cases	All cases	Uncommon	Variable

Sample diagnosis on pathology report

Lung, right upper lobe, surgical biopsy – Smoking-related interstitial fibrosis (See comment).

Hypersensitivity pneumonitis

Hypersensitivity pneumonitis is a distinctive form of interstitial lung disease characterized by an immunologically mediated inflammatory response to inhaled organic antigens in susceptible individuals. It is also known as *hypersensitivity pneumonia* or *extrinsic allergic alveolitis*. In contrast to allergic conditions such as asthma and hay fever, this condition does not feature type I hypersensitivity. Instead, the inflammatory response is a type III (immune-complex mediated) or type IV (T-cell mediated) hypersensitivity response. This explains why the inflammatory infiltrate in hypersensitivity pneumonitis is composed of lymphocytes, not eosinophils.

The disease can be triggered by a wide range of antigens, some of which are listed in Table 5.11. Exposure to pet birds at home is by far the most common cause of biopsy-proven hypersensitivity pneumonitis. The condition is also known as *bird fancier's lung*, and the inciting antigen is thought to be related to bloom, a waxy protein that coats bird feathers. Less commonly, mycobacterial antigens in aerosols derived from hot tub water are implicated in a form of hypersensitivity pneumonitis known as *hot tub lung*. *Farmer's lung* is perhaps the best known form of hypersensitivity pneumonitis, but it is seldom biopsied because the relationship between exposure and disease is usually obvious. It is important to remember that a source of antigen exposure cannot be identified in 25 to 38% of cases of biopsy-proven hypersensitivity pneumonitis.

Hypersensitivity pneumonitis has been traditionally classified on clinical grounds into acute, subacute and chronic types. Acute hypersensitivity pneumonitis is diagnosed clinically and rarely biopsied. In contrast, subacute and chronic hypersensitivity pneumonitis may mimic other interstitial lung diseases, requiring lung biopsy for diagnosis. Lung biopsies are especially important in atypical clinical settings, such as when an inciting antigen cannot be identified. Biopsies may also be required when radiologic and BAL findings do not allow a confident diagnosis, or in patients who do not respond to therapy.

The diagnosis can be suggested in transbronchial biopsies (Chapter 1, Figure 1.36), although diagnostic areas are not always sampled. Therefore, surgical lung biopsies may be required to establish the diagnosis in some cases.

Major diagnostic findings

The most consistent pathologic feature of hypersensitivity pneumonitis is the presence of a *cellular chronic interstitial pneumonia* characterized by slight expansion of the alveolar septa by an inflammatory infiltrate consisting mainly of lymphocytes (Figures 5.70 to 5.74, and Figure 5.1a). A few scattered plasma cells, histiocytes or multinucleated giant cells may also be present within the interstitial inflammatory infiltrate. The interstitial expansion is usually mild and diffuse.

Variable pathologic findings

- A characteristic but subtle feature of hypersensitivity pneumonitis is *peribronchiolar accentuation of the inflammatory infiltrate*. The infiltrate is most prominent in the walls of respiratory bronchioles and alveolar ducts (Figure 5.70a), and decreases in intensity in alveoli distal to these structures. Inflammation of small bronchioles, also referred to as *cellular chronic bronchiolitis*, may be subtle and is not always readily appreciated.

Table 5.11. Sources of antigen exposure in hypersensitivity pneumonitis

Name of syndrome	Inciting antigen	Antigen source
Bird fancier's lung	Avian proteins	Pet birds (parakeets, pigeons, canaries, cockatiels, hens, parrots, doves, budgerigars, goldfinches, ducks, turtledoves, chickens, partridges, storks, quails)
Hot tub lung	Non-tuberculous mycobacteria, almost always *M. avium complex* (MAC)	Aerosolized warm water from hot tubs contaminated with mycobacteria
Feather duvet lung	Avian antigens	Raw goose or duck feathers in feather duvets or pillows
Humidifier lung	Thermophilic actinomycetes (bacteria)	Warm water
Farmer's lung, mushroom worker's lung, bagassosis	Thermophilic actinomycetes (bacteria) such as *Saccharopolyspora rectivirgula* (formerly *Micropolyspora faeni*)	Moldy hay, moldy mushroom compost, moldy sugarcane
Maple bark strippers' lung	*Cryptostroma corticale*	Moldy maple bark
Cheese workers' lung	*Penicillium* (fungus)	Moldy cheese
Summer-type hypersensitivity pneumonitis (Japan)	*Trichosporon asahii, Trichosporon mucoides, Cryptococcus albidus* (fungi)	Home environment
Wind-instruments lung	*Candida albicans*, Phoma, *Ulocladium* (fungi), *Mycobacterium abscessus/chelonae*	Mycobacteria or fungi in wind instruments such as saxophones or trombones

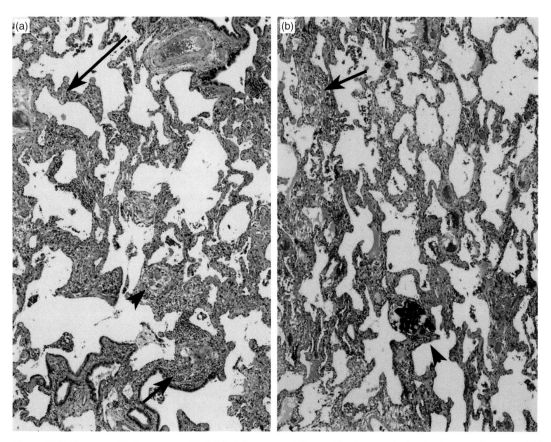

Figure 5.70. Hypersensitivity pneumonitis. (a) An inflammatory infiltrate diffusely expands the alveolar septa (long arrow). The infiltrate is accentuated in the walls of small bronchioles (short arrow). Granulomas are tiny and inconspicuous (arrowhead). **(b)** Diffuse interstitial expansion resembling the cellular variant of NSIP. The tip-off to the correct diagnosis is the presence of an occasional loose granuloma within the interstitial infiltrate (arrow). A microcalcification can be seen at low magnification (arrowhead). Such structures typically form within multinucleated giant cells and are a clue to the diagnosis.

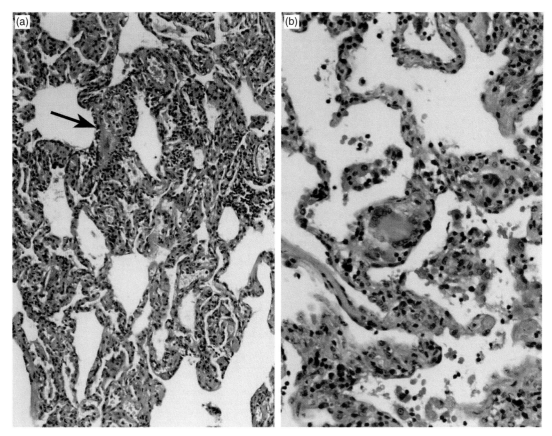

Figure 5.71. Hypersensitivity pneumonitis. (a) Lymphocytes are seen within the alveolar septa. They are slightly more prominent in the wall of an alveolar duct (arrow) **(b)** A single multinucleated giant cell is seen within this interstitial infiltrate, which is composed mainly of lymphocytes and plasma cells.

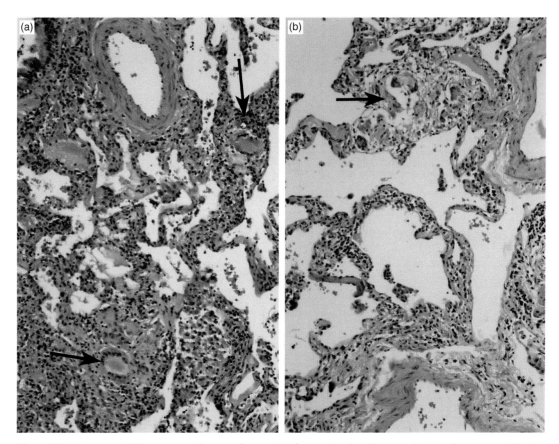

Figure 5.72. Hypersensitivity pneumonitis: granulomas. (a) A few scattered multinucleated giant cells are seen within this interstitial inflammatory infiltrate (arrows). The giant cell at top is located in peribronchiolar interstitium. **(b)** This tiny poorly formed granuloma (arrow) is located in the interstitium adjacent to a small pulmonary artery, suggesting that it involves a small bronchiole or alveolar duct. It is a rather loose aggregate of a few histiocytes and multinucleated giant cells.

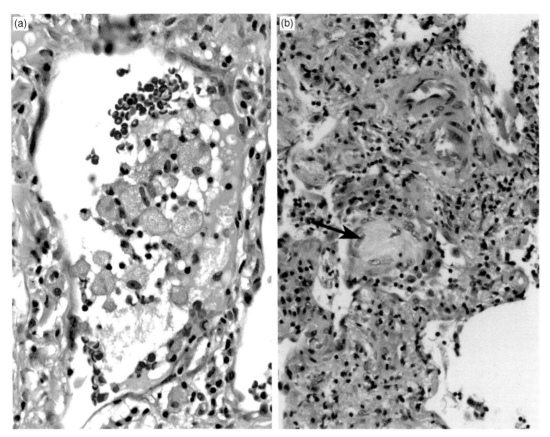

Figure 5.73. Hypersensitivity pneumonitis. (a) Foamy macrophages within an airspace. **(b)** A tiny fibroblast plug (organizing pneumonia).

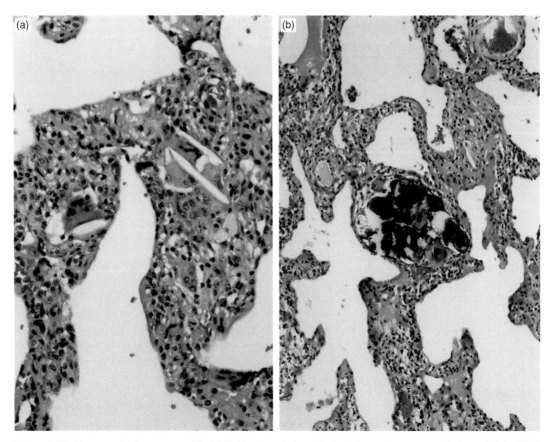

Figure 5.74. Hypersensitivity pneumonitis. (a) Multinucleated giant cells in the interstitium contain cholesterol clefts. **(b)** This calcific structure is probably a Schaumann body.

- Although hypersensitivity pneumonitis is an interstitial disease, secondary changes are common within the airspaces. They include rare tiny fibroblast plugs (*organizing pneumonia*) and clusters of *foamy macrophages* within peribronchiolar airspaces (Figure 5.73). The latter is thought to be a post-obstructive phenomenon caused by bronchiolar narrowing.
- Eosinophils are absent in hypersensitivity pneumonitis because it is not a type I (allergic) hypersensitivity response. In rare cases where eosinophils are present, they are few in number.
- Granulomas can be seen in some but not all cases of hypersensitivity pneumonitis. They are usually found within the inflammatory infiltrate in alveolar septa or bronchiolar walls (Figure 5.72). They are tiny, poorly formed and non-necrotizing. Multinucleated giant cells are also common. They may contain microcalcifications, Schaumann bodies, cholesterol clefts or other endogenous products of macrophage metabolism (Figure 5.74). These inclusions are of no significance. They are often misinterpreted as exogenous (foreign) particles, leading to the erroneous conclusion that they are derived from the source of exposure.
- The classic triad of hypersensitivity pneumonitis consists of (1) cellular chronic interstitial pneumonia, (2) poorly formed interstitial granulomas and (3) tiny foci of organizing pneumonia. Unfortunately this triad is identified in only 9% of transbronchial lung biopsies and 50% of surgical lung biopsies. Organizing pneumonia is the least common and least significant part of this triad, and its absence does not significantly impact interpretation. However, the absence of granulomas is more problematic. In cases with a cellular chronic interstitial pneumonia but no granulomas or giant cells, the diagnosis can still be suggested by the pathologist, especially if there is evidence of peribronchiolar accentuation. The differential diagnosis in such cases also includes some drug reactions, connective tissue diseases and cellular NSIP.

Clinical profile

Hypersensitivity pneumonitis occurs in adults of both sexes, although there is a predilection for women. Most patients are never-smokers. In fact, cigarette smoking is thought to be "protective". Hypersensitivity pneumonitis is classified clinically according to the onset and duration of symptoms as acute (developing within hours of exposure and lasting hours to days), subacute (lasting for up to 4 to 6 months) or chronic (lasting for more than 4 to 6 months). Recent data suggest that this classification is less than ideal.

Patients with acute hypersensitivity pneumonitis (e.g., farmer's lung) develop symptoms within 2 to 9 hours of exposure to the antigen. Systemic symptoms or influenza-like symptoms such as chills, fever, sweating, myalgias, body aches, headache and nausea are common. Some patients present with cough and dyspnea. Subacute hypersensitivity pneumonitis usually presents with cough, dyspnea or fever over a period of weeks to months. Patients with chronic hypersensitivity pneumonitis present predominantly with dyspnea and cough. Fever, fatigue, weight loss, flu-like symptoms and chest discomfort are less common. A history of episodic exacerbation of symptoms in certain locations or situations is a clue to the diagnosis of hypersensitivity pneumonitis. The most common physical findings are inspiratory crackles and squeaks. Wheezing, cyanosis and digital clubbing are present only in a minority of cases.

The diagnosis can be difficult because there is no well-defined gold standard. Key investigations include bronchoalveolar lavage (BAL), pulmonary function tests and high-resolution computed tomography (HRCT). BAL usually shows lymphocytosis with a predominance of CD8-positive T-lymphocytes over CD4-positive T-lymphocytes (reversal of the normal CD4:CD8 ratio). Pulmonary function tests most often show restrictive changes with a decrease in the diffusing capacity of carbon monoxide (DL_{CO}). Some patients show obstructive changes. Other investigations include serologic tests for antibodies to a variety of antigens, skin hypersensitivity tests or antigen challenge tests. The specificity of serologic tests is questionable.

Radiologic findings

Radiographs may be normal or may show bilateral interstitial infiltrates. HRCT is more sensitive than chest X-rays. In classic cases, they show bilateral ground-glass opacities with fine centrilobular nodules and *air trapping*, manifested by *mosaic attenuation* on expiratory films. Some patients may have normal findings even on HRCT. Radiologic abnormalities are said to be more pronounced in the upper lobes, although a recent large study challenges this assumption. Honeycombing may be present on HRCT in a small minority of patients; these represent cases in which fibrosis has supervened and progressed, and can be radiologically indistinguishable from usual interstitial pneumonia/idiopathic pulmonary fibrosis.

Differential diagnosis

- Organizing pneumonia may enter the differential diagnosis but most cases feature several prominent fibroblast plugs, and interstitial inflammation, when present, is generally less conspicuous. In contrast, interstitial inflammation is the predominant finding in hypersensitivity pneumonitis, and fibroblast plugs, if present, are rare and tiny (Figure 5.73b).
- UIP enters the differential diagnosis when fibrosis is prominent, and features such as scarring and honeycombing are present. Distinguishing UIP from chronic hypersensitivity pneumonitis in such cases can be challenging. The most reliable histologic indicator of hypersensitivity pneumonitis in such cases is the presence of a cellular chronic interstitial pneumonia (typical of subacute hypersensitivity pneumonitis) away from the areas of scarring and honeycomb lung. In other words, at

least some areas in the biopsy should show interstitial chronic inflammation with peribronchiolar accentuation and scattered loose granulomas or giant cells. It is important to remember that granulomas can also be found in UIP. They may be related to poor clearance of debris from areas of scarring and honeycomb change, or superimposed infection or aspiration of particulate matter from gastric contents (food/pill fragments). Therefore, granulomas do not necessarily negate the diagnosis of UIP or establish a diagnosis of chronic hypersensitivity pneumonitis.

- An entity that can be difficult to separate from hypersensitivity pneumonitis is the cellular variant of non-specific interstitial pneumonia (NSIP). Both feature interstitial chronic inflammation composed primarily of lymphocytes. Therefore, when a lung biopsy shows changes reminiscent of cellular NSIP, a careful search for multinucleated giant cells or tiny, loose granulomas within the inflamed interstitium should be performed. Cases without these findings may still represent hypersensitivity pneumonitis, provided that the clinical context is appropriate. Therefore, from the clinical standpoint, a pathologic diagnosis of cellular NSIP or a descriptive diagnosis of *cellular chronic interstitial pneumonia* should prompt a thorough history for a potential source of antigen exposure. A diagnosis of idiopathic NSIP should be made only after hypersensitivity pneumonitis has been excluded clinically.
- Hot tub lung. Pathologic features shared by hot tub lung and hypersensitivity pneumonitis include interstitial inflammation, granulomas and foci of organizing pneumonia. The distinction lies in the relative prominence of interstitial inflammation and granulomas, the morphologic characteristics of the granulomas and the history of hot tub use. While interstitial chronic inflammation is the predominant feature in hypersensitivity pneumonitis, granulomas dominate the histologic picture in hot tub lung. In classic cases of hot tub lung, granulomas are large, well-formed and present mainly within airspaces. In contrast, the granulomas of hypersensitivity pneumonitis are tiny and poorly formed and are located mainly within the interstitium. Regardless of the histologic findings, a clinical history of hot tub use is essential for a diagnosis of hot tub lung.
- MAC infection can cause dense chronic inflammation in airway walls with poorly formed granulomas, mimicking hypersensitivity pneumonitis. Identification of mycobacteria by special stains or cultures will resolve this problem, but organisms are seldom found in such cases. In the absence of an organism, significant extension of the inflammatory infiltrate into the alveolar septa favors hypersensitivity pneumonitis.
- The presence of non-necrotizing granulomas may raise the possibility of sarcoidosis. However, sarcoidosis is a predominantly granulomatous disease in which lung parenchyma away from the granulomas is normal. In contrast, hypersensitivity pneumonitis is predominantly

lymphocytic rather than granulomatous, and the interstitium is diffusely involved. The granulomas of sarcoidosis are large and prominent, whereas those of hypersensitivity pneumonitis are tiny and inconspicuous (Chapter 2, Figure 2.49).

Treatment and prognosis

Hypersensitivity pneumonitis is usually responsive to therapy, which includes identification of the source of exposure and removal of the patient from it or vice versa. Corticosteroids are used in many patients, most of whom show an excellent response. In a recent large series, 29 of 57 (51%) patients were completely symptom free at a median of 8 months of follow-up and 32% showed improvement; only 18% did not improve.

Chronic hypersensitivity pneumonitis has a worse prognosis than acute or subacute hypersensitivity pneumonitis. This is thought to be due to the development of fibrosis, which probably accounts for the small number of patients that die of this disease. In one study, median survival in patients with fibrosis was 7.1 years while median survival in those without fibrosis was at least 20.9 years (in fact, it could not be accurately calculated since more than 85% of patients were still alive at last follow-up). In the same study, the overall 5-year mortality was 27% and the median survival was 12.8 years.

Sample diagnosis on pathology report

Lung, right upper lobe, transbronchial biopsy – Cellular chronic interstitial pneumonia with poorly formed granulomas consistent with hypersensitivity pneumonitis (See comment).

Non-specific interstitial pneumonia

Non-specific interstitial pneumonia (NSIP) is an uncommon form of interstitial lung disease if strict criteria are followed. It can be encountered as an idiopathic condition, or can occur in patients with clinical evidence of hypersensitivity pneumonitis, connective tissue diseases or drug toxicity. Currently, NSIP is thought to be the most common histologic finding in connective tissue diseases and their forme frustes. It is also seen as a focal finding in cases of UIP, either in the same lobe or in different lobes. This last point is very significant, because it throws doubt on the accuracy of the diagnosis of NSIP, even when it is "confirmed" by a surgical lung biopsy. It is likely that many cases currently diagnosed as NSIP actually represent sampling error in UIP.

Major diagnostic findings

- Uniform and diffuse alveolar septal expansion by collagen or lymphocytes or both (Figures 5.75 and 5.76). Significant collagen deposition defines the *fibrosing variant of NSIP*. In the *cellular variant of NSIP*, alveolar septal expansion is purely cellular without significant fibrosis.
- No patchwork pattern (see section on UIP for explanation).

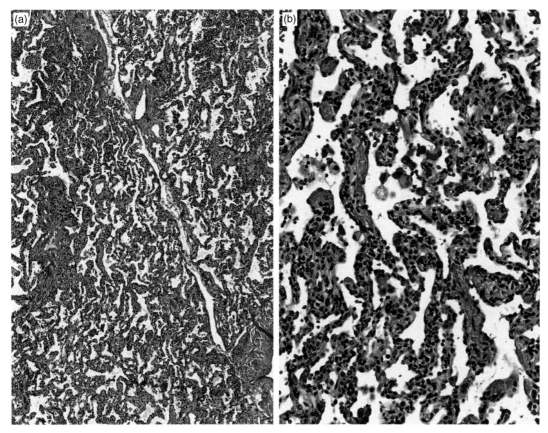

Figure 5.75. NSIP, cellular variant. (a) Diffuse cellular interstitial infiltrate without scarring or architectural distortion. **(b)** The infiltrate is almost entirely cellular, with no significant fibrosis.

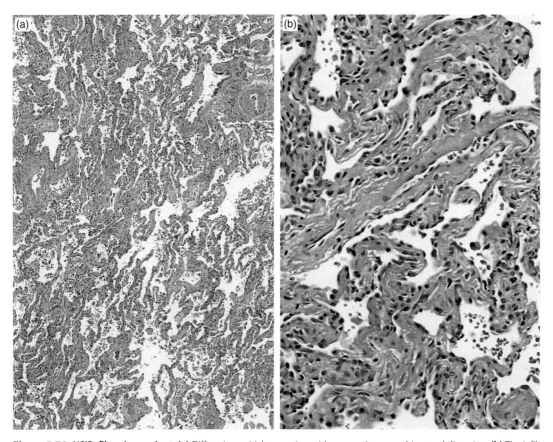

Figure 5.76. NSIP, fibrosing variant. (a) Diffuse interstitial expansion without scarring or architectural distortion. **(b)** The infiltrate is cellular but there is also mild collagen deposition.

- No intervening islands of normal lung between fibrotic areas.
- No significant scarring or honeycomb change on pathologic examination.
- No honeycomb change on radiologic examination.
- Surgical lung biopsy.
- No features to suggest an alternative diagnosis, the most important of which are UIP, hypersensitivity pneumonitis, organizing DAD, organizing pneumonia and SRIF.

Variable pathologic findings

A few fibroblast foci may be present. Minimal scarring and minimal, focal honeycomb change is also acceptable. Tiny foci of organizing pneumonia may also be present.

Diagnostic work-up

No special stains are required. The diagnosis can be made on H&E-stained sections.

Clinical profile

The clinical presentation of NSIP is similar to that of UIP. Although individuals with NSIP tend to be younger than those with UIP, this distinction is not useful in an individual case. As with UIP, many patients present with cough or progressive dyspnea. Patients with NSIP may have a known history of underlying connective tissue disease, but in some cases the diagnosis of a specific connective tissue disease is made months to years after the pathologic diagnosis of NSIP. This latter phenomenon has led to the clinical hypothesis that in many cases NSIP is a manifestation of "lung-dominant connective tissue disease".

Radiologic findings

NSIP manifests radiologically as bilateral interstitial infiltrates, often with an apicobasal gradient. Honeycomb change prominent enough to be visible radiologically excludes NSIP. Unlike UIP, the radiologic diagnosis of NSIP is notoriously inaccurate. This is because cases that lack honeycomb change radiologically frequently show microscopic honeycomb change. Thus, a large proportion of cases that meet radiologic criteria for fibrosing NSIP prove to be UIP on biopsy.

Differential diagnosis

The differential diagnosis of NSIP includes UIP, organizing DAD, organizing pneumonia and SRIF. These entities are compared and contrasted in Tables 5.6 and 5.10. The differential diagnosis with UIP is discussed in detail in the section on UIP. The differential diagnosis with hypersensitivity pneumonitis is discussed in that section.

Treatment and prognosis

Unlike UIP, NSIP is occasionally responsive to immunosuppressant therapy, including corticosteroids, azathioprine, cyclophosphamide and mycophenolate mofetil. Not surprisingly, treatment is more likely to be of benefit in the cellular variant than in the fibrosing variant. The clinical course is generally more indolent than UIP, with longer survival. In a recent study from Europe (published in 2015), 2-year survival was 89%, 5-year survival was 66% and 10-year survival was 50%.

Sample diagnosis on pathology report

Lung, right lower lobe and right middle lobe, surgical biopsies – Cellular chronic interstitial pneumonia (See comment).
   or
Lung, right lower lobe and right middle lobe, surgical biopsies – Chronic fibrosing interstitial pneumonia most consistent with non-specific interstitial pneumonia, fibrosing variant (See comment).

Connective tissue disease-related interstitial lung disease (CTD-ILD)

Connective tissue diseases of many types can involve the lung. The lung manifestations are variable, but NSIP, UIP, organizing pneumonia and DAD are common to many of these diseases. Other findings such as follicular bronchiolitis or lymphoid interstitial pneumonia may rarely be present. The most common connective tissue diseases associated with interstitial lung disease and their common manifestations are listed in Table 5.12.

Major diagnostic findings

The diagnosis of a connective tissue disease-related interstitial lung disease cannot be made on the basis of pathologic findings alone, as there are no specific or pathognomonic findings. Compared to idiopathic interstitial lung disease, connective tissue disease-related cases tend to show greater inflammation, pleuritis and lymphoid aggregates. None of these findings is specific enough to allow a confident pathologic diagnosis of connective tissue disease. The most the pathologist can do is raise the possibility of an underlying connective tissue disease, or (if the patient has a known connective tissue disease) state whether the findings are consistent with connective tissue disease. This dubious exercise is highly subjective, and of questionable accuracy.

The most common findings are UIP, NSIP, organizing pneumonia and DAD. The pathologic findings are frequently unclassifiable (Figure 5.77), and this has been cited as a tip-off that one may be dealing with a connective tissue disease.

Sample diagnosis on pathology report

With known history:
   Lung, right lower lobe and right middle lobe, surgical biopsies – Usual interstitial pneumonia, consistent with rheumatoid arthritis-associated interstitial lung disease (See comment).
Without known history:
   Lung, right lower lobe and right middle lobe, surgical biopsies – Usual interstitial pneumonia (See comment).

Table 5.12. Connective tissue diseases and interstitial lung disease

Connective tissue disease	Most common manifestations (interstitial lung disease)	Other manifestations in the lung
Rheumatoid arthritis	NSIP UIP Organizing pneumonia	Follicular bronchiolitis Pleuritis Rheumatoid nodules (see Chapter 2) Constrictive bronchiolitis Pulmonary hypertension Secondary amyloidosis
Progressive systemic sclerosis (scleroderma)	NSIP UIP	Pulmonary vascular changes, including pulmonary hypertension Aspiration pneumonia
Polymyositis and dermatomyositis	NSIP DAD UIP	Aspiration pneumonia Organizing pneumonia
Sjögren syndrome	NSIP UIP	LIP Follicular bronchiolitis MALT lymphoma Secondary amyloidosis Light chain deposition disease
Systemic lupus erythematosus	NSIP Pleuritis	Capillaritis Organizing pneumonia DAD Vascular changes, including pulmonary hypertension

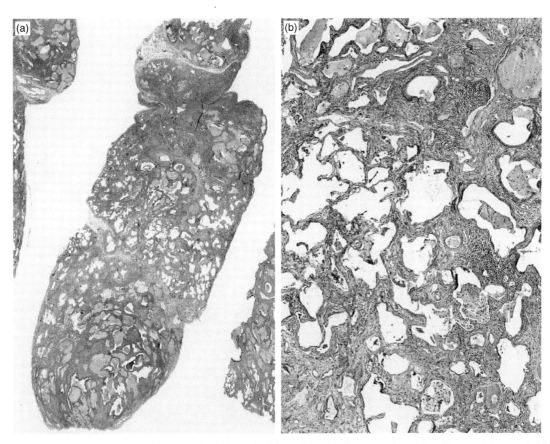

Figure 5.77. Connective tissue disease-related interstitial lung disease (Sjögren syndrome in a 49-year-old woman). (a) Interstitial fibrosis with honeycomb change. The degree of honeycomb change was judged to be too excessive for NSIP. **(b)** Unlike UIP, there is no patchwork pattern, and fibroblast foci are absent. Note lymphoid aggregates. The case was considered unclassifiable.

Table 5.13. Drugs commonly implicated in interstitial lung disease

Drug	Pathologic manifestations
Amiodarone	DAD with foamy macrophages Organizing pneumonia with foamy macrophages Cellular chronic interstitial pneumonia with foamy macrophages Eosinophilic pneumonia with foamy macrophages Pleuritis Mass-like lesions
Nitrofurantoin	UIP-like interstitial changes Cellular chronic interstitial pneumonia DAD Organizing pneumonia
Methotrexate	Cellular chronic interstitial pneumonia (with or without poorly formed granulomas) (Figure 5.78) Organizing pneumonia DAD

Drug-related lung disease

Many drugs have been linked to interstitial lung disease, acute lung injury and other types of non-neoplastic lung disease (see references for an exhaustive list). The most common drugs seen in practice and their associated lung manifestations are shown in Table 5.13. Drugs associated with eosinophilic pneumonia are listed in Chapter 4.

Major diagnostic findings

There are no pathognomonic pathologic findings for any type of drug-related lung disease, and lung biopsies do not "confirm" drug toxicity. The main requirements for a diagnosis of drug-related lung disease are:

- Onset of symptoms or radiologic findings after starting the drug (interval may be many years in some cases).
- Exclusion of alternative etiologies by clinical investigation and pathologic examination, the most important of which is infection.
- Pathologic findings consistent with drug toxicity (acute lung injury, cellular chronic interstitial pneumonia, etc.).
- Clinical response to cessation of drug therapy.

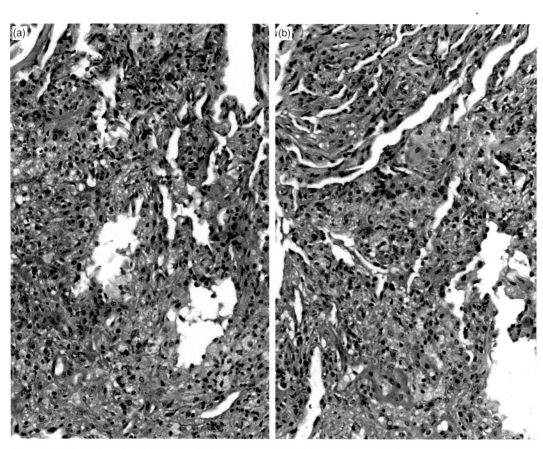

Figure 5.78. Methotrexate-related interstitial lung disease. (a) Cellular chronic interstitial pneumonia characterized by expansion of the interstitium by lymphocytes and histiocytes. **(b)** Poorly formed aggregates of histiocytes within the interstitium.

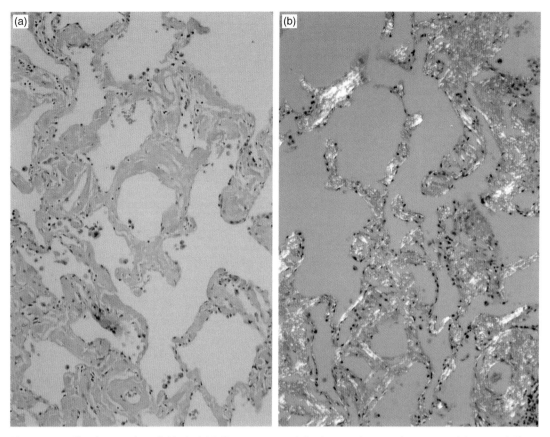

Figure 5.79. Alveolar septal amyloidosis. (a) Diffuse expansion of alveolar septa by amorphous eosinophilic material. The process can mimic interstitial fibrosis. **(b)** Apple-green birefringence on Congo red staining (polarized light).

Sample diagnosis on pathology report

Lung, right middle lobe, transbronchial biopsies – Cellular chronic interstitial pneumonia (See comment).

Miscellaneous and rare causes of interstitial lung disease

Alveolar septal amyloidosis is one of the three major forms of amyloidosis in the lung, the others being nodular amyloidosis (addressed in Chapter 6) and tracheobronchial amyloidosis (discussed in Chapter 9). Alveolar septal amyloidosis is discussed here since it is an interstitial process that can be mistaken for interstitial fibrosis. It is typically seen in surgical lung biopsies or at autopsy, but it may be encountered in transbronchial lung biopsies. The condition is characterized by diffuse expansion of alveolar septa by amyloid deposits and is easily confirmed by Congo red staining (Figure 5.79). The prognosis is very poor because patients almost invariably have systemic amyloidosis and frequently show evidence of cardiac involvement.

Hard metal lung disease is an uncommon form of interstitial lung disease caused by occupational exposure to an alloy known as "hard metal" in susceptible or hypersensitive individuals. Hard metal is formed when tungsten carbide powder and cobalt are heated together at high temperatures and high pressure. Occasionally, titanium and tantalum are also present. It is approximately (95%) as hard as diamond, making it useful for cutting other hard substances such as metals, stones and concrete. Hard metal is used in cutting, drilling, grinding and polishing hard materials, as well as production of electrical parts, drill tips, tool edges, machinery and nuclear armament components. Affected individuals are typically exposed to hard metal in the form of a dust or aerosol, and usually do not use a mask or respirator at work. Prior to the knowledge that this condition was caused by exposure to hard metal, it was known as *giant cell interstitial pneumonia* (GIP), a term coined by Averill Liebow in 1968, based on the most striking histologic feature. Most patients with classic histologic features of GIP have a history of exposure to hard metal. Cases of GIP without documented hard metal exposure have been described, but are thought to be rare. The most characteristic finding is the presence of multinucleated giant cells within the alveoli (airspaces), admixed with macrophages (Figure 5.80). These giant cells typically show emperipolesis ("cellular cannibalism"), a phenomenon in which macrophages engulf other cells. The chief difference between emperipolesis and phagocytosis is that in phagocytosis the engulfed cells are destroyed, whereas in emperipolesis they are viable and simply "passing through". Another example of this phenomenon is Rosai–Dorfman disease. In hard metal disease, the engulfed cells are usually macrophages, lymphocytes or neutrophils.

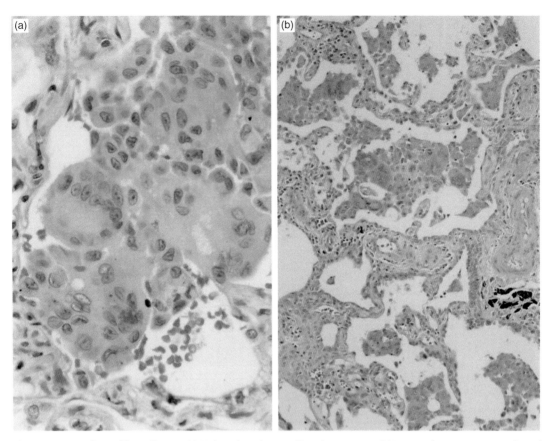

Figure 5.80. Hard metal lung disease. (a) Multinucleated giant cells within airspaces. **(b)** Interstitial pneumonia in peribronchiolar lung parenchyma.

The interstitium is thickened by a variable combination of chronic inflammation, fibrosis and lymphoid aggregates. The chronic inflammation is composed predominantly of lymphocytes and a few plasma cells. The process is usually accentuated around bronchioles (bronchiolocentric). A history of exposure to hard metal dust is the key to establish that a case that shows histologic features of GIP represents hard metal lung disease. A history of working in a tungsten carbide plant, machine shop, tool manufacturing plant, drilling, grinding or lathing, or mixing powders should be sought. Tungsten can be detected in formalin-fixed paraffin-embedded lung tissue by energy-dispersive X-ray spectroscopy (EDS), helping to confirm the diagnosis. In addition to tungsten, titanium, aluminum, silicon and iron are often detected by this method. Cobalt is soluble and not detected, although is thought to be important in the pathogenesis of the disease, perhaps even more so than tungsten.

Lymphoid interstitial pneumonia (LIP) is a vanishingly rare entity that has been largely supplanted by other well-defined causes of interstitial lymphocytic infiltrates, including MALT lymphoma, follicular bronchiolitis, NSIP and hypersensitivity pneumonitis. In modern times, this term should not be used unless low-grade lymphoma has been carefully excluded. The diagnosis requires a striking interstitial lymphoplasmacytic infiltrate (Figure 5.81). Intra-alveolar eosinophilic material is a characteristic but underappreciated finding.

Pleuroparenchymal fibroelastosis is a rare entity in which elastotic fibrosis envelops the lung. The condition overlaps in many ways with UIP, and its existence as a discrete entity has been questioned.

References

Usual interstitial pneumonia

American Thoracic Society; European Respiratory Society. American Thoracic Society/European Respiratory Society international multidisciplinary consensus classification of the idiopathic interstitial pneumonias. *Am J Respir Crit Care Med* 2002;**165**:277–304.

Flaherty KR, Toews GB, Travis WD, *et al.* Clinical significance of histological classification of idiopathic interstitial pneumonia. *Eur Respir J* 2002;**19**:275–83.

Flaherty KR, Travis WD, Colby TV, *et al.* Histopathologic variability in usual and nonspecific interstitial pneumonias. *Am J Respir Crit Care Med* 2001;**164**:1722–7.

Gruden JF, Panse PM, Leslie KO, Tazelaar HD, Colby TV. UIP diagnosed at surgical lung biopsy, 2000–2009: HRCT patterns and proposed classification system. *AJR Am J Roentgenol* 2013;**200**:W458–67.

Katzenstein AA, Mukhopadhyay S, Myers JL. Diagnosis of usual interstitial pneumonia and distinction from other fibrosing interstitial lung diseases. *Hum Pathol* 2008;**39**:1275–94.

Katzenstein AA, Myers JL, Prophet WD, Corley LS III, Shin MS. Bronchiolitis obliterans organizing pneumonia and usual interstitial pneumonia. A comparative

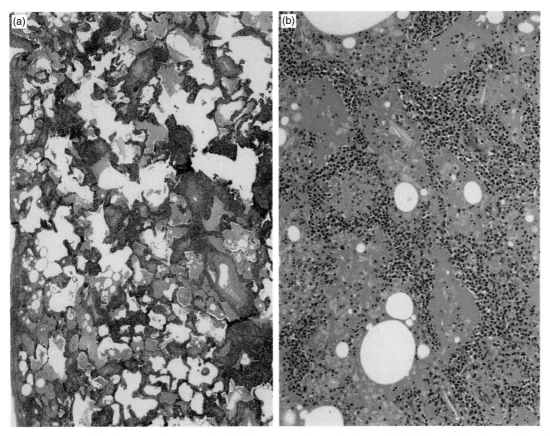

Figure 5.81. Lymphoid interstitial pneumonia. (a) Diffuse interstitial expansion by a cellular infiltrate. **(b)** The degree of interstitial expansion is greater than cellular NSIP or hypersensitivity pneumonitis. Note intra-alveolar eosinophilic material resembling edema fluid.

clinicopathologic study. *Am J Surg Pathol* 1986;**10**:373–81.

Katzenstein AA, Zisman DA, Litzky LA, Nguyen BT, Kotloff RM. Usual interstitial pneumonia: Histologic study of biopsy and explant specimens. *Am J Surg Pathol* 2002;**261**:1567–77.

Nadrous HF, Myers JL, Decker PA, Ryu JH. Idiopathic pulmonary fibrosis in patients younger than 50 years. *Mayo Clin Proc* 2005;**80**:37–40.

Park JH, Kim DS, Park IN, *et al*. Prognosis of fibrotic interstitial pneumonia: idiopathic versus collagen vascular disease-related subtypes. *Am J Respir Crit Care Med* 2007;**175**:705–11.

Sverzellati N, Wells AU, Tomassetti S, *et al*. Biopsy-proved idiopathic pulmonary fibrosis: spectrum of non-diagnostic thin-section CT diagnoses. *Radiology* 2010;**254**;957–64.

The concept of acute lung injury

American Thoracic Society; European Respiratory Society. American Thoracic Society/European Respiratory Society international multidisciplinary consensus classification of the idiopathic interstitial pneumonias. *Am J Respir Crit Care Med* 2002;**165**:277–304.

Bulmer SR, Lamb D, McCormack RGM, Walbaum PR. Aetiology of unresolved pneumonia. *Thorax* 1978;**33**:307–14.

Cordier JF. Cryptogenic organizing pneumonia. *Eur Respir J* 2006;**28**:422–46.

Epler GR, Colby TV, McLoud TC, Carrington CB, Gaensler EA. Bronchiolitis obliterans organizing pneumonia. *N Engl J Med* 1985;**312**:152–8.

Godoy MCB, Viswanathan C, Marchiori E, *et al*. The reversed halo sign: update and differential diagnosis. *Br J Radiol* 2012;**85**:1226–35.

Johkoh T, Müller NL, Cartier Y, *et al*. Idiopathic interstitial pneumonia: diagnostic accuracy of thin-section CT in 129 patients. *Radiology* 1999;**211**:555–60.

Katzenstein AA, Mukhopadhyay S, Myers JL. Diagnosis of usual interstitial pneumonia and distinction from other fibrosing interstitial lung diseases. *Hum Pathol* 2008;**39**:1275–94.

Katzenstein AA, Myers JL, Prophet WD, Corley LS III, Shin MS. Bronchiolitis obliterans organizing pneumonia and usual interstitial pneumonia. A comparative

clinicopathologic study. *Am J Surg Pathol* 1986;**10**:373–81.

Mukhopadhyay S, Katzenstein AL. Pulmonary disease due to aspiration of food and other particulate matter: a clinicopathologic study of 59 cases diagnosed on biopsy or resection specimens. *Am J Surg Pathol* 2007;**31**:752–9.

Myers JL, Katzenstein AL. Ultrastructural evidence of alveolar epithelial injury in idiopathic bronchiolitis obliterans-organizing pneumonia. *Am J Pathol* 1988;**132**:102–9.

Diffuse alveolar damage

Askin FB, Katzenstein AL. Pneumocystis infection masquerading as diffuse alveolar damage: a potential source of diagnostic error. *Chest* 1981;**79**:420–2.

de Hemptinne Q, Remmelink M, Brimioulle S, Salmon I, Vincent JL. ARDS: a clinicopathological confrontation. *Chest* 2009;**135**:944–9.

Katzenstein AL, Myers JL, Mazur MT. Acute interstitial pneumonia. A clinicopathologic, ultrastructural, and cell kinetic study. *Am J Surg Pathol* 1986;**10**:256–67.

Mukhopadhyay S, Parambil JG. Acute interstitial pneumonia (AIP): relationship to Hamman-Rich syndrome, diffuse alveolar damage (DAD) and acute respiratory distress syndrome (ARDS). *Semin Respir Crit Care Med* 2012;**33**:476–85.

Parambil JG, Myers JL, Ryu JH. Diffuse alveolar damage: uncommon manifestation of pulmonary involvement in patients with connective tissue diseases. *Chest* 2006;**130**:553–8.

Parambil JG, Myers JL, Aubry MC, Ryu JH. Causes and prognosis of diffuse alveolar damage diagnosed on surgical lung biopsy. *Chest* 2007;**132**:50–7.

Patel SR, Kampaliotis D, Ayas NT, et al. The role of open-lung biopsy in ARDS. *Chest* 2004;**125**:197–202.

Schwarz MI, Albert RK. "Imitators" of the ARDS. Implications for diagnosis and treatment. *Chest* 2004;**125**:1530–5.

Yousem SA, Gibson K, Kaminski N, Oddis CV, Ascherman DP. The pulmonary histopathologic manifestations of the anti-Jo-1 tRNA synthetase syndrome. *Mod Pathol* 2010;**23**:874–80.

Yousem SA, Faber C. Histopathology of aspiration pneumonia not associated with food or other particulate matter: a clinicopathologic study of 10 cases diagnosed on biopsy. *Am J Surg Pathol* 2011;**35**:426–31.

Pulmonary Langerhans cell histiocytosis

Delobbe A, Durieu J, Duhamel A, et al. Determinants of survival in pulmonary Langerhans' cell granulomatosis (histiocytosis X). *Eur Respir J* 1996;**9**:2002–6.

Friedman PJ, Liebow AA, Sokoloff J. Eosinophilic granuloma of lung. Clinical aspects of primary pulmonary histiocytosis in the adult. *Medicine (Baltimore)* 1981;**60**:385–96.

Kambouchner M, Basset F, Marchal J, Uhl JF, Hance AJ, Soler P. Three-dimensional characterization of pathologic lesions in pulmonary Langerhans cell histiocytosis. *Am J Respir Crit Care Med* 2002;**166**:1483–90.

Mukhopadhyay S, Eckardt S, Scalzetti EM. Diagnosis of pulmonary Langerhans cell histiocytosis by CT-guided core biopsy of lung: a report of 3 cases. *Thorax* 2010;**65**:833–5.

Roden AC, Hu X, Kip S, et al. BRAF V600E expression in Langerhans cell histiocytosis. Clinical and immunohistochemical study on 25 pulmonary and 54 extrapulmonary cases. *Am J Surg Pathol* 2014;**38**:548–51.

Tazi A, de Margerie C, Naccache JM, et al. The natural history of adult pulmonary Langerhans cell histiocytosis. *Orphanet J Rare Dis* 2015;**10**:30 Epub ahead of print.

Travis WD, Borok Z, Roum JH, et al. Pulmonary Langerhans cell granulomatosis (Histiocytosis X). A clinicopathologic study of 48 cases. *Am J Surg Pathol* 1993;**17**:971–86.

Vassallo R, Jensen EA, Colby TV, et al. The overlap between respiratory bronchiolitis and desquamative interstitial pneumonia in pulmonary Langerhans cell histiocytosis: high-resolution CT, histologic, and functional correlations. *Chest* 2003;**124**:1199–205.

Vassallo R, Ryu JH, Schroeder DR, et al. Clinical outcomes of pulmonary Langerhans'-cell histiocytosis in adults. *N Engl J Med* 2002;**346**:484–90.

Yousem SA, Dacic S, Nikiforov YE, Nikiforova M. Pulmonary Langerhans cell histiocytosis: profiling of multifocal tumors using next-generation sequencing identifies concordant occurrence of BRAF V600E mutations. *Chest* 2013;**143**:1679–84.

Smoking-related interstitial fibrosis

Auerbach O, Garfinkel L, Hammond EC. Relation of smoking and age to findings in lung parenchyma: A microscopic study. *Chest* 1974;**65**:29–35.

Hogg J, Wright J, Wiggs B, et al. Lung structure and function in cigarette smokers. *Thorax* 1994;**49**:473–8.

Katzenstein AL, Mukhopadhyay S, Zanardi C, Dexter EE. Clinically occult interstitial fibrosis in smokers: classification and significance of a surprisingly common finding in lobectomy specimens. *Hum Pathol* 2010;**41**:316–25.

Katzenstein AL. Smoking-related interstitial fibrosis (SRIF), pathogenesis and treatment of usual interstitial pneumonia (UIP), and transbronchial biopsy in UIP. *Mod Pathol* 2012;**25**:S68–78.

Katzenstein AL. Smoking-related interstitial fibrosis (SRIF): pathologic findings and distinction from other chronic fibrosing lung diseases. *J Clin Pathol* 2013;**66**:882–7.

Kawabata Y, Hoshi E, Murai K, et al. Smoking-related changes in the background lung of specimens resected for lung cancer: a semiquantitative study with correlation to postoperative course. *Histopathology* 2008;**53**:707–14.

Lederer DJ, Enright PL, Kawut SM, et al. Cigarette smoking is associated with subclinical parenchymal lung disease. The multi-ethnic study of atherosclerosis (MESA)-lung study. *Am J Respir Crit Care Med* 2009;**180**:407–14.

Primiani A, Dias-Santagata D, Iafrate AJ, Kradin RL. Pulmonary adenocarcinoma mutation profile in smokers with smoking-related interstitial fibrosis. *Int J COPD* 2014;**9**:525–31.

Snider G, Kleinerman J, Thurlbeck W, Bengali Z. The definition of emphysema. Report of a national heart, lung and blood institute, division of lung diseases workshop. *Am Rev Respir Dis* 1985;**132**:182–5.

Yousem SA. Respiratory bronchiolitis-associated interstitial lung disease with fibrosis is a lesion distinct from fibrotic nonspecific interstitial pneumonia: a proposal. *Mod Pathol* 2006;**19**:1474–9.

Hypersensitivity pneumonitis

Barrios RJ. Hypersensitivity pneumonitis: histopathology. *Arch Pathol Lab Med* 2008;**132**:199–203.

Coleman A, Colby TV. Histologic diagnosis of extrinsic allergic alveolitis. *Am J Surg Pathol* 1988;**12**:514–18.

Emanuel DA, Wenzel FJ, Bowerman CI, Lawton BR. Farmer's lung: clinical, pathologic and immunologic study of twenty-four patients. *Am J Med* 1964;**37**:392–401.

Hirschmann JV, Pipavath SN, Godwin JD. Hypersensitivity pneumonitis: a historical, clinical, and radiologic review. *Radiographics* 2009;**29**:1921–38.

Katzenstein AL, Mukhopadhyay S, Myers JL. Diagnosis of usual interstitial pneumonia and distinction from other fibrosing interstitial lung diseases. *Hum Pathol* 2008;**39**:1275–94.

Metersky ML, Bean SB, Meyer JD, et al. Classification of hypersensitivity pneumonitis: a hypothesis. *Int Arch Allergy Immunol* 2009;**149**:161–6.

Morell F, Roger A, Reyes L, Cruz MJ, Murio C, Muñoz X. Bird fancier's lung: a series of 86 patients. *Medicine (Baltimore)* 2008;**87**:110–30.

Mukhopadhyay S, Gal AA. Granulomatous lung disease: an approach to the differential diagnosis. *Arch Pathol Lab Med* 2010;**134**:667–90.

Mukhopadhyay S. Pathology of hypersensitivity pneumonitis. Medscape Reference. Updated March 31, 2015. Available at: http://emedicine.medscape.com/article/2078434-overview.

Reyes CN, Wenzel FJ, Lawton BR, Emanuel DA. The pulmonary pathology of farmer's lung disease. *Chest* 1982;**81**:142–6.

Non-specific interstitial pneumonia

American Thoracic Society; European Respiratory Society. American Thoracic Society/European Respiratory Society international multidisciplinary consensus classification of the idiopathic interstitial pneumonias. *Am J Respir Crit Care Med* 2002;**165**:277–304.

Bjoraker JA, Ryu JH, Edwin MK, et al. Prognostic significance of histopathologic subsets in idiopathic pulmonary fibrosis. *Am J Respir Crit Care Med* 1998;**157**:199–203.

Flaherty KR, Toews GB, Travis WD, et al. Clinical significance of histological classification of idiopathic interstitial pneumonia. *Eur Respir J* 2002;**19**:275–83.

Flaherty KR, Travis WD, Colby TV, et al. Histopathologic variability in usual and nonspecific interstitial pneumonias. *Am J Respir Crit Care Med* 2001;**164**:1722–27.

Katzenstein AL, Fiorelli RF. Nonspecific interstitial pneumonia/fibrosis. *Am J Surg Pathol* 1994;**18**:136–47.

Katzenstein AA, Mukhopadhyay S, Myers JL. Diagnosis of usual interstitial pneumonia and distinction from other fibrosing interstitial lung diseases. *Hum Pathol* 2008;**39**:1275–94.

Katzenstein AA, Zisman DA, Litzky LA, Nguyen BT, Kotloff RM. Usual interstitial pneumonia: Histologic study of biopsy and explant specimens. *Am J Surg Pathol* 2002;**261**:1567–77.

Nunes H, Schubel K, Piver D, et al. Nonspecific interstitial pneumonia: survival is influenced by the underlying cause. *Eur Respir J* 2015;**45**:746–55.

Schneider F, Hwang DM, Gibson K, Yousem SA. Nonspecific interstitial pneumonia: a study of 6 patients with progressive disease. *Am J Surg Pathol* 2012;**36**:89–93.

Travis WD, Matsui K, Moss J, Ferrans VJ. Idiopathic nonspecific interstitial pneumonia: prognostic significance of cellular and fibrosing patterns. Survival comparison with usual interstitial pneumonia and desquamative interstitial pneumonia. *Am J Surg Pathol* 2000;**24**:19–33.

Ctd-Ild

American Thoracic Society; European Respiratory Society. American Thoracic Society/European Respiratory Society international multidisciplinary consensus classification of the idiopathic interstitial pneumonias. *Am J Respir Crit Care Med* 2002;**165**:277–304.

Bouros D, Wells AU, Nicholson AG, et al. Histopathologic subsets of fibrosing alveolitis in patients with systemic sclerosis and their relationship to outcome. *Am J Respir Crit Care Med* 2002;**165**:1581–6.

Douglas WW, Tazelaar HD, Hartman TE, et al. Polymyositis-dermatomyositis-associated interstitial lung disease. *Am J Respir Crit Care Med* 2001;**164**:1182–5.

Katzenstein AA, Mukhopadhyay S, Myers JL. Diagnosis of usual interstitial pneumonia and distinction from other fibrosing interstitial lung diseases. *Hum Pathol* 2008;**39**:1275–94.

Kim EJ, Elicker BM, Maldonado F, et al. Usual interstitial pneumonia in rheumatoid arthritis-associated interstitial lung disease. *Eur Respir J* 2010;**35**:1322–28.

Nunes H, Schubel K, Piver D, et al. Nonspecific interstitial pneumonia: survival is influenced by the underlying cause. *Eur Respir J* 2015;**45**:746–55.

Parambil JG, Myers JL, Lindell RM, Matteson EL, Ryu JH. Interstitial lung disease in primary Sjögren syndrome. *Chest* 2006;**130**:1489–95.

Park JH, Kim DS, Park IN, et al. Prognosis of fibrotic interstitial pneumonia: idiopathic versus collagen vascular disease-related subtypes. *Am J Respir Crit Care Med* 2007;**175**:705–11.

Song JW, Do KH, Kim MY, Jang SJ, Colby TV, Kim DS. Pathologic and radiologic differences between idiopathic and collagen vascular disease-related usual interstitial pneumonia. *Chest* 2009;**136**:23–30.

Strange C, Highland KB. Interstitial lung disease in the patient who has connective tissue disease. *Clin Chest Med* 2004;**25**:549–59.

Drug-related lung disease

Camus P, Kudoh S, Ebina M. Interstitial lung disease associated with drug therapy. *Br J Cancer* 2004;**91**(Suppl 2):S18–23.

Hayes D Jr, Anstead MI, Kuhn RJ. Eosinophilic pneumonia induced by daptomycin. *J Infect* 2007;**54**:e211–3.

Imokawa S, Colby TV, Leslie KO, Helmers RA. Methotrexate pneumonitis: review of the literature and histopathological findings in nine patients. *Eur Respir J* 2000;**15**:373–81.

Kennedy JI, Myers JL, Plumb VJ, Fulmer JD. Amiodarone pulmonary toxicity. Clinical, radiologic, and pathologic correlations. *Arch Intern Med* 1987;**147**:50–5.

Lal Y, Assimacopoulos AP. Two cases of daptomycin-induced eosinophilic

pneumonia and chronic pneumonitis. *Clin Infect Dis* 2010;**50**:737–40.

Larsen BT, Vaszar LT, Colby TV, Tazelaar HD. Lymphoid hyperplasia and eosinophilic pneumonia as histologic manifestations of amiodarone-induced lung toxicity. *Am J Surg Pathol* 2012;**36**:509–16.

Leduc D, De Vuyst P, Lhereux P, Gevenois PA, Jacobovitz D, Yernault JC. Pneumonitis complicating low-dose methotrexate therapy for rheumatoid arthritis. Discrepancies between lung biopsy and bronchoalveolar lavage findings. *Chest* 1993;**104**:1620–3.

Magee F, Wright JL, Chan N, et al. Two unusual pathological reactions to nitrofurantoin: case reports. *Histopathology* 1986;**10**:701–6.

Rossi SE, Erasmus JJ, McAdams HP, Sporn TA, Goodman PC. Pulmonary drug toxicity: radiologic and pathologic manifestations. *RadioGraphics* 2000;**20**:1245–59.

Mendez JL, Nadrous HF, Hartman TE, Ryu JH. Chronic nitrofurantoin-induced lung disease. *Mayo Clin Proc* 2005;**80**:1298–1302.

Miscellaneous and rare causes of interstitial lung disease

Becker CD, Gil J, Padilla ML. Idiopathic pleuroparenchymal fibroelastosis: an unrecognized or misdiagnosed entity? *Mod Pathol* 2008;**21**:784–7.

Cottin V, Cordier JF. Interstitial pulmonary amyloidosis. *Respiration* 2008;**75**:210.

Davison AG, Haslam PL, Corrin B, et al. Interstitial lung disease and asthma in hard-metal workers: bronchoalveolar lavage, ultrastructural, and analytic findings and results of bronchial provocation tests. *Thorax* 1983;**38**:119–28.

Frankel SK, Cool CD, Lynch DA, Brown KK. Idiopathic pleuroparenchymal fibroelastosis: description of a novel clinicopathologic entity. *Chest* 2004;**126**:2007–13.

Hui AN, Koss MN, Hochholzer L, Wehunt WD. Amyloidosis presenting in the lower respiratory tract. Clinicopathologic, radiologic, immunohistochemical and histochemical studies on 48 cases. *Arch Pathol Lab Med* 1986;**110**:212–8.

Koss MN, Hochholzer L, Langloss JM, Wehunt WD, Lazarus AA. Lymphoid interstitial pneumonia: clinicopathological and immunopathological findings in 18 cases. *Pathology* 1987;**19**:178–85.

Naqvi AH, Hunt A, Burnett BR, Abraham JL. Pathologic spectrum and lung dust burden in giant cell interstitial pneumonia (hard metal lung disease/cobalt pneumonitis):

review of 100 cases. *Arch Environ Occup Health* 2008;**63**:51–70.

Ohori NP, Sciurba FC, Owens GR, Hodgson MJ, Yousem SA. Giant-cell interstitial pneumonia and hard-metal pneumoconiosis. A clinicopathologic study of four cases and review of the literature. *Am J Surg Pathol* 1989;**13**:581–7.

Smith RRL, Hutchins GM, Moore GW, Humphrey RL. Type and distribution of pulmonary parenchymal and vascular amyloid. Correlation with cardiac amyloidosis. *Am J Med* 1979;**66**:96–104.

Swigris JJ, Berry GJ, Raffin TA, Kuschner WG. Lymphoid interstitial pneumonia: a narrative review. *Chest* 2002;**122**:2150–64.

Non-neoplastic lung nodules and masses

Lung nodules and masses are among the most common indications for lung biopsies. After a neoplasm has been excluded by histologic examination, the next question is whether a specific non-neoplastic diagnosis can be made. This chapter addresses such lesions, and discusses the histologic approach to the diagnosis. Pathologists interpreting core needle biopsies of lung nodules will also benefit from reading the relevant section in Chapter 1.

Many pathologic conditions form masses, mass-like lesions, nodules or nodular opacities on chest radiographs or CT scans of the chest. The nodular nature of many of these lesions can also be appreciated on pathologic examination. However, some lesions that feature nodules or nodular areas radiologically may not be clearly nodular pathologically (e.g., talc granulomatosis or hypersensitivity pneumonitis). Conversely, some lesions that are clearly nodular on pathologic examination may be too tiny to be seen on chest imaging (e.g., meningothelial-like nodules). The focus of this chapter is on entities that appear nodular on pathologic examination.

A potpourri of non-neoplastic lung nodules is shown in Figure 6.1, and an algorithmic approach to the diagnosis is presented in Figure 6.2. Table 6.1 lists the common lesions that pathologists need to consider in the differential diagnosis. For convenience, the entities are listed in decreasing order of frequency from the pathologist's perspective. Some of the most common non-neoplastic causes of lung nodules such as necrotizing granulomas, sarcoidosis and organizing pneumonia are discussed in other chapters based on other prominent pathologic findings (Table 6.2).

Nodular amyloidosis

Amyloidosis occurs in the lung in many forms, including nodular, tracheobronchial and alveolar septal. Alveolar septal amyloidosis is usually a manifestation of systemic AL amyloidosis, and is discussed in Chapter 5. Tracheobronchial amyloidosis involves the airways and is discussed in Chapter 9. This section focuses on the nodular form of amyloidosis, which is usually an isolated finding limited to the lungs. Nodular amyloidosis is also known as *amyloidoma*, a term that highlights the mass-like appearance of the lesion. To date, there are no reports of an association with or progression to systemic amyloidosis. Nodular amyloidosis is thought to be a result of localized production of clonal immunoglobulins by plasma cells restricted to the lung. In the vast majority of cases, the amyloid is composed of light chains, thus representing a localized form of AL amyloidosis. Cases related to deposition of serum

amyloid A protein or transthyretin have been reported but are exceedingly rare.

The diagnosis can be made in needle biopsies as well as surgical (wedge) biopsies of the lung.

Major diagnostic findings

- Mass-like deposition of amyloid in the lung parenchyma, forming a nodule (Figure 6.3). The appearance of the amyloid itself is identical to other forms of amyloidosis. That is, the material is amorphous, eosinophilic and acellular or paucicellular. It stains light orange ("salmon-pink") on Congo red and shows apple-green birefringence when examined under polarized light.
- Multinucleated giant cells are an important clue to the diagnosis of nodular amyloidosis, since they are almost always found in this form of the disease and are generally absent in other forms of pulmonary amyloidosis. They are usually found at the periphery of the amyloid deposits.

Variable pathologic findings

- Sheets of plasma cells are often present in and around the amyloid deposits. By immunohistochemistry or in situ hybridization, the plasma cells in nodular amyloidosis are light chain restricted (monotypic) in most cases (78%). There may also be evidence of heavy chain restriction. The plasma cells have been reported to express CD19.
- Lymphocytes may be admixed with the plasma cells. The lymphocytic infiltrate is reactive and polytypic.
- As in other forms of amyloidosis, secondary calcification and ossification of the amyloid deposits is common and is a helpful feature in the differential diagnosis with pulmonary hyalinizing granuloma (see below).

Diagnostic work-up

- A Congo red stain should be performed in all cases, since positive staining is the hallmark of amyloidosis. The ideal thickness of the section for Congo red staining is 6 microns. It is thought that sections thinner than this may fail to stain appropriately.
- Other stains occasionally used to identify amyloid include crystal violet, thioflavin T and thioflavin S. In the era prior to immunohistochemistry and mass spectrometry, potassium permanganate pre-treatment was used to differentiate AL amyloid (which retains apple-green birefringence after permanganate pre-treatment) from AA

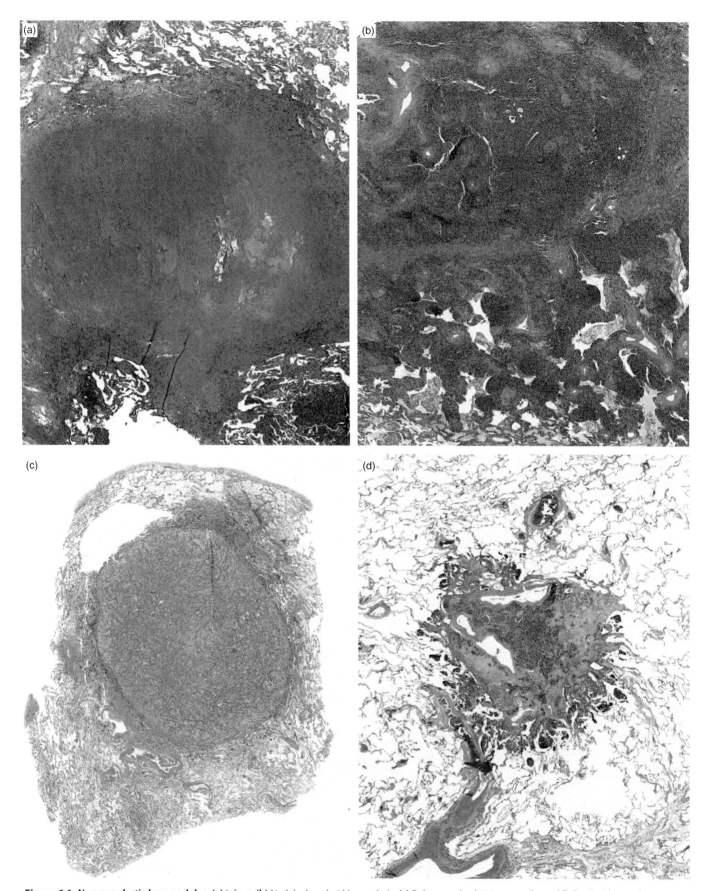

Figure 6.1. Non-neoplastic lung nodules. (a) Infarct. **(b)** Nodular lymphoid hyperplasia. **(c)** Pulmonary hyalinizing granuloma. **(d)** Carcinoid tumorlet.

Table 6.1. Pearls and pitfalls in the diagnosis of non-neoplastic lung nodules

Any pathologic finding that destroys alveolar architecture can potentially form a nodule

Neoplastic nodules can mimic non-neoplastic disease histologically: e.g., solitary fibrous tumor, epithelioid hemangioendothelioma, epithelioid angiosarcoma

Necrotizing granulomas are the most common cause of non-neoplastic lung nodules (see Chapter 2)

Core needle biopsies often provide specific benign diagnoses for lung nodules (see Chapter 1)

In core needle biopsies, the most common non-neoplastic causes of lung nodules are granulomas, scars and organizing pneumonia

Most non-neoplastic lung lesions with abundant necrosis are necrotizing granulomas; a small minority are infarcts

Think of nodular amyloidosis, light chain deposition disease and pulmonary hyalinizing granuloma in the differential diagnosis of nodules composed of densely eosinophilic pink material

Pulmonary hyalinizing granuloma is a misnomer (it is not granulomatous)

Pulmonary hyalinizing granuloma can be positive for Congo red

If a reactive lymphoid infiltrate forms a nodule in the lung, think nodular lymphoid hyperplasia, not LIP

The presence of multiple carcinoid tumorlets does not necessarily imply diffuse idiopathic pulmonary neuroendocrine cell hyperplasia (DIPNECH)

If the center of a "granuloma" contains lamellated collagen bundles, consider silicosis

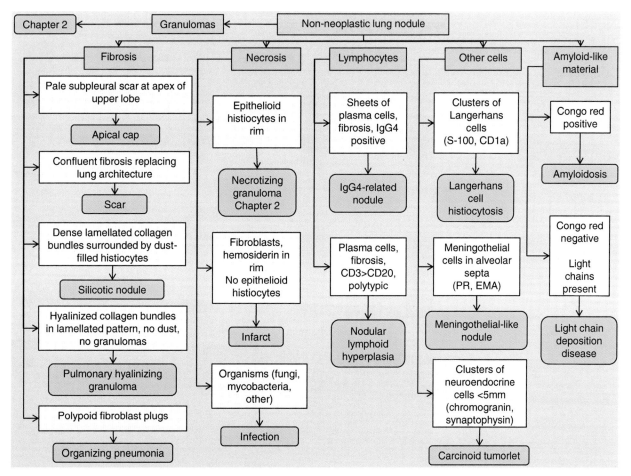

Figure 6.2. Algorithmic approach to nodular non-neoplastic lung lesions.

Table 6.2. Non-neoplastic causes of lung nodules

Diagnosis	Main histologic feature	Where to find the entity in this book	Typical setting in which this lesion is diagnosed
Necrotizing granulomas	Necrosis with epithelioid histiocytes	Chapter 2	Radiologic finding of lung nodule or nodules. Small lung biopsies, surgical (wedge) biopsies, resections
Sarcoidosis	Non-necrotizing granulomas	Chapter 2	Radiologic finding of bilateral lung nodules or hilar adeno-pathy. Transbronchial or endobronchial biopsy. Lymph node biopsies. Occasionally surgical lung biopsy
Organizing pneumonia	Fibroblast plugs within airspaces	Chapter 5	Radiologic finding of nodule or opacity. Transbronchial or needle biopsy, surgical lung biopsy
Scars (including pulmonary apical caps)	Replacement of lung architecture by fibrosis	This chapter	Incidental finding in lobectomy specimen. Needle biopsy of lung nodule or mass
Abscess	Localized area of suppurative necrosis	Chapter 4	Radiologic finding of lung mass. Resection specimen
Silicotic nodules	Fibrous nodules with a lamellated, hyalinized center and a cellular rim	This chapter	Incidental finding in hilar nodes
Langerhans cell histiocytosis	Stellate interstitial nodules containing sheets of Langerhans cells	Chapter 5	Surgical lung biopsy in smoker with multiple bilateral tiny lung nodules (common). Small lung biopsies (uncommon)
Infarct	Localized focus of necrosis	This chapter	Surgical lung biopsy for ill-defined peripheral opacity
Nodular amyloidosis	Localized deposit of amyloid containing multinucleated giant cells	This chapter	Surgical lung biopsy or needle biopsy for radiologic finding of solitary or multiple lung nodules
Pulmonary hyalinizing granuloma	Bundles of hyalinized collagen forming a parenchymal lung nodule	This chapter	Surgical lung biopsy or needle biopsy for radiologic finding of multiple lung nodules
IgG4-related lung nodule	Fibrosis and chronic inflammation with numerous IgG4-positive plasma cells	This chapter	Surgical lung biopsy for radiologic finding of solitary or multiple lung nodules
Round atelectasis	Thickened pleura invaginated into lung, causing a mass-like lesion	This chapter	Lung resection for radiologic finding of solitary mass. Incidental finding
Light chain deposition disease	Amyloid-like nodule containing light chains, Congo red negative	This chapter	Lung biopsy for radiologic finding of solitary or multiple lung nodules
Carcinoid tumorlets	Tiny focus of neuroendocrine proliferation in bronchiolar wall	This chapter	Incidental finding (common). Biopsies performed for radiologic nodules (uncommon)
Meningothelial-like nodule	Minute proliferation of meningothelial-like cells within alveolar septa	This chapter	Incidental finding (very common). Biopsies performed for radiologic nodules (very uncommon)

(a)

(b)

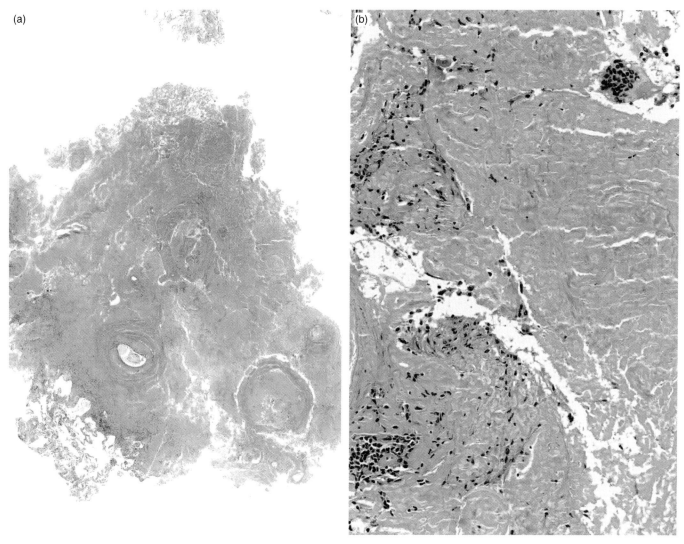

Figure 6.3. Nodular amyloidosis (amyloidoma). (a) Low magnification, showing parenchymal nodule. **(b)** Amyloid deposits associated with multinucleated giant cells.

amyloid (which loses birefringence after permanganate pre-treatment).

- Amyloid subtyping. It is often stated that amyloid subtyping is very important for appropriate management, but the clinical impact of amyloid subtyping is unclear, especially in nodular amyloidosis of the lung, a benign lesion with no relation to systemic amyloidosis and no need for further therapy regardless of amyloid subtype.

- Laser microdissection and tandem mass spectrometry (LDMS) has been shown to have superior sensitivity when compared with immunohistochemistry. However, this technique is available only at a few centers worldwide and requires expensive specialized equipment and expertise in data analysis. This technique provides confirmation that the amyloid is immunoglobin-derived and also accurately determines the predominant light chain (kappa or lambda). It also provides evidence of the absence of other types of amyloid-forming proteins such as serum amyloid A (SAA) or transthyretin (TTR). Most cases of nodular amyloidosis are kappa-predominant, but lambda-predominant or

mixed cases have also been described. Heavy chains such as gamma-heavy chain and alpha-heavy chain are often co-deposited along with light chains, a finding that is uncommon in alveolar septal or tracheobronchial amyloidosis associated with systemic AL amyloidosis.

- Immunohistochemistry has been the traditional method for amyloid subtyping, and has the advantage of being widely available and easy to perform. The ideal section thickness for immunohistochemical staining of amyloid is 2 μ. In expert hands, it has been shown that immunohistochemistry alone can accurately identify the type of amyloid in 76% of cases. In practice, however, its utility is severely limited by high background staining in amyloid deposits, or by lack of staining in some cases. Antibodies directed against several amyloidogenic proteins are available for immunohistochemistry. They include kappa and lambda light chains, serum amyloid A protein, serum amyloid P component, transthyretin, lysozyme, fibrinogen alpha chain, insulin, apoA1, β2 microglobulin and Lect2. Although immunohistochemistry is suboptimal

261

for amyloid subtyping, it can be used for establishing light chain restriction in plasma cells. Even in this setting, however, immunohistochemistry is being superseded by in situ hybridization for light chains, which is easier to interpret because of a cleaner signal.

- Clonal immunoglobulin gene rearrangements have been detected by the polymerase chain reaction in approximately 50% of cases of nodular amyloidosis. There is no evidence of translocations involving the *MALT1* gene region.

Clinical profile

The age at diagnosis ranges from 48 to 80 years, with a mean in the 60s. There is no sex predilection. The nodules of nodular amyloidosis are usually discovered incidentally in asymptomatic individuals. Cough and hemoptysis have been reported in a few patients.

A history of collagen vascular disease may be present in a subset of patients (36%). The most commonly reported underlying collagen vascular disease is Sjögren syndrome, but other conditions have also been reported, including undifferentiated connective tissue disease, Hashimoto thyroiditis and polymyalgia rheumatica.

Approximately one-fourth of patients have a monoclonal serum protein. However, laser microdissection and tandem mass spectrometry have been useful in demonstrating that the circulating protein is not always related to the amyloid deposits in the lung. In one case of nodular amyloidosis, the patient was found to have κ light chains in the serum and an IgM κ-secreting lymphoplasmacytic lymphoma in the bone marrow. However, the pulmonary amyloid was IgG κ, unrelated to the circulating monoclonal κ light chains derived from the lymphoma. In another case, a circulating monoclonal gammopathy of undetermined significance was IgG λ, but the lung amyloid was unrelated (IgA λ).

Radiologic findings

The most common radiologic presentation is a solitary pulmonary nodule. Approximately a third of cases present with multiple lung nodules. The nodules may be PET-positive (FDG-avid).

Differential diagnosis

- Pulmonary hyalinizing granuloma is a fibrosing, nodule-forming process of the lung that can closely mimic nodular amyloidosis. Both entities feature nodules formed by paucicellular eosinophilic material. Although one might expect that Congo red staining would easily resolve this problem, pulmonary hyalinizing granulomas can be Congo red positive, a pitfall first described by Dr. Averill Liebow in 1957 (please see the section on pulmonary hyalinizing granuloma later on in this chapter). A key feature that helps to differentiate between the two lesions is that the collagen in pulmonary hyalinizing granulomas has a lamellar pattern, while amyloid does not. Additionally, amyloid deposits are frequently associated with multinucleated giant cells, calcification or ossification, whereas pulmonary hyalinizing granuloma is not.

- Light chain deposition disease, described in detail in the next section in this chapter, is a condition in which circulating light chains deposit in tissues but do not form true amyloid. On H&E, these non-amyloid light chain deposits are amorphous, eosinophilic and acellular, and may be strikingly similar to true amyloid. The main differentiating feature is that true amyloid is Congo red positive whereas non-amyloid light chain deposits are not. By electron microscopy, amyloid is fibrillar whereas non-amyloid light chain deposits are electron dense, electron dense and fibrillar, or crystalline. Laser microdissection and tandem mass spectrometry can also be helpful in this situation by demonstrating the presence of amyloid-associated proteins, such as serum amyloid P component, which are absent in non-amyloid light chain deposits. It is obvious from the preceding discussion that the presence of light chains is common to both entities, and is therefore not helpful in the differential diagnosis.

- Systemic amyloidosis. Although the amyloid deposits in alveolar septal amyloidosis and nodular amyloidosis of the lung are morphologically similar and are mostly composed of immunoglobulins, there are several significant differences. Systemic amyloidosis manifests in the lung as diffuse alveolar septal amyloid deposition (see section on alveolar septal amyloidosis in the chapter on interstitial lung disease), is mostly composed of lambda light chains, rarely contains heavy chains or CD19-positive plasma cells, and has a dismal prognosis. In contrast, nodular amyloidosis is characterized by nodular amyloid deposits associated with multinucleated giant cells, is mostly composed of kappa light chains, frequently contains heavy chains and CD19-positive plasma cells, and has an excellent prognosis.

Treatment and prognosis

Nodular amyloidosis does not require specific treatment and the prognosis is excellent. In most patients, the nodules do not recur. There are no reports of pulmonary nodular amyloidosis evolving into systemic amyloidosis. On long-term follow-up, some patients develop new infiltrates or small bilateral nodules in the lungs (36 to 50 months later), marginal zone lymphoma in the skin (1 to 4 years later) or marginal zone lymphoma in the parotid gland (6 years later). There are no reports of death from disease, even in patients with recurrences.

Sample diagnosis on pathology report

Lung, right upper lobe, surgical biopsy – Nodular amyloidosis (See comment).

Light chain deposition disease ("amyloid-like nodules")

Pulmonary light chain deposition disease is characterized by the deposition of an amyloid-like material in lung tissues that is virtually identical to amyloid except that it does not show apple-green birefringence with a Congo red stain. Since Congo

Table 6.3. Pulmonary amyloidosis vs. light chain deposition disease

	Pulmonary amyloidosis	Pulmonary light chain deposition disease
Amorphous eosinophilic material on H&E	Yes	Yes
Apple-green birefringence when stained with Congo red and examined under polarized light	Yes	No
Electron microscopy	Fibrillar meshwork	Granular deposits; crystalline deposits reported
Serum amyloid P component and apolipoprotein E	Present	Absent
Material composed of light chains	Yes	Yes
Usual light chain	Kappa (nodular form) Lambda (alveolar septal form)	Kappa
Light chains in serum	In some cases	In some cases
Lymphoplasmacytic infiltrate	Yes	Yes
Multinucleated giant cells	Yes (nodular form)	Yes
Lung cysts	Rare	Common
Lung nodules	Yes (nodular form)	Yes (common)
Systemic involvement	May occur (alveolar septal form)	May occur
Association with lymphoproliferative disorders	Some cases	Some cases
Association with Sjögren syndrome	Yes	Yes
Prognosis	Good in nodular form; poor in diffuse alveolar septal form	Good in nodular form; poor in diffuse alveolar septal form
Treatment	None (nodular form) Melphalan-stem cell rescue (alveolar septal form)	Unclear. Probably none for nodules. Lung transplantation for progressive cysts

red staining is the defining feature of amyloid, it is felt that the term "amyloidosis" should not be used for this condition. There has been justifiable skepticism that some cases of this type simply represent amyloid that does not stain for Congo red for technical reasons, and such cases have been referred to as "amyloid-like nodules". However, with the increasing use of mass spectrometry, it is now clear that the material in light chain deposition disease is a non-amyloid substance. Overall, it is useful to think of light chain deposition in the lung as occurring in two forms, one characterized by positive Congo red staining (amyloidosis), the other by negative staining (light chain deposition disease). The differences between amyloidosis and light chain deposition disease are summarized in Table 6.3.

Pulmonary light chain deposition disease is rare and probably under-recognized. At the time of this writing (2015), approximately 45 well-documented cases have been reported in the literature, including a series of nine cases (Sheard *et al*). The most common cause of light chain deposition in the lung is an underlying lymphoproliferative disorder, but there is also an association with Sjögren syndrome. Many cases are idiopathic. Light chain deposits may also occur in organs other than the lungs, such as the kidneys, liver and heart. Lung

involvement can occur as part of systemic light chain deposition or isolated pulmonary disease.

Light chain deposition disease is usually diagnosed in surgical lung biopsies, but the diagnosis can also be made in core needle biopsies.

Major diagnostic findings

- Deposition of amorphous eosinophilic amyloid-like material in the lung (Figure 6.4). The material may be present in the interstitium or vessel walls.
- Demonstration that the material is composed of light chains. This can be accomplished by immunohistochemistry or mass spectrometry.
- Despite the resemblance to amyloid, the material does not show apple-green birefringence on Congo red when examined under polarized light, and therefore does not fulfil criteria for amyloid.

Variable pathologic findings

- As in the nodular form of pulmonary amyloidosis, multinucleated giant cells are a common finding in

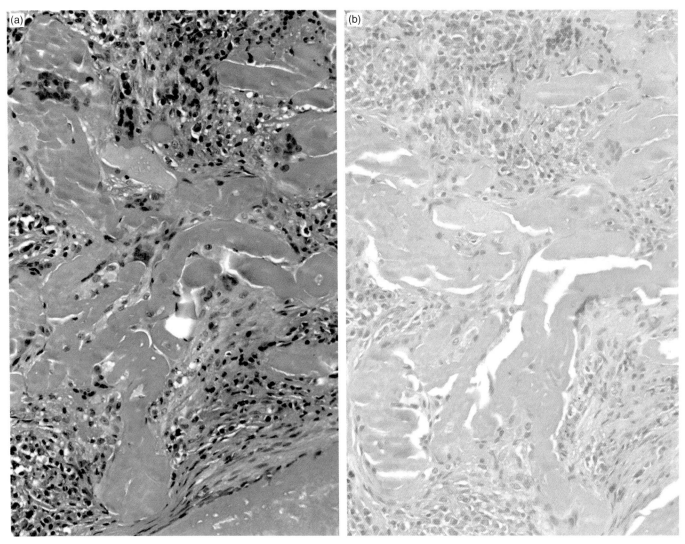

Figure 6.4. Light chain deposition disease. (a) Core needle biopsy of a lung nodule from a 58-year-old woman with multiple nodules. Note amorphous eosinophilic material resembling amyloid, plasma cell infiltrate in background and scattered multinucleated giant cells. The plasma cells were predominantly kappa light chain-positive (not shown). **(b)** Congo red stain. The usual salmon-pink color is absent. There was no apple-green birefringence upon polarization (not shown).

pulmonary light chain deposition disease. They are present in virtually all cases. Small poorly formed non-necrotizing granulomas are common, and may contain Schaumann bodies.

- Lymphocytes and plasma cells may be present adjacent to amyloid deposits as well as in the adjacent lung. Lymphoid infiltrates are present in nearly every case, and may be dense. The distribution may be peri-lymphatic (lymphangitic), with involvement of bronchovascular bundles and interlobular septa, or interstitial. The plasma cells may be monotypic.
- Cysts are appreciable in histologic specimens in some cases. The wall of the cysts may contain eosinophilic material, lymphoplasmacytic infiltrates or poorly formed granulomas.
- As in amyloidosis, secondary calcification and ossification can occur.
- Concurrent leukemia (CLL) has been reported in one case.

Diagnostic work-up

- A Congo red stain should be performed in all cases, since negative staining is the hallmark of the disease. It is thought that thin sections less than 6 μ in thickness may fail to stain appropriately with Congo red.
- Electron microscopy shows granular, electron-dense material. Crystalline structures have also been reported.
- Laser microdissection and tandem mass spectrometry (LDMS) provides confirmation that the material is light chain-derived and accurately determines the predominant light chain, which is usually kappa. It also shows that proteins associated with true amyloidosis, such as serum amyloid P component and apolipoprotein E, are absent.
- Immunohistochemistry can be used to show that the amyloid-like material is composed of light chains. It has the advantage of wide availability but is limited by high background staining (as in amyloidosis). It can also be used

for establishing light chain restriction in the accompanying plasma cells.

- Clonality of the plasma cells has been shown by PCR in some cases.

Clinical profile

The age range in cases of pulmonary light chain deposition disease reported thus far is 28 to 84 years, with a mean in the 60s. Cases have been reported in both sexes, but there is a definite female predilection. Most cases are discovered when lung nodules are found incidentally during a work-up for other reasons. Cases have also been found in patients presenting with recurrent lower respiratory tract infection, fever, night sweats and shortness of breath. Contrary to what has been stated in the past, most patients with pulmonary light chain deposition disease have no history of renal involvement. The most commonly reported underlying disease is Sjögren's syndrome, but other conditions have also been reported, including lymphoproliferative disorders. A monoclonal serum protein may be present.

Radiologic findings

The most common radiologic findings are lung cysts or nodules. Both nodules *and* cysts are present in some patients, this combination being a clue to the diagnosis. The cysts are thin-walled and predominantly spherical. They may be present in any lobe, do not appear to have a zonal distribution, and may be central or peripheral. Both upper lobe- and lower lobe-predominant cases have been reported. They are usually multiple but may be solitary. In cases with multiple cysts, the number varies from 2 to greater than 16. They vary in size from 3 to 35 mm. One or more blood vessels are usually present in the cyst wall, and central traversing vessels may be present inside the cyst in some cases.

Lung nodules are present in nearly every case. They are regular, non-cavitary, and more often multiple than solitary. In cases with multiple nodules, the number varies from 2 to greater than 15. They appear to have no constant distribution. The radiologic impression is usually that of a neoplasm.

Differential diagnosis

- Amyloidosis is obviously the main differential diagnostic consideration since the H&E appearance of the deposits is identical and most cases of pulmonary amyloid are light chain-derived. The main differentiating feature is apple-green birefringence on Congo red staining, which is the hallmark of amyloidosis but is absent in light chain deposition disease. Electron microscopy can also be helpful, since amyloid is fibrillar whereas non-amyloid light chain deposits are granular or crystalline. Laser microdissection and tandem mass spectrometry is perhaps the most useful modality in this situation since it can demonstrate the presence of light chains as well as the absence of amyloid-associated proteins such as serum amyloid P component and apolipoprotein E.

- Other diseases characterized by lung cysts or nodules enter the radiologic differential diagnosis but are easily distinguished from light chain deposition disease by their H&E features. The combination of lung nodules and cysts also occurs in pulmonary Langerhans cell histiocytosis.

Treatment and prognosis

Treatment of light chain deposition disease is directed at the underlying condition. In the largest series, on radiologic follow-up most cases showed no appreciable change in the size or number of cysts or nodules. In one patient with 63 months of follow-up, several new large cysts developed at the lung bases, along with two new nodules, also at the lung bases. Despite the apparently indolent nature of the disease in this report, some patients in other series have developed respiratory failure requiring lung transplantation 3, 10 and 11 years after the onset of symptoms. It has been suggested that nodular disease has a better prognosis than diffuse interstitial disease.

Sample diagnosis on pathology report

If the amyloid-like material can be shown to be composed of light chains and is Congo red negative:

Lung, right middle lobe, surgical biopsy – Light chain deposition disease (See comment).

or

If the amyloid-like material is not clearly light chain-derived, and is Congo red negative:

Lung, right middle lobe, surgical biopsy – Amyloid-like nodule (See comment).

Pulmonary hyalinizing granuloma

The term "pulmonary hyalinizing granuloma" is a misnomer because the lesion is not granulomatous. Instead, it is characterized by a distinctive type of keloid-like hyalinized collagen that forms nodules within lung parenchyma. The morphology is identical to the fibrosing lesion of the mediastinum known as sclerosing mediastinitis, and the pathogenesis is also thought to be similar, i.e., it may be related to prior histoplasmosis, tuberculosis or an unknown immunologic mechanism. Some cases may be IgG4-related.

Major diagnostic findings

- Nodules formed by thick bundles of dense, ropy, keloid-like hyalinized collagen arranged in a lamellar or whorled pattern separated by clear spaces ("cracks", Figure 6.5). The collagen bundles have an amorphous appearance that closely mimics amyloid.
- Lymphocytes, plasma cells, histiocytes and fibroblasts are commonly interspersed between the collagen bundles, but collagen deposition is the predominant abnormality.

Variable pathologic findings

- Dense lymphoid aggregates may be present within and at the edge of the lesion. The edge of the lesion may be more cellular than the center.

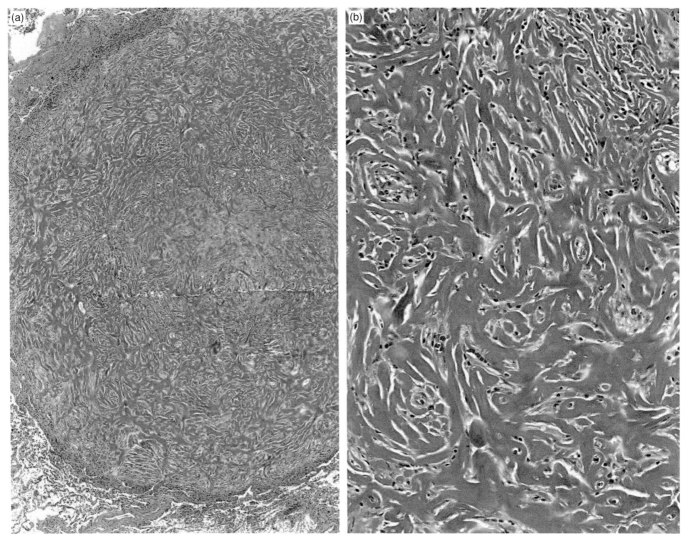

Figure 6.5. Pulmonary hyalinizing granuloma. (a) Well-circumscribed pink nodule. **(b)** High magnification, showing thick bundles of hyalinized collagen arranged in a lamellar pattern. The spaces between the collagen bundles contain a few inflammatory cells.

- Blood vessels can be prominent within the hyalinized fibrosis. They may show intimal fibrosis and medial hyalinization. Occasionally, they may be obliterated. Endothelialitis, if present, is a clue to IgG4-related disease.
- Small foci of necrosis occur in some cases. They appear as eosinophilic debris that insinuates between collagen bundles. Neutrophils and karyorrhectic debris may be present within the necrosis.
- Scattered eosinophils are seen in a few cases. They may occasionally be present in substantial numbers.
- There should be no evidence of granulomatous inflammation, multinucleated giant cells or calcification.
- Grossly, the nodules are well-circumscribed, firm and white or grayish-white.

Diagnostic work-up

The diagnosis of pulmonary hyalinizing granuloma does not require special stains. Interestingly, Congo red staining can be a pitfall for the unwary. In Engleman's original report, 11 of 18

cases of pulmonary hyalinizing granuloma were positive for Congo red and showed apple-green birefringence. This phenomenon can lead to a mistaken diagnosis of amyloidosis. A recent case report suggests that pulmonary hyalinizing granuloma may be positive for IgG4.

Clinical profile

Pulmonary hyalinizing granuloma is typically found in middle-aged adults. Symptoms are mild, or the lesion is found incidentally in asymptomatic individuals. Reported symptoms include cough, dyspnea, hemoptysis, fatigue and chest pain. The reported age range is 13 to 77 years, with a mean in the 40s. There is no sex predilection. Concurrent sclerosing mediastinitis is present in 20% of cases, and may be a clue to the correct diagnosis. Concurrent autoimmune diseases are also common. Serum titers of antinuclear antibody (ANA), anti-smooth muscle antibodies and anti-microsomal antibodies may be elevated. A single case with elevated serum IgG4 levels has been reported.

Radiologic findings

Pulmonary hyalinizing granuloma most commonly presents as multiple bilateral lung nodules mimicking metastatic malignancy. Cases with multiple unilateral nodules or a solitary nodule have also been reported. The nodules are randomly distributed and are well circumscribed. The borders may be well defined or irregular. The reported size range is 2–9 cm, with an average of 2.8 cm. On follow-up, the nodules either remain stable or slowly enlarge over a period of years. PET positivity (SUV 5.1 to 7.1) has been reported.

Differential diagnosis

- Nodular amyloidosis appears very similar to pulmonary hyalinizing granuloma. Both processes are characterized by nodules formed by paucicellular eosinophilic material. Amyloid is Congo red positive and pulmonary hyalinizing granuloma may be too. However, the collagen bundles in pulmonary hyalinizing granuloma are arranged in a lamellar or whorled pattern, while amyloid is not. Further, nodular amyloidosis is frequently associated with multinucleated giant cells, calcification or ossification, whereas pulmonary hyalinizing granuloma is not.
- Light chain deposition disease, described in detail in a prior section in this chapter, can appear similar to pulmonary hyalinizing granuloma. Light chain deposition disease is Congo red negative, and usually pulmonary hyalinizing granuloma is too. However, the eosinophilic material in pulmonary hyalinizing granuloma is collagen as opposed to light chains in light chain deposition disease. The matter can be resolved by immunohistochemistry or laser microdissection and tandem mass spectrometry.
- Sclerosing mediastinitis is identical in appearance to pulmonary hyalinizing granuloma and is commonly found concurrently in the same patient. The main difference between the two is that sclerosing mediastinitis is a mediastinal process while pulmonary hyalinizing granuloma occurs within the lung parenchyma.
- Silicotic nodules are composed of hyalinized, lamellar fibrosis with "cracks" similar to pulmonary hyalinizing granuloma. However, the presence of numerous dust-laden macrophages around the nodules should be a tip-off to the correct diagnosis. Silica and silicates are present within the dust; they are needle-shaped and birefringent when viewed under polarized light.
- Fungal and mycobacterial granulomas can "burn out" with lamellar fibrosis similar to pulmonary hyalinizing granuloma. However, in these lesions, the lamellar fibrosis is usually at the periphery of the nodule, whereas it comprises the entire nodule in pulmonary hyalinizing granuloma. The presence of granulomatous inflammation, central necrosis or calcification argues against pulmonary hyalinizing granuloma.
- Neoplasms such as solitary fibrous tumor and inflammatory myofibroblastic tumor commonly contain collagen bundles, mimicking the appearance of pulmonary hyalinizing granuloma. However, they also have a prominent spindle cell component in addition to collagen, while pulmonary hyalinizing granuloma does not. Immunohistochemistry for CD34 and STAT6 aids in the diagnosis of solitary fibrous tumor, while fluorescence in-situ hybridization (FISH) or immunohistochemistry for anaplastic lymphoma kinase (ALK) aids in the diagnosis of inflammatory myofibroblastic tumor.
- IgG4-related lung disease shares several features with pulmonary hyalinizing granuloma, including dense fibrosis and lymphoplasmacytic inflammatory infiltrates. One case of pulmonary hyalinizing granuloma with elevated tissue and serum IgG4 has been reported, and it is likely that some cases will fall under the spectrum of IgG4-related disease. The diagnosis of IgG4-related disease requires immunohistochemistry for IgG4 and, ideally, elevated IgG4 levels in the serum.

Treatment and prognosis

There is no specific medical therapy. The prognosis is good, although the nodules may slowly enlarge. No deaths have been recorded.

Sample diagnosis on pathology report

Lung, right lower lobe, needle biopsy – Pulmonary hyalinizing granuloma (See comment).

Nodular lymphoid hyperplasia

Nodular lymphoid hyperplasia is an uncommon cause of benign lung nodules. It is defined by the presence of a reactive lymphoplasmacytic infiltrate combined with fibrosis, presenting radiologically as a solitary lung mass or multiple lung nodules. This type of lesion has been called "pseudo-lymphoma" in the past, but the term "pulmonary nodular lymphoid hyperplasia" has gained acceptance as the clinical, radiologic and pathologic findings of this lesion have been better described. Most recently, it has been shown that pulmonary nodular lymphoid hyperplasia contains increased numbers of IgG4-positive plasma cells in the majority of cases.

Major diagnostic findings

- Nodular lesion in the lung parenchyma composed of lymphocytes, plasma cells and fibrosis (Figure 6.6). Sheets of plasma cells may be present as is the case in other IgG4-related diseases. Fibrosis is present in most cases and usually takes the form of a central scar. The lymphoid infiltrate often includes lymphoid follicles with prominent germinal centers.
- The diagnosis requires exclusion of low-grade lymphoma (especially marginal zone lymphoma) (see differential diagnosis, below).

Variable pathologic findings

- In most cases, the lesion is adjacent to the pleura.
- Focal extension of lymphocytes from the nodule into adjacent bronchovascular bundles or

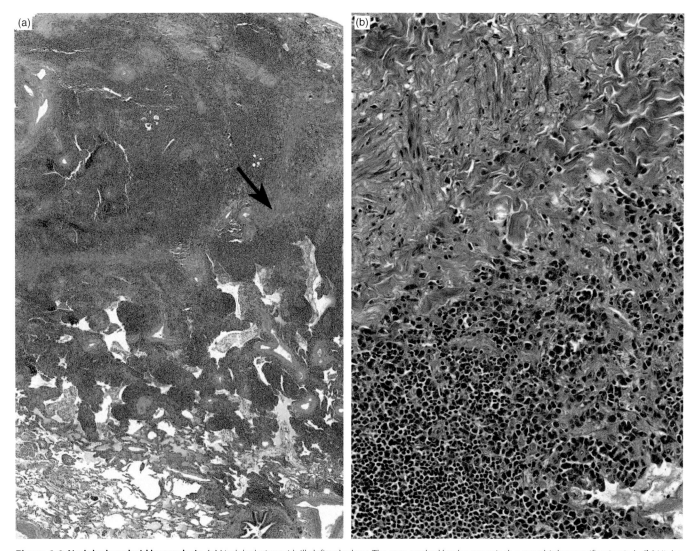

Figure 6.6. Nodular lymphoid hyperplasia. (a) Nodular lesion with ill-defined edges. The area marked by the arrow is shown at high magnification in b. **(b)** Higher magnification, showing characteristic admixture of fibrosis (top), lymphocytes (bottom left) and plasma cells (bottom right). The lesion was T-cell predominant and negative for B-cell gene rearrangements. The plasma cells were positive for IgG4 (not shown).

interlobular septa may occur but extensive tracking along lymphatic routes is absent.

- Immunohistochemistry usually shows a mix of CD3-positive T-cells and CD20-positive B-cells, with the former predominating. The B-cell component commonly forms lymphoid follicles with reactive germinal centers.
- Kappa and lambda light chains show a polytypic expression pattern.
- Immunohistochemical staining for IgG4 may show large numbers of IgG4-positive plasma cells, ranging from 32 to 167 IgG4-positive plasma cells per high-power field.
- Foci of lymphoplasmacytic intimal endothelial inflammation of small veins have been described in some cases, but this finding is usually focal and subtle. This finding is a clue to the presence of IgG4-related disease.
- Russell bodies have been described in a few cases.

Diagnostic work-up

- As described above, the pathologic work-up should focus on exclusion of low-grade lymphoma using morphology, immunohistochemistry and/or PCR. The most helpful antibodies to start with are CD3 and CD20.
- Special stains for IgG4 can be performed. Positive IgG4-positive plasma cells provide additional support for the diagnosis of nodular lymphoid hyperplasia.

Clinical profile

Nodular lymphoid hyperplasia is often found incidentally in patients being investigated for other reasons. The patients range in age from 19 to 80 years with a mean in the 50s. Taken as a group, patients with nodular lymphoid hyperplasia are slightly younger than those with MALT lymphoma. There is no sex predilection. In most cases, the process is discovered when lung nodules are identified incidentally on radiographs performed for other reasons. Occasional patients may have non-specific symptoms such as cough, dyspnea or chest pain. In most cases, there are no underlying or associated autoimmune diseases.

Radiologic findings

Nodular lymphoid hyperplasia can present as solitary or multiple lung nodules. Solitary nodules are more common in most series. Multiple nodules are usually 2 to 3 in number. Multiple bilateral nodules have also been reported. The nodules range in size from 0.6 to 6 cm. Concomitant hilar or mediastinal adenopathy has been described.

Differential diagnosis

- Low-grade lymphoma. The most important entity in the differential diagnosis is low-grade lymphoma, especially extranodal marginal zone lymphoma (MALT lymphoma) of the lung, which can form solitary or multiple nodules and frequently contains a mix of small lymphocytes, numerous plasma cells and reactive germinal centers. Cytologic features are not helpful in the distinction between these entities since the tumor cells in low-grade lymphomas are deceptively bland. The diagnosis of lymphoma is generally based on a combination of morphology, immunohistochemistry and B-cell gene rearrangements by PCR. Features that favor low-grade lymphoma include dense lymphoid infiltrates tightly cuffing the pleura, interlobular septa and bronchovascular bundles (peri-lymphatic or lymphangitic distribution) and B-cell predominant infiltrates by immunohistochemistry. Some authors claim that lymphoepithelial lesions may be present in nodular lymphoid hyperplasia whereas others state that they are absent. We do not find this feature helpful in the differential diagnosis. Similarly Dutcher bodies (intranuclear inclusions) are said to be present in MALT lymphomas and absent in nodular lymphoid hyperplasia, but we do not find this to be a helpful feature in practice. CD43 expression in the B-cells allegedly favors MALT lymphoma. PCR for B-cell gene rearrangements is helpful in difficult cases since lymphomas are usually monoclonal while nodular lymphoid hyperplasia is polyclonal.
- IgG4-related lung disease is in the differential diagnosis since pulmonary nodular lymphoid hyperplasia shares several morphologic features with IgG4-related diseases and contains large numbers of IgG4-positive plasma cells. Whether to label such cases as nodular lymphoid hyperplasia or IgG4-related disease is an arbitrary decision. Since nodular lymphoid hyperplasia is a discrete, well-defined entity with known clinical implications whereas IgG4-related disease is an ever-expanding mish-mash of various entities, we favor the former term until the significance of IgG4 positivity is better defined.

- Theoretically, other reactive lymphoid proliferations such as follicular bronchiolitis and lymphoid interstitial pneumonia enter the differential diagnosis. Although the reactive nature of the lymphoid infiltrate and the cellular composition is similar, the distribution of disease is not. Follicular bronchiolitis is limited to the walls of bronchioles. Lymphoid interstitial pneumonia is a diffuse interstitial process that thickens alveolar septa. Neither of these entities features architecture-distorting lung nodules.
- Organizing pneumonia typically contains a few lymphocytes and plasma cells, but does not form well-defined lymphoplasmacytic nodules with central scarring. The main finding in organizing pneumonia is the presence of fibroblast plugs within airspaces. Fibroblast plugs are absent in nodular lymphoid hyperplasia.

Treatment and prognosis

Nodular lymphoid hyperplasia does not require any additional treatment. No evidence of recurrence or evolution to lymphoma has emerged on long-term follow-up (up to 6 years). No deaths have been reported.

Sample diagnosis on pathology report

Lung, right middle lobe, surgical biopsy – Nodular lymphoid hyperplasia (See comment).

IgG4-related disease

In recent years, a wide variety of pathologic findings in the lung has been attributed to IgG4-related disease, including interstitial lung disease, pleural disease and lung nodules. This section focuses on nodules that fall under the spectrum of IgG4-related disease. Some degree of healthy skepticism is in order before accepting this premise. The most common justifications cited in favor of considering IgG4-related disease a valid clinico-pathologic entity include raised IgG4 levels in the serum, multi-system involvement, response to corticosteroids, and distinctive pathologic features, including lymphoplasmacytic infiltrates, storiform fibrosis and obliterative phlebitis. However, many cases that have been labeled as IgG4-related disease in the literature have normal serum IgG4 levels, show no evidence of multi-system involvement, do not require corticosteroid therapy because they are completely resected solitary lesions, and lack one or more of the typical pathologic features. The inclusion of such cases under the umbrella of IgG4-related disease based solely on an arbitrary immunohistochemical cut-off for IgG4 staining is dubious. Irrespective of the precise terminology applied to such lesions, they are essentially benign fibroinflammatory nodules of unknown etiology and pathogenesis.

Major diagnostic findings

- Benign nodule composed of a reactive lymphoplasmacytic infiltrate, prominent plasma cells and fibrosis (Figure 6.7).
- Positive staining for IgG4 in the plasma cells. In surgical lung biopsies, current criteria require (1) ≥ 50

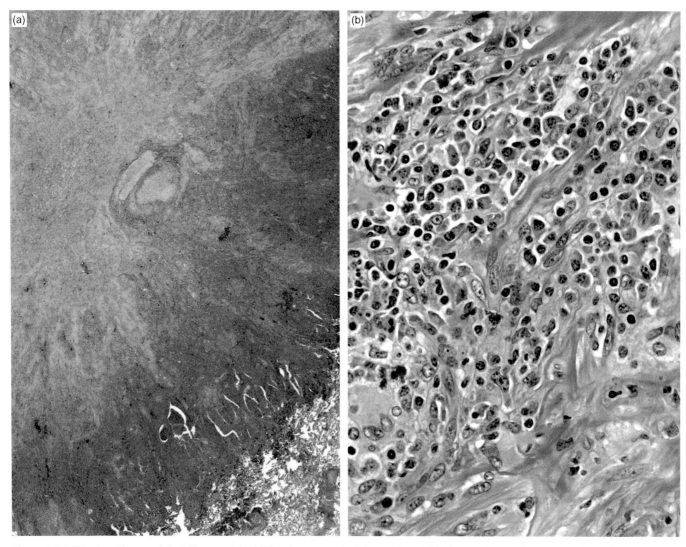

Figure 6.7. IgG4-related lung nodule. (a) Lung nodule with fibrotic center and cellular periphery. **(b)** High magnification, showing typical mix of sheets of plasma cells, dense hyalinized fibrosis and scattered eosinophils. Most of the plasma cells were positive for IgG4 by immunohistochemistry (not shown).

IgG4-positive plasma cells per high-power field or (2) ratio of IgG4-positive plasma cells/IgG-positive plasma cells ≥ 40%. The recommendations suggest counting three fields with the highest number of IgG4-positive plasma cells, and reporting the average. In biopsy specimens, the requirement is relaxed to ≥ 20 IgG4-positive plasma cells per high-power field

Variable pathologic findings

- *Storiform fibrosis* is a characteristic feature of IgG4-related disease in other sites but may or may not be present in IgG4-related lung nodules. It is characterized by the presence of dense collagen bundles with a whorled appearance and intervening "cracks". Even in the absence of storiform fibrosis, most IgG4-related lung nodules feature dense fibrosis intimately admixed with lymphoplasmacytic infiltrates.
- *Obliterative phlebitis* has been reported in the lung but may be absent in some cases. Lung involvement is also unique in

that obliterative arteritis may occur, rather than phlebitis. It is characterized by a lymphoplasmacytic infiltrate within arterial walls with or without luminal obliteration. Necrotizing vasculitis is thought to be rare.
- A few eosinophils are often present in IgG4-related disease in other organs, and this is also true in IgG4-related lung disease.
- Findings away from the main mass include lymphoplasmacytic infiltrates in airway walls, arteries, veins, interlobular septa and the pleura. These infiltrates often follow a lymphangitic distribution.
- Granulomas and prominent neutrophilic infiltrates are thought to be inconsistent with a diagnosis of IgG4-related disease. However, small aggregates of neutrophils may be present within airspaces.
- Other reported findings include lymphoid follicles with germinal centers, prominent lymphatic dilatation and emperipolesis in S-100-positive histiocytes.

Diagnostic work-up

- CD3-positive T-lymphocytes should outnumber CD20-positive B-cells. Immunohistochemistry or in situ hybridization for kappa and lambda light chains should reveal polytypic plasma cells.
- Either IgG4 alone or a combination of IgG4 and IgG can be used for the diagnosis. Most centers use a monoclonal IgG4 antibody which shows strong cytoplasmic staining in lesional plasma cells. The diagnostic criteria have been listed previously under "Major diagnostic findings".

Clinical profile

The reported age in patients with IgG4-related lung nodules or masses ranges from 42 to 82 years. Men outnumber women by approximately 2 to 1. In many instances, lung nodules are discovered incidentally in asymptomatic individuals, or on chest imaging studies performed during the work-up of extra-pulmonary manifestations of IgG4-related disease. Other cases are discovered when imaging is performed for non-specific respiratory symptoms such as cough or dyspnea. Many but not all patients show elevated serum IgG4 levels. An elevated serum IgG4 level is not mandatory for the diagnosis.

The most compelling case for bona fide IgG4-related lung nodules can be made in patients who show evidence of prior, concurrent or subsequent IgG4-related disease in other organs, including autoimmune pancreatitis, orbital pseudotumor, chronic sclerosing sialadenitis, retroperitoneal fibrosis, nephritis, lymphadenopathy, or involvement of the gallbladder, bile duct or prostate.

Radiologic findings

Lung nodules, consolidated lesions or masses attributed to IgG4-related disease have ranged from 0.9 to 6 cm in size. They may be solitary or multiple, can slowly enlarge in size, and may be spiculated and PET-positive. Concurrent interlobular septal thickening and ground-glass opacities are common, and mimic lymphangitic spread of lung carcinoma.

Differential diagnosis

- The main entity in the differential diagnosis is nodular lymphoid hyperplasia. There are several similarities between the two entities, including reactive lymphoplasmacytic inflammatory infiltrates with prominent plasma cells, fibrosis, nodule formation and positivity for IgG4. It is likely that many cases described in the past as "plasma cell granuloma" or "inflammatory pseudotumor" of the lung would today fit into one of these two categories. In cases with convincing IgG4 positivity, differentiation between nodular lymphoid hyperplasia and IgG4-related disease can be arbitrary. It has been suggested that in comparison to IgG4-related disease, nodular lymphoid hyperplasia is more cellular with florid follicular hyperplasia and relatively little fibrosis. The presence of IgG4-related disease elsewhere in the body, prominent fibrosis or obliterative phlebitis would favor an IgG4-related lung nodule over nodular lymphoid

hyperplasia. By definition, negative staining for IgG4 excludes IgG4-related disease.
- Lymphomatoid granulomatosis can enter the differential diagnosis in elderly patients with multiple lung nodules, especially if vascular infiltration is prominent. In such cases, positivity for EBER will help to diagnose lymphomatoid granulomatosis. In contrast, the presence of extrapulmonary IgG4-related disease, prominent plasma cell infiltrates, scattered eosinophils and serum or tissue positivity for IgG4 favor IgG4-related disease. However, occasional cases with necrosis can be very challenging.

Treatment and prognosis

The treatment implications of this diagnosis are unclear. Solitary nodules probably do not require therapy but often undergo wedge resection or lobectomy for suspected lung cancer. Most do not recur. Multiple lung nodules occurring in patients with IgG4-related disease may respond to corticosteroid therapy. Rituximab has been tried recently for IgG4-related disease, but its effects on lung nodules have not been specifically reported.

Sample diagnosis on pathology report

Lung, right lower lobe, wedge resection – Benign fibroinflammatory nodule with increased IgG4-positive plasma cells highly suggestive of IgG4-related disease (See comment).

Pulmonary apical cap

Pulmonary apical cap is a distinctive fibroelastotic scar that occurs in the apices of the upper lobes and forms a mass-like lesion. The etiology remains uncertain despite much angst and numerous hypotheses over the years. An ischemic basis seems most plausible. Apical caps are most commonly seen as an incidental finding in lobectomies of upper lobes, but may also be seen in core needle biopsies or wedge resections of masses in the apices, or surgical biopsies of the upper lobes.

Major diagnostic findings

The main finding is the presence of a wedge-shaped fibroelastotic scar in the periphery of the lung parenchyma (Figure 6.8). The wedge is pleura-based and its apex faces inwards, towards the lung parenchyma. The pleural aspect is typically gently curved while the parenchymal aspect has an irregular contour. A characteristic feature is the very pale, light-staining color of the scar, similar to solar elastosis of the skin. This "fibroelastotic" appearance is caused by the presence of wavy, lightly basophilic elastic fibers within the lesion.

Variable pathologic findings

- Lymphoid follicles may be present within apical caps. These may have prominent germinal centers.
- Lung epithelium may be entrapped within the scar. Entrapped epithelium at the periphery of the scar may be hyperplastic and quite worrisome in appearance. However,

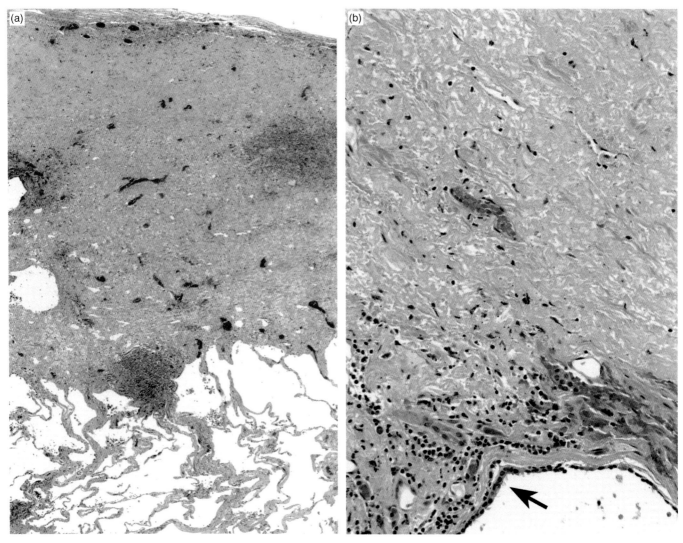

Figure 6.8. Pulmonary apical cap. (a) Pleura-based fibroelastotic scar within the lung parenchyma. Note lymphoid aggregates and undulating border. **(b)** High magnification, showing light-staining scar composed of wavy elastic fibers. Entrapped lung epithelium is at the bottom of the picture. Note cilia (arrow).

the cells are usually cuboidal in shape and lack the degree of cytologic atypia typically seen in adenocarcinoma.

- Dust-laden macrophages can be scattered within the scar. The dust is usually black and carbonaceous ("anthracotic").
- A wide variety of vascular changes have been reported, including thrombosis of pulmonary arteries and arterioles, focal recanalization, and hyalinized sclerosis involving pulmonary veins.
- In some cases a hyalinized pleural plaque identical to an asbestos-related pleural plaque can be seen on the surface of the apical scar. This type of plaque is densely collagenized and strongly eosinophilic.
- If elastic stains are performed, one can appreciate the remnants of residual lung architecture in the elastic stain, and it becomes apparent that the air spaces are filled with loose connective tissue.
- Metaplastic calcification and ossification are fairly common in apical caps.

- Occasional granulomas or meningothelial-like nodules may be present within the lesion.
- Iron stains fail to reveal asbestos bodies in most cases.

Diagnostic work-up

- In most cases, no special stains are required for the diagnosis.
- An elastic stain such as an EVG or Movat can highlight the collapsed lung architecture and the filling of air spaces with connective tissue matrix.

Clinical profile

Apical caps are encountered in adults of all ages and both sexes. Patients range in age from 16 to 94 years and include both men and women. The lesion appears to be more common with advancing age. In the vast majority of cases, apical caps are an incidental finding on a chest radiograph, or an incidental finding in lobectomies of upper lobes performed for lung cancer. Increasingly, they are seen in CT-guided core needle biopsies performed for lesions that are detected incidentally in the course of a radiographic examination for other reasons.

Radiologic findings

Radiographs show a mass-like shadow in the left upper lobe, right upper lobe or rarely the apices of the lower lobes. The lesion may be unilateral or bilateral. The size ranges from 0.7 to 5 cm. The lesions are often described as spiculated, pleura-based parenchymal masses associated with pleural thickening. Many are non-calcified, but occasionally focal coarse calcifications may be present. Emphysematous changes with bullae are often noted in the adjacent lung on chest radiographs. On chest CT, the lesion has extensive contact with the pleura of the apex of the upper lobe. The edge of the mass is relatively sharply defined but has undulating or irregular borders. Apical caps can be PET-positive (FDG-avid), which is surprising considering their hypocellular nature.

Differential diagnosis

- Pleural plaques. Pleural plaques are characterized by dense hyalinized (pink) fibrosis. In contrast, the fibrosis in apical caps is pale and light staining.
- Non-specific parenchymal scars are distinguished from apical caps mainly by their location. While apical caps are present at the apices of the lobes, parenchymal scars typically occur randomly in other locations.
- Radiation-related scars may have an appearance similar to apical caps. They may be predominantly collagenous, but predominantly elastotic examples have also been described. They are said to have more pronounced vascular changes than apical caps. The diagnosis requires a history of prior irradiation to the area.

Treatment and prognosis

Apical caps are benign. They do not require resection or any other specific therapy.

Sample diagnosis on pathology report

Lung, right upper lobe, needle biopsy – Pulmonary apical cap (See comment).

Round atelectasis

Round atelectasis (also known as rounded atelectasis, atelectatic pseudotumor, shrinking pleuritis with atelectasis, asbestos pseudotumor, or Blesovsky syndrome) is a mass-like lesion caused by the invagination of fibrotic pleura into the underlying lung causing focal atelectasis. It is most likely related to prior pleural inflammation and fibrosis. Many cases are associated with asbestos exposure. The lesion is infrequently resected since it is usually identified correctly on the basis of its characteristic radiologic findings.

Major diagnostic findings

- The diagnostic feature is an invaginated focus of thickened pleura covered by a pleural plaque (Figure 6.9). The plaque is composed of dense collagen bundles with a paucicellular appearance, separated by clear spaces with a "cracked" appearance. The underlying invaginated pleura is also thickened and bulges downwards into the underlying lung parenchyma, causing atelectasis of the adjacent lung. The entire process results in the formation of a mass-like lesion.
- Other than the focus of atelectasis underlying the invaginated pleura, there is no other abnormality in the lung parenchyma that could account for the formation of a mass.

Variable pathologic findings

- The invaginated pleura under the fibrous plaque may be thickened by a combination of loose fibrosis, edema, a few scattered inflammatory cells and dilated capillaries. Pleural adhesions are often present. The pleura often shows wrinkling and folding, appreciated best on elastic stains.
- Pleural plaques are present in most cases, but sometimes there is simply residual fibrosis without plaque formation. Plaques may also be found on the costal or diaphragmatic pleura, and may be grossly visible to the prosector.
- Lymphoid aggregates are common in the invaginated pleura as well as the junction between the pleura and the underlying lung.
- Mild non-specific fibrosis of the alveolar septa and patchy organizing pneumonia may be seen in the underlying lung.
- Asbestos bodies may be identifiable in the lung parenchyma in some cases.

Diagnostic work-up

- Elastic stains such as EVG, VVG or Movat help to highlight the various layers of the process, the architectural distortion, and the wrinkling and folding of the pleura. However, they are not necessary for the diagnosis.
- A Movat stain is particularly helpful, since it highlights fibrosis (yellow) and elastic tissue (black) in the same slide.
- Iron stains can be helpful to find asbestos bodies.

Clinical profile

Round atelectasis has been documented in patients ranging from 20 to 92 years of age with a mean in the 60s. Males predominate in most descriptions, with a male to female ratio of 8:2 in some studies. The lesion is usually discovered in chest radiographs performed for other reasons in asymptomatic individuals, but some patients may have minimal symptoms. A history of asbestos exposure is present in approximately 70% of cases.

Radiologic findings

The radiologic findings of round atelectasis are well described. The most common finding is a round or oval peripheral mass that abuts thickened pleura. A concomitant

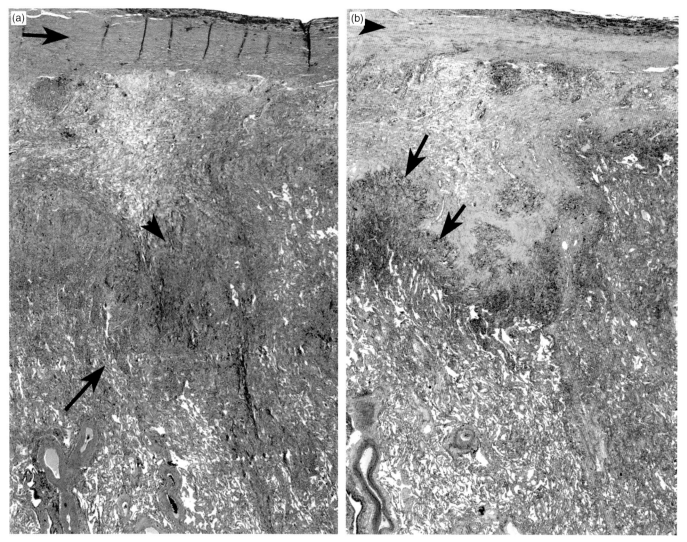

Figure 6.9. Round atelectasis. (a) A hyalinized pleural plaque (short arrow) sits atop a round area of fibrotic invaginated pleura (arrowhead). The underlying lung is atelectatic (long arrow). The combination of changes forms a mass-like lesion. **(b)** The architecture of the lesion is easier to appreciate on a Movat pentachrome stain, which highlights wrinkled elastic laminae in the invaginated pleura (arrows), as well as dense fibrosis in the overlying plaque (arrowhead).

pleural effusion may be present. Pleural thickening leads to collapse of the underlying parenchyma forming a mass-like lesion that can vary from 2.5 to 8 cm in size. The lesion can enhance uniformly with contrast. An important clue to the diagnosis is the "comet tail" sign, which is caused by the distortion of bronchial and vascular structures leading to the appearance of a tail that leads into the rounded opacity. This sign is thought to represent distortion of bronchial and vascular structures in the region of atelectasis and can be recognized on CT scans. Homogeneous contrast enhancement is seen. The lesion can be found in any lobe, but is most common in the lower lobes, particularly the right lower lobe.

Differential diagnosis

Clinically, the most important consideration is a malignant neoplasm, and this is usually easy to rule out pathologically. Pathologically, the most important differential diagnosis is

pleural fibrosis and parenchymal scars. The key to the diagnosis is recognizing that the mass is formed by invaginated pleura rather than a parenchymal abnormality.

Treatment and prognosis

No treatment or surgical intervention is required if the diagnosis is made on the basis of radiologic findings. However, if the diagnosis is unclear, the lesion may be surgically resected. Recognition of the lesion at the time of frozen section may avert lobectomy. In the majority of cases, the lesion remains stable over time. Occasional spontaneous regression has been reported.

Sample diagnosis on pathology report

Lung, right lower lobe, wedge resection – Pleural plaque, and changes consistent with round atelectasis (See comment).

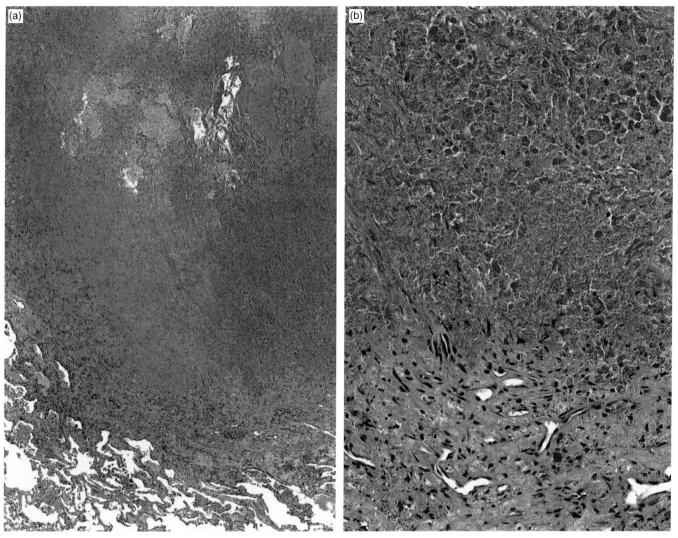

Figure 6.10. Infarct. (a) The necrotic center of this nodule occupies the top half of the picture. The cellular rim is at the bottom. Note hemosiderin-laden macrophages within adjacent lung. The appearance at this magnification is very similar to that of a necrotizing granuloma. **(b)** Higher magnification, showing necrosis and the cellular rim containing fibroblasts, granulation tissue and hemosiderin. Note the absence of granulomatous inflammation.

Infarct

Infarcts are under-recognized as a cause of lung nodules and infiltrates. Since the lung has a dual circulation (derived from bronchial arteries and pulmonary arteries), infarcts occur only if there is significant compromise of both components. This typically involves vascular occlusion accompanied by compromise of the cardiopulmonary system in the form of cardiac failure, shock or chronic lung disease. Obstruction of the pulmonary veins has been noted by several authors to be a major contributor to the formation of pulmonary infarcts. In some cases, the underlying cause cannot be determined.

Infarcts are usually diagnosed on the basis of clinical and radiologic findings. They may occasionally be biopsied or excised if the radiologic findings are atypical, including unusual nodules, masses or non-resolving infiltrates.

Infarcts may be encountered in core needle biopsy specimens, wedge resections, lobectomies and autopsies.

Major diagnostic findings

- Necrosis is the key diagnostic finding in infarcts (Figure 6.10). It is typically described as "bland", "ischemic" or "coagulative" and is eosinophilic in appearance. However, cases have been described in which the necrosis is basophilic or "dirty", at least focally, due to the presence of karyorrhectic debris derived from the necrotic, disintegrating nuclei. Typically, the necrosis of infarcts contains remnants or "ghosts" of alveolar septal architecture. Small islands of residual viable lung parenchyma may survive within this necrotic tissue.
- The rim of an infarct is quite characteristic (Figure 6.10). It is composed of fibroblasts, granulation tissue (capillaries), occasional foamy macrophages, hemosiderin-laden macrophages and variable amounts of collagen. Fibroblasts may be oriented perpendicularly, with a palisaded appearance mimicking granulomatous inflammation ("pseudo-granulomatoid").

Variable pathologic findings

- Infarcts are usually located in subpleural lung parenchyma. Venous infarcts tend to be located adjacent to interlobular septa. Radiologically, up to 89% of infarcts are subpleural in location.
- The lesion is often described as wedge-shaped or triangular, but this characteristic shape is seen in only 26% of cases examined histologically. The remainder have a variety of shapes, including "geographic" (irregular), round or mixed.
- Hemorrhage is a prominent feature in most infarcts and is a clue to the diagnosis. It is characterized by red blood cells, hemosiderin and hematoidin pigment at the edge of the lesion itself, as well as in the lung parenchyma surrounding the lesion. Hemosiderin is brown and coarsely granular, and is often present within macrophages. Like hemosiderin, hematoidin is a red cell breakdown product. It appears as a bright yellow pigment.
- Thrombi or emboli within pulmonary arteries are common in the lung adjacent to infarcts. They may be fresh (recent), organizing or recanalized.
- Inflammation within the walls of blood vessels has been described and can mimic vasculitis, especially Wegener's granulomatosis. However, true granulomatous inflammation and necrotizing vasculitis are not seen in infarcts.
- Squamous metaplasia is a frequent finding, noted in up to 35% of cases.
- Reactive epithelial changes are common in the alveolar pneumocytes at the edge of the lesion. In needle biopsy or fine-needle aspiration samples, this may raise the possibility of a malignancy.
- Multinucleated giant cells within the airspaces have been described. This can raise the possibility of granulomatous inflammation or Wegener's granulomatosis.
- Cholesterol clefts may be present.
- Plugs of organizing pneumonia may be seen in the air spaces surrounding the infarct.
- Calcification is seen in a small minority of cases.

Diagnostic work-up

- No specific work-up required in typical cases, but special stains for elastic tissue, such as Verhoeff–Van Gieson (VVG) or Movat pentachrome can be helpful in highlighting the loss of normal architecture and vascular abnormalities.
- An iron stain helps to document the presence of hemosiderin in the surrounding parenchyma.

Clinical profile

The age range is 22 to 85 years with median ages ranging from 48 to 55 years. There is a slight predilection for men in most series. The clinical triad of lung infarction consists of hemoptysis, chest pain and "pleurisy"; however, these typical findings are usually absent in cases that come to biopsy. Most patients that undergo biopsy have non-specific symptoms such as cough and shortness of breath. Infarcts are often discovered incidentally on radiographs performed for other reasons. In one large series, this type of incidental presentation accounted for 65% of all cases. Other common presenting symptoms include chest pain, hemoptysis and pleural effusion. Many patients (up to 43%) have a history of prior surgery. In one study, 8% had a history of deep vein thrombosis, and 8% had a history of congestive heart failure. Clinical work-up after a pathologic diagnosis of lung infarcts may lead to the discovery of right atrial thrombi, pulmonary thromboemboli or thrombi of the distal extremities. Work-up for an underlying malignancy may also be productive. Overall, the most common underlying finding in patients with lung infarcts is the presence of venous thromboembolism.

Radiologic findings

The classic radiologic manifestation of a lung infarct is a peripheral opacity that abuts the pleura, with a cardiac margin that is sharp and convex or hump-shaped ("Hampton's hump"). However, in pathologically confirmed cases, the most common radiologic finding is a solitary lung nodule. Nodules may also be bilateral, or there may be unilateral or bilateral consolidation. Although any lobe may be involved, the right lower lobe appears to be the most common site. Infarcts are seldom included in the radiologic differential diagnosis in cases that come to biopsy.

Differential diagnosis

- Histologically, infarcts are most commonly mistaken for necrotizing granulomas. Although the distinction can be challenging at times, the key to the diagnosis is recognizing that the palisading cells at the edge of the necrosis are fibroblasts, not epithelioid histiocytes. Other clues that favor an infarct over a granuloma include hemorrhagic necrosis, abundant hemosiderin deposition at the periphery of the lesion, and vascular thrombi.
- The presence of airspace giant cells, vascular inflammation, hemosiderin and occasional "dirty" necrosis may raise the specter of vasculitis, especially Wegener's granulomatosis. However, necrotizing vasculitis and granulomatous inflammation are absent.

Treatment and prognosis

There is no specific treatment, and the prognosis is that of the underlying disease. Most lung infarcts resolve with scarring, although cavitation has also been described.

Sample diagnosis on pathology report

Lung, right lower lobe, wedge resection – Infarct (See comment).

Silicosis

Silicosis is a pneumoconiosis caused by the deposition of *silica* and *silicates* within lung parenchyma. Crystalline silica is

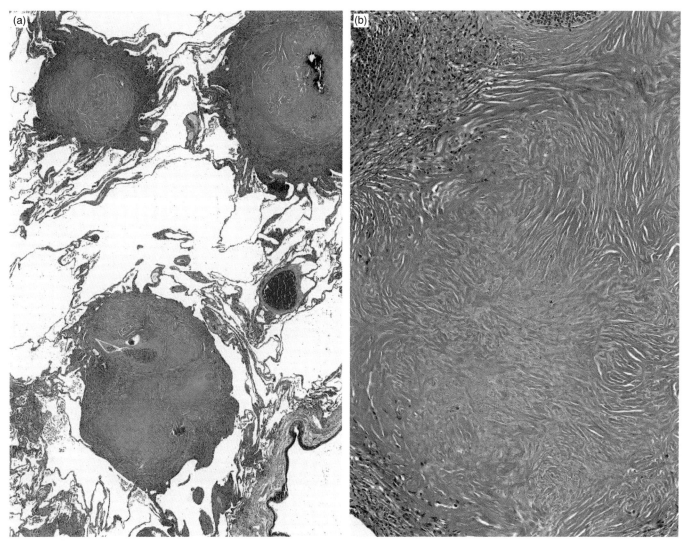

Figure 6.11. Silicosis. (a) Multiple lung nodules superficially resembling necrotizing granulomas. The nodule at the bottom is shown at higher magnification in b. **(b)** The center of this nodule shows lamellated bundles of hyalinized collagen with a cracked appearance. The degenerative appearance seen in the middle of the image is often misinterpreted as necrosis. The cellular rim is at top left and bottom left. Case courtesy of Dr. AV Arrossi.

strongly fibrogenic, i.e., it induces the deposition of collagen in the lung. In contrast, silicates (minerals composed of silica plus another element) are not fibrogenic. Exposure to inhaled crystalline silica occurs chiefly through occupational exposure to *quartz*, mainly by disruption of quartz-rich rocks in road construction, tunneling, mining, sandblasting, rock drilling, quarry work, stone masonry, pottery making and stonecutting. Crystalline silica can also be a component of carbonaceous dusts such as coal dust, asbestos, iron or clay. Since coal dust contains crystalline silica, coal workers may develop silicosis instead of classic coal workers' pneumoconiosis. Silicosis has also been reported in denim jean sandblasters. Finally, exposure to silica may occur in a domestic setting in a condition known as *hut lung* or *domestically acquired particulate lung disease* (see section on mixed-dust pneumoconiosis in Chapter 8).

Major diagnostic findings

- The hallmark of silicosis is the presence of *silicotic nodules* within lung parenchyma. These are small, round,

well-circumscribed, discrete fibrous nodules that at first glance resemble granulomas (Figure 6.11). They are usually found in peribronchiolar parenchyma, but they may also be randomly distributed. The H&E appearance of silicotic nodules is quite distinctive. It is characterized by a fibrotic center composed of lamellated and whorled bundles of dense hyalinized collagen with distinctive "cracks", surrounded by a cellular rim containing fibroblasts and dust-laden macrophages (Figure 6.11). A few lymphocytes or plasma cells may occasionally be present. The dust within the macrophages is a mix of tiny dark brown or black carbonaceous particles, crystalline silica and silicates, and is usually inconspicuous. Silica and silicates are tiny, needle-shaped or acicular particles. Black dust is visible by standard light microscopy, whereas silica and silicates are difficult to see. Their identification is greatly facilitated by examination under polarized light, where silica particles appear weakly birefringent, whereas silicates are strongly birefringent (Figure 6.12). Black dust is not birefringent. In most silicotic

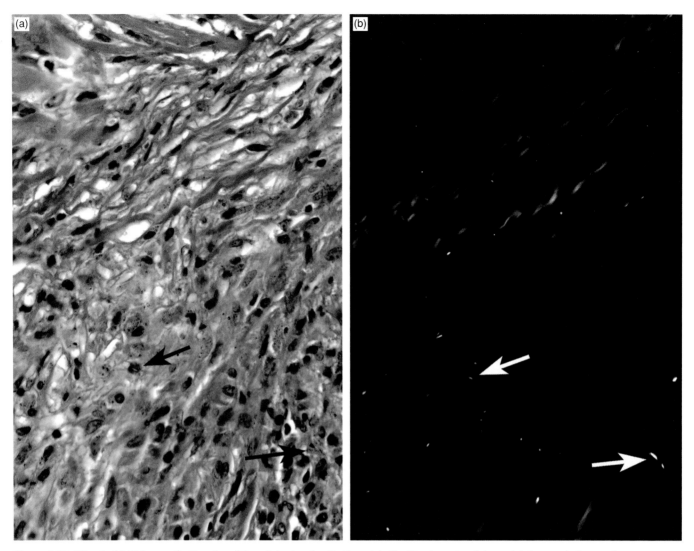

Figure 6.12. Silicosis. (a) High magnification view of the cellular rim of a silicotic nodule. The fibrotic center of the nodule is towards the top of the picture. Tiny dark-brown and black dust particles are visible within macrophages, but needle-shaped silica/silicate particles are very difficult to visualize (black arrows). **(b)** Under polarized light, needle-shaped particles are easier to see (white arrows). Strongly birefringent particles are silicates, while weakly birefringent particles represent silica. In retrospect, some of these are just barely visible on H&E (black arrows in part a), but many remain impossible to visualize. Case courtesy of Dr. AV Arrossi.

nodules, non-birefringent dust particles are more abundant than birefringent silica or silicate particles.

- Silicotic nodules are a common incidental finding in lymph nodes (hilar or peribronchial) in lobectomy specimens as well as in mediastinal lymph node dissections for lung cancer. Although a diagnosis of *silicotic nodule* can be given to lesions in lymph nodes solely on the basis of pathologic features, the diagnosis of *silicosis* requires the presence of silicotic nodules within lung parenchyma and an appropriate exposure history. Defined in this way, silicosis is a very uncommon diagnosis in routine surgical pathology practice. Most individuals with silicosis are not biopsied because the condition is easily recognized on the basis of occupational history and clinical and radiologic features.

- The pathologic diagnosis of silicosis requires silicotic nodules to be the predominant finding in the lung. If black carbonaceous dust predominates over silicotic nodules, the lesion is classified as *mixed-dust pneumoconiosis* rather than silicosis.

Variable pathologic findings

- The fibrous centers of silicotic nodules often show degenerative changes that mimic necrosis. They are light-staining and often calcify. True necrosis or granulomatous inflammation does not occur in uncomplicated silicotic nodules. The presence of either of these features should raise the possibility of superimposed tuberculosis or non-tuberculous mycobacterial infection. Areas of necrosis surrounded by palisading histiocytes, lymphocytes and plasma cells (resembling rheumatoid nodules) have been described in coal workers, and have been termed *Caplan's lesion*. This type of lesion is uncommon in silicosis and exceedingly rare in North America.

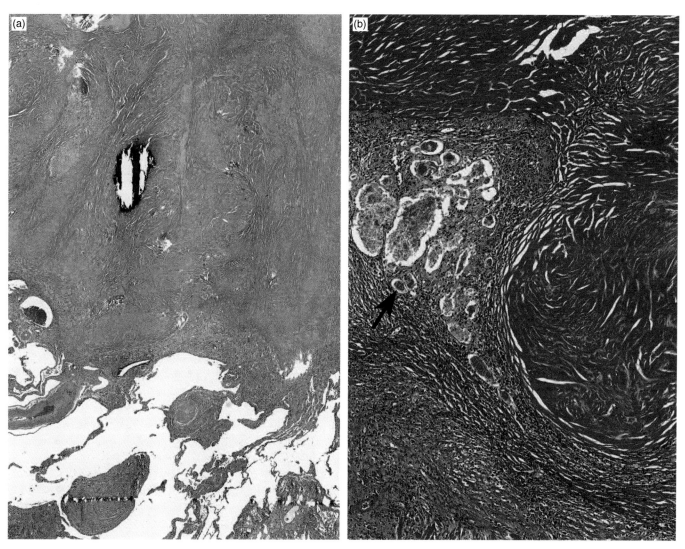

Figure 6.13. Silicosis. (a) Progressive massive fibrosis in silicosis. Small silicotic nodules (bottom) are coalescing to form a large confluent fibrotic mass (top). Note focus of calcification. The mass was grossly 5 cm in size. Case courtesy of Dr. AV Arrossi. **(b)** Silicoproteinosis. Eosinophilic material fills airspaces adjacent to a silicotic nodule (arrow). Case courtesy of Dr. Carol Farver.

- Dust-filled macrophages are often present in the lung parenchyma away from the silicotic nodules, usually within the interstitium. They are more prominent around respiratory bronchioles and alveolar ducts. They often form minute cellular lesions that lack the characteristic fibrosis of silicotic nodules, and are presumed to be early lesions that will eventually evolve into fibrous silicotic nodules.
- In silicosis, interstitial fibrosis is mainly caused by silicotic nodules. However, interstitial thickening of varying degrees is also caused by the presence of dust-filled histiocytes in lung parenchyma away from silicotic nodules, accompanied by a sparse infiltrate of lymphocytes and occasional plasma cells. Numerous cholesterol clefts may be present in these areas.
- Coalescence of silicotic nodules and the associated fibrosis into nodular parenchymal scars greater than 1 cm in diameter is termed *progressive massive fibrosis* (PMF,

Figure 6.13). This process corresponds to the presence of large opacities on chest radiographs.
- Alveolar proteinosis has been described in sandblasters with acute exposure to silica (acute silicoproteinosis). It is characterized by intra-alveolar accumulation of granular eosinophilic material similar to that seen in autoimmune pulmonary alveolar proteinosis (PAP) (Figure 6.13). However, it tends to be a focal finding and is usually overshadowed by silicotic nodules.
- Silicotic nodules are most numerous in the upper lobes and posterior aspects of the lungs, but middle lobe involvement has also been described, and the lower lobes may be involved by fibrosis. Silicotic nodules in the visceral pleura or subpleural lung have been described as *candle wax lesions* based on their waxy gross appearance.
- A florid spindle cell proliferation with a storiform pattern and an occasional infiltrative growth pattern has been described in mediastinal lymph nodes involved by silicosis. This cellular proliferation is an exaggerated form of the

usual fibrohistiocytic response seen at the edges of silicotic nodules. It must not be misinterpreted as neoplastic.

- Silicotic nodules with classic morphologic features and silica particles have also been reported in extrapulmonary lymph nodes, liver, spleen and bone marrow.

Diagnostic work-up

As described above, examination of silicotic nodules under polarized light is helpful. However, birefringent particles are not always present, even in classic silicotic nodules. Special stains for acid-fast bacteria (Ziehl-Neelsen) and fungi (GMS) should be performed when true necrosis or granulomatous inflammation is present. Although it is well established that silica and silicate particles can be *detected* by polarizing microscopy, *definitive identification* of these particles requires energy-dispersive X-ray spectroscopy (EDS), which can be combined with scanning electron microscopy (SEM). EDS determines the elemental composition of inorganic particles. Silica particles consist of the element silicon (Si) and oxygen, whereas silicate particles consist of a mix of Si and other elements (K-Al-Si or Mg-Al-Si, for example). Although SEM/EDS is not required for a pathologic diagnosis of silicosis, it can be helpful in difficult cases, or when mixed-dust pneumoconiosis is a consideration, by providing a precise assessment of the composition of the deposited dust. SEM/EDS can be performed on formalin-fixed paraffin-embedded material.

Clinical profile

Acute silicosis or silicoproteinosis – an acute illness that develops soon after exposure to high levels of silica – falls outside the purview of surgical pathologists. Chronic silicosis, which is the form most likely to be seen by pathologists, develops 10 to 30 years after exposure and has variable, non-specific clinical manifestations. Patients are usually adult men, but women may rarely be affected by domestically acquired variants of the disease. Patients with early stages of silicosis may be asymptomatic or may have minimal symptoms. Among symptomatic individuals, chronic cough and dyspnea are most common. Silicotic nodules limited to the hilar lymph nodes usually do not cause symptoms.

Radiologic findings

Like most other pneumoconioses, silicosis preferentially affects the upper lobes. As one would expect from the pathologic features described in the preceding paragraphs, multiple small nodules are the most common radiologic finding. On chest radiographs, these are termed *small rounded opacities* in the International Labor Office (ILO) scheme. It is well documented that pathologic evidence of silicosis in the lung parenchyma can occur in the absence of abnormalities on chest radiographs. On chest CT, silicotic nodules are typically multiple, small, and well defined, and have a predilection for the upper and posterior zones of the lungs. Subpleural nodules are common, and branching centrilobular structures have also been described. In patients who develop progressive massive fibrosis, the nodules coalesce, resulting in large, bilateral mass-like opacities.

Silicotic nodules are also common in hilar, intrapulmonary and mediastinal lymph nodes. On chest CT, calcification in the involved nodes is common, and is classically peripheral, an appearance described as *eggshell calcification*. Punctate calcification is also common.

Differential diagnosis

- Since they have a pink center and a cellular periphery, silicotic nodules are often misinterpreted as necrotizing granulomas. Unlike true granulomas, however, the center consists of hyalinized collagen with a "cracked" appearance rather than true necrosis. Although histiocytes and fibroblasts in the cellular periphery can mimic epithelioid histiocytes, they do not form a palisade. The presence of birefringent needle-shaped particles does not reliably differentiate the two entities since dust-filled histiocytes do occasionally coalesce around true necrotizing granulomas.
- As mentioned above, silicosis should be diagnosed only if silicotic nodules are the predominant finding in the lungs. If deposition of black dust is the main finding, and silicotic nodules are relatively few in number, the diagnosis should be mixed-dust pneumoconiosis.
- Nodules may also develop in coal workers' pneumoconiosis, and these too contain collagen and dust-filled macrophages. However, they lack the characteristic lamellated appearance of silicotic nodules.
- Sarcoidosis is occasionally mistaken for silicosis on clinical and radiologic grounds, but the two have little in common pathologically. The granulomatous nature of sarcoidosis is usually clearly apparent, whereas silicotic nodules do not contain true epithelioid histiocytes or multinucleated giant cells. When fibrosis occurs in sarcoidosis, it usually starts at the periphery of the granulomas and proceeds inwards. In contrast, the fibrosis in silicotic nodules is most prominent in the center. The presence of a lymphangitic distribution or granulomatous vasculitis further supports the diagnosis of sarcoidosis.
- Autoimmune pulmonary alveolar proteinosis (PAP). The presence of silicotic nodules adjacent to the involved airspaces easily excludes autoimmune PAP.

Treatment and prognosis

There is no effective treatment. Patients with advanced disease may be considered for lung transplantation. Progression of silicosis can occur many years after occupational exposure ceases. Silicosis is thought to predispose to tuberculosis. If progressive massive fibrosis develops, the prognosis is poor.

Sample diagnosis on pathology report

Lymph nodes, station 7, excision – Silicotic nodules. Negative for tumor (See comment).

Lung, right, explant pneumonectomy – Parenchymal silicotic nodules consistent with silicosis (See comment).

Meningothelial-like nodules

Meningothelial-like nodules of the lung were first described as "multiple minute pulmonary tumors resembling chemodectomas" in 1960 by Korn, Bensch, Liebow and Castleman. These authors described many of the salient features of this curious lesion that hold true to this day, including the female predilection, minute size, nodular morphology and interstitial location. However, the authors' central assertion – that these lesions were chemodectomas – was subsequently shown to be incorrect by electron microscopy and immunohistochemistry. These techniques demonstrated that the cells in these nodules are ultrastructurally and immunohistochemically identical to the cells found in meningiomas, and do not show standard features of neuroendocrine differentiation such as positivity for synaptophysin or chromogranin. Therefore, the outmoded term *chemodectoma* is inappropriate. The reason for the existence of meningothelial-like cells in the lung remains unknown despite extensive investigation over the years.

In the vast majority of cases, meningothelial-like nodules are incidental findings of no significance. For this reason, they are discussed in the section on artifacts in Chapter 1. They are also included here since they rarely present as radiologically evident nodules. Meningothelial-like nodules are commonly seen in surgical lung biopsies and lobectomies, and may occasionally be encountered in small biopsies.

Major diagnostic findings

Meningothelial-like nodules are minute proliferations of cytologically bland cells found exclusively within alveolar septa (Figure 6.14, and Chapter 1, Figures 1.31 and 1.32). They are separated from the airspaces by alveolar pneumocytes. These cellular proliferations thicken the involved alveolar septa, usually resulting in the formation of a tiny nodule containing uninvolved airspaces within it. As the name suggests, meningothelial-like nodules are composed of cells resembling meningothelial cells. The "meningothelial-like" features include a streaming arrangement in syncytial sheets (Figure 6.14), occasional whorls, bland nuclear features and occasional intranuclear pseudoinclusions. Nucleoli are usually absent. The cytoplasm is eosinophilic and abundant with indistinct borders, which can result in misinterpretation as granulomas. Pleomorphism is minimal, and mitoses are absent.

Variable pathologic findings

- Most meningothelial-like nodules are too tiny to be seen on gross examination or on radiologic studies. The tiniest lesions are composed of just a few cells and measure well under 1 mm in size. The largest measure up to 6 mm, and are then appreciable grossly as tiny tan nodules.
- The cells may contain hemosiderin in the cytoplasm. There is no admixed inflammatory component. Fibrosis may be present in the background.

- Meningothelial-like nodules may be found within alveolar septa in the peripheral parenchyma (abutting interlobular septa or within subpleural alveolar septa), in lung parenchyma in the center of the lobule, or within scars. Unlike carcinoid tumorlets, they are uncommon in peribronchiolar interstitium or bronchiolar walls.
- The nodules are usually solitary but may be multiple. In the rare condition known as *diffuse pulmonary meningotheliomatosis*, nodules are multiple by definition, and are numerous in most cases (Figure 6.15). We have seen a case with more than 150 meningothelial-like nodules in a surgical lung biopsy, most slides containing more than 10 nodules each.
- The original description of meningothelial-like nodules claimed that they were "always centered upon pulmonary venules and consequently upon the septums, especially where the latter inserted upon the pleura". This observation was intended to bolster the theory that these lesions were minute chemodectomas, emptying their secretions into adjoining venules. Although the incorrect hypothesis that they are chemodectomas has been laid to rest, the concept of an alleged relationship to venules persists. When this question was specifically re-examined in a recent detailed study, no consistent relationship was found between meningothelial-like nodules and venules. The absence of a venule within an otherwise typical meningothelial-like nodule should not deter its recognition.
- Meningothelial-like nodules can be encountered in association with virtually any form of lung disease, including various types of chronic interstitial lung disease, organizing pneumonia, diffuse alveolar damage, granulomatous inflammation, malignant tumors and vascular disease. In surgical biopsies, the highest incidence is in cases of thromboembolic disease/infarcts (42%) and RBILD/DIP (26%).
- In autopsy studies, the incidence of meningothelial-like nodules is 0.7–4.9% and in resections for cancer it varies from 1.1% to 9.5%. However, a higher incidence (13.8%) has been reported recently in surgical biopsies and in extensive sampled lobectomy specimens (48% when 27 sections were sampled per lobe). One might speculate that if such lobes were sampled in their entirety, meningothelial-like nodules might be found in virtually every case.

Diagnostic work-up

- No immunohistochemical stains are required for the diagnosis. However, the immunoprofile has been extensively studied (see below).
- Meningothelial-like nodules are invariably positive for progesterone receptors (PR), epithelial membrane antigen (EMA), vimentin and CD56 (Figure 6.16). Staining for PR and vimentin tends to be strong, while CD56 staining is usually weak and patchy. EMA is weaker than the staining

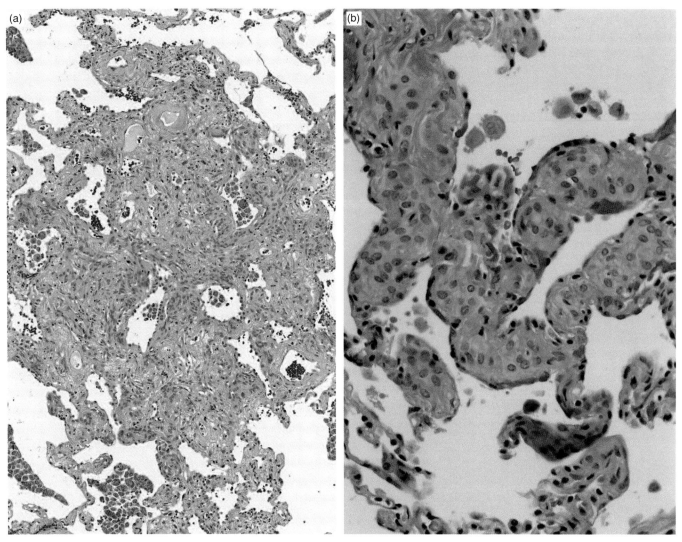

Figure 6.14. Meningothelial-like nodule. (a) Tiny irregular nodule formed by alveolar septa thickened by a cellular proliferation. Note uninvolved airspaces. **(b)** The cells within the alveolar septa resemble meningothelial cells. They are cytologically bland and lack clear cell borders.

in adjacent lung epithelium. Although CD56 is generally used as a neuroendocrine marker or as a marker of plasma cell myeloma, it has also been reported in meningiomas. Therefore, CD56 positivity further supports the theory of meningothelial differentiation in these lesions. The negative staining for estrogen receptors also parallels the pattern in meningiomas, which are typically PR-positive and ER-negative.

- Meningothelial-like nodules do not stain for neuroendocrine markers (synaptophysin and chromogranin), muscle markers (myosin, myoD1, myogenin, desmin and smooth muscle actin (SMA)), vascular markers (CD34, CD31, Factor VIII-related antigen, D2–40), markers of alveolar epithelium (TTF-1, keratin AE1/AE3, CK7), melanocytic markers (S-100, HMB-45), CD99, HER2/neu, CD68, E-cadherin, CA19–9, CD57, GFAP or inhibin.

- Molecular studies have found both monoclonal and polyclonal examples. Although meningothelial-like

nodules do occasionally show loss of heterozygosity (LOH) in the same loci as meningiomas, the frequency is much lower than in meningiomas. Specifically, LOH at the 22q, 14q and 1p loci is found in 10%, 0% and 0% of solitary meningothelial-like nodules and 4.7%, 0% and 4.7% of multiple meningothelial-like nodules compared with 60%, 43% and 44% of meningiomas.

Clinical profile

- Most meningothelial-like nodules are encountered in adults older than 40 years of age, with a mean in the 60s. The oldest reported patient to date was 91 years old. Cases in younger patients are uncommon. Less than 10 patients younger than 30 have been reported in the literature thus far out of a total of greater than 350 cases. Meningothelial-like nodules are rare in children. No cases have been reported in lungs from fetuses and infants.

- The predilection of meningothelial-like nodules for females has been confirmed in every study thus far, the female to

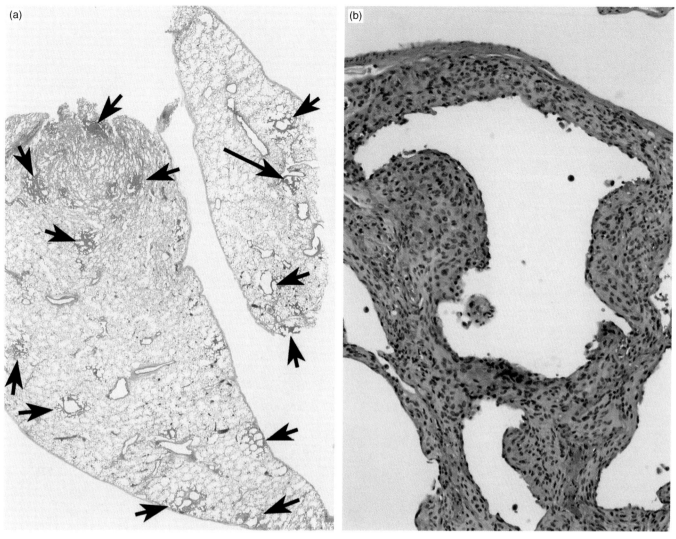

Figure 6.15. Diffuse pulmonary meningotheliomatosis. (a) Numerous tiny nodules (arrows) are seen in this surgical lung biopsy, taken from a 47-year-old woman who was found to have multiple bilateral lung nodules on chest CT. The lesion indicated by the long arrow is shown at high magnification in b. **(b)** Typical morphology and interstitial location of a meningothelial-like nodule.

male ratio ranging from 1.6:1 to 9:1. The reason for this is unknown, although it is tempting to speculate that there is some relation to PR positivity. Interestingly, intracranial meningiomas also show a slight female predilection (3:2).

- In the vast majority of cases, pulmonary meningothelial-like nodules are incidental findings of no clinical significance, encountered in lung biopsies or resections performed for other reasons. Rarely, they are sufficiently numerous to cause clinical symptoms and/or to allow their detection as tiny bilateral nodules on radiographs. The rare condition in which patients with innumerable meningothelial-like nodules present with clinical and radiologic evidence of interstitial lung disease has been termed "diffuse pulmonary meningotheliomatosis". Symptoms include dyspnea and cough. Pulmonary function tests may show mild restrictive changes. Histologically, the condition is characterized by numerous meningothelial-like nodules, the lung being otherwise normal. No cut-off has been defined for the number of nodules required to make this diagnosis.

Radiologic findings

Most meningothelial-like nodules are too tiny to be visible on radiographs. In diffuse pulmonary meningotheliomatosis, radiographs show multiple bilateral reticulonodular infiltrates.

Differential diagnosis

- Carcinoid tumorlets resemble meningothelial-like nodules since they form tiny clusters of bland cells. The reader will recall that authorities like Liebow and Castleman – and many after them – erroneously considered meningothelial-like nodules to be neuroendocrine in nature. Useful features that aid in the recognition of carcinoid tumorlets are their location within the walls of bronchioles, the appearance of "falling into" airspaces, the nested arrangement and the salt-and-pepper nuclear chromatin. In contrast to meningothelial-like nodules, carcinoid tumorlets stain with synaptophysin and chromogranin. The use of CD56 as a neuroendocrine marker in this setting may be a pitfall,

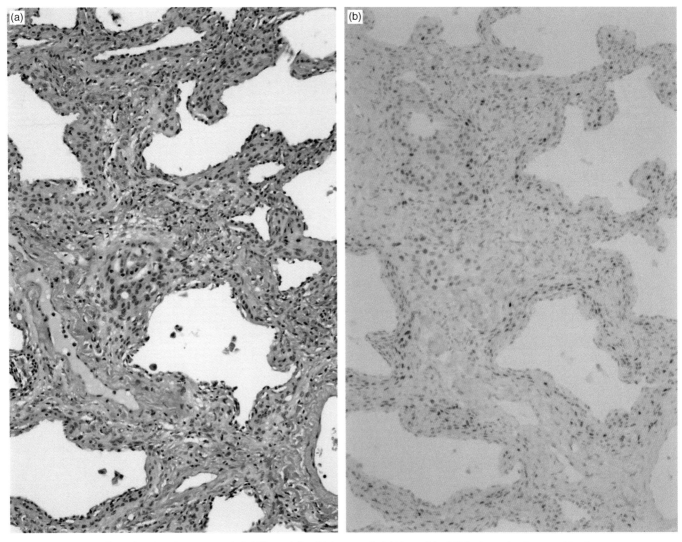

Figure 6.16. Immunohistochemistry in meningothelial-like nodules. (a) Meningothelial-like nodule. **(b)** The lesional cells are positive for progesterone receptors (PR).

since CD56 also stains meningothelial-like nodules. However, CD56 staining in meningothelial-like nodules is typically weak and patchy, whereas it is usually strong and diffuse in carcinoid tumorlets. Synaptophysin or chromogranin staining should easily resolve this issue.

- Granulomatous inflammation. Because of their bland cytology, abundant cytoplasm and clustered growth pattern, meningothelial-like nodules are often mistaken for granulomas. However, epithelioid histiocytes in granulomas usually have reniform, slightly folded or sole-of-a-slipper-shaped nuclei while the nuclei in meningothelial-like nodules do not. An admixed inflammatory component in granulomas and the characteristic streaming appearance of meningothelial-like nodules are also helpful differentiating features. EMA and PR staining can resolve the issue in difficult cases.
- Langerhans cell histiocytosis is characterized by interstitial nodules with irregular edges that may be mistaken for meningothelial-like nodules. Both are common in smokers

and may present radiographically as multiple bilateral tiny nodules. However, in addition to Langerhans cells, the nodules of Langerhans cell histiocytosis contain numerous inflammatory cells, while inflammation is not a feature of meningothelial-like nodules. Here too, immunohistochemical stains can be useful if the diagnosis is in doubt.

Treatment and prognosis

Meningothelial-like nodules do not require treatment. The prognosis is that of the underlying disease. Data regarding the natural history of diffuse pulmonary meningotheliomatosis is minimal. In Suster and Moran's report, the only patient with long-term follow-up (more than 8 years) developed metastases to non-pulmonary sites from her uterine leiomyosarcoma but did not show evidence of radiologic progression of her meningothelial-like nodules. Whether patients with diffuse pulmonary meningotheliomatosis require therapy is unknown.

Sample diagnosis on pathology report

In most cases, meningothelial-like nodules do not need to be mentioned in the main diagnosis. If multiple nodules are present and there is a possibility of diffuse pulmonary meningotheliomatosis, the diagnosis may read as follows:

Lung, right lower lobe, surgical biopsy – Multiple meningothelial-like nodules (See comment).

Carcinoid tumorlets

Carcinoid tumorlets are tiny microscopic proliferations of neuroendocrine cells occurring in the walls of small bronchioles. They are a common incidental finding in lung biopsies and resections performed for other reasons, most commonly chronic lung diseases such as small airway disease, bronchiectasis, granulomatous lung diseases and interstitial fibrosis. In these settings, carcinoid tumorlets are thought to be a reactive, secondary phenomenon. Carcinoid tumorlets are also common in the background lung in cases of carcinoid tumor, the incidence in this setting being as high as 76%. Rarely, multiple carcinoid tumorlets and other forms of neuroendocrine cell hyperplasia are found in biopsies lacking an underlying chronic lung disease in patients with evidence of airway obstruction. This condition has been termed "diffuse idiopathic pulmonary neuroendocrine cell hyperplasia" (DIPNECH). DIPNECH is currently thought to be preneoplastic (for carcinoid tumors), although, as pointed out recently by Marchevsky *et al*, most carcinoid tumors reported in patients with DIPNECH have been found synchronously along with tumorlets, and there are no reports of carcinoid tumor developing subsequently (metachronously) in patients initially diagnosed with DIPNECH.

Since most carcinoid tumorlets are incidental findings, they are also discussed in the section on artifacts in Chapter 1. They may be encountered in any type of lung specimen.

Major diagnostic findings

- Microscopic collection of neuroendocrine cells forming a minute nodule in the wall of a small bronchiole (Figure 6.17, and Chapter 1, Figure 1.25). The cells are cytologically bland and contain nuclei with granular chromatin, often with a "salt-and-pepper" quality. Other than the minute size, the morphology is identical to carcinoid tumors, from which tumorlets are separated by an arbitrary size cut-off set by the WHO. According to the current definition, carcinoid tumorlets measure less than 5 mm in size, while identical lesions that measure 5 mm or greater are carcinoid tumors.
- Carcinoid tumorlets may involve small membranous bronchioles, respiratory bronchioles or alveolar ducts. The cells may be present in the bronchiolar wall or lumen or both, and often spill into peribronchiolar airspaces.

Variable pathologic findings

- A closely related form of neuroendocrine proliferation is known as "neuroendocrine cell hyperplasia". It is characterized by proliferation of neuroendocrine cells in the form of tiny linear strands located between the bronchiolar epithelium and basement membrane, or tiny polyp-like protrusions into bronchiolar lumens. By definition, neuroendocrine cell hyperplasia does not extend beyond the basement membrane while carcinoid tumorlets do. Both forms of neuroendocrine cell proliferation are often seen together in the same specimen and likely constitute part of the same spectrum.
- As highlighted recently by Marchevsky *et al*, criteria for the diagnosis of DIPNECH are not clearly defined. Specifically, the minimum amount of neuroendocrine cell hyperplasia that needs to occur and the number of carcinoid tumorlets that need to be identified before the process can be considered "diffuse" have not been specified. It is also unclear whether DIPNECH can or should be diagnosed purely on the basis of pathologic findings in the absence of clinical features of obstructive lung disease or radiologic evidence of multiple lung nodules. Finally, the term "idiopathic" requires a subjective judgement that the tumorlets are not a secondary phenomenon related to an underlying chronic lung disease such as small airway disease or interstitial fibrosis. In most cases, the presence of such abnormalities argues against DIPNECH.
- Tumorlets are often found within scars and some degree of peribronchiolar fibrosis is often present within or around the lesion. As in carcinoid tumors, the cells often replace the involved bronchiole. This phenomenon should not be misinterpreted as constrictive bronchiolitis, a process that involves extrinsic luminal compression and eventual luminal replacement by fibrous scar tissue. Reported rates of "constrictive bronchiolitis" in DIPNECH are inconsistent, varying from none to strikingly high (44%). Some of these reports may represent the type of misinterpretation discussed above, especially in cases where the "constrictive bronchiolitis" did not predict a rapid decline in FEV1. Alternatively, it is possible that constrictive bronchiolitis is one of the many small airway abnormalities that can be associated with secondary neuroendocrine cell hyperplasia.

Diagnostic work-up

- No immunohistochemical stains are required for the diagnosis. However, neuroendocrine markers such as synaptophysin and chromogranin can be helpful in confirming the H&E impression of a neuroendocrine proliferation. The use of CD56 in this setting is a potential pitfall since meningothelial-like nodules (see prior section) can also be positive.

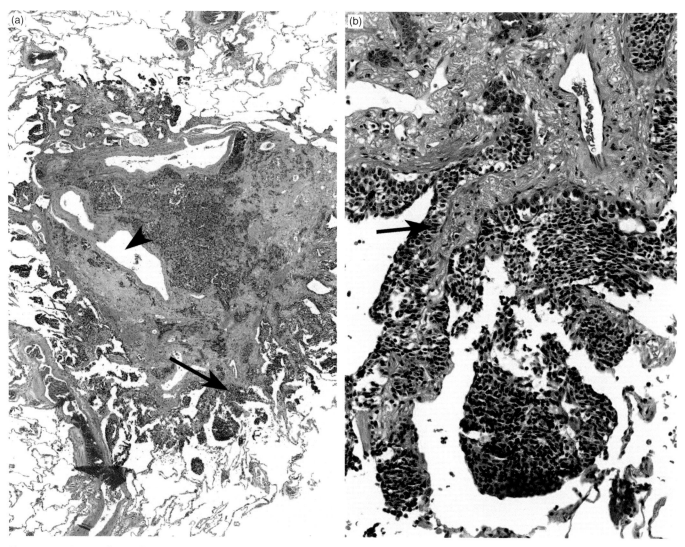

Figure 6.17. Carcinoid tumorlet. (a) Tiny cellular proliferation "obliterating" a bronchiole. A clue to the bronchiolar location is the presence of an adjacent pulmonary artery (arrowhead). Arrow indicates area shown at higher magnification in part b. **(b)** The morphology of the cells is identical to carcinoid tumors. Note spillage of cells into airspaces, at bottom. Linear subepithelial neuroendocrine hyperplasia is also present (arrow).

Clinical profile

- Incidental carcinoid tumorlets may be found at any age and in both sexes. The clinical features are those of the underlying disease.
- DIPNECH has been reported in patients ranging from 36 to 76 years with a mean of approximately 60 years. The majority of cases occur in middle-aged women. Slightly more than 60% are never-smokers. Most have active pulmonary symptoms, often for many years prior to diagnosis. Some are diagnosed with asthma, bronchiolitis or COPD on clinical grounds. A small minority of cases have been diagnosed in biopsies of incidentally discovered pulmonary nodules. Common symptoms attributed to DIPNECH include cough (71%), dyspnea (63%) and wheezing (25%). On pulmonary function tests, approximately half the patients show evidence of severe obstruction (FEV1 < 50%) but some have restrictive or mixed abnormalities. Only 10% have reversible airflow limitation. In general, residual volume and total lung capacity are increased.

Radiologic findings

In the vast majority of cases, carcinoid tumorlets are incidental pathologic findings, and are too tiny to be seen on imaging studies. The radiologic findings of DIPNECH on high-resolution CT scans include air trapping (mosaic attenuation on expiratory images, seen in 96% of cases), multiple lung nodules and bronchial wall thickening (80%). Nodules are greater than 20 in number in 60% of cases, and innumerable in one-third. By definition, nodules 5 mm or larger in size are diagnosed as carcinoid tumors. Synchronous carcinoid tumors are found in approximately 25% of cases of DIPNECH.

Differential diagnosis

- Meningothelial-like nodules enter the differential diagnosis of carcinoid tumorlets because they too are tiny proliferations of cytologically bland epithelioid cells. The most useful differentiating feature on H&E is that carcinoid tumorlets occur in bronchiolar walls and often spill into airspaces whereas meningothelial-like nodules occur exclusively within alveolar septa. Immunohistochemically, carcinoid tumorlets stain for synaptophysin and chromogranin while meningothelial-like nodules are positive for progesterone receptors, epithelial membrane antigen (EMA) and vimentin. As mentioned in the section on meningothelial-like nodules, CD56 is not helpful in this differential diagnosis since both lesions can be positive.

- Carcinoid tumor. Differentiation between carcinoid tumorlet and carcinoid tumor is based on an arbitrary size cut-off set by the WHO. Lesions less than 5 mm are labeled as carcinoid tumorlets, whereas identical lesions that measure 5 mm or greater are diagnosed as carcinoid tumor.

- DIPNECH. The key features that differentiate DIPNECH from incidental carcinoid tumorlets are the presence of multiple lesions and the absence of associated pathologic findings that might induce secondary neuroendocrine cell hyperplasia. Most authors agree that the diagnosis of DIPNECH requires pathologic evidence of neuroendocrine cell proliferation (neuroendocrine cell hyperplasia and/or multiple carcinoid tumorlets), usually in a surgical lung biopsy. In the appropriate clinical setting, transbronchial biopsies can also be used. As mentioned in the introduction, criteria for the final diagnosis of DIPNECH are currently unclear. In our practice, we do not diagnose DIPNECH solely on the basis of pathologic findings. The pathologic diagnosis documents the presence of multiple carcinoid tumorlets and/or neuroendocrine cell

hyperplasia, and a comment lists the presence or absence of associated findings. The final diagnosis of DIPNECH is thus left to the clinician, who is best placed to apply this label based on clinical evidence of airflow obstruction and multiple lung nodules.

Treatment and prognosis

- It is unclear whether any therapy is effective. Options include observation, octreotide, inhaled or systemic corticosteroids, and bronchodilators. Octreotide is increasingly used, although there is no evidence that it reverses lung function abnormalities. Lung resection or transplantation may be considered for patients with severe symptoms. One case of single lung transplantation was reported in 1995, and two cases of double lung transplantation have been reported recently in patients with COPD of unknown cause. These two patients were diagnosed with DIPNECH on the basis of pathologic findings in the explanted lungs.

- Most patients diagnosed with DIPNECH have remained stable over many years. The reported 5-year survival is 83%. Only a few patients have progressed to develop severe airflow obstruction.

Sample diagnosis on pathology report

Lung, right lower lobe, surgical biopsy – Multiple carcinoid tumorlets (See comment).

   or

Lung, right lower lobe, surgical biopsy – Multiple carcinoid tumorlets and neuroendocrine cell hyperplasia (See comment).

References

Nodular amyloidosis

Berk JL, O'Regan A, Skinner M. Pulmonary and tracheobronchial amyloidosis. *Semin Respir Crit Care Med* 2002;**23**:155–65.

Cordier JF, Loire R, Brune J. Amyloidosis of the lower respiratory tract. Clinical and pathologic features in a series of 21 patients. *Chest* 1986;**90**:827–31.

Gilbertson JA, Theis JD, Vrana JA, et al. A comparison of immunohistochemistry and mass spectrometry for determining the amyloid fibril protein from formalin-fixed biopsy tissue. *J Clin Pathol* 2015; Epub ahead of print.

Grogg KL, Aubry MC, Vrana JA, Theis JD, Dogan A. Nodular pulmonary amyloidosis is characterized by localized immunoglobulin deposition and is frequently associated with an indolent B-cell lymphoproliferative disorder. *Am J Surg Pathol* 2013;**37**:406–12.

Howard ME, Ireton J, Daniles F, et al. Pulmonary presentations of amyloidosis. *Respirology* 2001;**6**:61–4.

Hui AN, Koss MN, Hochholzer L, Wehunt WD. Amyloidosis presenting in the lower respiratory tract. Clinicopathologic, radiologic, immunohistochemical and histochemical studies on 48 cases. *Arch Pathol Lab Med* 1986;**110**:212–8.

Miyamoto T, Kobayashi T, Makiyama M, et al. Monoclonality of infiltrating plasma cells in primary pulmonary nodular amyloidosis: detection with polymerase chain reaction. *J Clin Pathol* 1999;**52**:464–7.

Smith RRL, Hutchins GM, Moore GW, Humphrey RL. Type and distribution of pulmonary parenchymal and vascular amyloid. Correlation with cardiac amyloidosis. *Am J Med* 1979;**66**:96–104.

Urban BA, Fishman EK, Goldman SM, et al. CT evaluation of amyloidosis: spectrum of disease. *Radiographics* 1993;**13**:1295–1308.

Utz JP, Swensen SJ, Gertz MA. Pulmonary amyloidosis. The Mayo Clinic experience from 1980 to 1993. *Ann Intern Med* 1996;**124**:407–13.

Light chain deposition disease ("amyloid-like nodules")

Arrossi AV, Merzianu M, Farver CF, et al. Nodular pulmonary nodular light chain deposition disease: an entity associated with Sjögren Syndrome or marginal zone lymphoma. *J Clin Pathol* 2015; Oct 26; Epub ahead of print.

Bhargava P, Rushin JM, Rusnock EJ, et al. Pulmonary light chain deposition disease: report of five cases and review of the literature. *Am J Surg Pathol* 2007;**31**:267–76.

Buxbaum JN, Chuba JV, Hellman GC, Solomon A, Gallo GR. Monoclonal immunoglobulin deposition disease: light chain and light and heavy chain deposition diseases and their relation to light chain amyloidosis. Clinical features, immunopathology, and molecular analysis. *Ann Intern Med* 1990;**112**:455–64.

Colombat M, Holifanjaniaina S, Guillonneau F, et al. Mass spectrometry-based proteomic analysis: a good diagnostic tool for cystic lung light chain deposition disease. *Am J Respir Crit Care Med* 2013;**188**:404–5.

Colombat M, Stern M, Groussard O, *et al.* Pulmonary cystic disorder related to light chain deposition disease. *Am J Respir Crit Care Med* 2006;**173**:777–80.

Hirschi S, Colombat M, Kessler R, *et al.* Lung transplantation for advanced cystic lung disease due to nonamyloid light chain deposits. *Ann Am Thorac Soc* 2015;**11**:1025–31.

Khoor A, Myers JL, Tazelaar HD, Kurtin PJ. Amyloid-like pulmonary nodules, including localized light-chain deposition. *Am J Clin Pathol* 2004;**121**:200–4.

Kijner CH, Yousem SA. Systemic light chain deposition disease presenting as multiple pulmonary nodules. A case report and review of the literature. *Am J Surg Pathol* 1988;**12**:405–13.

Rostagno A, Frizzera G, Ylagan L, Kumar A, Ghiso J, Gallo G. Tumoral non-amyloidotic monoclonal immunoglobulin light chain deposits ("aggregoma"): presenting feature of B-cell dyscrasia in three cases with immunohistochemical and biochemical analyses. *Br J Haematol* 2002;**119**:62–9.

Sheard S, Nicholson AG, Edmunds L, Wotherspoon AC, Hansell DM. Pulmonary light-chain deposition disease: CT and pathology findings in nine patients. *Clin Radiol* 2015; **70**:515–22.

Pulmonary hyalinizing granuloma

Chalaoui J, Gregoire P, Sylvestre J, Lefebvre R, Amyot R. Pulmonary hyalinizing granuloma: a cause of pulmonary nodules. *Radiology* 1984;**152**:23–6.

Chapman EM, Gown A, Mazziotta R, Churg A. Pulmonary hyalinizing granuloma with associated elevation in serum and tissue IgG4 occurring in a patient with a history of sarcoidosis. *Am J Surg Pathol* 2012;**36**:774–8.

Dent RG, Godden DJ, Stovin PGI, Stark JE. Pulmonary hyalinizing granuloma in association with retroperitoneal fibrosis. *Thorax* 1983;**38**:955–6.

Engleman P, Liebow AA, Gmelich J, Friedman PJ. Pulmonary hyalinizing granuloma. *Am Rev Respir Dis* 1977;**115**:997–1008.

Guccion JG, Rohatgi PK, Saini N. Pulmonary hyalinizing granuloma. Electron microscopic and immunologic studies. *Chest* 1984;**85**:571–3.

Lien CT, Yang CJ, Yang SF, Chou SH, Huang MS. Pulmonary hyalinizing granuloma mimicking multiple lung metastases. *J Thorac Imaging* 2010;**25**:W36–9.

Schlosnagle DC, Check IJ, Sewell CW, Plummer A, York RM, Hunter RL. Immunologic abnormalities in two patients with pulmonary hyalinizing granuloma. *Am J Clin Pathol* 1982;**78**:231–5.

Shibata Y, Kobayashi T, Hattori Y, *et al.* High-resolution CT findings in pulmonary hyalinizing granuloma. *J Thorac Imaging* 2007;**22**:374–7.

Ussavarungsi K, Khoor A, Jolles HI, Mira-Avendano I. A 40-year-old woman with multiple pulmonary nodules. Pulmonary hyalinizing granuloma. *Chest* 2014;**146**: e198–203.

Yousem SA, Hochholzer L. Pulmonary hyalinizing granuloma. *Am J Clin Pathol* 1987;**87**:1–6.

Nodular lymphoid hyperplasia

Abbondanzo SL, Rush W, Bijwaard KE, Koss MN. Nodular lymphoid hyperplasia of the lung. A clinicopathologic study of 14 cases. *Am J Surg Pathol* 2000;**24**:587–97.

Bégueret H, Vergier B, Parrens M, *et al.* Primary lung small B-cell lymphoma versus lymphoid hyperplasia. Evaluation of diagnostic criteria in 26 cases. *Am J Surg Pathol* 2002;**26**:76–81.

Carrillo J, Restrepo CS, Rosado-de-Christenson M, Leon PO, Rivera AL, Koss MN. Lymphoproliferative lung disorders: a radiologic-pathologic overview. Part 1: reactive disorders. *Semin Ultrasound CT MRI* 2013;**34**:525–34.

Guinee DG Jr, Franks DJ, Gerbino AJ, Murakami SS, Acree SC, Koss MN. Pulmonary nodular lymphoid hyperplasia (pulmonary pseudo-lymphoma). The significance of increased numbers of IgG4-positive plasma cells. *Am J Surg Pathol* 2013;**37**:699–709.

Koss MN, Hochholzer L, Nichols PW, Wehunt WD, Lazarus AA. Primary non-Hodgkin's lymphoma and pseudolymphoma of lung: a study of 161 patients. *Hum Pathol* 1983;**14**:1024–38.

Kradin RL, Mark EJ. Benign lymphoid disorders of the lung, with a theory regarding their development. *Hum Pathol* 1983;**14**:857–67.

Sakurai H, Hada M, Oyama T. Nodular lymphoid hyperplasia of the lung: a very rare disease entity. *Ann Thorac Surg* 2007;**83**:2197–9.

Shrestha B, Sekiguchi H, Colby TV, *et al.* Distinctive pulmonary histopathology with increased IgG4-positive plasma cells in patients with autoimmune pancreatitis. Report of 6 and 12 cases with similar histopathology. *Am J Surg Pathol* 2009;**33**:1450–62.

Yi E, Aubry MC. Pulmonary pseudoneoplasms. *Arch Pathol Lab Med* 2010;**134**:417–26.

Zen Y, Inoue D, Kitao A, *et al.* IgG4-related lung and pleural disease: a clinicopathologic study of 21 cases. *Am J Surg Pathol* 2009;**33**:1886–93.

IgG4-related disease

Deshpande V, Zen Y, Chan JK, *et al.* Consensus statement on the pathology of IgG4-related disease. *Mod Pathol* 2012;**25**:1181–92.

Deshpande V, Chicano S, Finkelberg D, *et al.* Autoimmune pancreatitis: a systemic immune complex mediated disease. *Am J Surg Pathol* 2006;**30**:1537–45.

Fujiu K, Sakuma H, Miyamoto H, Yamaguchi B. Immunoglobulin G4-related inflammatory pseudotumor of the lung. *Gen Thorac Cardiovasc Surg* 2010;**58**:144–8.

Guinee DG Jr, Franks DJ, Gerbino AJ, Murakami SS, Acree SC, Koss MN. Pulmonary nodular lymphoid hyperplasia (pulmonary pseudo-lymphoma). The significance of increased numbers of IgG4-positive plasma cells. *Am J Surg Pathol* 2013;**37**:699–709.

Hamed G, Tsushima K, Yasuo M, *et al.* Inflammatory lesions of the lung, submandibular gland, bile duct and prostate in a patient with IgG4-associated multifocal systemic fibrosclerosis. *Respirology* 2007;**12**:455–7.

Khan ML, Colby TV, Viggiano RW, Fonseca R. Treatment with bortezomib of a patient having hyper IgG4 disease. *Clin Lymphoma Myeloma Leuk* 2010;**10**:217–9.

Shrestha B, Sekiguchi H, Colby TV, *et al.* Distinctive pulmonary histopathology with increased IgG4-positive plasma cells in patients with autoimmune pancreatitis. Report of 6 and 12 cases with similar histopathology. *Am J Surg Pathol* 2009;**33**:1450–62.

Yamashita K, Haga H, Kobashi Y, Miyagawa-Hayashino A, Yoshizawa A, Manabe T. Lung involvement in IgG4-related lymphoplasmacytic vasculitis and interstitial fibrosis. Report of 3 cases and review of the literature. *Am J Surg Pathol* 2008;**32**:1620–6.

Zen Y, Inoue D, Kitao A, *et al.* IgG4-related lung and pleural disease: a clinicopathologic study of 21 cases. *Am J Surg Pathol* 2009;**33**:1886–93.

Zen Y, Kitagawa S, Minato H, *et al.* IgG4-positive plasma cells in inflammatory pseudotumor (plasma cell granuloma) of the lung. *Hum Pathol* 2005;**36**:710–17.

Pulmonary apical cap

Butler C II, Kleinerman J. The pulmonary apical cap. *Am J Pathol* 1970;**60**:205–16.

Butnor KJ, Sporn TA, Roggili VL. Pulmonary apical cap. *Am J Surg Pathol* 2001;**25**:1344.

Dail DH. Pulmonary apical cap. *Am J Surg Pathol* 2001;**25**:1344.

Doxtader EE, Mukhopadhyay S, Katzenstein AL. Core needle biopsy in benign lung lesions: pathologic findings in 159 cases. *Hum Pathol* 2010;**41**:1530–5.

Hirami Y, Nakata M, Maeda A, Yukawa T, Shimizu K, Tanemoto K. Pulmonary apical mass, the so-called pulmonary apical cap, in a 43-year-old women. *Ann Thorac Cardiovasc Surg* 2010;**16**:122–4.

Mugler K. Pathologic quiz case: bilateral apical lung masses in an autopsy patient. Pulmonary apical cap. *Arch Pathol Lab Med* 2004;**128**:E35–6.

McLoud DC, Isler RJ, Novellini RA, Putman C, Simeone J, Stark P. The apical cap. *AJR Am J Roentgenol* 1981;**137**:299–306.

Renner RR, Bernice NJ. The apical cap. *Semin Roentgenol* 1977;**12**:299–302.

Renner RR, Markarian B, Pernice NJ, Heitzman ER. The apical cap. *Radiology* 1974;**110**:569–73.

Yousem SA. Pulmonary apical cap: a distinctive but poorly recognized lesion in pulmonary surgical pathology. *Am J Surg Pathol* 2001;**25**:679–83.

Round atelectasis

Blesovsky A. The folded lung. *Br J Dis Chest* 1966;**60**:19–22.

Hillerdal G. Rounded atelectasis. Clinical experience with 74 patients. *Chest* 1989;**95**:836–41.

McHugh K, Blaquiere RM. CT features of round atelectasis. *Am J Roentgenol* 1989;**153**:257–60.

Menzies R, Fraser R. Round atelectasis. Pathologic and pathogenetic features. *Am J Surg Pathol* 1987;**11**:674–81.

Partap VA. The comet tail sign. *Radiology* 1999;**213**:553–4.

Roach HD, Davies GJ, Attanoos R, Crane M, Adams H, Phillips S. Asbestos: when the dust settles – an imaging review of asbestos-related disease. *Radiographics* 2002;**22**:S167–84.

Schneider HJ, Felson B, Gonzalez LL. Rounded atelectasis. *Am J Roentgenol* 1980;**134**:225–32.

Smith LS, Schillaci RF. Rounded atelectasis due to acute exudative effusion. *Chest* 1984;**85**:830–2.

Szydlowsky GW, Cohn HE, Steiner RM, *et al.* Rounded atelectasis: a pulmonary pseudotumor. *Ann Thorac Surg* 1992;**53**:817–21.

Voisin C, Fisekci S, Voisin-Saltiel S, Ameille J, Brochard P, Pairon J-C. Asbestos-related rounded atelectasis. Radiologic and mineralogic data in 23 cases. *Chest* 1995;**107**:477–81.

Infarct

Bray TJ, Mortensen KH, Gopalan D. Multimodality imaging of pulmonary infarction. *Eur J Radiol* 2014;**83**:2240–54.

Dalen JE, Haffajee CI, Alpert JS 3rd, Howe JP, Ockene IS, Paraskos JA. Pulmonary embolism, pulmonary hemorrhage and pulmonary infarction. *N Engl J Med* 1977;**296**:1431–5.

Dalen JE. Pulmonary embolism: what have we learned since Virchow? Natural history, pathophysiology and diagnosis. *Chest* 2002;**122**:1440–56.

Hampton AO, Castleman B. Correlation of postmortem chest teleroentgenograms with autopsy findings with special reference to pulmonary embolism and infarction. *Am J Roentgenol* 1940;**43**:305–26.

Katzenstein AL, Mazur MT. Pulmonary infarct: an unusual manifestation of fibrosing mediastinitis. *Chest* 1980;**77**:521–4.

Nelson WP, Lundberg GD, Dickerson RB. Pulmonary artery obstruction and cor pulmonale due to chronic fibrous mediastinitis. *Am J Med* 1965;**38**:279–85.

Parambil JG, Savci CD, Tazelaar HD, Ryu JH. Causes and presenting features of pulmonary infarctions in 43 cases identified by surgical lung biopsy. *Chest* 2005;**127**:1178–83.

Wagenvoort CA. Pathology of pulmonary thromboembolism. *Chest* 1995;**107**:10S–17S.

Williamson WA, Tronic BS, Levitan N, Webb-Johnson DC, Shahian DM, Ellis FH Jr. Pulmonary venous infarction. *Chest* 1992;**102**:937–40.

Yousem FA. The surgical pathology of pulmonary infarcts: diagnostic confusion with granulomatous disease, vasculitis, and neoplasia. *Mod Pathol* 2009;**22**:679–85.

Silicosis

Antao VC, Pinheiro GA, Terra-Filho M, Kawakama J, Müller NL. High-resolution CT in silicosis: correlation with radiographic findings and functional impairment. *J Comput Assist Tomogr* 2005;**29**:350–6.

Argani P, Ghossein R, Rosai J. Anthracotic and anthracosilicotic spindle cell pseudotumors of mediastinal lymph nodes: report of five cases of a reactive lesion that simulates malignancy. *Hum Pathol* 1988;**29**:851–5.

Castranova V, Vallyathan V. Silicosis and coal workers' pneumoconiosis. *Environ Health Perspect* 2000;**108**:675–84.

Craighead JE, Vallyathan NV. Cryptic pulmonary lesions in workers exposed to dust containing silica. *JAMA* 1980;**244**:1939–41.

Craighead JE, Kleinerman J, Abraham JL, *et al.* Diseases associated with exposure to silica and nonfibrous silicate minerals. *Arch Pathol Lab Med* 1988;**112**:673–720.

Honma K, Abraham JL, Chiyotani K, *et al.* Proposed criteria for mixed-dust pneumoconiosis: Definition, descriptions, and guidelines for pathologic diagnosis and clinical correlation. *Hum Pathol* 2004;**35**:1515–23.

McDonald JW, Roggli VL. Detection of silica particles in lung tissue by polarizing light microscopy. *Arch Pathol Lab Med* 1995;**119**:242–6.

Murray J, Webster I, Reid G, Kielkowski D. The relation between fibrosis of hilar lymph glands and the development of parenchymal silicosis. *Br J Ind Med* 1991;**48**:267–9.

Slavin RE, Swedo JL, Brandes D, Gonzalez-Vitale JC, Osornio-Vargas A. Extrapulmonary silicosis: a clinical, morphologic and ultrastructural study. *Hum Pathol* 1985;**16**:393–412.

Ziskind M, Jones RM, Weill H. Silicosis. State of the art. *Am Rev Respir Dis* 1976;**113**:643–65.

Meningothelial-like nodules

Churg AM, Warnock ML. So-called "minute pulmonary chemodectoma": a tumor not related to paragangliomas. *Cancer* 1976;**37**:1759–69.

Gaffey MJ, Mills SE, Askin FB. Minute pulmonary meningothelial-like nodules. A clinicopathologic study of so-called minute pulmonary chemodectoma. *Am J Surg Pathol* 1988;**12**:167–75.

Ionescu DN, Sasatomi E, Aldeeb D, *et al.* Pulmonary meningothelial-like nodules: a genotypic comparison with meningiomas. *Am J Surg Pathol* 2004;**28**:207–14.

Korn D, Bensch K, Liebow AA, Castleman B. Multiple minute pulmonary tumors resembling chemodectomas. *Am J Pathol* 1960;**37**:641–72.

Kuhn C 3rd, Askin FB. The fine structure of so-called minute pulmonary chemodectomas. *Hum Pathol* 1975;**6**:681–91.

Mukhopadhyay S, El-Zammar OA, Katzenstein AL. Pulmonary meningothelial-like nodules: new insights into a common but poorly understood entity. *Am J Surg Pathol* 2009;**33**:487–95.

Niho S, Yokose T, Nishiwaki Y, Mukai K. Immunohistochemical and clonal analysis of minute pulmonary meningothelial-like nodules. *Hum Pathol* 1999;**30**:425–9.

Pelosi G, Maffini F, Decarli N, Viale G. Progesterone receptor immunoreactivity in minute meningothelioid nodules of lung. *Virchows Arch* 2002;**440**:543–6.

Spain DM. Intrapulmonary chemodectomas in subjects with organizing pulmonary thromboemboli. *Am Rev Respir Dis* 1967;**96**:1158–64.

Suster S, Moran CA. Diffuse pulmonary meningotheliomatosis. *Am J Surg Pathol* 2007;**31**:624–31.

Carcinoid tumorlets

Aguayo SM, Miller YE, Waldron JA Jr., *et al.* Brief report: idiopathic diffuse hyperplasia of pulmonary neuroendocrine cells and airways disease. *N Engl J Med* 1992;**327**:1285–8.

Armas OA, White DA, Erlandson RA, Rosai J. Diffuse idiopathic pulmonary neuroendocrine cell proliferation presenting as interstitial lung disease. *Am J Surg Pathol* 1995;**19**:963–70.

Aubry MC, Thomas CS Jr., Jett JR, Swensen LJ, Myers JL. Significance of multiple carcinoid tumors and tumorlets in surgical lung specimens: analysis of 28 patients. *Chest* 2007;**131**:1635–43.

Carr LL, Chung JH, Achcar RD, *et al.* The clinical course of diffuse idiopathic pulmonary neuroendocrine cell hyperplasia. *Chest* 2015;**147**:415–22.

Davies SJ, Gosney JR, Hansell DM, *et al.* Diffuse idiopathic pulmonary neuroendocrine cell hyperplasia: an under-recognized spectrum of disease. *Thorax* 2007;**62**:248–52.

Gorshtein A, Gross DJ, Barak D, *et al.* Diffuse idiopathic pulmonary neuroendocrine cell hyperplasia and the associated lung neuroendocrine tumors: clinical experience with a rare entity. *Cancer* 2012;**118**:612–9.

Koo CW, Baliff JP, Torigian DA, Litzky LA, Gefter WB, Akers SR. Spectrum of pulmonary neuroendocrine cell proliferation: diffuse idiopathic pulmonary neuroendocrine cell hyperplasia, tumorlet, and carcinoids. *AJR Am J Roentgenol* 2010;**195**:661–8.

Marchevsky AM, Wirtschafter E, Walts AE. The spectrum of changes in adults with multifocal pulmonary neuroendocrine proliferations: what is the minimum set of pathologic criteria to diagnose DIPNECH? *Hum Pathol* 2015;**46**:176–81.

Miller RR, Muller NL. Neuroendocrine cell hyperplasia and obliterative bronchiolitis in patients with peripheral carcinoid tumors. *Am J Surg Pathol* 1995;**19**:653–8.

Nassar AA, Jaroszewski DE, Helmers RA, Colby TV, Patel BM, Mookadam F. Diffuse idiopathic pulmonary neuroendocrine cell hyperplasia: a systematic overview. *Am J Respir Crit Care Med* 2011:**184**:8–16.

Cysts and cyst-like lesions of the lung in children and adults

This chapter deals with non-neoplastic lung lesions that are cystic, or are characterized histologically by cyst-like lesions (Figure 7.1). One entity traditionally considered non-neoplastic but for which a neoplastic etiology has been proposed recently (lymphangioleiomyomatosis) is also included. Although these lesions are etiologically diverse, and constitute a mix of developmental, congenital and acquired entities, they are discussed together because of the common pathologic finding of a cyst-like lesion. An algorithmic approach to cystic or cyst-like lesions of the lung is outlined in Figure 7.2. A few pearls and pitfalls related to these lesions are listed in Table 7.1.

Non-neoplastic cystic lesions are usually encountered as congenital anomalies in children, but they may occasionally present in adulthood. Although several conditions enter the differential diagnosis, only a few are seen commonly by surgical pathologists. These include pulmonary sequestration, congenital cystic adenomatoid malformation (CCAM) and bronchogenic cyst. The first half of this chapter is devoted to these entities. The second half of the chapter addresses lesions that are potential causes of pneumothorax (emphysema, lymphangioleiomyomatosis, and Birt–Hogg–Dubé syndrome). A general approach to wedge resections of the lung from patients with pneumothorax is also outlined.

Intralobar sequestration

A pulmonary sequestration (also known as bronchopulmonary sequestration) is a mass of lung tissue that lacks a connection to (i.e., is sequestered from) the vasculature and bronchial tree of the normal lung. In contrast to the normal lung, which is supplied by pulmonary arteries, the blood supply of sequestrations is derived from one or several systemic arteries, which are usually branches of the lower thoracic or upper abdominal aorta. The absence of a well-formed connection to the bronchial tree is often difficult to appreciate, but may manifest as bronchial atresia.

Pulmonary sequestrations can be located within (intralobar sequestration) or outside (extralobar sequestration) the lung. Sequestrations located outside the lung contain their own pleural covering. In contrast, intralobar sequestrations – being intraparenchymal – are covered by the pleura of the normal lung. Most sequestrations (75–85%) are intralobar.

Major diagnostic findings

- Localized mass-like lesion within a lobe of the lung. The lesion may be a solitary cyst, a multi-cystic mass, a multi-cystic mass with a solid component or an ill-defined solid lesion demarcated from the surrounding normal lung. In most cases, the histologic findings include variable combinations of cystic change, chronic inflammation and/or fibrosis. Any one of these may predominate in a given case. These changes are thought to be secondary to bronchial obstruction caused by bronchial atresia. The combination of fibrosis and inflammation can mimic interstitial lung disease, bronchiectasis or honeycombing. Cysts are often present and may be the most prominent finding (Figure 7.3a). They range from dilated bronchioles to areas resembling honeycomb change to larger mucin-filled cysts lined by ciliated columnar (respiratory-type) epithelium. Some sequestrations show only subtle histologic abnormalities that are difficult to distinguish from normal lung parenchyma.

- A systemic artery always supplies the lesion, and its recognition is the key to the diagnosis (Figure 7.3). This type of artery is a branch of the aorta rather than the pulmonary artery. It often reaches the lesion sequestered within the lung by running within the pulmonary ligament (a pleural sheath that connects the mediastinum to the lower lobes). The most convenient way for the pathologist to confirm that the lesion is supplied by a systemic artery is to check the surgeon's note, which will usually mention that a systemic artery was ligated in order to resect the mass.

- Histologically, the abnormal systemic arteries that supply pulmonary sequestrations have a distinctive appearance. Normal pulmonary arteries are elastic-type arteries proximally but turn into muscular-type arteries distally. Although normal branches of the aorta are muscular-type arteries, the anomalous feeding vessels that supply sequestrations have an elastic structure typical of large arteries (pulmonary artery or aorta), characterized by multiple concentric layers of elastic fibers alternating with smooth muscle fibers (Figure 7.4). The main difference between these vessels and normal pulmonary arteries is the absence of a partner bronchus (i.e., there is no bronchovascular bundle). The structure of the anomalous systemic artery also differs from smaller pulmonary arteries, which are muscular-type arteries containing only two elastic layers sandwiching a well-defined layer of smooth muscle. In summary, the presence of elastic-type arteries within lung parenchyma without partner bronchi is an important histologic tip-off to the diagnosis.

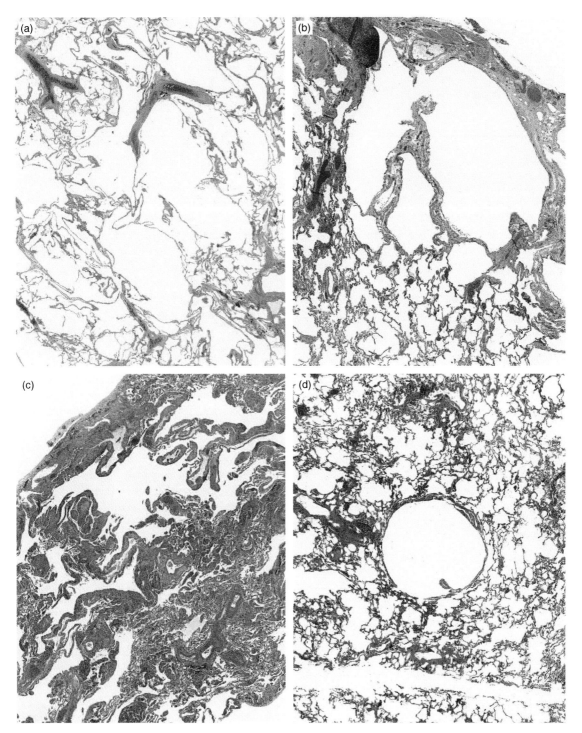

Figure 7.1. Cysts and cyst-like spaces in the lung. (a) Emphysema, smoking-related. **(b)** Emphysema, distal acinar, with blebs (pneumothorax specimen). **(c)** Lymphangioleiomyomatosis. **(d)** Birt–Hogg–Dubé syndrome.

Variable pathologic findings

- Most intralobar sequestrations are resected in a lobectomy or segmentectomy specimen. Grossly, they may appear as a solitary cyst, a multi-cystic mass bordered by consolidated or spongy lung, or a solid, poorly circumscribed spongy mass without an obvious cystic component. The cyst or cysts often contain mucoid material. The solid areas often have a yellow hue.

The systemic artery supplying the lesion may be grossly identifiable.
- There is considerable variation from case to case in the amount of inflammation in intralobar sequestrations. Some cases, especially in young children, show no significant inflammation. In others, especially in adults, superimposed areas of acute bronchopneumonia (neutrophils within airspaces) and/or organizing pneumonia (plugs of fibroblasts within airspaces) may be

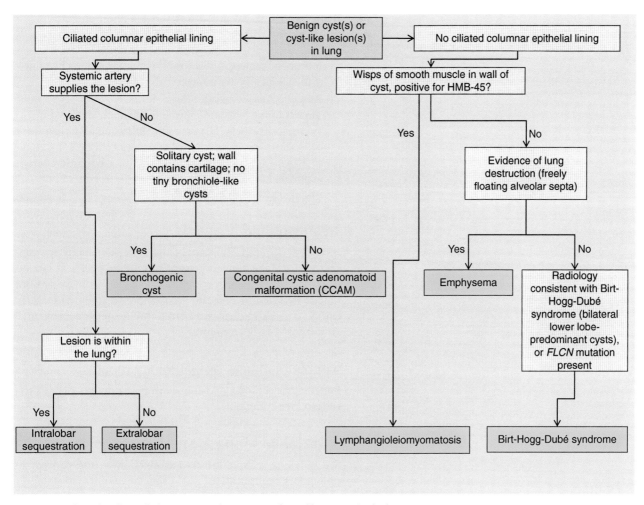

Figure 7.2. Algorithm for pathologic approach to cysts and cyst-like spaces in the lung.

present. These likely represent superimposed infection. Multinucleated giant cells or granulomas have also been described in some cases, likely representing superimposed infection. Microorganisms reported within sequestrations include *Aspergillus* and *Nocardia*, suggesting that some sequestrations retain a partial connection to the bronchial tree.

- Foamy macrophages or amorphous debris may fill airspaces or cysts.
- Although intralobar sequestrations do not communicate with the normal bronchial tree, bronchi may be present within the lesional tissue. Peribronchiolar metaplasia and multiple mucin-filled, respiratory epithelium-lined spaces resembling honeycomb change may also be seen.
- Thick-walled small arteries can often be found within the lesion. These are thought to be a consequence of pulmonary hypertension caused by the systemic arterial blood supply.
- Pleural adhesions are a common finding in the area overlying the sequestration.
- Atherosclerotic changes may be present in the systemic arterial blood supply.

Diagnostic work-up

- Special stains for elastic tissue (elastic Van Gieson, Verhoeff–Van Gieson or Movat pentachrome) can be helpful in identifying a systemic elastic-type artery, but are not always required. It may be more practical to check the operative note or ask the surgeon if a systemic artery supplied the lesion.
- Radiologic correlation can be helpful to determine if the lesion was inside the lung or was found in an extrapulmonary location.

Clinical profile

Intralobar sequestrations usually present in young adults or older children, although the reported age range is wide (newborns to 61 years). In contrast to extralobar sequestrations (see next section), intralobar sequestrations are rare in infants. Half the patients are more than 20 years old at the time of diagnosis. Many cases are discovered incidentally in asymptomatic individuals. Those with symptoms present with cough, hemoptysis or chest pain. A history of recurrent respiratory infections (bronchitis or pneumonia) is common.

Table 7.1. Pearls and pitfalls in non-neoplastic cystic lung lesions

Always consider the possibility of a pulmonary sequestration in any type of non-neoplastic mass in the left lower lobe

The key finding in pulmonary sequestrations is a systemic artery. The tip-off is the presence of an elastic-type artery in peripheral lung. Ask the surgeon if the arterial supply to the lesion was from a systemic artery

Congenital cystic adenomatoid malformations can present in adulthood

Most congenital cystic adenomatoid malformations are type 1 or type 2

The absence of fibrosis is part of the definition of emphysema. If you see significant fibrosis with emphysema, consider smoking-related interstitial fibrosis (SRIF) or combined pulmonary fibrosis and emphysema (CPFE)

Lymphangioleiomyomatosis is a cystic lesion. Do not expect to see lymphatics

HMB-45 staining in lymphangioleiomyomatosis is usually weak and focal

Consider the possibility of lymphangioleiomyomatosis or Birt–Hogg–Dubé syndrome if you receive a lower lobe specimen from a patient with pneumothorax

Consider the possibility of lymphangioleiomyomatosis or Birt–Hogg–Dubé syndrome in any woman with pneumothorax

Radiologic findings

A consistent and striking feature of intralobar sequestrations is their predilection for the lower lobes, which are affected in 97% of cases. The left side is more commonly involved, the left lower lobe being the most common site. Intralobar sequestration should be part of the differential diagnosis in any patient with recurrent pneumonia localized to a lower lobe.

Radiographs typically show consolidation or a solid mass, but a solitary cyst or multi-cystic mass may be present, or the lesion may appear as an ill-defined opacity. Cavitation is not uncommon. Air–fluid levels are seen within a third of cases, mimicking the radiologic appearance of an abscess. The systemic arterial supply of pulmonary sequestrations can be demonstrated radiologically, either by computed tomography (CT) after contrast enhancement, or by angiography (arteriography/aortography).

Differential diagnosis

- Congenital cystic adenomatoid malformation. Cystic change within an intralobar sequestration can raise the possibility of CCAM. Once a systemic artery is identified, the lesion is by definition a sequestration regardless of the presence and morphology of cystic changes.
- Non-specific chronic inflammation and/or fibrosis. This is the most likely interpretation if the pathologist is unaware

of the radiologic and intra-operative findings. Pathologists faced with this morphology in a benign lesion resected from a lower lobe must consider the possibility of an intralobar sequestration, and look for clinical or histologic evidence of a systemic artery.

- Abscess. Abscesses can present in the superior segment of the left lower lobe and may be incidentally detected in young individuals. The extensive inflammatory changes can mimic the secondary inflammatory changes in sequestrations. Again, identification of a systemic arterial supply is key, and a quick review of the operative note usually suffices to exclude this possibility.

Treatment and prognosis

Intralobar sequestrations are benign. They are cured by surgical excision; lobectomy is generally preferred over sequestrectomy. It remains unclear whether surgery is indicated for lesions detected incidentally in asymptomatic individuals. In contrast to extralobar sequestrations, associated congenital anomalies are not common.

Sample diagnosis on pathology report

Lung, left lower lobe, excision – Intralobar pulmonary sequestration (See comment).

Extralobar sequestration

See previous section for an introduction to the concept of pulmonary sequestration.

Major diagnostic findings

- Benign but abnormal (maldeveloped) mass of lung tissue, located outside the confines of the normal lung. Encountering lung tissue in an extrapulmonary location can be a disorienting experience, but is the mainstay of the diagnosis. We have seen cases in which pathologists have hesitated to identify lung tissue at frozen section when faced with a "mass" in an unusual location such as the paraspinal region. Diagnosis can also be difficult when the sequestration is located immediately adjacent to the normal lung.
- The lung tissue in an extralobar sequestration may superficially resemble normal lung, but is never entirely normal. In some cases the only abnormality is the presence of slightly dilated alveoli. Variable degrees of cystic change are present in other cases. The cyst contents may be mucoid, resembling a mucocele.
- Identifying a systemic arterial supply is the key to the diagnosis. A systemic arterial blood supply to the lesion is most reliably identified by the operating surgeon, but the pathologist can also help to confirm the presence of a systemic artery. Please see the preceding section on intralobar sequestration for details on pathologic identification of systemic arteries in pulmonary sequestrations.

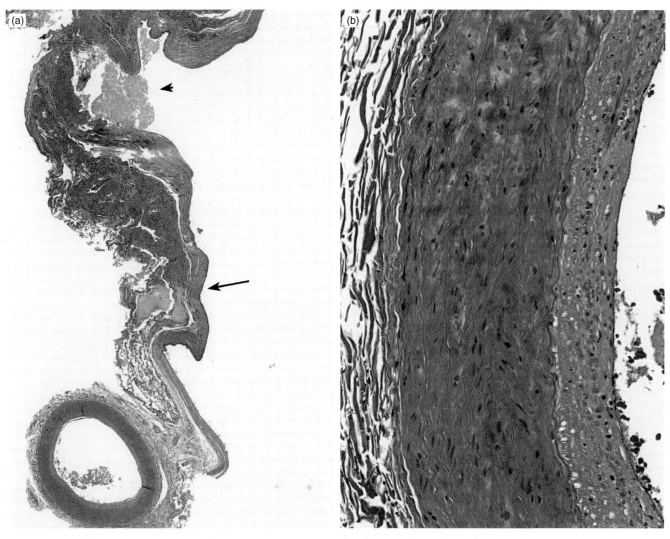

Figure 7.3. Intralobar sequestration. (a) Cystic lesion containing mucin (arrowhead). Arrow indicates lumen of cyst. Note systemic artery at bottom. **(b)** Systemic artery shown at high magnification. Note multiple elastic layers. A pulmonary artery would be expected to show two well-defined elastic layers at this level in the lung.

Variable pathologic findings

- Grossly, extralobar sequestrations may appear solid, sponge-like or multi-cystic. The classic gross appearance is that of a small purple pyramidal mass resembling a piece of spleen or liver. If the lesion is cystic, the cyst contents may be mucoid.
- Congenital cystic adenomatoid malformations, usually type 2, arise within approximately half of all extralobar sequestrations (Figures 7.5 and 7.6). These are proliferations of small, irregular, bronchiole-like structures lined by ciliated columnar epithelium, separated by variable amounts of normal alveolated lung. At first glance, these structures resemble normal bronchioles. Unlike normal bronchioles, however, they are closely packed, have irregular shapes and are not paired with a pulmonary artery branch. The lumens may be empty or filled with mucin. Some authors refer to such CCAM-like changes as "microcystic maldevelopment", which is thought to be a consequence of bronchial atresia.

- Cartilage may be present around the abnormal bronchiole-like structures.
- Adipose tissue may be present within the sequestered lung tissue (Figure 7.5).
- Scattered skeletal muscle fibers can be found within extralobar sequestrations. This bizarre finding – disconcerting because skeletal muscle is not normally found within the lung – has been termed "rhabdomyomatous dysgenesis" (Figure 7.6).
- Small thick-walled branches of the supplying systemic artery are often scattered within the lesion. They may be clustered together.
- Small, scattered foci of chronic inflammation composed mainly of lymphocytes are not uncommon.
- Granulomas may occasionally be found within the lesion.

Diagnostic work-up

See previous section on "Intralobar sequestration".

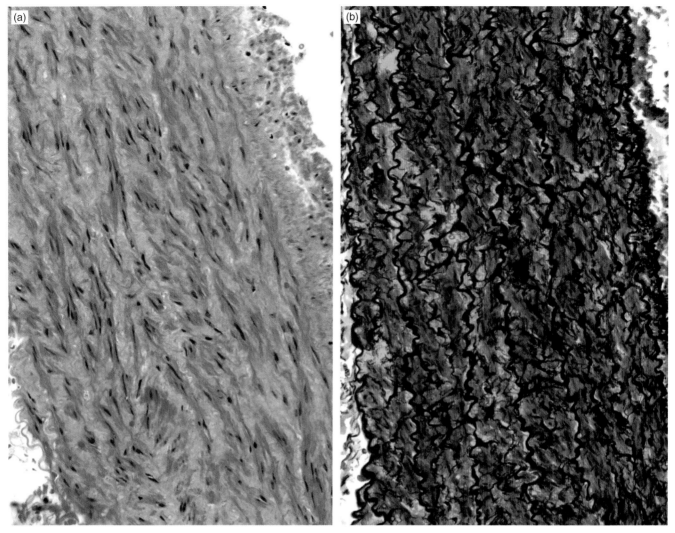

Figure 7.4. Systemic artery in intralobar sequestration. (a) The wall of this artery shows a lamellated appearance characterized by multiple elastic tissue layers alternating with fragmented muscle fibers, an arrangement typical of systemic elastic arteries. **(b)** Movat pentachrome stain. The typical lamellar alternation of elastic fibers (black) and smooth muscle fibers (red) is better appreciated. The green color, corresponding to the blue myxoid background in part A, is a result of the high mucopolysaccharide content.

Clinical profile

Extralobar pulmonary sequestrations are usually encountered in infants (most commonly in neonates) and young children. Approximately 60% of cases occur in infants under 6 months of age. However, cases are well documented in adults, including rarely in older individuals up to the age of 65. The reported male to female ratio is 4:1.

Most extralobar sequestrations are detected incidentally on routine prenatal ultrasounds between the third and eighth months of gestation. Many infants with these lesions are asymptomatic. However, some cases are found on chest radiographs obtained in newborns presenting with respiratory distress, cyanosis or feeding difficulties. Associated congenital anomalies are present in approximately half, the most common being congenital diaphragmatic hernia and congenital heart disease.

Radiologic findings

Extrapulmonary sequestrations are usually first detected on prenatal ultrasound. They appear as cystic, solid or mixed solid–cystic lesions, usually occurring just under the lung (between a lower lobe and the diaphragm, typically near the medial left costophrenic sulcus), but they may present as a mass within or under the diaphragm, the hilum, posterior or anterior mediastinum, pericardium, paraspinal region or retroperitoneum (above the kidney or adjacent to the adrenal gland). They can occur on either side of the midline, but are slightly more common on the left (65%). Many are found between the lower lobes and the diaphragm (63%).

The systemic artery supplying the lesion (usually arising from the aorta) can often be identified radiologically on chest CT. However, in some cases, the systemic artery may not be identifiable, leading to misinterpretation. The clinical and

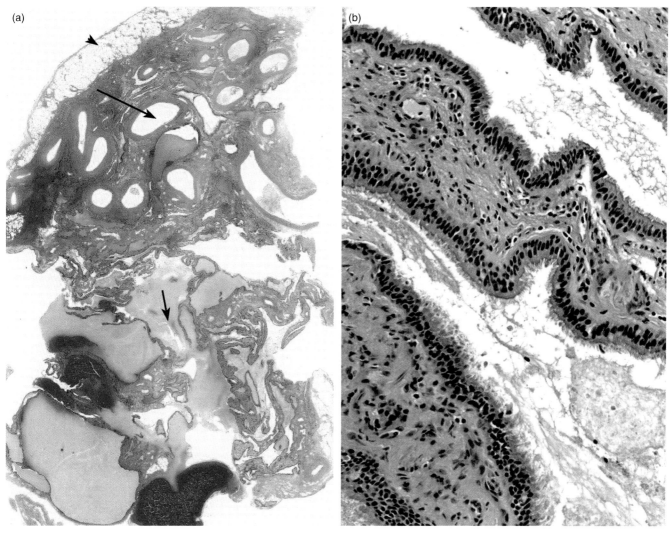

Figure 7.5. Extralobar sequestration. (a) Low magnification, showing numerous mucin-filled cysts resembling type 2 CCAM (short arrow, bottom) and systemic artery (long arrow, top). Note adipose tissue within lesion (arrowhead, top edge). **(b)** High magnification, showing closely packed bronchiole-like structures, lined by ciliated columnar epithelium.

radiologic differential diagnosis depends on the location of the lesion. Sequestrations located in the abdomen often raise clinical concern for neuroblastoma.

Differential diagnosis

- Congenital cystic adenomatoid malformation (CCAM), not associated with sequestration. Proliferations of small, variably dilated bronchiole-like structures identical to type 2 CCAM are common within extralobar sequestrations. Thus, the histologic features of an extralobar sequestration can be very similar to those of a CCAM. The main differentiating feature between the two entities is the presence of a systemic arterial supply (Figure 7.7). Although systemic arteries can be identified histologically, speaking with the surgeon or checking the intra-operative note is the easiest and most reliable way to determine if a systemic artery did indeed supply the lesion. Lesions that have a systemic arterial supply should be diagnosed as "extralobar sequestration", and the

presence of type 2 CCAM within the lesion should be documented.
- Bronchogenic cyst. These lesions are usually extrapulmonary (mediastinal) cysts with a cartilage-containing wall, histologically resembling a normal bronchus. Since extralobar sequestrations occasionally occur in the mediastinum, there is some scope for misdiagnosis. Bronchogenic cysts can be differentiated from sequestrations by their lack of a systemic arterial supply.
- Bronchopulmonary foregut malformation. This is a piece of lung with a patent connection to the gastrointestinal tract.

Treatment and prognosis

Extralobar sequestrations are benign. There is a small risk of infection or hemorrhage within the lesion. Spontaneous regression has been reported. Treatment consists of surgical excision, although the rationale for resecting these lesions

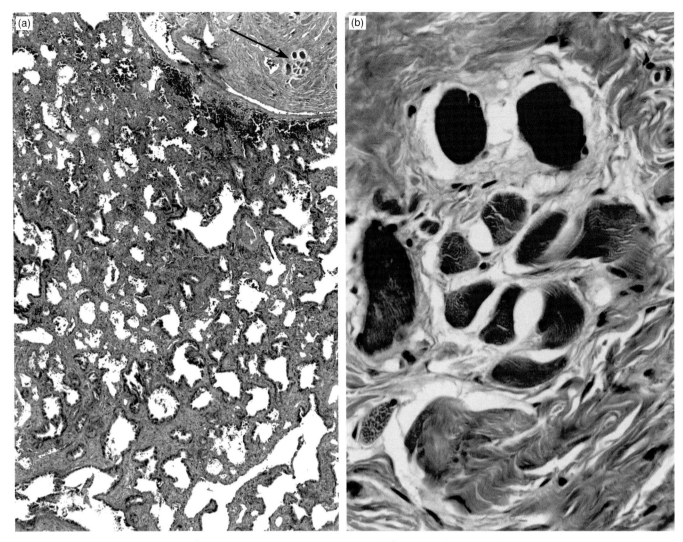

Figure 7.6. Extralobar sequestration with type 2 CCAM. (a) Type 2 CCAM composed of back-to-back bronchiole-like structures with minimal intervening normal lung. Arrow indicates area magnified in b. **(b)** High magnification, showing a focus of skeletal muscle fibers ("rhabdomyomatous dysgenesis").

remains unclear. The prognosis is usually favorable, unless there are associated congenital anomalies.

Sample diagnosis on pathology report

Paraspinal mass, excision – Extralobar pulmonary sequestration, with congenital cystic adenomatoid malformation, type 2 (See comment).

Congenital cystic adenomatoid malformation

Congenital cystic adenomatoid malformation (CCAM) is best known as a benign cystic lesion of fetuses and newborns. However, it occasionally presents in older children or adults, causing problems in diagnosis and classification. CCAMs were classified by Stocker into three types in 1977 and five types in 2001; the latter classification was accompanied by a proposal to change the designation of the lesion from CCAM to "congenital pulmonary airway malformation" (CPAM). These classifications can be difficult to apply in practice, and their alleged prognostic significance has been challenged. Although much

discussion and angst often surrounds classification, in routine surgical pathology practice the majority of CCAMs are type 1 (large cyst type) or type 2 (small cyst type). The other types are rare. Some cases of type 4 CCAM probably represent the cystic variant of pleuropulmonary blastoma, a neoplasm of childhood. Such cases may account for reports of rhabdomyosarcoma arising in CCAM.

A simplified classification of CCAM, based largely on Stocker's original classification, is presented in Table 7.2. The term CCAM will be used in this book since the majority of these lesions are cystic and because clinicians are generally familiar with this term.

Major diagnostic findings

- Cysts of various sizes. Most commonly, there are either a few large cysts (or a solitary large cyst) surrounded by multiple tiny cysts (type 1 CCAM), or a microscopic proliferation of several tiny cysts without a dominant large cyst (type 2 CCAM) (Figure 7.8). The arbitrary size cut-off that defines a large cyst is 2 cm.

Table 7.2. Simplified classification of congenital cystic adenomatoid malformations

Type	Key features
1 ("large cyst type")	Gross: one or more large cysts (at least one greater than 2 cm) Microscopic: there may be smaller microscopic cysts in the wall of the grossly visible cysts
2 ("small cyst type")	Gross: multiple small cysts, all less than 2 cm Microscopic: multiple bronchiole-like structures lined by ciliated columnar epithelium Variable amounts of intervening alveoli
3	Gross: solid or spongy Microscopic: immature-appearing lung microscopically lined by cuboidal epithelium

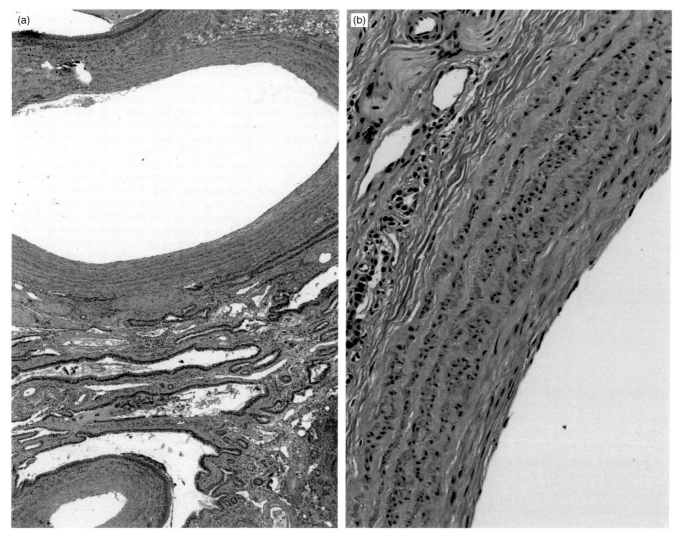

Figure 7.7. Systemic artery within an extralobar sequestration. (a) Systemic artery in an extralobar sequestration. Adjacent structures represent type 2 CCAM. **(b)** High magnification of wall of artery, showing alternation of elastic tissue and muscle typical of these abnormal systemic arteries.

- Microscopically, the cysts in most CCAMs are lined by ciliated columnar epithelium (Figure 7.9). In type 2 lesions, the cysts resemble bronchioles and often contain smooth muscle. However, unlike normal bronchioles, they are closely packed or arranged "back-to-back" with little intervening alveolated lung parenchyma, have irregular shapes and lack a partner artery (i.e., they do not occur in bronchovascular bundles).

- There should be no clinical or histologic evidence of a systemic arterial supply, this being a defining feature of pulmonary sequestrations.

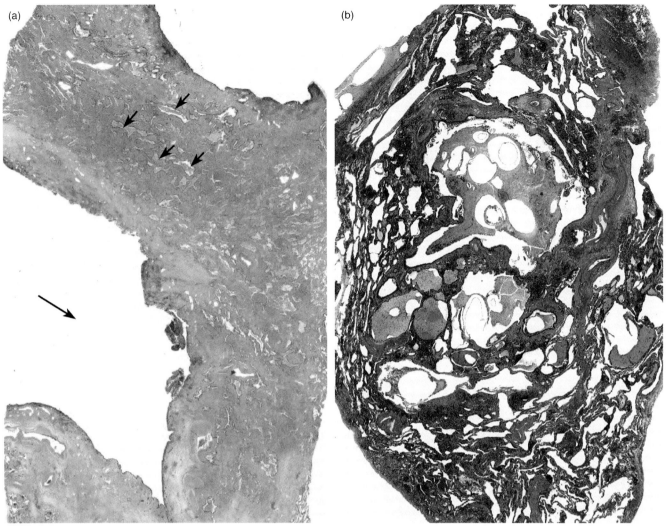

Figure 7.8. Congenital cystic adenomatoid malformation, microscopic features (low magnification). (a) Type 1 CCAM. Large cyst (long arrow in lumen) with several small cysts (short arrows) in its wall. **(b)** Type 2 CCAM. This multi-cystic mass is composed of several small mucin-filled cysts, none greater than 2 cm in size.

Variable pathologic findings

- Grossly, most CCAMs appear as a multi-cystic or spongy mass. Type 1 CCAMs have at least one large cyst greater than 2 cm, whereas in type 2 CCAMs none of the cysts is more than 2 cm in diameter (Figure 7.10). The smallest cysts in type 2 CCAMs may not be visible on gross examination and may impart a spongy appearance to the lesion. The lung surrounding the lesion is normal.
- Type 2 CCAMs arise within approximately half of all extralobar sequestrations (see previous section). The finding of a CCAM within a sequestration is of no prognostic significance. Some authors refer to CCAM-like changes in any setting as "microcystic maldevelopment", and have suggested that this is a consequence of bronchial atresia.
- Typically, most of the tiny bronchiole-like structures of type 2 CCAM lack smooth muscle and cartilage. However, smooth muscle is present in some cases, and cartilage, although less common, may also be present.
- The cysts may contain mucin in their lumens.

- Superimposed chronic inflammation may be present in some cases.
- Mucinous lining cells may be found in type 1 CCAMs, and should prompt a search for adenocarcinoma. Mucinous adenocarcinoma (previously known as mucinous bronchioloalveolar carcinoma) has been reported in some cases, mainly in type 1 CCAMs occurring in older children and adults.

Diagnostic work-up

- In most cases, no special stains are required for diagnosis. If a vascular structure within the lesion is suspected to be a systemic artery, a special stain for elastic tissue can be helpful.
- It is useful to verify that the lesion is a localized abnormality (i.e., limited to a single lobe) by checking the radiologic findings, and that there was no evidence of a systemic arterial supply (by talking to the surgeon or checking the operative note).

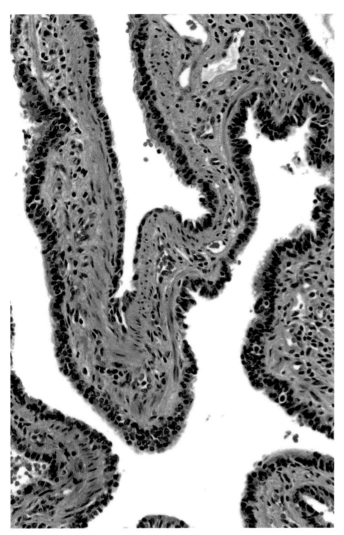

Figure 7.9. Congenital cystic adenomatoid malformation, microscopic features (high magnification). These tiny cysts in a type 2 CCAM are lined by ciliated columnar epithelium. A few wisps of smooth muscle are visible just under the epithelium.

Clinical profile

CCAM is usually diagnosed within the first 2 years of life. It is often detected incidentally on routine prenatal ultrasounds performed during pregnancy. Newborns may present with respiratory compromise or may not have any symptoms. Lesions that do not cause symptoms presumably account for CCAM that presents in older children and adults.

Although uncommon, CCAMs are well documented in older children and adults, including rarely in elderly individuals. Older children often present with a clinical picture suggesting pneumonia. Adults may present with cough, dyspnea, chest pain, hemoptysis or fever. A history of persistent or recurrent infection is common. Some cases are detected incidentally on chest radiographs performed for unrelated reasons.

Radiologic findings

CCAM is often detected on prenatal ultrasound. Small lesions may not be visible on chest X-rays. On chest CT, CCAM appears as a solitary cystic mass or multiple cysts with air–fluid levels. Some cases appear as an abnormal hyperlucent area on CT. Unlike pulmonary sequestrations, there is no predilection for any lobe or side. The radiologic differential diagnosis includes bronchial atresia and congenital lobar emphysema.

In older children and adults, most cases present radiologically as solitary or multilocular cystic lesions with air–fluid levels. Owing to the presence of air–fluid levels, abscess is frequently in the radiologic differential diagnosis.

Differential diagnosis

- Pulmonary sequestration. Since CCAM-like cystic changes can occur within intralobar sequestrations, differentiation between sequestration and CCAM rests on the demonstration of a systemic arterial supply, a defining feature of pulmonary sequestrations.
- Bronchogenic cyst. These lesions are very uncommon in the lung but have been reported. They enter the differential diagnosis of type 1 CCAM, since both may present as a solitary respiratory epithelium-lined cyst within the lung. Cartilage is usually present in the wall of bronchogenic cysts and is usually absent in the wall of a type 1 CCAM. However, the most reliable differentiating feature between the two is the presence of small bronchiole-like cysts in the wall of the main cyst in type 1 CCAM; in contrast, bronchogenic cysts are solitary.

Treatment and prognosis

Most CCAMs are benign, and surgical excision is curative. They do not recur if completely removed. A few cases of CCAM containing mucinous adenocarcinoma have been reported. Overall, the prognosis is good, although there are exceptional reports of recurrence and even death. This infrequent complication has been cited as one of the reasons for resecting these lesions; a lobectomy is often performed.

Sample diagnosis on pathology report

Lung, right lower lobe, lobectomy – Congenital cystic adenomatoid malformation, type 2 (See comment).

Bronchogenic cyst

Most bronchogenic cysts arise in the mediastinum. However, since rare cases of histologically documented bronchogenic cysts have been described within the lung parenchyma, the entity is discussed here in the differential diagnosis of a solitary intraparenchymal (intrapulmonary) lung cyst.

Major diagnostic findings

- Benign solitary unilocular cyst lined by ciliated columnar epithelium (respiratory epithelium). Most bronchogenic cysts contain cartilage in the cyst wall. Some authorities require that a definitive diagnosis of bronchogenic cyst should be made only in cases with cartilage in the wall, other cases being designated "foregut cyst". The cyst wall of a bronchogenic cyst resembles the wall of a normal

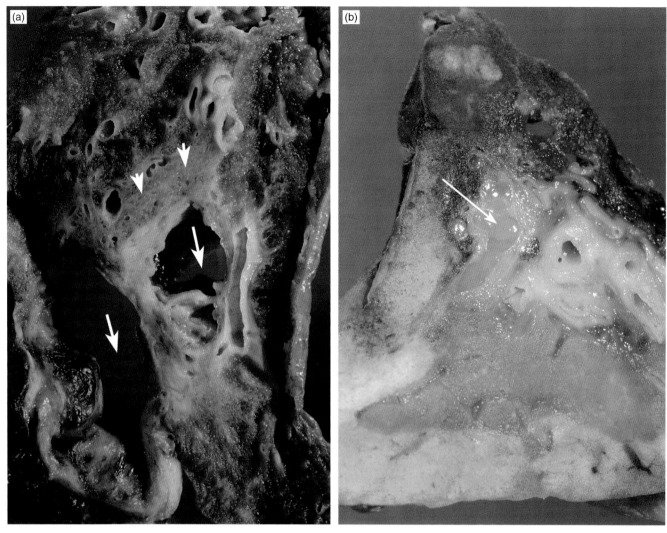

Figure 7.10. Congenital cystic adenomatoid malformation, macroscopic features. (a) Type 1 CCAM. Large cysts greater than 2 cm define a type 1 lesion (arrows), but there are also smaller cysts in the walls of the larger cysts (arrowheads). **(b)** Type 2 CCAM. Mucin-filled cysts, none greater than 2 cm in size. Smaller cysts were seen microscopically but are not visible on gross examination.

bronchus (Figure 7.11). Demonstration of cartilage is the key in differentiating bronchogenic cyst from its mimics, and its demonstration may require serial sectioning and examination of multiple deeper cuts.

- There should be no evidence of a systemic arterial supply (characteristic of pulmonary sequestrations) or smaller cysts adjacent to the wall of the main cyst (a feature of type 1 CCAM).

Variable pathologic findings

- Grossly, bronchogenic cyst is a solitary unilocular cyst. The cyst contents may be watery, mucoid or turbid, depending on the presence of superimposed infection.
- In addition to cartilage, the wall often contains bronchial submucosal (seromucous) glands and smooth muscle (Figure 7.11).
- The epithelial lining may be ulcerated, and there may be varying degrees of acute or chronic inflammation in the wall of the cyst.

- There may be squamous metaplasia of the epithelial lining. The lining cells may be focally attenuated (cuboidal).
- Microscopically, the cyst lumen may contain mucus, necrotic debris or purulent material (acute inflammatory exudate).

Diagnostic work-up

No special stains are required for this diagnosis.

Clinical profile

Bronchogenic cysts can occur at any age and affect either sex, but the majority of cases occur within the first four decades of life. Among adults, most patients present in the 20s and 30s. Presentation beyond the age of 50 is unusual, but rare cases have been documented up to the eighth decade of life. Bronchogenic cysts occur in children but are uncommon in infancy.

Symptoms are more common in children than in adults. They include cough, pain, dyspnea and wheezing or

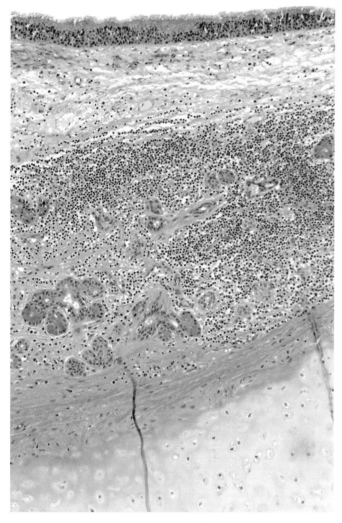

Figure 7.11. Bronchogenic cyst. Low-magnification view showing wall of cyst (lumen is at top). Note ciliated columnar (respiratory) lining at top and cartilage at bottom.

respiratory distress, presumably caused by mass effect, infection or rupture. Dysphagia may result if the mass compresses the esophagus. A significant proportion of cases – ranging from more than a third to slightly more than half – are detected incidentally in asymptomatic individuals on chest radiographs performed for other reasons.

Radiologic findings

Overall, more than three-fourths of bronchogenic cysts occur in the mediastinum. The classic location is in the middle mediastinum above, adjacent to or below the tracheal carina (subcarinal). Some cases are found in the posterior and anterior mediastinum. Bronchogenic cysts have also been reported in the paratracheal region, adjacent to the esophagus, in the hilum of the lung and beneath the diaphragm. Rare cases have also been reported within the lung parenchyma, although it is likely that some of these were type 1 CCAMs misinterpreted as bronchogenic cysts.

Radiographs show a mass with a thin wall, either with water- or soft tissue-attenuation on CT. The cystic nature of

the mass is not always apparent, even on contrast-enhanced CT, and bronchogenic cyst is not considered in the preoperative differential diagnosis in a significant proportion of cases. The diagnosis is more likely to be suspected in cases with water-attenuation, while soft tissue-attenuation lesions are likely to be mistaken for other entities. Even when a cyst is suspected, other cysts such as foregut duplication cysts enter the differential diagnosis. Air–fluid levels and calcification may be present. Bronchogenic cysts are often attached by a stalk to a nearby structure such as the trachea or esophagus, but do not communicate with the tracheobronchial tree.

Differential diagnosis

- Type 1 CCAM enters the differential diagnosis of intrapulmonary bronchogenic cyst since both have a ciliated columnar epithelial lining. Furthermore, type 1 CCAMs may have cartilage in their walls. In this differential diagnosis, the absence of cartilage favors type 1 CCAM. In fact, many cases of intrapulmonary bronchogenic cyst reported in the literature and illustrated in textbooks represent type 1 CCAM. Another important differentiating feature that helps to differentiate these two entities is the presence of small cysts adjacent to the wall of the main cyst in type 1 CCAM. Small cysts are absent in bronchogenic cysts.
- Teratoma enters the differential diagnosis, particularly in the mediastinum. Both lesions may contain cartilage and respiratory epithelium, but teratomas also contain tissues derived from other germ cell layers.
- Abscess. This can be a difficult problem when the lesion is within the lung in an adult patient. Infected bronchogenic cysts can contain purulent material and the epithelial lining may be extensively ulcerated and develop squamous metaplasia, changes that can also occur in abscesses. In the mediastinum, demonstration of cartilage and respiratory-type epithelium should be sufficient to differentiate between these entities. In the lung, since an epithelial lining and cartilage may be part of a bronchus, these features cannot be considered pathognomonic of a bronchogenic cyst. In this setting, demonstration of a communication with the bronchi favors an abscess. In contrast, bronchogenic cysts lack a patent connection to the tracheobronchial tree.
- Foregut duplication cyst. This is a major differential diagnostic consideration for bronchogenic cysts in the subcarinal region.
- Müllerian paravertebral cyst (of Hattori) should be considered in the differential diagnosis when no cartilage is found in an epithelium-lined posterior mediastinal or paravertebral cyst arising in a woman.

Treatment and prognosis

Bronchogenic cysts are benign. Surgical excision is curative, although post-operative complications have been reported. Some authorities argue for a "wait and watch" approach for asymptomatic patients, but others advocate surgery even in

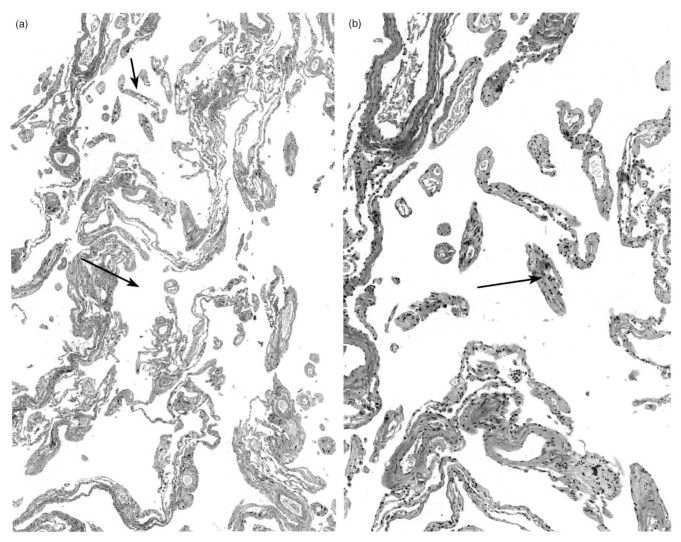

(a)

(b)

Figure 7.12. Emphysema. (a) Airspace enlargement (long arrow) and evidence of airspace destruction (floating alveolar septum, short arrow). This is an example of "centrilobular" emphysema. **(b)** High magnification. Arrow indicates floating alveolar septum.

this setting, citing data that such patients may develop symptoms on follow-up, and that post-operative complications are higher in symptomatic individuals.

Sample diagnosis on pathology report

Lung, right hilum, excision – Benign epithelium-lined cyst consistent with bronchogenic cyst (See comment).

Emphysema (including bullae and blebs)

Emphysema is defined as "a condition of the lung characterized by abnormal, permanent enlargement of airspaces distal to the terminal bronchiole, accompanied by the destruction of their walls, and without obvious fibrosis". Although emphysema is defined on the basis of pathologic findings, in practice most cases are diagnosed on the basis of clinical and radiologic features. Cigarette smoking is by far the most common cause. The umbrella term chronic obstructive pulmonary disease (COPD) includes chronic bronchitis and emphysema. A major feature of COPD is airflow limitation that is not fully reversible. Airflow limitation is defined (by spirometry) as a post-bronchodilator ratio of FEV1 to FVC (FEV1/FVC) of < 70%.

Emphysema is commonly encountered by pathologists in surgical lung biopsies, wedge resections from patients with spontaneous pneumothorax, lung volume reduction surgery specimens, lobectomies (in the background of lung cancer), pneumonectomies, explant pneumonectomies (emphysematous lungs removed prior to lung transplantation) and autopsies.

In addition to smoking-related emphysema, which accounts for the vast majority of cases seen in practice, the other settings in which emphysema occurs include α-1 antitrypsin deficiency (panacinar emphysema) and patients with spontaneous pneumothorax (paraseptal or distal acinar emphysema).

Major diagnostic findings

- In histologic sections, emphysema manifests as enlarged airspaces with evidence of alveolar septal destruction (Figure 7.12). Severe emphysema is easy to recognize, whereas milder forms are difficult to diagnose. Airspace

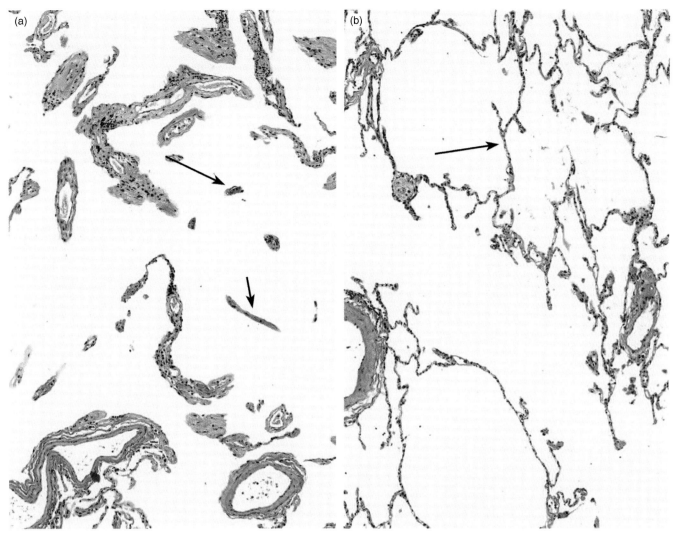

Figure 7.13. Emphysema vs. overinflation. (a) Emphysematous lung from a smoker showing airspace enlargement as well as alveolar septal destruction (arrows). **(b)** Overinflated lung from a never-smoker without emphysema. Airspaces are enlarged but alveolar walls are intact (arrow).

enlargement without evidence of alveolar septal destruction represents overinflation and should not be termed emphysema. The enlarged airspaces of emphysema are caused by destruction of lung parenchyma with resultant loss of alveolar septa. In contrast to normal alveoli, which contain intact walls all the way around, the walls of emphysematous spaces are not intact. Instead, they lose their connections to adjacent alveolar septa, and appear to "float" freely within the airspaces in the form of tiny linear nubbins (Figure 7.13).

- No significant fibrosis. Uncomplicated emphysema does not feature significant alveolar septal fibrosis. If significant interstitial fibrosis is present microscopically, the possibility of smoking-related interstitial fibrosis (SRIF) (Figure 7.14) or combined pulmonary fibrosis and emphysema (CPFE) should be considered. Radiologic or macroscopic evidence of fibrosis should also prompt consideration of a superimposed process.
- Emphysema does not account for the presence of interstitial lung disease, lung opacities, infiltrates or

nodules, and does not need to be diagnosed in most small biopsies.

Variable pathologic findings

- Air-filled spaces of various sizes (bullae and blebs) are frequently found in emphysematous lungs. There are no universally accepted definitions of bullae and blebs (see Table 7.3, and Figure 7.1b). However, most definitions specify that a bulla should be within the lung parenchyma and is greater than 1 cm in diameter, whereas a bleb should be located within the visceral pleura. In practice, the exact location of a peripheral air-filled space can be difficult to determine, and is of no clinical significance. Both bullae and blebs can occur as focal lesions in otherwise normal lungs.
- Placental transmogrification. This finding is a bizarre form of bullous emphysema, in which severely emphysematous lung tissue is so dramatically altered that it resembles placental tissue. The alveolar septa are widened by edema, fibrosis, blood vessels, inflammatory cells, clear cells and

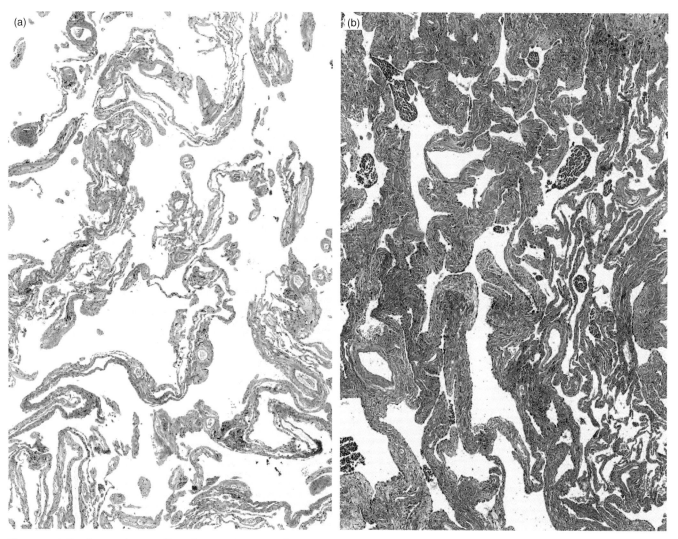

Figure 7.14. Emphysema (uncomplicated) vs. emphysema with smoking-related interstitial fibrosis. (a) Emphysema without interstitial fibrosis.
(b) Smoking-related interstitial fibrosis (SRIF) is characterized by the presence of hyalinized collagen (fibrosis) that widens the alveolar septa. This finding is usually superimposed on emphysematous lung.

occasionally adipose tissue, mimicking the appearance of placental villi. A radiologic finding that helps to avoid misdiagnosis is that these patients present with a large unilateral bulla or lucency. For reasons that remain unclear, many of these patients are young non-smokers with no evidence of emphysema in the remainder of the lung.

- The histologic distinction between the various forms of emphysema (centrilobular, panacinar, paraseptal, irregular) is difficult to apply in practice and is of no significance in most cases. The various forms of emphysema were originally described in paper-mounted whole lung sections (Gough–Wentworth sections), an obsolete practice of historical significance. The forms of emphysema have also been described as gross findings best appreciated in lungs that have been fixed upright and examined under water.

- Centrilobular emphysema is the most common type of emphysema (Figure 7.1a, Figures 7.12 to 7.15). It is related to cigarette smoking. The term centrilobular was used because it was felt that the lesions started in the centers of

lung lobules. This distribution is lost in severe emphysema, and overlaps greatly with panacinar emphysema (Figure 7.15).

- Panacinar emphysema is uncommon. It is characterized by airspace enlargement and alveolar septal destruction involving the entire lobule (Figure 7.15), and is mainly a consequence of α-1 antitrypsin deficiency. Detection of panacinar emphysema preferentially affecting the lower lobes should prompt consideration of α-1 antitrypsin deficiency; radiologists are best placed to detect this scenario. Interestingly, a significant proportion of individuals with homozygous α-1 antitrypsin deficiency either have no emphysema or apical-predominant emphysema.

- "Paraseptal (distal acinar) emphysema" is common. It is best seen by radiologists, but can also be appreciated on gross examination of surgically resected lungs. As the name suggests, the lesions in this form of emphysema abut the pleura and interlobular septa. Bullae and blebs in young smokers with spontaneous pneumothorax are considered by some to fall under this form of the disease.

Table 7.3. Bullae and blebs: definitions

Source	Definition
• Spencer's Pathology of the Lung, 2013	• Bleb: collections of air within the visceral pleura that probably result from rupture of subpleural alveoli • Bulla: bullous emphysema is a descriptive term for any form of emphysema that manifests with airspaces measuring greater than 1 cm
• Fleischner Society guidelines (for radiologists), 2008	• Bleb: small gas-containing space within the visceral pleura or in the subpleural lung, not larger than 1 cm • Bulla: little clinical importance, use discouraged
• Thurlbeck's Pathology of the Lung, 2005 (and Ciba Guest symposium, 1959)	• Bleb: a collection of air between the layers of the visceral pleura • Bulla: an emphysematous space with a diameter of more than 1 cm in the distended state
• Katzenstein and Askin's Surgical Pathology of Non-Neoplastic Lung Disease, 2006	• Bleb: collections of air within the visceral pleura • Bulla: large, air-filled spaces in the lung, by definition, greater than 1 cm in diameter • Bleb: localized collection of air within the pleura or immediate subpleural lung, usually less than 1 cm in diameter • Bulla: sharply demarcated air-containing space of 1 cm or more in diameter
• Ryu and Swensen, 2003	• Bleb: localized collection of air within the pleura or immediate subpleural lung, usually less than 1 cm in diameter • Bulla: sharply demarcated air-containing space of 1 cm or more in diameter

• In most cases of smoking-related emphysema, smoker's macrophages are present within the airspaces. For reasons explained in Chapter 4, this finding is termed "respiratory bronchiolitis".

• Fibrosis may be superimposed on emphysema. This may take the form of alveolar septal widening by hyalinized collagen, which has been termed smoking-related interstitial fibrosis (SRIF) (Figure 7.14). Alternatively, a well-defined form of interstitial fibrosis, most commonly usual interstitial pneumonia (UIP), may co-exist with emphysema. This combination is termed CPFE (Figure 5.33).

• Unrelated findings such as granulomatous inflammation or unsuspected small tumors may be found in emphysematous lungs in lung volume reduction specimens.

Diagnostic work-up

No special stains are required to diagnose emphysema.

Clinical profile

The vast majority of cases of emphysema seen by pathologists occur in adult smokers. Both sexes are affected. Most patients are more than 50 years old at diagnosis. Development of emphysema at a young age should trigger consideration of α-1 antitrypsin deficiency. The majority of patients are men; approximately 35% are women. Non-productive cough, chronic and progressive dyspnea, sputum production and wheezing are the most common symptoms. Symptoms may be present without airflow limitation, and vice versa. Some patients are asymptomatic. Exacerbations are common. Activity can be severely limited in advanced cases. Chronic respiratory failure may lead to right heart failure and cor pulmonale.

Radiologic findings

Centrilobular emphysema is characterized by centrilobular areas of decreased attenuation, with imperceptible walls and non-uniform distribution, and is found mainly in the upper lung zones. Paraseptal emphysema shows cystic low-attenuation areas with evident walls arrayed in a single subpleural tier.

Differential diagnosis

• Normal or overinflated lung. Pathologic over-diagnosis of emphysema is common and is the main pitfall to avoid. This can be avoided by strictly requiring evidence of alveolar septal destruction (incomplete, free floating alveolar septa) in addition to airspace enlargement.

• Lymphangioleiomyomatosis. In contrast to emphysema, the cysts of lymphangioleiomyomatosis are focal lesions in a background of relatively normal lung. Their walls contain wisps of abnormal smooth muscle, while the walls of emphysematous spaces do not.

• SRIF and CPFE. Obvious or significant interstitial fibrosis is not a feature of uncomplicated emphysema, and should prompt consideration of these entities.

Treatment and prognosis

Emphysema is treated symptomatically with inhaled long-acting beta agonists and inhaled corticosteroids. Many patients require home oxygen. Lung volume reduction surgery may be

(a)

(b)

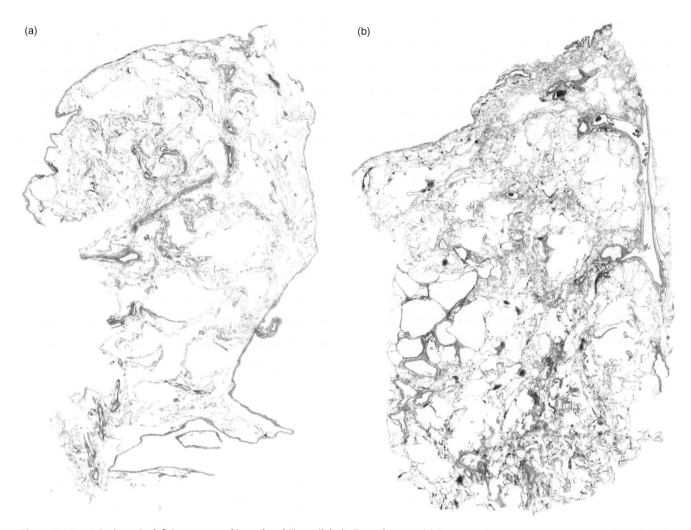

Figure 7.15. α-1 Antitrypsin deficiency vs. smoking-related ("centrilobular") emphysema. (a) Severe emphysema in a young never-smoker with PiZZ α-1 antitrypsin deficiency. **(b)** Severe emphysema in a smoker with COPD. The two forms of emphysema are essentially indistinguishable by routine histology.

an option for patients with severe upper lobe emphysema and low exercise capacity. Lung transplantation is an option for end-stage cases. Emphysema is one of the major indications for lung transplantation, the others being idiopathic pulmonary fibrosis and cystic fibrosis.

Sample diagnosis on pathology report

Emphysema is almost never the sole finding in a surgical (wedge) biopsy. The only specimens in which emphysema may be the predominant finding are explant pneumonectomies (in which the lungs are removed because of severe emphysema) and autopsies.

    Lung, right, explant pneumonectomy – Severe emphysema with bulla formation.

    Lung, right upper lobe, surgical biopsy – Emphysema, respiratory bronchiolitis and changes consistent with smoking-related interstitial fibrosis.

Pulmonary interstitial emphysema

Pulmonary interstitial emphysema is not true emphysema, but instead represents entry of air from ruptured alveoli into the

pulmonary interstitial tissues around the bronchovascular bundles, interlobular septa and pleura (lymphangitic distribution), a phenomenon that has been termed the "Macklin effect". In most cases, mechanical ventilation is thought to be the underlying cause, but a significant minority of cases develop in individuals who have never been ventilated. Other factors that have been implicated as the cause of initial alveolar rupture and air entry include blunt trauma, necrotizing pneumonia and repeated episodes of coughing.

    Pulmonary interstitial emphysema is best known to neonatal intensivists and radiologists in newborn (especially preterm) infants who have been mechanically ventilated for the respiratory distress syndrome. However, the condition also occurs in adults. A recent study found pulmonary interstitial emphysema in 36% of explanted lungs from adults who underwent lung transplantation for other reasons, the most common being usual interstitial pneumonia.

Major diagnostic findings

- Dilated air-filled spaces within the pulmonary interstitium, usually (but not always) lined by macrophages and

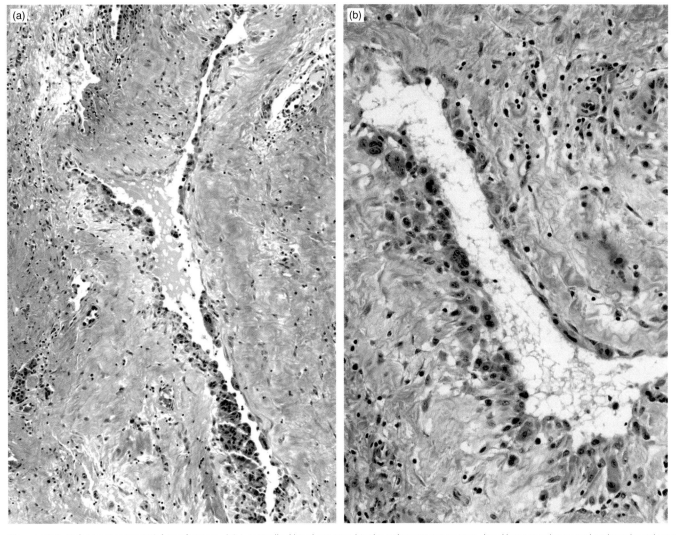

Figure 7.16. Pulmonary interstitial emphysema. (a) A cystically dilated space within the pulmonary interstitium, lined by macrophages and multinucleated giant cells. This lesion was located just beneath the pleura. **(b)** High magnification of another air-filled space from the same case. Macrophages and giant cells line the space, and there is fibrosis in the wall.

multinucleated giant cells (Figure 7.16). There is no epithelial lining. The spaces may be elongated, round, compressed or irregular (starfish-like). Some authors postulate that the giant cells are a marker of chronic, persistent disease, and use different terms for cases with ("persistent interstitial pulmonary emphysema") and without ("acute interstitial pulmonary emphysema") giant cells.

- The dilated spaces are most prominent around bronchovascular bundles but may also be seen in interlobular septa and pleura. This is the distribution in which lymphatics are found in the lung, hence the designation "lymphangitic". This distribution is not obvious in every case.

Variable pathologic findings

- Varying degrees of dense fibrosis may surround the dilated spaces (Figure 7.16). The fibrosis may contain plump fibroblasts as well as layers of dense collagen.
- Pulmonary interstitial emphysema can be localized, unilateral or diffuse and bilateral.

- Eosinophils may be present in the lumens of the spaces as well as in the surrounding fibrosis. This tissue eosinophilia in response to the presence of air within the tissues is reminiscent of the pleural eosinophilia that sometimes accompanies pneumothorax (reactive eosinophilic pleuritis).
- In explanted lungs in adults, pulmonary interstitial emphysema can be found in any lobe, and commonly involves more than one lobe.
- The air-filled spaces may be visible grossly under the pleura ("blebs") or as multiple cysts within the lung parenchyma.

Diagnostic work-up

Immunohistochemistry is not required for the diagnosis. However, it can be helpful in difficult cases. As expected, the lining cells are positive for CD68 and negative for keratin AE1/AE3. One potential pitfall is focal staining with D2–40. When present, staining with this marker is partial, differing from the complete, continuous staining characteristic of true lymphatics.

Clinical profile

Pulmonary interstitial emphysema can be seen in children as well as adults. Most affected children are premature, pre-term infants with a history of mechanical ventilation for respiratory distress syndrome. Others have a history of prior pneumonia (especially necrotizing pneumonia) or trauma. Mild cases can be asymptomatic but severe cases are commonly associated with respiratory distress, pneumothorax and pneumomediastinum.

In adults, the finding is common in lungs explanted for other reasons. In one study, 75% of adult patients with pulmonary interstitial emphysema in explant lungs had a history of prior mechanical ventilation and/or biopsy. The mechanical ventilation ranged from 2 days to 3 years prior to transplantation.

Radiologic findings

In neonates, most cases are diagnosed on the basis of radiologic findings, characterized by cyst-like lucencies or linear perivascular lucencies. These findings may be visible on chest X-rays. The lucencies may coalesce into larger spaces. In adults, the presence of multiple bilateral air lucencies along bronchovascular bundles ("ring around the artery" sign) on chest CT can be diagnostic; cases misinterpreted as pulmonary emphysema have been reported.

Differential diagnosis

- Granulomatous inflammation. The presence of macrophages and multinucleated giant cells may resemble granulomatous inflammation, but true granulomas are composed of epithelioid histiocytes and do not line air-filled spaces.
- Emphysema. True emphysema involves destruction of the alveolar septa, and lacks a peri-bronchovascular distribution, macrophages or giant cells.
- Lymphangiectasia. Congenital pulmonary lymphangiectasis can be a close mimic of pulmonary interstitial emphysema, especially if no giant cells are present in the latter. Staining for the lymphatic marker D2–40 can be very helpful in this situation. Staining should be complete and continuous in lymphangiectasis, and focal (incomplete) in pulmonary interstitial emphysema.
- CCAM. CCAM enters the differential diagnosis of localized pulmonary interstitial emphysema. However, the cysts of CCAM are lined by epithelial (ciliated columnar) cells, whereas the spaces of pulmonary interstitial emphysema lack an epithelial lining.

Treatment and prognosis

In children, the incidence of pulmonary interstitial emphysema can be decreased by surfactant treatment. Once pulmonary interstitial emphysema has developed, treatment involves changing ventilation settings to minimize airway pressures ("high-frequency ventilation", lateral decubitus positioning, and inhalation of helium or nitric oxide). For localized pulmonary interstitial emphysema, lobectomy and even pneumonectomy has been successfully performed.

Mild cases of pulmonary interstitial emphysema resolve completely without sequelae, but more extensive disease frequently results in pneumothorax, and may cause pneumomediastinum and pneumopericardium. The clinical implications of a pathologic diagnosis of pulmonary interstitial emphysema in lungs explanted for other diseases in adults are unknown.

Sample diagnosis on pathology report

In most cases in adults, pulmonary interstitial emphysema is an incidental finding and does not need to be mentioned in the main diagnosis. In neonatal autopsies, and in individuals in whom surgical resection was performed for cystic disease, a sample diagnosis is as follows:

Lung, left upper lobe, lobectomy – Pulmonary interstitial emphysema (See comment).

Lymphangioleiomyomatosis

The term "lymphangioleiomyomatosis" is misleading because it emphasizes a feature that is almost never seen in the lung (lymphatic involvement) and does not communicate the most striking pathologic finding in this disease in the lung (lung cysts). The prefix "lymphangio" refers to lymphatic obstruction (e.g., of the thoracic duct) that is frequently a clinically significant problem but is seldom visible in lung specimens, where the characteristic cysts and smooth muscle cells usually have no obvious relation to lymphatics.

Lymphangioleiomyomatosis (LAM) has traditionally been considered a form of non-neoplastic cystic "interstitial" lung disease. However, accumulation of evidence over the years has led to the recent claim that LAM is actually a low-grade metastasizing destructive neoplasm, a view that has been challenged. Further discussion of this complicated issue is outside the scope of this book, but interested readers are referred to the articles by McCormack *et al* and Glassberg for an interesting debate on this issue (see references). Although it is possible that LAM may one day fall outside the scope of a textbook of non-neoplastic lung disease, it is included here since it is currently considered in the differential diagnosis of benign cystic lung lesions.

Major diagnostic findings

- Cysts and abnormal smooth muscle fibers. In most cases, each slide contains a few small air-filled cysts randomly distributed within the lung parenchyma. The cyst wall consists mainly of normal lung tissue, along with a few wisps of smooth muscle fibers best appreciated at high magnification (Figure 7.17). The smooth muscle in LAM is abnormal since it is not associated with the usual smooth muscle-containing structures (arteries, bronchioles or alveolar ducts), appears "immature" and stains for human melanin black-45 (HMB-45). The smooth muscle cells are spindly and have eosinophilic cytoplasm. In most cases, the histologic diagnosis of LAM is fairly straightforward if the pathologist is aware that the smooth muscle proliferation can be focal and subtle (Figure 7.18). In classic cases, the diagnosis of LAM can be made on H&E alone.
- Immunohistochemistry for smooth muscle actin and/or HMB-45 may be used as a diagnostic adjunct. The abnormal smooth muscle cells in LAM cysts are positive for

(a)

(b)

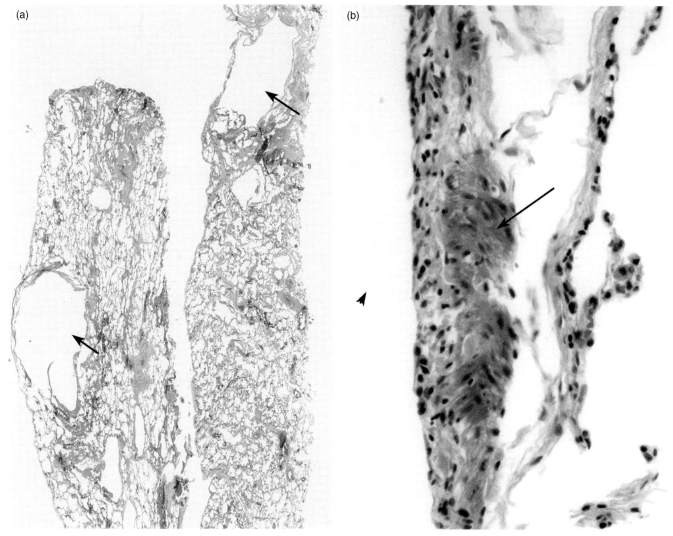

Figure 7.17. Lymphangioleiomyomatosis. (a) Low magnification, showing two cysts within lung parenchyma (arrows). **(b)** High magnification, showing smooth muscle in wall of cyst (arrow). Arrowhead is in cyst lumen.

smooth muscle actin (SMA). They are also usually positive for HMB-45, a marker that is also expressed in melanomas and a variety of tumors allegedly derived from "perivascular epithelioid cells" ("PEComas"). HMB-45 staining in LAM is typically weak and focal (Figure 7.19), and may not be positive in every cyst or every smooth muscle fiber in a given focus. The percentage of HMB-45-positive cells per case has been reported to range from 17 to 67%. Most cases are at least focally HMB-45-positive.

- In the vast majority of cases, the patient is a woman with bilateral lung cysts on chest CT.

Variable pathologic findings

- The smooth muscle proliferation may occasionally be very striking, forming sheets or tiny nodules (Figure 7.20). Nodule formation, especially in the absence of cysts, should prompt consideration of other diagnoses such as benign metastasizing leiomyoma. Abnormal smooth muscle can occasionally be found in the walls of bronchioles.

- Hemosiderin-laden macrophages may be found within alveoli in the vicinity of the cyst or smooth muscle.
- Non-specific changes attributable to pneumothorax may be present (see section on pneumothorax for details).
- Micronodular pneumocyte hyperplasia, which has been described as a feature of LAM in tuberous sclerosis patients, is rarely seen in practice. It is a localized nodular proliferation of benign cuboidal epithelial cells (type 2 pneumocytes) lining alveolar walls.
- We have seen florid capillary proliferation mimicking pulmonary capillary hemangiomatosis, and multiple meningothelial-like nodules mimicking LAM smooth muscle co-existing with typical LAM cysts. The relationship between these lesions is unclear, but all are potentially hormone-driven.
- Unrelated pathologic processes may be found in addition to the cysts, resulting in unusual radiologic findings and prompting lung biopsy. One example is the presence of foamy macrophages within airspaces.

311

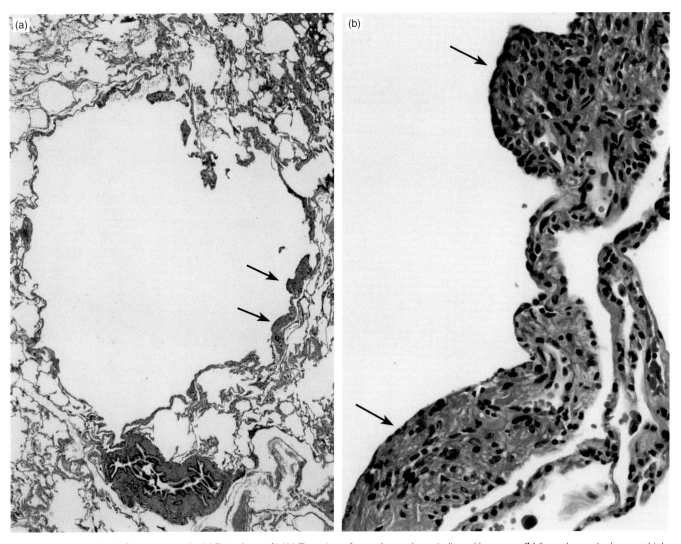

Figure 7.18. Lymphangioleiomyomatosis. (a) Typical cyst of LAM. Tiny wisps of smooth muscle are indicated by arrows. **(b)** Smooth muscle shown at high magnification. The abnormal smooth muscle proliferation is patchy and subtle (arrows).

- It is well established that LAM can be diagnosed on transbronchial lung biopsies if the abnormal smooth muscle fibers are included in the sample.
- Advanced cases of LAM may show extensive cystic change with large "bullous" cysts that can replace the normal lung parenchyma.
- Angiomyolipomas can be found in the hilum of the lung in patients with tuberous sclerosis.
- Estrogen receptors (ER) and progesterone receptors (PR) are expressed by the smooth muscle cells in the majority of cases.

Diagnostic work-up

Immunohistochemical staining is not mandatory for the diagnosis; however, HMB-45 staining is commonly performed, as discussed in the previous sections. In our experience, occasional cases are HMB-45 negative. Cathepsin K, a marker of PEComas, can be very helpful in such cases, since staining is stronger and more diffuse than HMB-45.

Clinical profile

LAM is almost exclusively a disease of women in the reproductive age group. The mean age at presentation is in the 30s, with a range of 21–62 years. Well-documented cases in men are exceedingly rare, and have usually occurred in the setting of tuberous sclerosis. Patients with LAM usually present with dyspnea, cough or symptoms attributable to spontaneous pneumothorax or recurrent pneumothoraces. Less common symptoms include hemoptysis, wheezing and chyloptysis. Chylous pleural effusions develop in some patients.

The association of LAM with tuberous sclerosis receives much attention, but is seldom an issue in routine surgical pathology practice since most cases of LAM are sporadic (i.e., not associated with a syndrome). The diagnosis of tuberous sclerosis is a complex topic outside the scope of this book. Overall, 13% of patients with lymphangiomyomatosis have tuberous sclerosis, and 30–40% of patients with tuberous sclerosis have lymphangiomyomatosis. When LAM occurs in the context of tuberous sclerosis, it is most often associated

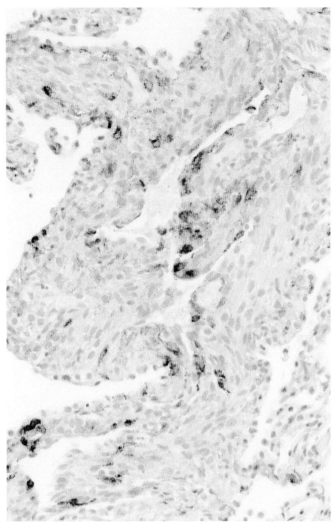

Figure 7.19. Lymphangioleiomyomatosis. Patchy weak staining for HMB-45 in the abnormal smooth muscle cells is typical.

with renal angiomyolipomas. In contrast, renal angiomyolipomas are less common in patients with sporadic LAM.

Radiologic findings

The radiologic findings of LAM, especially on chest CT, are characteristic, usually allowing a diagnosis to be made without a lung biopsy. They are characterized by the presence of numerous bilateral randomly distributed thin-walled cysts that are usually present within the lung parenchyma in all zones. Pleural effusions and interstitial reticular opacities are described in many patients. Patchy areas of ground-glass attenuation can be seen; these likely represent foci of intra-alveolar hemorrhage manifesting pathologically as hemosiderin-laden macrophages. Other entities such as pulmonary Langerhans cell histiocytosis, Birt–Hogg–Dubé syndrome and metastatic endometrial stromal sarcoma can present as multiple bilateral lung cysts and may mimic LAM radiologically.

Differential diagnosis

- Benign metastasizing leiomyoma. Diagnostic overlap with LAM occurs only in cases where smooth muscle proliferation

is florid. Benign metastasizing leiomyoma is characterized by solid nodules composed of smooth muscle, which are HMB-45-negative. They often contain entrapped lung epithelium.
- Metastatic endometrial stromal sarcoma. The metastatic lesions of this tumor in the lung have a peculiar tendency for cystic change and can mimic LAM closely. Immunohistochemical stains for CD10 and HMB-45 help to differentiate these lesions.
- Birt–Hogg–Dubé syndrome. These patients have cysts superficially resembling LAM, but they lack HMB-45-positive smooth muscle in their walls.
- Emphysema. Emphysema typically features lung destruction with freely floating alveolar septa. There is no HMB-45-positive smooth muscle.

Treatment and prognosis

The prognosis of LAM is variable. Most cases are characterized by slowly declining lung function despite therapy, with eventual respiratory failure and cor pulmonale. Reported survival rates at 10 years range from 79 to 91%.

A variety of anti-estrogen therapies such as oophorectomy, tamoxifen and progesterone have been tried, but their efficacy is questionable. Some patients are candidates for lung transplantation; a survival rate of 69% at 5 years after transplantation has been reported. However, it is unclear whether these results are superior to conventional medical therapy. The disease is known to recur after transplantation. The mTOR inhibitor sirolimus (rapamycin) has emerged in recent years as an alternative therapeutic option. Pneumothorax in LAM is treated as in other conditions.

Sample diagnosis on pathology report

Lung, right upper lobe, surgical biopsy – Lymphangioleiomyomatosis (See comment).

Birt–Hogg–Dubé syndrome

Birt–Hogg–Dubé syndrome is a rare autosomal dominant genodermatosis (inherited single gene disorder with skin manifestations) characterized by hair follicle hamartomas of the skin, spontaneous pneumothorax and renal tumors. The syndrome is caused by germline mutations in the folliculin (*FLCN*) gene, located on chromosome 17. This gene codes for the folliculin protein whose function has not yet been fully characterized. It is involved in the mTOR pathway and may be a regulator of cell-to-cell adhesion.

Major diagnostic findings

- Cysts within the lung parenchyma. These cysts appear as randomly distributed, air-filled, punched-out "holes" within the lung, resembling bullae or blebs (Figure 7.21 and Figure 7.1d). The surrounding lung is normal in most cases. The cyst walls show no evidence of a respiratory (ciliated) lining, and there is no widespread lung destruction. Importantly, there should be no evidence of HMB-45-positive abnormal smooth muscle in the wall of the cysts.

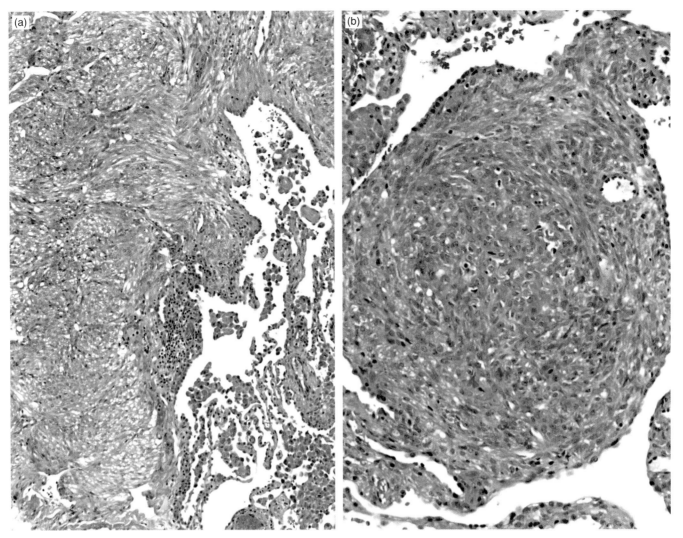

Figure 7.20. Lymphangioleiomyomatosis. (a) Florid proliferation of abnormal smooth muscle. Note hemosiderin-laden macrophages within airspaces at bottom right. **(b)** The abnormal smooth muscle forms a tiny nodule.

The cyst wall consists of normal alveolar septa lined by unremarkable alveolar pneumocytes (Figure 7.21). The overall appearance is rather non-distinctive. The possibility of Birt–Hogg–Dubé syndrome should always be considered when a cyst is found in a lung specimen from a lower lobe.

- The diagnosis can only be made in the following circumstances: (1) the radiologic findings are consistent with Birt–Hogg–Dubé syndrome, (2) there is a germline *FLCN* mutation, or (3) there is a history of skin or renal findings of Birt–Hogg–Dubé syndrome.

- The role of the pathologist is not to make a definitive diagnosis based on histologic findings, but to communicate the possibility of the syndrome to the clinician, who should then look for typical radiologic features and/or perform genetic testing for *FLCN* mutations. The diagnosis is best confirmed by genetic testing.

Variable pathologic findings

- The cysts may be subpleural, adjacent to bronchovascular bundles or located randomly deeper within the lung parenchyma. They often abut interlobular septa.

- There may be superimposed changes attributable to pneumothorax, such as subpleural fibrosis, chronic inflammation, scattered hemosiderin-laden macrophages, and reactive eosinophilic pleuritis. Such changes can be seen in any patient with a pneumothorax regardless of the underlying etiology. The cysts do not show inflammatory changes.

- The lung surrounding the cysts may occasionally show unrelated findings such as chronic inflammation, granulomas, or smoker's macrophages. Since the cysts are usually in the lower lobes, subpleural fibroelastotic scars (usually seen at the lung apices) are generally absent.

- "Intra-cystic septa" and "protruding venules", thought to represent residual interlobular septa, are present within the cysts in some cases.

Diagnostic work-up

No special stains are required. Immunohistochemistry reflects the fact that the cyst walls are made of normal alveolar septa, lined by alveolar pneumocytes.

(a)

(b)

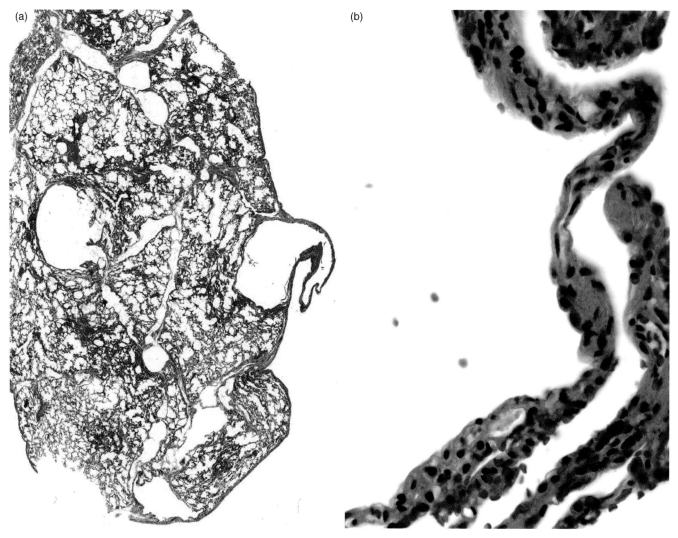

Figure 7.21. Birt–Hogg–Dubé syndrome. (a) Punched-out cysts in lung parenchyma. Most are subpleural or located adjacent to interlobular septa. **(b)** High magnification, showing unremarkable alveolar septa in the wall of a cyst.

Clinical profile

The reported age range is wide (7 to 83 years), but most patients present in the 20- to 40-year-old age group. A family history of similar clinical findings may be present, but is not mandatory, since the causative mutation can arise *de novo*. Pneumothoraces and skin manifestations tend to occur earlier than renal tumors. The disease occurs in both sexes without a consistent sex predilection, and in never-smokers as well as smokers. The characteristic triad (lung cysts, skin papules, renal tumors) is not present in all patients. Pulmonary cysts and skin lesions occur in more than 80% of patients, whereas renal tumors are seen in about a third.

The most common pulmonary manifestation of Birt–Hogg–Dubé syndrome is spontaneous pneumothorax. A history of recurrent and/or spontaneous pneumothoraces is common, and a history of spontaneous pneumothorax in family members may be present. Some patients do not have lung cysts. Even when cysts are present, lung function is usually unaffected. In some cases, spontaneous pneumothorax is the first manifestation of the disease. The age at which

pneumothorax can first occur is wide (7 to 71 years), with a median in the 30s. A few cases have been reported in which histologic examination of a lung specimen for spontaneous pneumothorax was the first clue to the presence of the syndrome. *FLCN* mutations have been documented in some patients with familial pneumothorax without skin or renal manifestations of Birt–Hogg–Dubé syndrome.

The skin lesions (fibrofolliculomas or trichodiscomas) typically present as multiple tiny white or skin-colored papules on the face, head, neck, upper trunk or arms. In most cases, skin lesions precede pulmonary manifestations and the diagnosis of Birt–Hogg–Dubé syndrome is made prior to pneumothorax. In the original report from Canada by Birt (a dermatologist), Hogg (a pathologist) and Dubé (an internist) in 1977, skin lesions usually appeared around age 25.

Renal tumors include oncocytoma, chromophobe renal cell carcinoma, clear cell carcinoma and/or peculiar hybrid tumors, which may be multifocal and/or bilateral. Multiple histologic types may occur in the same patient.

Radiologic findings

Radiologically, the lung cysts of Birt–Hogg–Dubé syndrome are typically bilateral, thin-walled, variably sized (2 mm to 8 cm), and randomly distributed. They are predominantly found within the lower lobes. They can vary in number from a few (5 to 10) to multiple (greater than 20) to innumerable.

Differential diagnosis

- Lymphangioleiomyomatosis (LAM). The finding of bilateral lung cysts in a young woman should raise the possibility of LAM. Renal tumors and skin manifestations can occur in both conditions. Histologic differentiation between the cysts of Birt–Hogg–Dubé syndrome and LAM should be straightforward since the former do not contain HMB-45-positive smooth muscle fibers in their walls. Radiologic findings help to differentiate the two in many cases, since LAM affects all lobes whereas Birt–Hogg–Dubé syndrome affects mainly the middle and lower lobes. In equivocal cases, definitive diagnosis requires mutation testing.
- Emphysema, blebs and bullae. Grossly and microscopically, the cysts of Birt–Hogg–Dubé syndrome may resemble blebs and bullae. In some cases, the clinical and radiologic setting – lower lobe cysts in a young never-smoker – may be a clue to the correct diagnosis. In contrast, blebs and bullae usually occur in the upper lobes of young men. Pathologically, in contrast to emphysema, there is no evidence of widespread alveolar septal destruction in Birt–Hogg–Dubé syndrome.
- Spontaneous pneumothorax. The most common differential diagnosis is idiopathic spontaneous pneumothorax. Changes related to pneumothorax, and other findings such as smoker's macrophages, may be present in both groups. The presence of punched-out cysts within the lung is the most important differentiating feature. As mentioned previously, since most cases of spontaneous pneumothorax occur in the apices of young men, a pneumothorax in the lower lobe of a woman should prompt a careful search for the cysts of Birt–Hogg–Dubé syndrome.

Treatment and prognosis

There is currently no effective treatment for the pulmonary cysts of Birt–Hogg–Dubé syndrome. Treatment for pneumothoraces in this disease is identical to that for pneumothorax in a sporadic setting. The diagnosis should prompt genetic counseling to identify affected family members and radiologic surveillance aimed at early identification of renal tumors. Morbidity is related mainly to the development of spontaneous recurrent pneumothoraces and renal tumors. There is no evidence that the syndrome leads to progressive respiratory impairment. In some cases, the lung cysts have remained stable for 4 years.

Sample diagnosis on pathology report

Lung, right lower lobe, surgical biopsy – Intraparenchymal cysts (See comment).

Approach to lung resections for pneumothorax

Wedge resections or resections of blebs and bullae from patients with pneumothorax are a common source of lung specimens for surgical pathologists. The approach to such cases is discussed in this chapter since some of the abnormalities that may be found in such specimens fall under the category of cystic lung disease. This section provides practical tips regarding expected pathologic findings, microscopic examination (what are we looking for?), and wording/diagnostic terminology in pathology reports.

Major diagnostic findings

There are no consistent or pathognomonic findings in pneumothorax specimens. Pathologic findings include changes caused by the pneumothorax, blebs or bullae (Figure 7.22), other abnormalities such as emphysema and fibrosis, and clues to the underlying etiology.

Variable pathologic findings

- The best known histologic finding in pneumothorax specimens is "reactive eosinophilic pleuritis", an inflammatory reaction to the presence of air in the pleura. It consists of a mix of eosinophils, macrophages, mesothelial cells and fibrin (Figure 7.23). Eosinophils may be strikingly increased in number, and may rarely involve the lung parenchyma and vessel walls, giving rise to a wide differential diagnosis. Knowledge of the clinical setting (pneumothorax) and the characteristic mix of cells should exclude these possibilities. Although it is reasonable to put this finding in the diagnostic line, it may be preferable instead to state "changes consistent with pneumothorax" and explain the details in a comment, since surgeons may not be familiar with this term.
- Variable degrees of pleural and subpleural fibrosis and scarring are common in pneumothorax specimens. The fibrosis may be subpleural and fibroelastotic in the apex of the lung (apical cap), or be composed of dense collagen. Localized areas of dome-shaped fibroblast proliferation (fibroblast foci) are common. These changes can be non-specific (common) or related to underlying interstitial lung disease (uncommon). A specific form of interstitial fibrosis, such as usual interstitial pneumonia, should not be diagnosed unless the fibrosis is extensive and the radiologic findings fit with underlying interstitial lung disease.
- Marked medial hypertrophy and intimal fibrosis can be present, resulting in thickened blood vessels. These findings should not be misinterpreted as evidence of pulmonary hypertension.

(a)

(b)

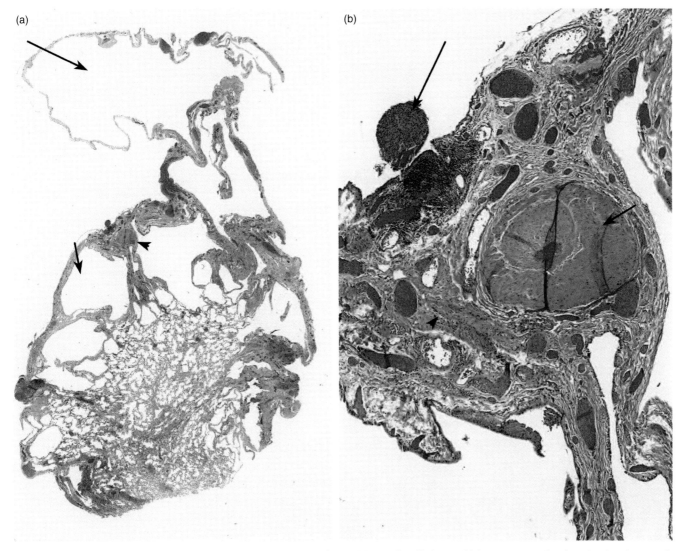

Figure 7.22. Bleb resection from a patient with spontaneous pneumothorax. (a) A small air-filled space (bleb) is seen protruding from the pleural aspect of the specimen (long arrow). Small air-filled spaces also abut the pleura (blebs or "distal acinar emphysema", short arrow). The area indicated by the arrowhead is magnified in b. **(b)** Reactive eosinophilic pleuritis (long arrow), thick-walled artery (short arrow) and non-specific fibrosis (arrowhead) are common findings in pneumothorax specimens.

- Exuberant type 2 pneumocyte hyperplasia mimicking adenocarcinoma has been described.
- The pathologic findings in blebs and bullae are discussed elsewhere (see "Emphysema"). In practice, a bleb or bulla cannot be found grossly or microscopically in many cases of spontaneous pneumothorax. This may be related to collapse of the bleb/bulla or the fact that some cases of pneumothorax may be caused by air leaks unrelated to blebs/bullae.
- Other than emphysema, blebs and bullae, clues to the underlying etiology are uncommon. These include well-documented causes of pneumothorax such as Birt–Hogg–Dubé syndrome, lymphangioleiomyomatosis and endometriosis, as well as findings whose relationship to pneumothorax is murky, such as bong lung. In the majority of specimens from patients with spontaneous pneumothorax, no specific etiology is found histologically (so-called "primary" spontaneous pneumothorax).

Table 7.4 lists the histologic findings to look for in these specimens.

Diagnostic work-up

No special stains are required unless changes suspicious for LAM or tumor are found.

Clinical profile

Pneumothorax can occur spontaneously in previously healthy individuals without an obvious cause (primary) or in patients with an underlying lung disease known to predispose to pneumothorax (such as emphysema or lymphangioleiomyomatosis). Indications for surgery in both situations include persistent air leak despite medical measures, and recurrent pneumothoraces. Primary pneumothorax can occur at any age and in both sexes. For reasons that remain unclear, many cases occur in tall, thin men in their 20s and 30s, and in smokers.

317

Table 7.4. Histologic findings in specimens from patients with spontaneous or recurrent pneumothorax

Findings caused by pneumothorax	Reactive eosinophilic pleuritis Fibrosis and chronic inflammation Type 2 pneumocyte hyperplasia Blood vessels: medial hypertrophy, intimal fibrosis, inflammation Pleural adhesions Small foci of acute lung injury (including organizing pneumonia)
Incidental or superimposed findings	Non-specific fibrosis and scarring Pulmonary apical cap (subpleural fibroelastotic scar in specimens from apices of upper lobes) Specific form of interstitial lung disease Smoker's macrophages (respiratory bronchiolitis) Macrophages with dark pigment in marijuana smokers (bong lung) Peribronchiolar chronic inflammation Malignant tumor
Histologic findings that may indicate the cause of pneumothorax*	Bullae or blebs Emphysema Placental transmogrification (bullous emphysema resembling placental tissue) Lymphangioleiomyomatosis Lung cysts of Birt–Hogg–Dubé syndrome Endometriosis *Paragonimus* organisms Pulmonary Langerhans cell histiocytosis

* Some low-grade metastatic sarcomas, most notoriously metastatic low-grade endometrial stromal sarcoma, may also cause pneumothorax, but these lesions are outside the scope of this book

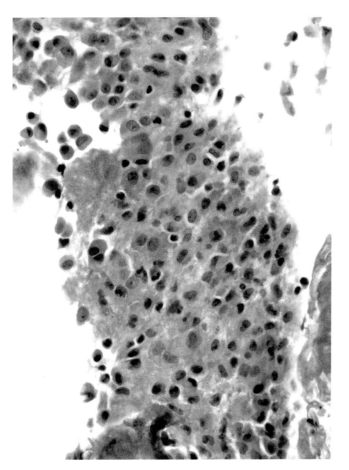

Figure 7.23. Reactive eosinophilic pleuritis. Note the characteristic mix of eosinophils, macrophages and reactive mesothelial cells in a fibrinous background.

Radiologic findings

These include features of the pneumothorax itself (air in the pleural cavity) and changes related to underlying etiology (blebs, bullae, emphysema, lymphangioleiomyomatosis, Birt–Hogg–Dubé syndrome).

Treatment and prognosis

Surgery for pneumothorax is generally performed for therapy, not for diagnostic purposes. The goal of the surgery is to close the air leak, fuse the pleural surfaces (typically with talc) and resect blebs or bullae. Subsequent treatment is not impacted by the pathologic diagnosis, unless a specific etiology is found. The rate at which a clinically significant diagnosis is made in a pneumothorax-related lung specimen varies from 0 to 8.3% (the latter using generous standards of clinical significance).

Sample diagnosis on pathology report

Lung, left upper lobe, bleb resection – Bleb, focal subpleural fibrosis, and changes consistent with pneumothorax (See comment).

Lung, right upper lobe, wedge resection – Features consistent with pneumothorax (See comment).

Lung, left upper lobe, wedge resection – Focal subpleural fibrosis and emphysema (See comment).

References

Intralobar sequestration

DeParedes CG, Pierce WS, Johnson DG, Waldhausen JA. Pulmonary sequestration in infants and children: a 20-year experience and review of the literature. *J Pediatr Surg* 1970;**5**:136–47.

Frazier AA, Rosado-de-Christenson ML, Stocker JT, Templeton PA. Intralobar sequestration: radiologic-pathologic correlation. *Radiographics* 1997;**17**:725–45.

Gompelmann D, Eberhardt R, Heubel C-P, *et al.* Lung sequestration: a rare cause for pulmonary symptoms in adulthood. *Respiration* 2011;**82**:445–50.

Nicolette LA, Kosloske AM, Bartow SA, Murphy S. Intralobar pulmonary sequestration: a clinical and pathological spectrum. *J Pediatr Surg* 1993;**28**:802–5.

Pryce DM. Lower accessory pulmonary artery with intralobar sequestration of lung: a report of seven cases. *J Pathol Bacteriol* 1946;**58**:457–67.

Riedlinger WFJ, Vargas SO, Jennings RW, *et al.* Bronchial atresia is common to extralobar sequestration, intralobar sequestration, congenital cystic adenomatoid malformation, and lobar emphysema. *Pediatr Dev Pathol* 2006;**9**:361–73.

Savic B, Birtel FJ, Tholen W, Funke HD, Knoche R. Lung sequestration: report of seven cases and review of 540 published cases. *Thorax* 1979;**34**:96–101.

Stocker JT, Malczak HT. A study of pulmonary ligament arteries. Relationship to intralobar pulmonary sequestration. *Chest* 1984;**86**:611–5.

Stocker JT. Sequestrations of the lung. *Semin Diagn Pathol* 1986;**3**:106–21.

Van Raemdonck D, De Boeck K, Devlieger H, *et al.* Pulmonary sequestration: a comparison between pediatric and adult patients. *Eur J Cardiothorac Surg* 2001;**19**:388–95.

Extralobar sequestration

Conran RM, Stocker JT. Extralobar sequestration with frequently associated congenital cystic adenomatoid malformation, type 2: report of 50 cases. *Pediatr Dev Pathol* 1999;**2**:454–63.

DeParedes CG, Pierce WS, Johnson DG, Waldhausen JA. Pulmonary sequestration in infants and children: a 20-year experience and review of the literature. *J Pediatr Surg* 1970;**5**:136–47.

Fraggetta F, Davenport M, Magro G, Cacciaguerra S, Nash R. Striated muscle cells in non-neoplastic lung tissue: a clinicopathologic study. *Hum Pathol* 2000;**31**:1477–81.

Laje P, Martinez-Ferro M, Grisoni E, Dudgeon D. Intraabdominal pulmonary sequestration. A case series and review of the literature. *J Pediatr Surg* 2006;**41**:1309–12.

Nijagal A, Jelin E, Feldstein VA, *et al.* The diagnosis and management of intradiaphragmatic extralobar pulmonary sequestrations: a report of 4 cases. *J Pediatr Surg* 2012;**47**:1501–5.

Recio Rodríguez M, Martínez de Vega V, Cano Alonso R, Carrascoso Arranz J, Martínez Ten P, Pérez Pedregosa J. MR imaging of thoracic abnormalities in the fetus. *Radiographics* 2012;**32**:E305–E321.

Riedlinger WFJ, Vargas SO, Jennings RW, *et al.* Bronchial atresia is common to extralobar sequestration, intralobar sequestration, congenital cystic adenomatoid malformation, and lobar emphysema. *Pediatr Dev Pathol* 2006;**9**:361–73.

Rosado-de-Christenson ML, Frazier AA, Stocker JT, Templeton PA. From the archives of the AFIP. Extralobar sequestration: radiologic-pathologic correlation. *Radiographics* 1993;**13**:425–41.

Savic B, Birtel FJ, Tholen W, Funke HD, Knoche R. Lung sequestration: report of seven cases and review of 540 published cases. *Thorax* 1979;**34**:96–101.

Stocker JT. Sequestrations of the lung. *Semin Diagn Pathol* 1986;**3**:106–21.

Congenital cystic adenomatoid malformation

Avitabile AM, Hulnick DH, Greco MA, Feiner HD. Congenital cystic adenomatoid malformation of the lung in adults. *Am J Surg Pathol* 1984;**8**:193–202.

Conran RM, Stocker JT. Extralobar sequestration with frequently associated congenital cystic adenomatoid malformation, type 2: report of 50 cases. *Pediatr Dev Pathol* 1999;**2**:454–63.

Lai PS, Cohen DW, Decamp MM, Fazio S, Roberts DH. A 40-year-old woman with an asymptomatic cystic lesion in her right lung. *Chest* 2009;**136**:622–7.

Langston C. New concepts in the pathology of congenital lung malformations. *Semin Pediatr Surg* 2003;**12**:17–37.

Luján M, Bosque M, Mirapeix RM, Marco MT, Asensio O, Domingo C. Late-onset congenital cystic adenomatoid malformation of the lung. Embryology, clinical symptomatology, diagnostic procedures, therapeutic approach and clinical follow-up. *Respiration* 2002;**69**:148–54.

MacSweeney F, Papagiannopoulos K, Goldstraw P, Sheppard MN, Corrin B, Nicholson AG. An assessment of the expanded classification of congenital cystic adenomatoid malformations and their relationship to malignant transformation. *Am J Surg Pathol* 2003;**27**:1139–46.

Oh BJ, Lee JS, Kim J-S, Lim C-M, Koh Y. Congenital cystic adenomatoid malformation of the lung in adults: clinical and CT evaluation of seven patients. *Respirology* 2006;**11**:496–501.

Riedlinger WFJ, Vargas SO, Jennings RW, *et al.* Bronchial atresia is common to extralobar sequestration, intralobar sequestration, congenital cystic adenomatoid malformation, and lobar emphysema. *Pediatr Dev Pathol* 2006;**9**:361–73.

Stocker JT. Cystic lung disease in infants and children. *Fetal Pediatr Pathol* 2009;**28**:155–84.

Stocker JT, Madewell JE, Drake RM. Congenital cystic adenomatoid malformation of the lung. Classification and morphologic spectrum. *Hum Pathol* 1977;**8**:155–71.

Bronchogenic cyst

Aktoğu S, Yuncu G, Halilçolar H, Ermete S, Buduneli T. Bronchogenic cysts: clinicopathological presentation and treatment. *Eur Respir J* 1996;**9**:2017–21.

Cioffi U, Bonavina L, De Simone M, *et al.* Presentation and surgical management of bronchogenic and esophageal duplication cysts in adults. *Chest* 1998;**113**:1492–6.

Langston C. New concepts in the pathology of congenital lung malformations. *Semin Pediatr Surg* 2003;**12**:17–37.

McAdams HP, Kirejczyk WM, Rosado-de-Christenson ML, Matsumoto S. Bronchogenic cyst: imaging features with clinical and histopathologic correlation. *Radiology* 2000;**217**:441–6.

Patel SR, Meeker DP, Biscotti CV, Kirby TJ, Rice TW. Presentation and management of bronchogenic cysts in the adult. *Chest* 1994;**106**:79–85.

Ribet ME, Copin MC, Gosselin B. Bronchogenic cysts of the mediastinum. *J Thorac Cardiovasc Surg* 1995;**109**:1003–10.

Salyer DC, Salyer WR, Eggleston JC. Benign developmental cysts of the mediastinum. *Arch Pathol Lab Med* 1977;**101**:136–9.

Stocker JT. Cystic lung disease in infants and children. *Fetal Pediatr Pathol* 2009;**28**:155–84.

St-Georges R, Deslauriers J, Duranceau A, *et al.* Clinical spectrum of bronchogenic cysts of the mediastinum and lung in the adult. *Ann Thorac Surg* 1991;**52**:6–13.

Zaugg M, Kaplan V, Widmer U, Baumann PC, Russi EW. Fatal air embolism in an airplane passenger with a giant intrapulmonary bronchogenic cyst. *Am J Respir Crit Care Med* 1998;**157**:1686–9.

Emphysema (including bullae and blebs)

Cavazza A, Lantuejoul S, Sartori G, *et al.* Placental transmogrification of the lung: clinicopathologic, immunohistochemical and molecular study of two cases, with particular emphasis on the interstitial clear cells. *Hum Pathol* 2004;**129**:686–9.

Fidler ME, Koomen M, Sebek B, Greco MA, Rizk CC, Askin FB. Placental transmogrification of the lung, a histologic variant of giant bullous emphysema. Clinicopathological study of three further cases. *Am J Surg Pathol* 1995;**19**:563–70.

Gough J. The pathological diagnosis of emphysema. *Proc Roy Soc Med* 1952;**45**:576–7.

Hansell DM, Bankier AA, MacMahon H, McLoud TC, Müller NL, Remy J. Fleischner society: glossary of terms for thoracic imaging. *Radiology* 2008;**246**;697–722.

Katzenstein A-L A, Mukhopadhyay S, Zanardi C, Dexter EE. Clinically occult interstitial fibrosis in smokers: classification and significance of a surprisingly common finding in lobectomy specimens. *Hum Pathol* 2010;**41**:316–25.

Keller CA, Naunheim KS, Osterloh J, Espiritu J, McDonald JW, Ramos RR. Histopathologic diagnosis made in lung tissue resected from patients with severe emphysema undergoing lung volume reduction surgery. *Chest* 1997;**111**:941–7.

Leopold JG, Gough J. The centrilobular form of hypertrophic emphysema and its relation to chronic bronchitis. *Thorax* 1957;**12**:219–35.

Rabe KF, Hurd S, Anzueto A, *et al.* Global strategy for the diagnosis, management and prevention of chronic obstructive pulmonary disease. GOLD executive summary. *Am J Respir Crit Care Med* 2007;**176**:532–55.

Snider GL, Kleinerman J, Thurlbeck WM, Bengali ZH. The definition of emphysema. Report of a National Heart, Lung and Blood Institute, Division of Lung Diseases Workshop. *Am Rev Resp Dis* 1985;**132**:182–5.

Stoller JK, Aboussouan LS. A review of α-1 antitrypsin deficiency. *Am J Respir Crit Care Med* 2012;**185**:246–59.

Pulmonary interstitial emphysema

Barcia SM, Kukreja J, Jones KD. Pulmonary interstitial emphysema in adults: a clinicopathologic study of 53 lung explants. *Am J Surg Pathol* 2014;**38**:339–45.

Belcher E, Abbasi MA, Hansell DM, *et al.* Persistent interstitial pulmonary emphysema requiring pneumonectomy. *J Thorac Cardiovasc Surg* 2009;**138**:237–9.

Campbell RE. Intrapulmonary interstitial emphysema: a complication of hyaline membrane disease. *Am J Roentgenol* 1970;**110**:449–56.

Demura Y, Ishizaki T, Nakanishi M, Ameshima S, Itoh H. Persistent diffuse pulmonary interstitial emphysema mimicking pulmonary emphysema. *Thorax* 2007;**62**:652.

Guo HH, Sweeney RT, Regula D, *et al.* Best cases from the AFIP: fatal 2009 influenza A (H1N1) infection, complicated by acute respiratory distress syndrome and pulmonary interstitial emphysema. *Radiographics* 2010;**30**:327–33.

Keszler M, Donn SM, Bucciarelli RL, *et al.* Multicenter controlled trial comparing high-frequency jet ventilation and conventional mechanical ventilation in newborn infants with pulmonary interstitial emphysema. *J Pediatr* 1991;**119**:85–93.

Macklin CC. Transport of air along sheaths of pulmonic blood vessels from alveoli to mediastinum. Clinical implications. *Arch Intern Med* 1939;**64**:913–26.

Macklin MT, Macklin CC. Malignant interstitial emphysema of the lungs and mediastinum as an important occult complication in many respiratory diseases and other conditions: an interpretation of the clinical literature in light of laboratory experiment. *Medicine* 1944;**23**:281–358.

Stocker JT, Madewell JE. Persistent interstitial pulmonary emphysema: another complication of the respiratory distress syndrome. *Pediatrics* 1977;**59**:847–57.

Wintermark M, Schnyder P. The Macklin effect. A frequent etiology for pneumomediastinum in blunt chest trauma. *Chest* 2001;**120**:543–7.

Lymphangioleiomyomatosis

Abbott GF, Rosado-de-Christenson ML, Frazier AA, Franks TJ, Pugatch RD, Galvin JR. From the archives of the AFIP: lymphangioleiomyomatosis: radiologic-pathologic correlation. *Radiographics* 2005;**25**:803–28.

Aubry MC, Myers JL, Ryu JH, *et al.* Pulmonary lymphangioleiomyomatosis in a man. *Am J Respir Crit Care Med* 2000;**162**:749–52.

Bonetti F, Chiodera PL, Pea M, *et al.* Transbronchial biopsy in lymphangiomyomatosis of the lung. HMB45 for diagnosis. *Am J Surg Pathol* 1993;**17**:1092–102.

Chu SC, Horiba K, Usuki J, *et al.* Comprehensive evaluation of 35 patients with lymphangiomyomatosis. *Chest* 1999;**115**:1041–52.

Cohen MM, Pollock-BarZiv S, Johnson SR. Emerging clinical picture of lymphangioleiomyomatosis. *Thorax* 2005;**60**:875–9.

Corrin B, Liebow AA, Friedman PJ. Pulmonary lymphangiomyomatosis. A review. *Am J Pathol* 1975;**79**:348–82.

Glassberg MK. To be or not to be a neoplasm: what is lymphangioleiomyomatosis? Are we calling it what it really is? *Am J Respir Crit Care Med* 2013;**188**:397–8.

Hayashi T, Kumasaka T, Mitani K, *et al.* Prevalence of uterine and adnexal involvement in pulmonary lymphangioleiomyomatosis: a clinicopathologic study of 10 patients. *Am J Surg Pathol* 2011;**35**:1776–85.

Kitaichi M, Nishimura K, Itoh H, Izumi T. Pulmonary lymphangioleiomyomatosis: a report of 46 patients including a clinicopathologic study of prognostic factors. *Am J Respir Crit Care Med* 1995;**151**:527–33.

McCormack FX, Travis WD, Colby TV, Henske EP, Moss J. Lymphangioleiomyomatosis: calling it what it is: a low-grade, destructive, metastasizing neoplasm. *Am J Respir Crit Care Med* 2012;**186**:1210–2.

Birt–Hogg–Dubé syndrome

Ayo DS, Aughenbaugh GL, Yi ES, Hand JL, Ryu JH. Cystic lung disease in Birt-Hogg-Dubé syndrome. *Chest* 2007;**132**:679–84.

Butnor KJ, Guinee DG Jr. Pleuropulmonary pathology of Birt-Hogg-Dubé syndrome. *Am J Surg Pathol* 2006;**30**:395–9.

Faber A, Borie R, Debray MP, Crestani B, Danel C. Distinguishing the histological and radiological features of cystic lung disease in Birt-Hogg-Dubé syndrome from those of tobacco-related spontaneous pneumothorax. *Histopathology* 2014;**64**:741–9.

Furuya M, Tanaka R, Koga S, *et al.* Pulmonary cysts of Birt-Hogg-Dubé syndrome: a clinicopathologic and immunohistochemical study of 9 families. *Am J Surg Pathol* 2012;**36**:589–600.

Graham RB, Nolasco M, Peterlin B, Garcia CK. Nonsense mutations in folliculin presenting as isolated familial spontaneous pneumothorax in adults. *Am J Respir Crit Care Med* 2005;**172**:39–44.

Kumasaka T, Hayashi T, Mitani K, *et al.* Characterization of pulmonary cysts in Birt-Hogg-Dubé syndrome: histopathologic and morphometric analysis of 229 pulmonary cysts from 50 unrelated patients. *Histopathology* 2014;**65**:100–10.

Menko FH, van Steensel MAM, Giraud S, *et al.* Birt-Hogg-Dubé syndrome: diagnosis and management. *Lancet Oncol* 2009;**10**:1199–206.

Nickerson ML, Warren MB, Toro JR, *et al.* Mutations in a novel gene lead to kidney tumors, lung wall defects, and benign tumors of the hair follicle in patients with the Birt-Hogg-Dubé syndrome. *Cancer Cell* 2002;**2**:157–64.

Painter JN, Tapanainen H, Somer M, Tukiainen P, Aittomaki K. A 4-bp deletion in the Birt-Hogg-Dubé gene (FLCN) causes dominantly inherited spontaneous pneumothorax. *Am J Hum Genet* 2005;**76**:522–7.

Sauter JL, Butnor KJ. Pathological findings in spontaneous pneumothorax specimens: does the incidence of unexpected clinically significant findings justify routine histological examination? *Histopathology* 2014; Epub ahead of print.

Approach to lung resections for pneumothorax

Askin FB, McCann BG, Kuhn C. Reactive eosinophilic pleuritis: a lesion to be distinguished from pulmonary eosinophilic granuloma. *Arch Pathol Lab Med* 1977;**101**:187–91.

Cyr PV, Vincic L, Kay JM. Pulmonary vasculopathy in idiopathic spontaneous pneumothorax in young subjects. *Arch Pathol Lab Med* 2000;**124**:717–20.

Faber A, Borie R, Debray MP, Crestani B, Danel C. Distinguishing the histological and radiological features of cystic lung disease in Birt-Hogg-Dubé syndrome from those of tobacco-related spontaneous pneumothorax. *Histopathology* 2014;**64**:741–9.

Fraire A. Histopathology of pneumothorax: potential diagnostic pitfalls. *Arch Pathol Lab Med* 2007;**131**:848–9.

Luna E, Tomashefski JF Jr, Brown D, Clarke RE. Reactive eosinophilic pulmonary vascular infiltration in patients with spontaneous pneumothorax. *Am J Surg Pathol* 1994;**18**:195–9.

Khan OA, Tsang GM, Barlow CW, Amer KM. Routine histological analysis of resected lung tissue in primary spontaneous pneumothorax: is it justified? *Heart Lung Circ* 2006;**15**:137–8.

Noppen M. Spontaneous pneumothorax: epidemiology, pathophysiology and cause. *Eur Respir Rev* 2010;**19**:217–9.

Sauter JL, Butnor KJ. Pathological findings in spontaneous pneumothorax specimens: does the incidence of unexpected clinically significant findings justify routine histological examination? *Histopathology* 2014; Epub ahead of print.

Schneider F, Murali R, Veraldi KL, Tazelaar HD, Leslie KO. Approach to lung biopsies from patients with pneumothorax. *Arch Pathol Lab Med* 2014;**138**:257–65.

Shilo K, Colby TV, Travis WD, Franks TJ. Exuberant type 2 pneumocyte hyperplasia associated with spontaneous pneumothorax: secondary reactive change mimicking adenocarcinoma. *Mod Pathol* 2007;**20**:352–6.

Pigment-laden macrophages in the lung

This chapter discusses diseases in which the presence of pigment (or dust) within macrophages is a prominent histologic feature. Some conditions in which this finding occurs are *occupational lung disease*s, including *pneumoconioses* caused by exposure to mineral dusts. In others, the presence of pigment within macrophages is related to cigarette smoking or prior hemorrhage. Figure 8.1 shows a few of these conditions side-by-side at identical magnification. Figure 8.2 presents an algorithm for the differential diagnosis. Table 8.1 lists a few pearls and pitfalls related to the evaluation of these diseases. Smoking-related diseases are discussed in Chapters 4 and 5, and the differential diagnosis of hemosiderin-laden macrophages is addressed in Chapter 4. Asbestosis is included here rather than in the chapter on interstitial diseases because a few scattered dust-laden macrophages are often a clue to the presence of nearby asbestos bodies (Figure 8.1a).

Coal workers' pneumoconiosis

Coal workers' pneumoconiosis is a well-known occupational lung disease of coal miners caused by excessive deposition of coal mine dust in the lungs. It is important to emphasize at the outset that coal miners may also develop other pneumoconioses such as silicosis, and are susceptible to other infectious, inflammatory and malignant diseases that occur in the general population. In the vast majority of cases, the diagnosis of coal workers' pneumoconiosis is based on radiologic findings on chest radiographs, an occupational history of exposure to coal dust for an appropriate duration, appropriate latency between exposure and disease manifestations, and reasonable exclusion of alternative etiologies. Pathologic input is seldom if ever required. Rarely, the pathologic findings of this disease may be encountered serendipitously by surgical pathologists in lungs resected for other reasons, or at autopsy.

Major diagnostic findings

- The hallmark of coal workers' pneumoconiosis is the presence of numerous macrophages laden with black dust in the walls of small airways, including small non-respiratory bronchioles, respiratory bronchioles and alveolar ducts (Figures 8.3 and 8.4, Figure 8.1b). Traditional descriptions of these dust-filled interstitial lesions are based on whether they are grossly palpable. Grossly non-palpable lesions are termed *macules* and palpable lesions are known as *nodules*. Grossly palpable lesions tend to be microscopically fibrotic. Thus, macules

are interstitial deposits of dust-laden macrophages without associated fibrosis, whereas dust-filled lesions with fibrosis are nodules (Figure 8.5). Macules usually have irregular or stellate outlines, and are typically centered on respiratory bronchioles. As with other lesions centered on distal small airways, the presence of an adjacent artery is a clue to the anatomic location of the lesion. Nodules tend to be slightly more rounded in shape than macules.
- An occupational history of exposure to coal dust is mandatory for the diagnosis. An element of subjective judgement is required to determine whether the duration of exposure and latency are appropriate.

Variable pathologic findings

- The term *progressive massive fibrosis* is used by pathologists as well as radiologists. Pathologically, progressive massive fibrosis is defined as a fibrotic mass measuring > 1 cm, formed by the coalescence of multiple smaller fibrotic nodules. Since chest radiographs cannot definitively differentiate fibrotic masses from other inflammatory or neoplastic masses, the radiologic designation of progressive massive fibrosis is based primarily on size (> 1 cm). The large fibrotic masses formed by progressive massive fibrosis distort lung architecture, destroy and obliterate normal structures and cause considerable morbidity. The term is also applied to large fibrotic masses formed by confluent fibrosis in other pneumoconioses such as silicosis. See Figure 6.13a in Chapter 6 for an example of this phenomenon.
- Another form of fibrosis known as *diffuse interstitial fibrosis* may occur in coal workers' pneumoconiosis. In contrast to progressive massive fibrosis, it is characterized by expansion of alveolar septa without significant distortion of lung architecture.
- Concurrent emphysema is common, and may contribute significantly to the clinical, radiologic and pathologic manifestations (Figure 8.3). It may appear as alveolar distension adjacent to macules or nodules ("focal emphysema"), or true emphysema related to cigarette smoking.
- Dust-laden macrophages also accumulate in the pleura, lymphatics and interlobular septa, resulting in extensive black discoloration of the affected lungs on gross examination. Dust-laden macrophages are also common within alveoli. The black color and coarse nature of the dust helps to differentiate these macrophages from

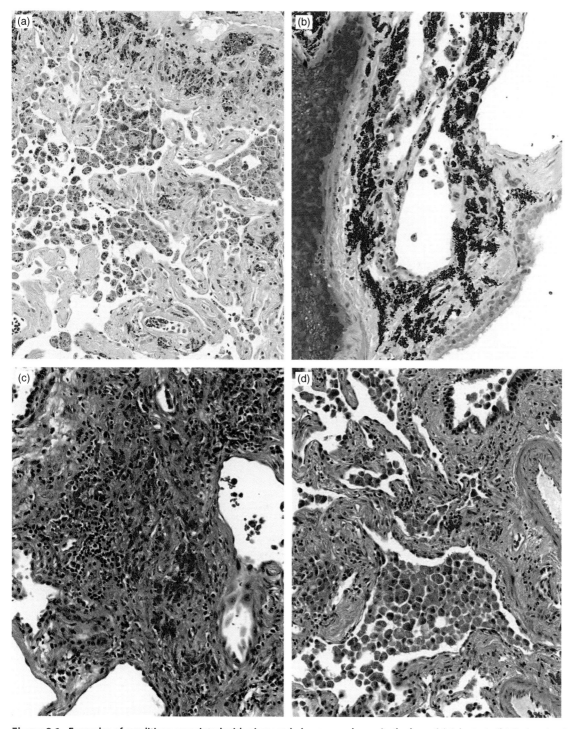

Figure 8.1. Examples of conditions associated with pigment-laden macrophages in the lung. (a) Asbestosis. **(b)** Coal workers' pneumoconiosis. **(c)** Mixed-dust pneumoconiosis. **(d)** Respiratory (smoker's) bronchiolitis. All images are shown at identical magnification.

smoker's macrophages and hemosiderin-laden macrophages.
- Peribronchial and hilar lymph nodes in coal workers' pneumoconiosis are often black on gross examination due to the presence of large numbers of pigmented macrophages within the sinusoids. Silicotic nodules are commonly found in these lymph nodes, even in the absence of silicotic nodules in the lung.

- Silicotic nodules identical to those seen in silicosis may also occur in the lungs of coal workers (see differential diagnosis).

Diagnostic work-up

A trichome or Movat pentachrome stain can highlight collagen deposition and may help to differentiate between macules and nodules.

Clinical profile

By definition, coal workers' pneumoconiosis is a disease of coal miners. The mean age is 62 years, and most patients are men. The average duration of work in mines prior to disease is 26 years. The clinical presentation is non-specific. Miners with mild forms of the disease can be asymptomatic. However, as the lesions become fibrotic and coalesce into progressive massive fibrosis, they are associated with respiratory symptoms and pulmonary function abnormalities. Chronic cough, black-tinged sputum and dyspnea are the most common symptoms.

Table 8.1. Pearls and pitfalls related to the evaluation of pigment-laden macrophages in the lung

Pigment-laden macrophages within the airspaces are most commonly related to cigarette smoking or hemosiderin

Both smoker's macrophages and hemosiderin-laden macrophages are positive on iron stains; misinterpretation is common

Some pneumoconioses (silicosis, asbestosis) can be diagnosed on the basis of pathologic findings, but in others (coal workers' pneumoconiosis, mixed-dust pneumoconiosis) definitive diagnosis requires an occupational history

Not all ferruginous (iron-coated) bodies are asbestos bodies

Asbestos bodies are ferruginous bodies with a thin transparent core

Asbestos bodies are indicative of asbestos exposure but not necessarily asbestosis

A pathologic diagnosis of asbestosis requires asbestos bodies + diffuse interstitial fibrosis in the appropriate pattern

Look for asbestos bodies in cases of mesothelioma and lung cancer. They are mostly found in alveolated lung parenchyma

Radiologic findings

Chest radiographs (X-rays) play a vital role in the diagnosis of coal workers' pneumoconiosis. They typically show multiple and bilateral *small rounded opacities* located predominantly in the upper zones of the lungs. Traditionally, chest radiographs for pneumoconioses – including coal workers' pneumoconiosis, silicosis and asbestosis – are evaluated by the International Labor Organization (ILO) classification system, which categorizes opacities according to their shape and size. Coal workers' pneumoconiosis is classified into *simple* and *complicated* types depending on the size of the lesions. In simple coal workers' pneumoconiosis, the lesions are 1 cm or less in size. Lesions larger than 1 cm – generally thought to be caused by progressive massive fibrosis – are classified as complicated coal workers' pneumoconiosis. Such lesions can undergo cavitation or calcification. Other superimposed complications such as lung carcinoma and infection can mimic progressive massive fibrosis. Individuals with mild forms of the disease may have no abnormalities on chest X-ray. It is also important to recognize that the chest X-ray findings in coal workers' pneumoconiosis can be virtually identical to silicosis.

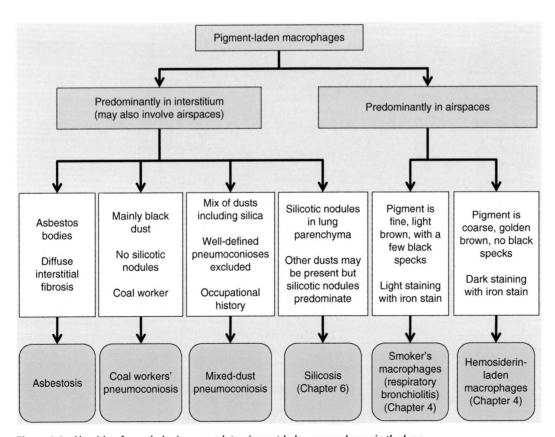

Figure 8.2. Algorithm for pathologic approach to pigment-laden macrophages in the lung.

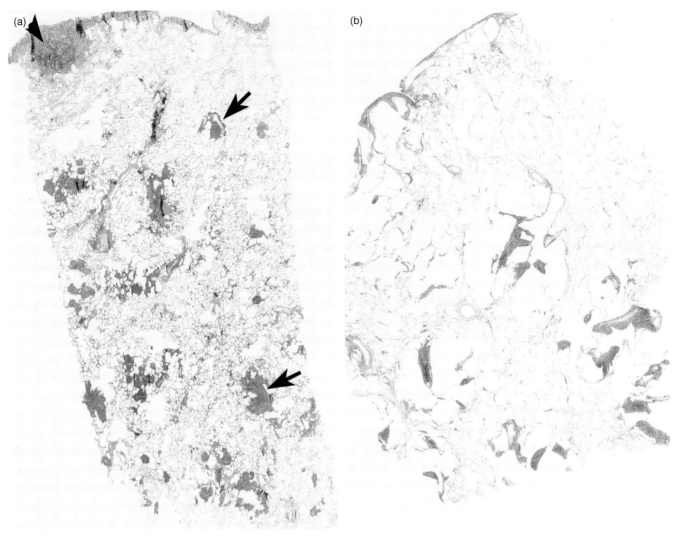

Figure 8.3. Coal workers' pneumoconiosis. (a) Scanning magnification, showing extensive deposition of black dust in the lung. Note deposition of dust in the pleura (arrowhead) and along bronchovascular bundles (arrows). **(b)** Another case shows areas of emphysema associated with dust deposits. Case courtesy of Dr. Jerrold Abraham.

Differential diagnosis

- From the pathologist's perspective, the main finding that can be mistaken for coal workers' pneumoconiosis is deposition of black dust (so-called "anthracotic pigment") in the bronchioles, presumably caused by usual, day-to-day exposure to environmental dust. Some degree of dust deposition in the walls of bronchi and bronchioles is not uncommon in the general population. In the hilar and peribronchial lymph nodes, dust-laden macrophages are so common as to be virtually a normal finding. The key to the diagnosis of coal workers' pneumoconiosis in such situations is *excessive* dust deposition combined with the appropriate occupational history.

- Mixed-dust pneumoconiosis shares certain features with coal workers' pneumoconiosis, including interstitial deposition of black dust and fibrotic lesions. Mixed-dust pneumoconiosis should be diagnosed if there is no history of exposure to coal dust and the dust deposits include silica or if silicotic nodules are present in the lung but are overshadowed by other types of dust deposition.

- As mentioned previously, silicosis does occasionally occur in coal workers. The main requirement for the diagnosis of silicosis is the same whether the individual is a coal miner or not, i.e., silicotic nodules must be present in the lung, and must be the predominant feature. Silicotic nodules must be distinguished from fibrotic nodules that occur in coal workers' pneumoconiosis. The whorled, lamellated appearance that characterizes silicotic nodules is not seen in the collagenized nodules of coal workers' pneumoconiosis.

Treatment and prognosis

There is no effective treatment. The prognosis depends on the extent of fibrosis.

Sample diagnosis on pathology report

Lung, right, pneumonectomy – Dust macules and nodules, consistent with coal workers' pneumoconiosis (See comment).

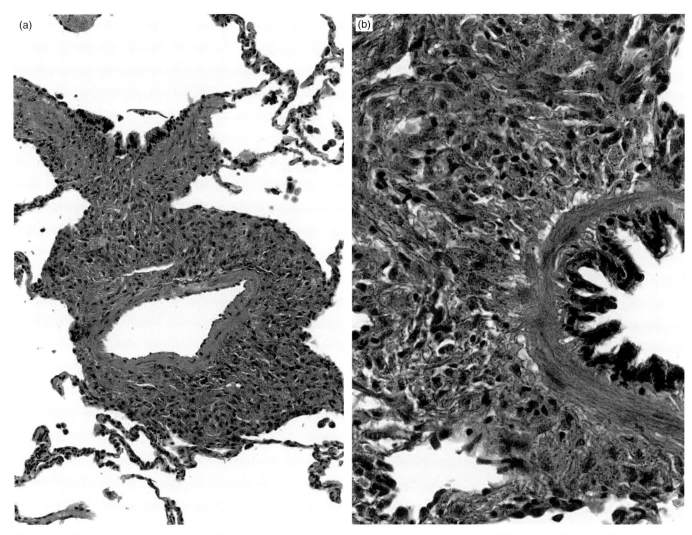

(a)

(b)

Figure 8.4. Coal workers' pneumoconiosis. (a) Dust-laden macrophages in the wall of a respiratory bronchiole. **(b)** Another small airway at higher magnification, showing black dust within macrophages.

Mixed-dust pneumoconiosis

Mixed-dust pneumoconiosis is a term used for any pneumoconiosis caused by exposure to a mix of crystalline silica and less fibrogenic dusts including silicates, carbon derived from coal, non-coal carbon, iron, kaolin and feldspar. Exposure to these types of mixed dusts does cause bona fide pneumoconiosis, but the findings may be difficult to classify since the affected individuals may not be coal miners, and diagnostic pathologic findings such as silicotic nodules or asbestos bodies may be absent. Such cases do not meet criteria for well-defined entities such as coal workers' pneumoconiosis, silicosis or asbestosis. The term *mixed-dust pneumoconiosis* provides a diagnostic label for these unclassifiable pneumoconioses. The precise mix of particles is variable but must include some amount of crystalline silica. The diagnostic criteria are summarized in Table 8.2.

Thus defined, mixed-dust pneumoconiosis results from a wide variety of exposures, including those traditionally associated with silicosis, such as pottery or foundry work. In addition, mixed-dust pneumoconiosis can occur in occupations unrelated to disruption of quartz-containing rocks, as well as in domestic settings that would not ordinarily be associated with pneumoconiosis. *Hut lung,* or *domestically acquired particulate lung disease,* is a form of mixed-dust pneumoconiosis caused by long-term exposure to smoke derived from biomass-fueled stoves in poorly ventilated domestic settings, most commonly huts. Biomass fuels are materials such as wood, charcoal, dung, crop residues, corn cobs and grass, all of which are used widely in developing countries as a source of fuel for cooking and other purposes. Hut lung is thought to be widespread in the developing world, although only a few pathologically confirmed cases have been reported. Potential sources of exposure to silica in the domestic setting include plant and charcoal combustion, as well as dust derived from grinding stones used in maize-grinding.

Major diagnostic findings

- The key histologic features in mixed-dust pneumoconiosis are *macules* and *mixed-dust fibrosis lesions*. These lesions are conceptually and morphologically similar to macules and nodules in coal workers' pneumoconiosis. Macules are interstitial accumulations of dust-laden macrophages

Table 8.2. Criteria for diagnosis of mixed-dust pneumoconiosis

Abnormal deposition of dust within the lung

Dust must contain at least some crystalline silica particles

Variable mix of macules (non-fibrous) and nodules (fibrous)

Silicotic nodules may be present but must not predominate

Criteria for asbestosis, silicosis or coal workers' pneumoconiosis must not be met

Occupational history of exposure to dust

Adapted from Honma *et al*, 2004 (see references).

without obvious collagenization, whereas mixed-dust fibrosis lesions are collagenized. The latter typically have a stellate shape and irregular contours. The deposited dust is a mix of crystalline silica and non-siliceous dusts, the latter often including black carbonaceous dust (Figures 8.6 to 8.8, Figure 8.1c).

- A definitive diagnosis of mixed-dust pneumoconiosis requires an appropriate exposure history, without which the pathologic diagnosis must be descriptive. The diagnosis of hut lung requires long-term exposure to biomass fuel-derived smoke in a domestic environment.

Variable pathologic findings

- Grossly, lungs with mixed-dust pneumoconiosis show evidence of excessive dust deposition. In some cases, gross examination shows features suggesting extensive fibrosis, including honeycomb change (Figure 8.9).
- Microscopically, interstitial fibrosis of varying degrees may be present. In some areas, the combination of patchy interstitial fibrosis and fibroblast foci may resemble UIP (Figure 8.10). As in other forms of pneumoconiosis,

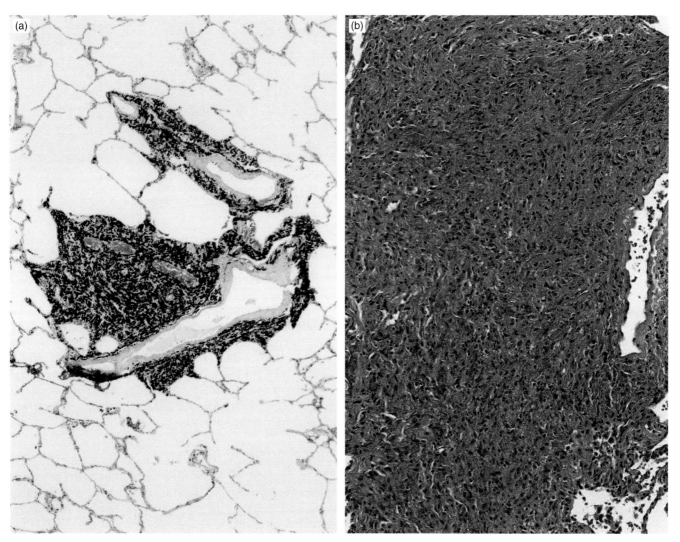

Figure 8.5. Coal workers' pneumoconiosis. (a) Non-fibrotic dust-filled lesion: macule. **(b)** Collagenized dust-filled lesion: nodule.

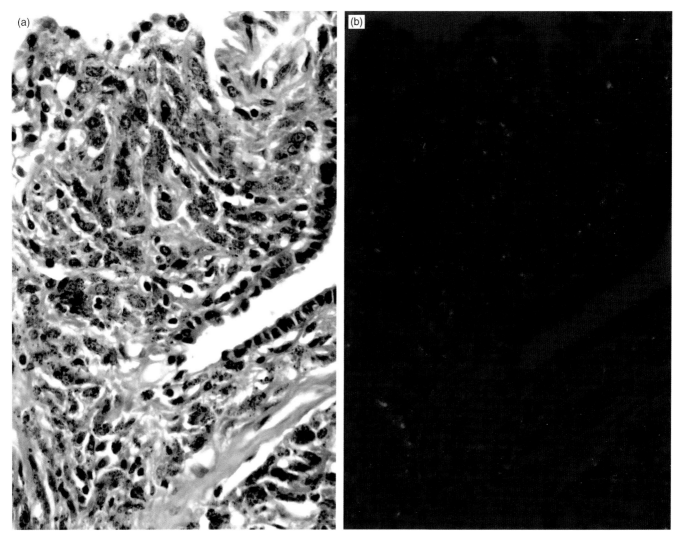

Figure 8.6. Mixed-dust pneumoconiosis. (a) Numerous dust-laden macrophages. **(b)** Examination under polarized light reveals admixed silica and silicate particles (weak or bright white), but also many other types of non-siliceous particles (non-birefringent or red). These images are from a steel foundry worker who was a core maker for 8 years. He developed end-stage fibrosis requiring lung transplantation. Energy-dispersive X-ray spectroscopy confirmed a mix of silica, silicates and many other types of particles including iron and zirconium.

coalescence of individual mixed-dust fibrosis lesions may lead to progressive massive fibrosis.

- Silicotic nodules may or may not be present. If present, they should be overshadowed by mixed-dust fibrosis lesions.
- Superimposed tuberculosis is thought to be less common in mixed-dust pneumoconiosis than in silicosis.
- Macrophages may be prominent within airspaces. They may show emperipolesis (Figure 8.10).
- Non-asbestos ferruginous bodies may be identified (Figure 8.8).

Diagnostic work-up

Polarizing microscopy helps to detect silica particles, supporting the diagnosis (Figures 8.6 and 8.7). See the section on silicosis in Chapter 6 for details of detection and identification of silica and silicate particles. Scanning electron microscopy

with energy-dispersive X-ray spectroscopy (SEM/EDS) of involved lung tissue reveals many more inorganic particles than are apparent under polarized light. Particle types detected include carbonaceous particles, silica, silicates and metallic particles containing iron or titanium (Figure 8.11). Very tiny or fine crystalline silica particles can be seen only by SEM/EDS because they are too small to be detected by polarized light microscopy. Special stains for collagen such as trichrome stains or the Movat pentachrome stain can help to differentiate macules from mixed-dust fibrotic lesions.

Clinical profile

The symptoms of mixed-dust pneumoconiosis are non-specific, and overlap greatly with other chronic fibrosing lung diseases. Pulmonary functions may be normal, obstructive, restrictive or mixed.

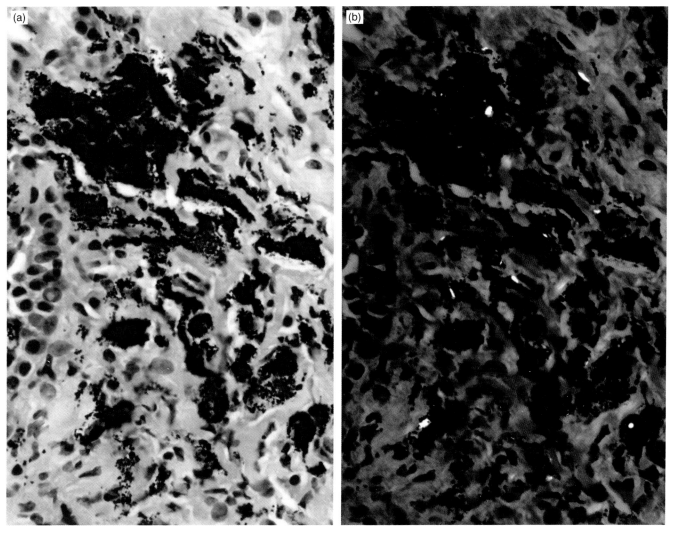

Figure 8.7. Mixed-dust pneumoconiosis (hut lung). (a) Extensive deposition of black dust within macrophages in the wall of a small bronchiole. **(b)** Under polarized light, a few birefringent silica and silicate particles are admixed with numerous particles of non-birefringent black dust. This woman used firewood and charcoal for cooking in a poorly ventilated hut for several years.

Radiologic findings

Chest radiographs may show a mix of small rounded and irregular opacities, but are normal in some cases. Small rounded nodules tend to have ill-defined contours. Chest CT findings include reticular or reticulonodular opacities.

Differential diagnosis

- The differential diagnosis with coal workers' pneumoconiosis is addressed in the preceding discussion on that topic.
- Silicotic nodules are the defining feature of silicosis but may also be present in mixed-dust pneumoconiosis. The principal difference between these entities is that silicotic nodules are the main pathologic abnormality in silicosis, whereas they are overshadowed by other types of dust in mixed-dust pneumoconiosis.
- The combination of asbestos bodies and diffuse interstitial fibrosis is diagnostic of asbestosis. However, if dust macules or mixed-dust fibrosis lesions are also present, the diagnosis should be *mixed-dust pneumoconiosis with asbestosis*.
- We have seen cases of mixed-dust pneumoconiosis that mimicked IPF clinically and radiologically. These patients underwent lung transplantation for end-stage fibrosis, at which time the true nature of the process became apparent only after pathologic examination of the explanted lungs. The history of significant occupational exposure to unusual dusts was obtained only in retrospect, prompted by the pathologic findings. Pathologically, mixed-dust pneumoconiosis can show some features of UIP such as patchy fibrosis, fibroblast foci and honeycomb change. However, the process is far more cellular, and the degree of dust deposition is greatly in excess of background levels expected in the general population. A detailed exposure history should be obtained in order to corroborate the pathologic impression.

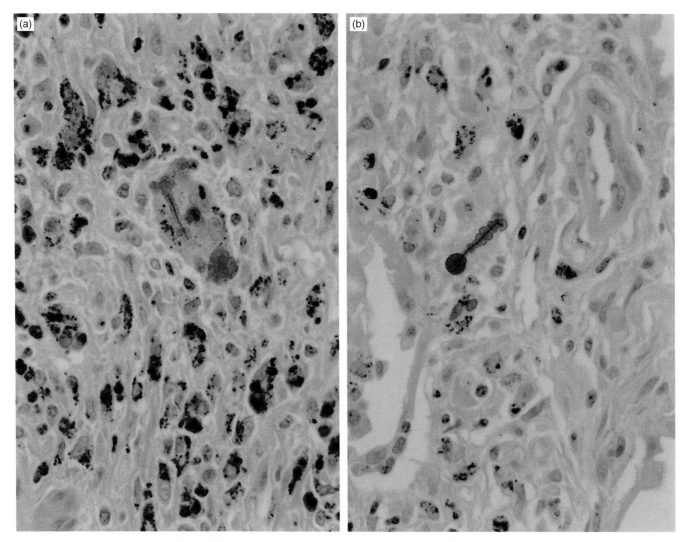

Figure 8.8. Mixed-dust pneumoconiosis. (a) Numerous dust-laden macrophages in a background of fibrosis. Note non-asbestos ferruginous body with a black core. **(b)** Another non-asbestos ferruginous body and interstitial dust deposition from the same case. The patient worked as a grinder in a motor works company, and underwent lung transplantation for end-stage fibrosis.

Treatment and prognosis

There is no effective therapy. The prognosis depends largely on the extent of fibrosis.

Sample diagnosis on pathology report

Without exposure history:

Lung, right upper lobe, transbronchial biopsy – Dust macules (See comment).

With exposure history:

Lung, right, explant pneumonectomy – Extensive interstitial mixed-dust deposition consistent with mixed-dust pneumoconiosis (See comment).

Asbestosis

Asbestosis is defined as *diffuse pulmonary fibrosis caused by the inhalation of excessive amounts of asbestos fibers*. Updated criteria for the pathologic diagnosis of asbestosis published in 2010 by the College of American Pathologists (CAP) and the

Pulmonary Pathology Society (PPS) require "an appropriate pattern of interstitial fibrosis plus the finding of asbestos bodies". This definition differs from the previous CAP/NIOSH definition published in 1982, which required "discrete foci of fibrosis in the walls of respiratory bronchioles associated with accumulation of asbestos bodies in histologic sections".

In practice, bona fide cases of asbestosis meeting the criteria listed above are infrequently seen by surgical pathologists. This is attributable to the fact that asbestosis generally requires heavy exposure to asbestos, and usually occurs after a long latency period. Thus, with the decreasing use of asbestos, asbestosis caused by recent exposure is likely to become increasingly uncommon. This situation was described by Gaensler *et al* as far back as 1991 in a landmark paper where the authors stated "in our own longitudinal studies of 1,764 asbestos-exposed workers we have not seen a single case of significant asbestosis with first exposure during the past 30 yr (sic)" (see references).

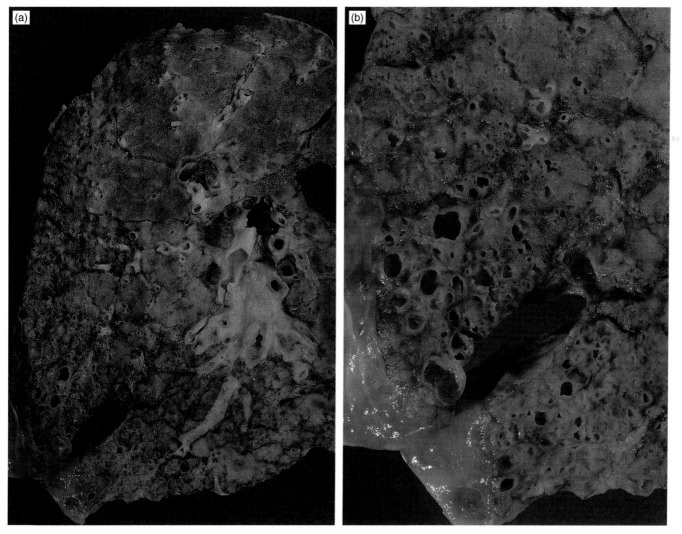

Figure 8.9. Mixed-dust pneumoconiosis. (a) Lung removed in the course of transplantation for end-stage fibrosis (explant pneumonectomy), showing extensive black discoloration, especially at the base. **(b)** Closer view shows extensive honeycomb change in the periphery of the lung. Same case as Figure 8.6. The clinical diagnosis was idiopathic pulmonary fibrosis (IPF). Details of the occupational history were not known prior to transplantation. The occupational history was obtained after pathologic examination.

The diagnosis of asbestosis is usually made presumptively on clinical and radiologic grounds, but pathologists still occasionally see lung biopsies with clinical requests to rule out asbestosis in individuals with a history of asbestos exposure. Additionally, pathologists will occasionally encounter asbestos bodies unexpectedly in lung specimens such as surgical biopsies or lobectomies.

Asbestos is the term applied to a group of six *silicate minerals* that occur naturally in a *fibrous* form, including chrysotile, crocidolite, anthophyllite, amosite, tremolite and actinolite. These are placed into two mineral groups known as serpentine and amphibole (Table 8.3). With the exception of chrysotile, the other types are all amphiboles. The type of asbestos fiber cannot be determined by routine light microscopy, and knowledge of the precise fiber type does not impact the pathologic diagnosis. However, the fiber type is thought to have implications for pathogenesis and potential carcinogenicity. A combination of fibrous shape, high surface area and

thin width is thought to be most carcinogenic. A non-asbestos mineral known as *erionite* is similar in size to amphibole asbestos, and causes a disease similar to asbestosis in the Cappadocia region in Turkey.

Details of specialized methods used to assess the burden of asbestos fibers and analyze mineral fiber content such as transmission electron microscopy (TEM), scanning electron microscopy (SEM) and energy-dispersive X-ray spectroscopy (EDS) are outside the scope of this book. Those interested in further details regarding these techniques are referred to the most recent CAP/PPS guidelines (Roggli *et al*, 2010 – see references).

Asbestos has been valued since ancient times for its high tensile strength and resistance to heat (it is famously fireproof). Until recently, it has been mined extensively for use in numerous industrial applications. At present, given widespread awareness of the association between asbestosis and lung disease, its use is strictly regulated. Even so, asbestos

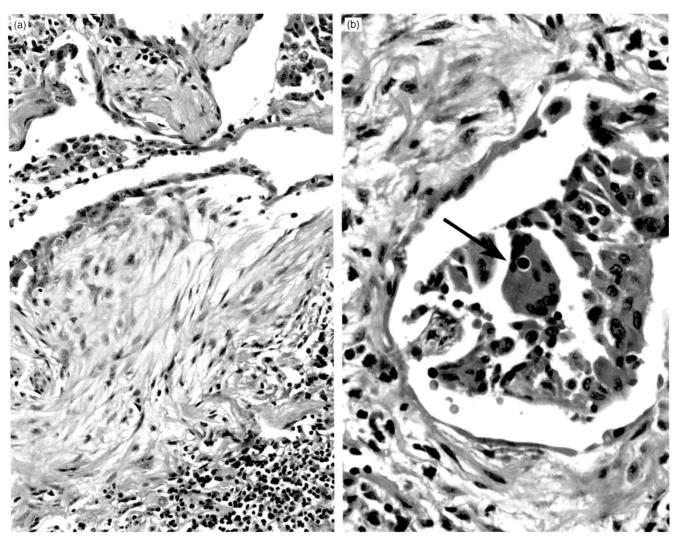

Figure 8.10. Mixed-dust pneumoconiosis. (a) Fibroblast focus, similar to UIP. **(b)** Macrophages fill this airspace. A multinucleated giant cell contains an intact eosinophil (emperipolesis, arrow). Same case as Figure 8.6.

continues to be used in many countries to this day, and it is estimated that asbestos persists in approximately 20% of buildings in the United States. Cases of asbestos-related disease – especially mesothelioma – stemming from prior exposure continue to be seen in practice. Asbestos exposure can occur in a wide variety of settings, some of which are listed in Table 8.4. Diseases of the lung and pleura associated with asbestos exposure are listed in Table 8.5.

Major diagnostic findings
- The two requirements for a pathologic diagnosis of asbestosis are *asbestos bodies* and *interstitial fibrosis*.
- Asbestos bodies are minute microscopic particles consisting of a *thin, transparent core* of asbestos covered by a golden yellow coat of iron and protein (Figures 8.12 and 8.13). The only other materials that have been reported to mimic the clear cores of asbestos bodies are refractory ceramic fibers (in Europe) and erionite (in Turkey). In North America, the light microscopic finding of

ferruginous bodies with thin transparent cores is considered specific for asbestos bodies. Uncoated asbestos fibers also exist in lung tissue. Although they are far more numerous than coated fibers, they cannot be seen with a light microscope. The significance of asbestos bodies is that they indicate higher-than-background levels of asbestos exposure. Current criteria require *two or more asbestos bodies* per square cm of a 5 μm thick lung section. Asbestos bodies should not be equated with asbestosis unless interstitial fibrosis of the appropriate pattern and distribution is also present. Although the finding of even a single asbestos body in a routine lung section is thought to indicate above-background exposure, it requires confirmation by other sophisticated techniques. Owing to their iron-rich coat, asbestos bodies are included under the umbrella of *ferruginous bodies*, a term that also includes non-asbestos fibers with iron-rich coats. The presence of iron in the coat can be confirmed by an iron stain such as the Perls' stain, which colors the coat deep blue

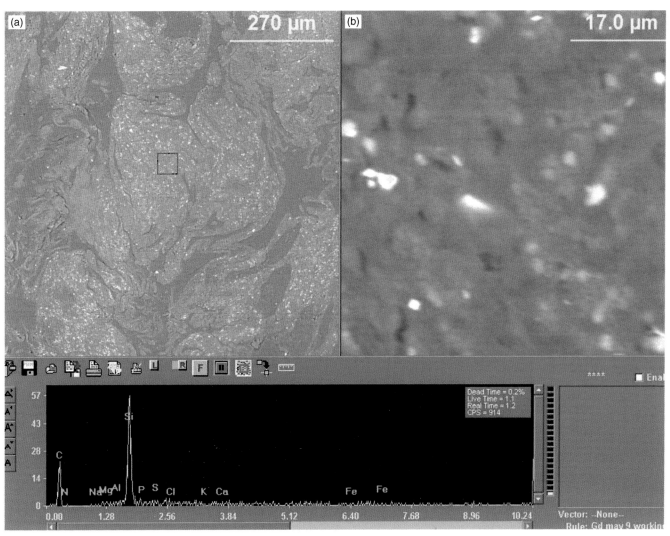

Figure 8.11. Energy-dispersive X-ray spectroscopy in mixed-dust pneumoconiosis. Energy-dispersive X-ray spectroscopy shows spikes for carbon and silicon, consistent with mixed-dust pneumoconiosis. The left-hand panel is the scanning electron microscope image. A blue box surrounds the particle being analyzed. In the right-hand panel, the same particle is seen at higher magnification, marked by a yellow plus sign. Image courtesy of Dr. Jerrold Abraham.

(Figure 8.13). Ferruginous bodies can also contain cores of coal ("coal bodies"), talc ("talc bodies"), aluminum silicate whiskers and other non-asbestos fibrous dusts. The color and shape of the core helps in distinguishing asbestos bodies from non-asbestos ferruginous bodies (Figures 8.8 and 8.14). For example, ferruginous bodies with black (coal) or thick yellow (talc) cores do not qualify as asbestos bodies. Asbestos bodies are invariably golden brown and beaded. Most are long, straight and slender with club-like, knobby ends, but some have curved or branching shapes (Figures 8.12 and 8.13). By light microscopy, asbestos bodies are found mainly within lung parenchyma, not in the pleura or pleural plaques. They have also been reported in extrapulmonary sites such as regional lymph nodes, liver and abdomen (omentum). In the lung, they may be found within airspaces or the interstitium, free or within fibrous tissue, alveolar macrophages or multinucleated giant cells. By special techniques, it has been shown that asbestos

bodies are found not only in asbestos handlers but also in urban dwellers without occupational exposure to asbestos, including women, blue-collar men and white-collar men.

- *Interstitial fibrosis.* This component of the diagnosis is more problematic because the type, distribution and degree of interstitial fibrosis in asbestosis vary considerably from case to case. The current definition only specifies that the fibrosis should be *diffuse* and should extend beyond the walls of respiratory bronchioles and alveolar ducts. It may be uniform, resembling NSIP or SRIF (Figure 8.15, Figure 8.1a), or patchy, resembling UIP. However, it may be difficult to establish with certainty that fibrosis in a given case is caused by asbestos exposure, especially when other etiologies are equally plausible. For example, individuals with asbestos exposure may also be cigarette smokers (as in Figure 8.15), and the latter is well known to cause diffuse interstitial fibrosis (see section on SRIF in Chapter 5). In such cases, it can be very difficult to determine whether the

Table 8.3. Types of asbestos fibers

	Serpentine	Amphibole
Shape/crystal structure	Snake-like	Straight, needle-like
Examples of asbestos fibers	Chrysotile	Amosite (used commercially) Crocidolite (used commercially) Actinolite (non-commercial) Anthophyllite (non-commercial) Tremolite (non-commercial)
How commonly used	> 90% of asbestos used in most countries	Minority of asbestos
Consistency	Softer	Harder
Stability in the lung	Unstable	Stable
Half-life	Short	Long
Ability to induce fibrosis in the lung (asbestosis)	Less	More
Incidence in ferruginous bodies with a thin core (asbestos bodies)	Low	High

Table 8.4. Occupations and other settings in which asbestos exposure can occur

Occupational	Asbestos miners and millers Asbestos textile workers Asbestos cement workers Asbestos insulators Pipefitters Shipyard workers Crocidolite-asbestos cigarette filter makers Electricians Construction workers
Non-occupational	Household contacts of asbestos workers Contact with contaminated clothes of asbestos workers Exposure to airborne dust from mines, quarries and roads Naturally occurring asbestos in rocks and soils: Turkey, southern Nevada, Libby (Montana)

Table 8.5. Diseases of the lung and pleura in which asbestos is thought to be causative or contributory

Site of pathology	Condition
Lung	Asbestosis Asbestos small airway disease Lung carcinoma
Pleura	Pleural plaques Diffuse pleural fibrosis Pleural effusion Mesothelioma

fibrosis is caused by cigarette smoking or asbestos exposure. Asbestos bodies without interstitial fibrosis cannot be diagnosed as asbestosis by pathologists.

Variable pathologic findings

- Asbestosis may be accompanied by pleural plaques. These lesions are thought to be caused mainly by asbestos exposure, and may serve as a clue to the diagnosis. Grossly, they are raised, waxy, knobby, plaque-like thickenings located mainly on the surface of the parietal pleura. They are often bilateral and may occasionally be extensive. Microscopically, they are composed of acellular or sparsely cellular dense hyalinized fibrosis. They are often calcified. Asbestosis can also cause diffuse pleural fibrosis that may mimic desmoplastic mesothelioma. Asbestos-induced pleural effusions are accompanied by fibrinous exudates on the pleura, chronic inflammation and fibrosis. Asbestos-induced pleural disease should not be labeled as asbestosis without evidence of parenchymal disease.
- Round atelectasis, a mass-like buckling of the pleura into the underlying lung, is also thought to be attributable to asbestos exposure. Is it discussed in detail in Chapter 6.

- The combination of asbestos bodies and interstitial fibrosis confined to the walls of respiratory bronchioles and alveolar ducts has been termed *asbestos small-airway disease* or small airway mineral dust disease. This limited form of fibrosis does not fulfil current criteria for asbestosis.
- Interstitial fibrosis with fibroblast foci, scarring and honeycomb change can occur in cases labeled as asbestosis. The fibrosis is said to be lower lobe predominant.
- A consensus report published in 2004 suggested that cases meeting criteria for asbestosis as well as mixed-dust pneumoconiosis be termed *mixed-dust pneumoconiosis with asbestosis.*

Diagnostic work-up

An iron stain is the most valuable stain in the work-up of asbestosis. It should be performed on blocks with lung parenchyma. It is more sensitive than H&E for detecting ferruginous bodies (Figure 8.13). However, it does not differentiate between asbestos bodies and non-asbestos ferruginous bodies. A trichrome or Movat pentachrome stain can be very helpful for documenting the presence of subtle interstitial fibrosis and assessing its distribution.

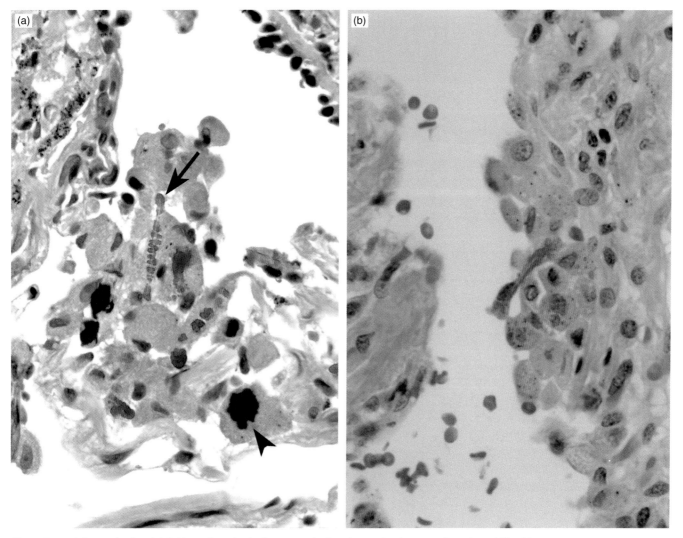

Figure 8.12. Asbestos bodies. (a) Golden yellow, slender ferruginous body within an alveolar macrophage (arrow). The thin transparent core identifies this as an asbestos body. Irregular black particles, likely carbonaceous, are also present within macrophages (arrowhead). **(b)** Asbestos body from a different case. Note the airspace location.

Clinical profile

Patients with asbestosis usually have a history of heavy occupational exposure to asbestos several years prior to presentation. The clinical picture is otherwise non-specific. The most common symptoms are shortness of breath and dry cough. Physical signs include dry rales and clubbing. Pulmonary function tests show restrictive changes and decreased DL_{CO}, but may be normal in some patients.

Radiologic findings

There are no specific radiologic findings. Typical cases show bilateral irregular interstitial opacities and pleural plaques. The latter are typically bilateral and calcified. They are most common in the middle to lower posterior parietal pleura and diaphragm. The interstitial opacities of asbestosis may be reticular or reticulonodular and often show a lower lobe predominance. The ILO scheme is used to describe the radiologic findings on chest X-rays. Chest CT findings of lower lobe predominance, reticular opacities and honeycomb change may be indistinguishable from UIP.

Differential diagnosis

- The most difficult entity to separate from asbestosis is UIP in the setting of IPF. This problem may be encountered when a lung biopsy shows UIP along with asbestos bodies. Since other idiopathic interstitial lung diseases can occur in asbestos-exposed persons, there is no reason why IPF, one of the most common forms of interstitial lung disease, should not occasionally occur in these individuals. However, current dogma dictates that the clinical, radiologic and pathologic findings in asbestosis can show a "UIP pattern" identical to IPF, and that the finding of asbestos bodies in such cases excludes IPF. This assertion is based on the questionable presumption that asbestos bodies, when present, are always the "cause" of lung fibrosis. There is no easy solution to this difficult (and fortunately uncommon) problem. One approach is to follow current guidelines and

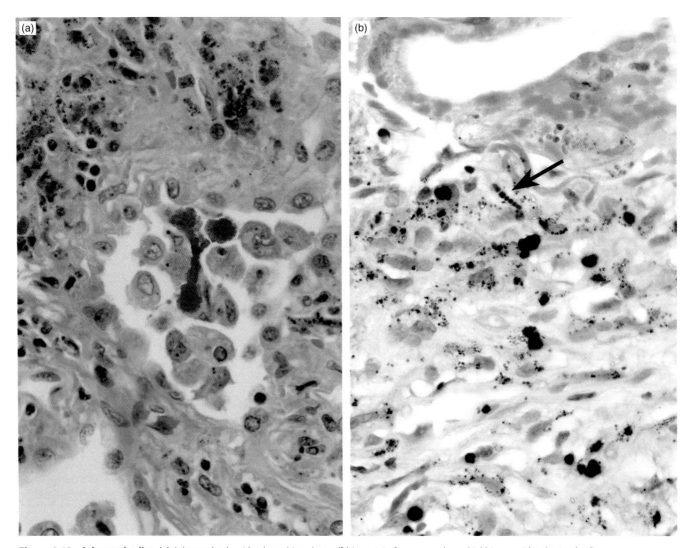

Figure 8.13. Asbestos bodies. (a) Asbestos body with a branching shape. **(b)** Iron stain from a transbronchial biopsy with asbestos bodies and other types of dust. The patient had pleural plaques and a history of possible asbestos exposure. Several ferruginous bodies are present. One of these is likely an asbestos body (arrow), but the core is not clearly seen. Visualization of the core in such cases is easier on the corresponding H&E-stained slide.

diagnose these cases as asbestosis. Another approach is to diagnose "UIP with asbestos bodies", and allow the clinician to decide whether or not the patient should be diagnosed with asbestosis. Although the distinction between end-stage asbestosis and IPF does have legal implications, its medical implications are minimal since both entities have a poor prognosis and lack effective therapies.

- Other pathologically distinctive forms of interstitial lung disease can occur in asbestos-exposed individuals and should be recognized as such by surgical pathologists. These include organizing pneumonia, diffuse alveolar damage, sarcoidosis and other granulomatous lung diseases. Most have been reported to occur in asbestos-exposed individuals, and there is widespread agreement that they do not represent asbestosis. The existence of such conditions explains why lung biopsies can be of value in asbestos-exposed individuals, and supports the contention that clinical or radiologic evidence of interstitial lung disease in an asbestos-exposed individual does not always represent asbestosis.

- Lung tissue in other pneumoconioses such as coal workers' pneumoconiosis or mixed-dust pneumoconiosis may contain numerous ferruginous bodies with golden yellow, beaded, iron-positive coats. These non-asbestos ferruginous bodies can be discriminated from asbestos bodies by the color (black, brown or yellow) and shape (round, broad or irregular) of their cores.

Treatment and prognosis

There is no effective treatment. The prognosis is poor. Morbidity and mortality may be related to severe pulmonary fibrosis. Asbestosis is associated with a well-documented increase in the risk of lung carcinoma as well as mesothelioma. Many patients subsequently develop lung cancer or mesothelioma.

Sample diagnosis on pathology report

Lung, right lower lobe, surgical biopsy – Asbestos bodies and interstitial fibrosis, consistent with asbestosis (See comment).

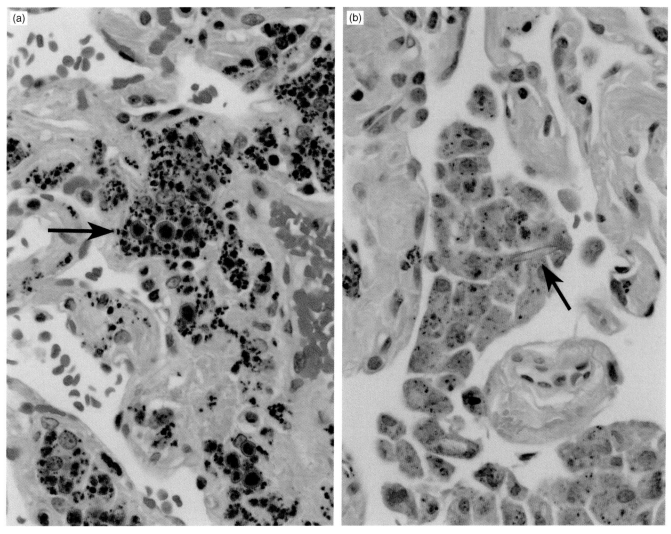

Figure 8.14. Non-asbestos ferruginous bodies. (a) These ferruginous bodies are not asbestos bodies because their cores are irregular and black. **(b)** This non-asbestos ferruginous body contains a lanceolate, pale yellow core, possibly talc. Compare with Figures 8.8 and 8.12.

or

Lung, right lower lobe, surgical biopsy – Usual interstitial pneumonia with asbestos bodies (See comment).

Miscellaneous pneumoconioses

Other rare occupational lung diseases and pneumoconioses such as *siderosis, silicate pneumoconiosis, rare earth pneumoconiosis, byssinosis* and *flock worker's lung* are outside the scope of this book. *Hard metal lung disease*, a well-recognized form of pneumoconiosis, is discussed in Chapter 5 along with other interstitial lung diseases. *Berylliosis* is discussed in Chapter 2 with other granulomatous diseases.

References

Coal workers' pneumoconiosis

Castranova V, Vallyathan V. Silicosis and coal workers' pneumoconiosis. *Environ Health Perspect* 2000;**108**:675–84.

Fisher ER, Watkins G, Lam NV, *et al.* Objective pathological diagnosis of coal workers' pneumoconiosis. *JAMA* 1981;**245**:1829–34.

Hu SN, Vallyathan V, Green FH, Weber KC, Laqueur W. Pulmonary arteriolar muscularization in coal workers' pneumoconiosis and its correlation with right ventricular hypertrophy. *Arch Pathol Lab Med* 1990;**114**:1063–70.

Kleinerman J, Green FHY, Laqueur WM, *et al.* Pathology standards for coal workers' pneumoconiosis. Report of the pneumoconiosis committee of the College of American Pathologists to the National Institute for Occupational Safety and Health. *Arch Pathol Lab Med* 1979;**103**:375–432.

Petsonk EL, Rose C, Cohen R. Coal mine dust lung disease. New lessons from an old exposure. *Am J Respir Crit Care Med* 2013;**187**:1178–85.

Pratt PC, Kilburn KH. Extent of pulmonary pigmentation as an indicator of particulate environmental air pollution. *Inhaled Part* 1970;**2**:661–70.

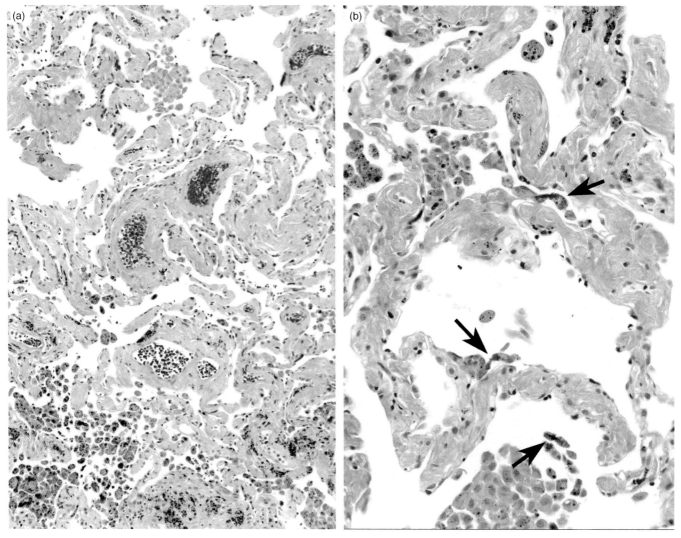

Figure 8.15. Interstitial fibrosis in asbestosis. (a) Diffuse alveolar septal fibrosis. Asbestos bodies are visible at bottom left. **(b)** Higher magnification, showing alveolar septal collagen deposition and asbestos bodies (arrows). The patient was a 30 pack-year cigarette smoker with emphysema, and it is possible that the fibrosis seen here represents SRIF in an individual with asbestos exposure.

Remy-Jardin M, Degreef JM, Beuscart R, Voisin C, Remy J. Coal workers' pneumoconiosis: CT assessment in exposed workers and correlation with radiographic findings. *Radiology* 1990;**177**:363–71.

Soutar CA. Update on lung disease in coal miners. *Br J Ind Med* 1987;**44**:145–8.

Vallyathan V, Brower PS, Green FHY, Attfield MD. Radiographic and pathologic correlation of coal workers' pneumoconiosis. *Am J Respir Crit Care Med* 1996;**154**:741–8.

Vallyathan V, Landsittel DP, Petsonk EL, *et al.* The influence of dust standards on the prevalence and severity of coal workers' pneumoconiosis at autopsy in the United States of America. *Arch Pathol Lab Med* 2011;**135**:1550–6.

Mixed-dust pneumoconiosis

Craighead JE, Kleinerman J, Abraham JL, *et al.* Diseases associated with exposure to silica and nonfibrous silicate minerals. *Arch Pathol Lab Med* 1988;**112**:673–720.

Diaz JV, Koff J, Gotway MB, Nishimura S, Balmes JR. Case report: a case of wood-smoke-related pulmonary disease. *Environ Health Perspect* 2006;**114**:759–62.

Fullerton DG, Bruce N, Gordon SB. Indoor air pollution from biomass fuel smoke is a major health concern in the developing world. *Trans R Soc Trop Med Hyg* 2008;**102**:843–51.

Gold JA, Jagirdar J, Hay JG, *et al.* Hut lung. A domestically acquired particulate lung disease. *Medicine* 2000;**79**:310–7.

Grobbelaar JP, Bateman ED. Hut lung: a domestically acquired pneumoconiosis of mixed etiology in rural women. *Thorax* 1991;**46**:334–40.

Honma K, Abraham JL, Chiyotani K, *et al.* Proposed criteria for mixed-dust pneumoconiosis: Definition, descriptions, and guidelines for pathologic diagnosis and clinical correlation. *Hum Pathol* 2004;**35**:1515–23.

Mukhopadhyay S, Gujral M, Abraham JL, Scalzetti EM, Iannuzzi MC. A case of hut lung: SEM/EDS analysis of a domestically acquired form of pneumoconiosis. *Chest* 2013;**144**:323–7.

Nasr MR, Savici D, Tudor L, Abou Abdallah D, Newman N, Abraham JL. Inorganic dust exposure causes pulmonary fibrosis in smokers: analysis using light microscopy, scanning electron microscopy and energy-dispersive X-ray spectroscopy. *Arch Envir Occup Health* 2007;**61**:53–60.

Shida H, Chiyotani K, Honma K, *et al.* Radiologic and pathologic characteristics of mixed dust pneumoconiosis. *Radiographics* 1996;**16**:483–98.

Torres-Duque C, Maldonado D, Perez-Padilla R, Ezzati M, Viegi G. Biomass fuels and respiratory diseases: a review of the evidence. *Proc Am Thorac Soc* 2008;**5**: 577–90.

Asbestosis

Churg A, Warnock M. Asbestos and other ferruginous bodies: their formation and clinical significance. *Am J Pathol* 1981;**102**:447–56.

Churg A, Warnock M. Analysis of the cores of ferruginous bodies from the general population. I. Patients with and without lung cancer. *Lab Invest* 1977;**37**:280–6.

Craighead JE, Abraham JL, Churg A, *et al.* The pathology of asbestos associated diseases of the lungs and pleural cavities: diagnostic criteria and proposed grading schema: report of the Pneumoconiosis Committee of the College of American Pathologists and the National Institute of Occupational Safety and Health. *Arch Pathol Lab Med* 1982;**106**:544–96.

Dodson RF, Hurst GA, Williams MG Jr., Corn C, Greenberg SD. Comparison of light and electron microscopy for defining occupational asbestos exposure in transbronchial lung biopsies. *Chest* 1988;**94**:366–70.

Gaensler EA, Jederlinic PJ, Churg A. Idiopathic pulmonary fibrosis in asbestos-exposed workers. *Am Rev Respir Dis* 1991;**144**:689–96.

Mårtensson G, Hagberg S, Pettersson K, Thiringer G. Asbestos pleural effusion: a clinical entity. *Thorax* 1987;**42**:646–51.

No authors listed. Diagnosis and initial management of nonmalignant diseases related to asbestos. *Am J Respir Crit Care Med* 2004;**170**:691–715.

Roggli VL, Gibbs AR, Attanoos R, *et al.* Pathology of asbestosis – update of the diagnostic criteria. Report of the Asbestosis Committee of the College of American Pathologists and Pulmonary Pathology Society. *Arch Pathol Lab Med* 2010;**134**:462–80.

Roggli VL, Vollmer R. Twenty-five years of fiber analysis. What have we learned? *Hum Pathol* 2008;**39**:307–15.

Schneider F, Sporn TA, Roggli VL. Asbestos fiber content of lungs with diffuse interstitial fibrosis. *Arch Pathol Lab Med* 2010;**134**:457–61.

Pathologic abnormalities in the airways (bronchi or bronchioles)

This chapter deals with non-neoplastic pathologic findings in the walls or lumens of bronchi and/or bronchioles, collectively known as *airways*. The goal is to provide pathologists with a menu of abnormalities to look for in airways in lung specimens. Examples of such abnormalities are shown in Figure 9.1, and an algorithmic approach to the diagnosis of airway abnormalities is suggested in Figure 9.2. Table 9.1 lists pearls and pitfalls associated with the pathologic assessment of airway lesions.

Conditions that involve the distal small bronchioles (respiratory bronchioles and alveolar ducts) often spill into the adjacent alveoli and thus fall in a gray zone between true airway disease and parenchymal lung disease. Therefore, they are discussed in the chapters on airspace or interstitial abnormalities (Chapters 4 and 5). Examples of such conditions include respiratory bronchiolitis, organizing pneumonia and hypersensitivity pneumonitis. The airways are frequently involved by a wide range of granulomatous processes, which are addressed in the chapter on granulomatous diseases (Chapter 2). Neuroendocrine proliferations that involve small bronchioles are discussed in the chapter on nodules (Chapter 6).

Bronchiectasis

Bronchiectasis is defined as *permanent and irreversible dilatation of the bronchi*. Since irreversibility is not a feature that can be assessed by pathologists, by necessity the pathologic definition of bronchiectasis differs from the clinical definition. It mainly requires marked bronchial dilatation accompanied by severe inflammation. In clinical practice, the diagnosis is usually based solely on radiologic findings.

The pathogenesis of bronchiectasis is thought to involve obstruction of the airways and/or repeated episodes of airway inflammation. Airway obstruction leads to impaired clearance of mucin, cell debris and pathogens, and predisposes to infection and inflammation. Clearance of debris is further impeded in inflamed airways, worsening the initial obstruction. Furthermore, repeated inflammation weakens the bronchial wall, leading to dilatation and predisposing to repeated infection. A vicious cycle ensues, the end-result being permanently inflamed, damaged and dilated bronchi.

The causes of bronchiectasis are listed in Table 9.2. Although well-defined etiologies receive the most attention in the literature, the cause of bronchiectasis remains unknown in at least half of all patients, even after extensive investigations are performed. In the remainder of cases, the most common etiologies in affluent countries are cystic fibrosis and non-

tuberculous mycobacterial disease, while tuberculosis is probably the leading cause in developing nations. Ciliary abnormalities such as the Kartagener syndrome or ciliary dyskinesia are less common, as are a variety of inflammatory disorders and rare immunodeficiency syndromes. Localized bronchiectasis develops secondary to airway obstruction by indolent tumors and non-neoplastic masses such as enlarged hilar lymph nodes.

In most cases, pathologic examination is not required for the diagnosis since bronchiectasis is easily identifiable on imaging studies. Bronchiectasis may be encountered by pathologists in resected lungs, either removed as part of a therapeutic procedure or as explanted lungs removed from patients with cystic fibrosis in the course of lung transplantation.

Major diagnostic findings

- The gross appearance is striking and can be virtually diagnostic. It is characterized by the presence of markedly dilated bronchi with thick walls, usually in all lobes of both lungs (Figure 9.3a). Unlike normal lungs, bronchi are visible even at the periphery of the lung. Localized bronchiectasis occurs distal to slow-growing hilar masses or neoplasms. The bronchiectasis in these cases is limited to airways distal to the point of obstruction (Figure 9.3b).
- Microscopically, the pathologic abnormalities primarily involve the bronchial tree beyond the main lobar bronchi. The bronchi show marked dilatation and distortion with severe chronic inflammation in the bronchial wall (Figure 9.4). The inflammatory infiltrate is composed mainly of lymphocytes and plasma cells. It is most dense in the mucosa/submucosa immediately beneath the respiratory epithelium. In general, the microscopic changes of bronchiectasis are similar regardless of the underlying etiology. For example, a diagnosis of cystic fibrosis cannot be made on the basis of pathologic findings alone.
- Although peribronchial fibrosis and parenchymal changes may supervene, the inflammatory changes in bronchiectasis are centered primarily on the bronchi. The combination of bronchiectasis and peribronchial fibrosis probably accounts for the origin of the term *cystic fibrosis*.

Variable pathologic findings

- The lumens of the inflamed bronchi and bronchioles are often filled with fibrinopurulent debris including mucin, necrosis, cell debris and an acute inflammatory exudate containing neutrophils.

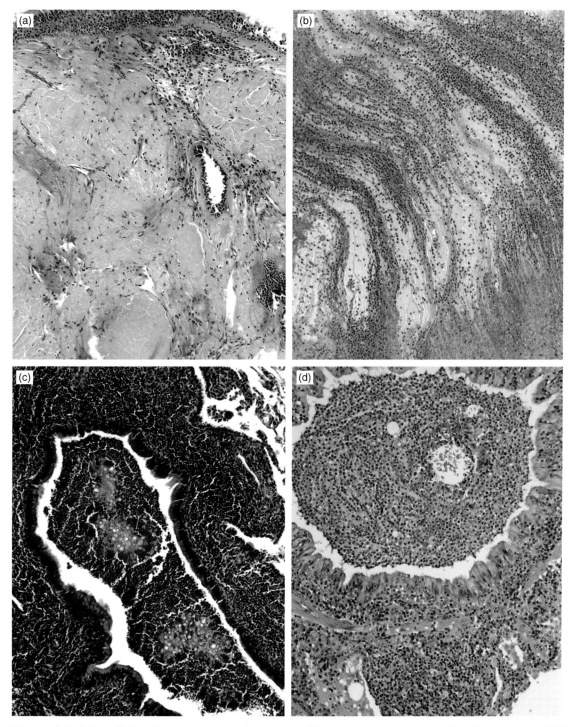

Figure 9.1. Pathologic findings involving airway walls or lumens. **(a)** Amyloid deposition in tracheobronchial amyloidosis. **(b)** Allergic mucin in mucoid impaction of bronchi. **(c)** Acute and chronic bronchiolitis in sporotrichosis. **(d)** Acute and chronic bronchiolitis in ulcerative colitis.

- Bronchioles distal to the inflamed bronchi show extensive acute and chronic inflammation identical to the changes seen in the bronchi. Lymphoid follicles with germinal centers are occasionally found in airway walls. In surgical biopsies that do not sample bronchi, it may be impossible to determine on histologic grounds whether small airway inflammation is primary, or represents changes secondary to bronchiectasis.

- Variable acute inflammation (neutrophilic) is usually present in the lumen as well as the airway wall. Neutrophils may also be present within epithelial cells.
- Granulomatous inflammation is not usually a feature of bronchiectasis unless the etiology is mycobacterial or fungal.
- The inflammatory infiltrate may erode into and destroy the bronchial cartilage and smooth muscle.

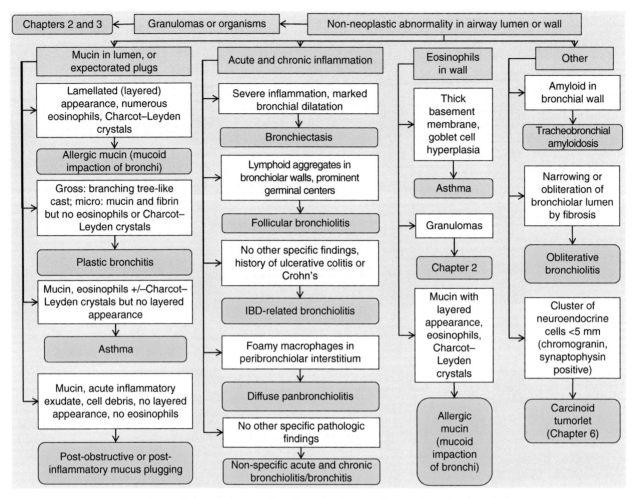

Figure 9.2. Algorithm. Approach to pathologic findings involving the walls or lumens of airways (bronchi or bronchioles).

- Mucosal ulceration is common in inflamed bronchi and bronchioles. The entire airway epithelium may be sloughed off, or portions of the epithelium may be ulcerated. The underlying stroma frequently contains granulation tissue.
- Non-specific peribronchial fibrosis and scarring may develop in long-standing bronchiectasis. It is usually limited to the lung immediately adjacent to the inflamed airways and the accompanying pulmonary arteries. Significant interstitial fibrosis away from airways is uncommon.
- Bronchial arteries may be prominent. They may show severe medial hypertrophy, intimal fibrosis and reactive endothelial cells. The reader will recall that in normal lungs bronchial arteries are present in bronchovascular bundles but are typically small and inconspicuous.
- Fibrinopurulent acute pleuritis can develop in some cases and may be accompanied by marked widening of interlobular septa.
- Chronic inflammation may extend down airway walls as far distally as the respiratory bronchioles and alveolar ducts.
- Lung parenchyma (alveolated lung) away from the inflamed airways is usually normal. However, peribronchiolar airspaces may show features of superimposed acute bronchopneumonia, characterized by filling of peribronchiolar airspaces by neutrophils accompanied by variable amounts of cellular debris, macrophages and fibrin. Other secondary changes in the peribronchiolar parenchyma are also common. They include foamy macrophages within peribronchiolar airspaces (post-obstructive changes, or *endogenous lipoid pneumonia*) and scattered fibroblast plugs (organizing pneumonia).
- Multiple carcinoid tumorlets may be present in the bronchioles. It is widely accepted that tumorlets arising in the context of inflamed airways are a secondary phenomenon, and should not be labeled DIPNECH (see Chapter 6).

Diagnostic work-up

No special stains are required unless there are features of a superimposed mycobacterial or fungal infection. Bacteria may be demonstrable within the acute inflammatory exudate within the bronchioles, but this finding is seldom of clinical significance since bacterial infections are usually well characterized by the time specimens are removed for pathologic examination.

Table 9.1. Pearls and pitfalls in the assessment of non-neoplastic bronchial and bronchiolar lesions

Endobronchial biopsies are performed to look for abnormalities located in airway walls or lumens. They do not include or assess lung parenchyma. In contrast, *transbronchial* biopsies should include alveolated lung because they are performed specifically for alveolar abnormalities

Centrilobular or tree-in-bud opacities on chest CT usually correspond to bronchiolar abnormalities such as infection, aspiration or non-specific inflammation

As currently defined, asthma is a clinical diagnosis that does not require pathologic input; however, it does have characteristic histologic findings

Not all "mucus" is the same. Pathologists should be able to recognize the characteristic layered appearance of *allergic mucin*. Its significance and differential diagnosis differs from that of ordinary mucin

Microscopic examination of mucus plugs is of value

Mucoid impaction of bronchi is a distinctive clinicopathologic entity that can present as a solitary mass mimicking lung cancer

Mucoid impaction of bronchi can occur in isolation or as part of the pathologic manifestations of allergic bronchopulmonary aspergillosis

Always consider the possibility of tracheobronchial amyloidosis in any endobronchial biopsy with pink material in the mucosa or submucosa

Tracheobronchial amyloidosis can be a serious and even life-threatening condition, but it is not associated with – and does not progress to – systemic amyloidosis

Consider the possibility of obliterative bronchiolitis if radiologic studies show air trapping or mosaic attenuation but the lung looks normal microscopically

Consider the possibility of obliterative bronchiolitis if there are tiny scars in the lung adjacent to arteries

Consider the possibility of obliterative bronchiolitis in any lung specimen from a lung transplant recipient that shows tiny scars

An elastic or Movat pentachrome stain is very helpful for identifying obliterated bronchioles

Table 9.2. Causes of bronchiectasis

Pathogenesis	Causes
Unknown	The cause in the majority of cases of bronchiectasis is unknown (50%)
Defective mucociliary clearance leading to repeated infection	Cystic fibrosis Ciliary dyskinesia Kartagener syndrome
Severe, persistent airway inflammation leading to bronchial weakening and dilatation	Allergic bronchopulmonary fungal disease/aspergillosis (proximal bronchiectasis) Inflammatory bowel disease Aspiration of gastric contents Rheumatoid arthritis Sjögren syndrome Ankylosing spondylitis Systemic lupus erythematosus Marfan syndrome Yellow nail syndrome Relapsing polychondritis
Destructive infection leading to weakening of bronchial walls and bronchial dilatation	Tuberculosis Adenovirus (childhood) Measles Pertussis Immunodeficiency
Congenital dilatation of bronchi (not bronchiectasis in the strict sense)	Williams–Campbell syndrome Mounier–Kuhn syndrome (tracheobronchomegaly)
Mechanical obstruction of a large airway, usually by a slow-growing mass, followed by dilatation of bronchi distal to the obstruction	Carcinoid tumor Endobronchial lipoma Enlarged hilar lymph nodes Right middle lobe syndrome Foreign body

Clinical profile

Bronchiectasis can occur at any age. Many patients are younger than 10 years of age at the onset of symptoms. There is no significant sex difference, although a female predilection has been suggested in some studies. Most patients with cystic fibrosis are in the 20- to 50-year-old age group. The first diagnosis is made at the time of newborn screening in 60% of cases. However, some children are diagnosed when they present with respiratory symptoms, meconium ileus or failure to thrive. A small minority of cases presents in adulthood with atypical presentations such as gastrointestinal symptoms, diabetes mellitus or infertility. In patients with established

bronchiectasis, cough with mucopurulent sputum, shortness of breath and hemoptysis are the most common symptoms. The clinical course is characterized by increasingly frequent hospitalizations for respiratory tract infections and exacerbations. Severe disease requires ICU stays, assisted ventilation, oxygen and intermittent courses of prednisone.

Patients with bronchiectasis are susceptible to various infections, including *Staphylococcus aureus, Pseudomonas aeruginosa, Hemophilus influenzae, Moraxella catarrhalis, Streptococcus pneumoniae, Achromobacter xylosoxidans, Pseudallescheria boydii*, MAC or *Burkholderia cepacia.*

Radiologic findings

Marked dilatation of the bronchi is the radiologic hallmark of bronchiectasis. The diagnosis has become easier with the widespread use of high-resolution CT scans. In cystic fibrosis, bronchiectatic changes are commonly seen throughout both

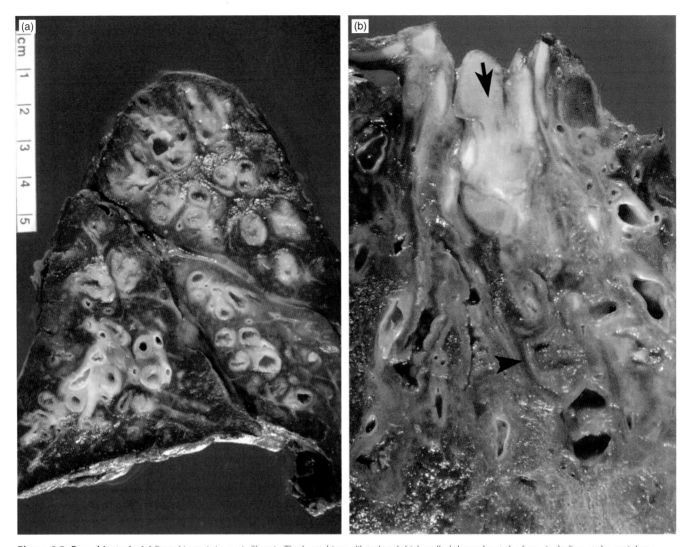

Figure 9.3. Bronchiectasis. (a) Bronchiectasis in cystic fibrosis. The bronchi are dilated and thick-walled throughout the lung, including at the periphery. **(b)** Post-obstructive bronchiectasis (arrowhead) distal to an endobronchial lipoma (arrow).

lungs and are often more prominent in the upper and perihilar lung zones, and in subsegmental and more peripheral bronchi. Associated bronchial wall thickening and retained secretions are commonly present. Numerous nodular densities may be seen. These are often centrilobular with a predominant tree-in-bud pattern, reflecting concurrent small airway disease. Airspace opacities correspond to parenchymal involvement. Mediastinal and bilateral hilar adenopathy may be present, reflecting reactive lymphadenopathy.

Differential diagnosis

The main entity that is commonly mistaken for bronchiectasis is honeycomb change, a common pathologic finding in fibrosing interstitial lung diseases such as usual interstitial pneumonia (Figure 5.12 in Chapter 5). Misinterpretation occurs because both entities feature dilated spaces filled with mucin and lined by respiratory epithelium. However, in contrast to bronchiectasis, in which respiratory epithelium lines dilated and inflamed bronchi, honeycomb change is characterized by extension of respiratory epithelium beyond normal bronchi

and into the surrounding lung parenchyma, forming clusters of cystic spaces (Figure 5.11 in Chapter 5). Another helpful feature in the differential diagnosis is the degree of inflammation, which is marked in bronchiectasis and generally minimal in fibrosing interstitial lung diseases. In the latter, the pathology is mainly parenchymal and fibrotic rather than bronchial and inflammatory. Bronchial dilatation does occur in fibrotic interstitial lung disease (traction bronchiectasis) but is not accompanied by significant inflammation (Figure 5.13 in Chapter 5).

Treatment and prognosis

Bronchiectasis is an irreversible process with no effective cure. Management is mainly supportive. It includes treatment of the underlying disease, treatment of exacerbations with appropriate antibiotic therapy, prevention of exacerbations, pulmonary rehabilitation, and occasionally surgery for intractable hemoptysis or other issues resistant to medical therapy. Patients with cystic fibrosis may be candidates for lung transplantation. Newer therapies for cystic fibrosis are currently in clinical

(a)

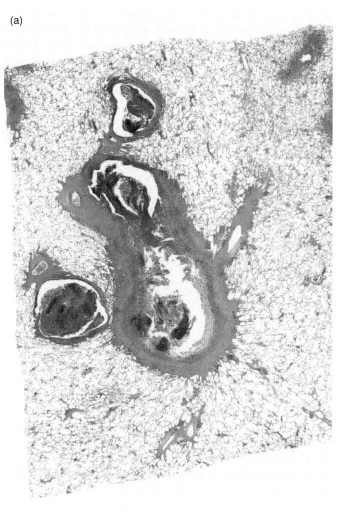

(b)

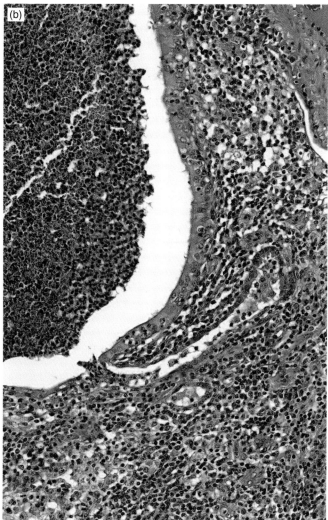

Figure 9.4. Bronchiectasis. (a) Dilated and inflamed airways. **(b)** High magnification, showing acute inflammatory exudate in the bronchial lumen and dense chronic inflammation in the bronchial wall.

trials, including the drugs ivacaftor and lumacaftor, which attempt to partially rectify dysfunction of the cystic fibrosis transmembrane regulator (CFTR) protein.

The prognosis of bronchiectasis depends on the underlying cause. In cystic fibrosis, progressive respiratory insufficiency ultimately causes death. The mean survival for cystic fibrosis patients is currently approximately 40 years but is expected to increase in coming years. Currently, the 5-year survival in cystic fibrosis after lung transplantation is approximately 50%. Post-transplant complications include infection, rejection and the need for lifelong immunosuppressive therapy with the attendant side effects. The prognosis of non-cystic fibrosis bronchiectasis varies considerably by etiology and severity of the disease. Some patients can survive for many years with appropriate supportive therapy.

Sample diagnosis on pathology report

Recipient lung, left, explant pneumonectomy – Bronchiectasis with severe acute and chronic bronchiolitis consistent with cystic fibrosis (See comment).

Bronchiolitis

Bronchiolitis, also known as *small airways disease*, is a common finding in surgical pathology of the lung. Broadly speaking, it encompasses any condition that predominantly involves small bronchioles including non-respiratory (membranous) bronchioles and respiratory bronchioles. See Chapter 1 for a more detailed description of these structures. Radiologists are unable to distinguish between these structures even on high-resolution CT scan, because they are all less than 2 mm in size. Therefore, diseases that involve the borderline between airways and parenchymal disease can only be accurately assessed by histopathology.

Etiologically, bronchiolitis is a mixed bag of inflammatory lesions, including those related to reactive lymphoid hyperplasia, infection, aspiration and systemic inflammatory diseases such as inflammatory bowel disease and rheumatoid arthritis. Some affect only bronchioles, while others spill into adjacent alveolated lung parenchyma. When alveolar involvement predominates over bronchiolar involvement, the term bronchiolitis fails to capture the essence of the lesion. Yet, the usage

Table 9.3. Causes of bronchiolitis

Type of bronchiolitis	Pathologic findings	Clinical associations
Follicular bronchiolitis	Lymphoid follicles with prominent germinal centers, limited exclusively to small bronchioles	Rheumatoid arthritis Sjögren syndrome Mixed connective tissue disease HIV/AIDS Immunodeficiency
Diffuse panbronchiolitis	Acute and/or chronic bronchiolitis mainly involving respiratory bronchioles Foamy macrophages in peribronchiolar alveolar septa	Reported mainly from Japan, rare in Western countries Concurrent chronic sinusitis, elevated cold agglutinins, *Hemophilus* or *Pseudomonas* in sputum Response to erythromycin therapy
Non-specific acute and/or chronic bronchiolitis	Chronic inflammation in bronchiolar wall, variable acute inflammation in lumen	Viral infection (influenza, RSV) Bacterial infection *Mycoplasma* infection Small airway inflammation in bronchiectasis Residuum of treated fungal infection Bronchiolitis associated with inflammatory bowel disease (ulcerative colitis and Crohn's disease)

persists in terms such as respiratory bronchiolitis, aspiration bronchiolitis and bronchiolitis obliterans-organizing pneumonia (BOOP).

In some cases of bronchiolitis, histologic findings such as organisms, granulomas or aspirated particulate material can be found, leading to a specific diagnosis. After such entities have been excluded (see Figure 9.2 for a helpful algorithm), there remain cases in which the main pathologic finding is acute and/or chronic inflammation involving small bronchioles. Although the features in most of these cases often appear hopelessly non-specific, there are a few findings that have been assigned specific nomenclature or are associated with particular clinical diseases. These forms of bronchiolitis are described in Table 9.3.

Bronchiolitis may be encountered in endobronchial biopsies, transbronchial biopsies or surgical lung biopsies.

Major diagnostic findings

- Acute and or chronic inflammation in the walls of bronchioles, with or without acute inflammatory exudate in the lumen (Figure 9.5). The inflammatory cells in the airway walls are mostly lymphocytes, with variable numbers of plasma cells or neutrophils. The luminal cells are usually neutrophils.
- No evidence of organisms, granulomas, numerous eosinophils, luminal obliteration or other findings suggesting an alternative diagnosis.

Variable pathologic findings

- Lymphoid follicles with prominent germinal centers raise the possibility of follicular bronchiolitis. The diagnosis requires that follicles be confined to bronchioles. Significant or diffuse involvement of the interstitium

excludes this diagnosis. Non-specific chronic bronchiolitis without prominent germinal centers should not be labeled follicular bronchiolitis.
- Other changes that commonly accompany bronchiolitis of any type include luminal dilatation (bronchiolectasis), mucus plugging (mucostasis), mild peribronchiolar fibrosis without luminal obliteration and mild squamous metaplasia.
- The diagnosis of inflammatory bowel disease-associated bronchiolitis is one of exclusion. The role of the surgical pathologist is to confirm the presence of severe inflammation in the airways or parenchyma, exclude other forms of lung disease such as organizing pneumonia, and, most importantly, exclude infection. The last is particularly important in this setting because patients with inflammatory bowel disease are often treated with immunosuppressants such as corticosteroids and TNF-α inhibitors. A diligent and exhaustive search for mycobacterial and fungal organisms is therefore mandatory before considering this possibility, and cultures should also be negative. There are no pathognomonic histologic features that separate infectious bronchiolitis from inflammatory bowel disease-associated bronchiolitis. In fact, the suppurative appearance of the inflammation can be so striking that it has been referred to as "sterile abscess".

Diagnostic work-up

No special stains are required unless granulomas or organisms are suspected. Extensive luminal acute inflammatory exudate or the presence of luminal necrosis should generally trigger special stains for microorganisms.

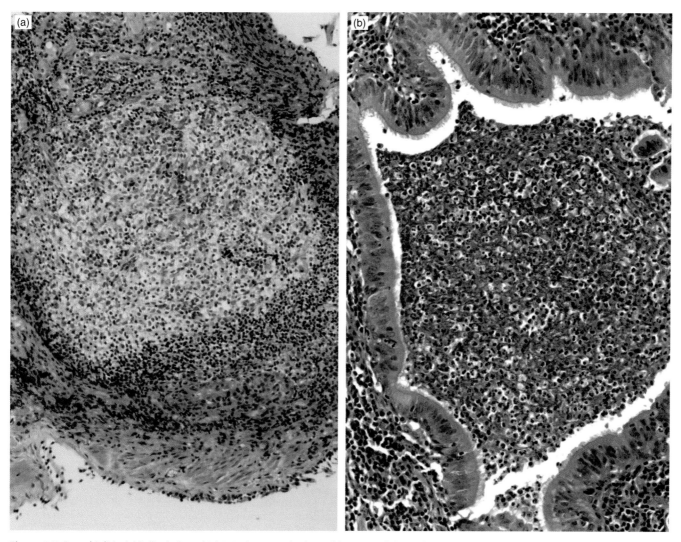

Figure 9.5. Bronchiolitis. (a) Follicular bronchiolitis in rheumatoid arthritis. **(b)** Acute and chronic bronchiolitis in ulcerative colitis.

Clinical profile

The clinical features of most forms of bronchiolitis are non-specific. They include cough, dyspnea and spirometric evidence of airway obstruction. Not surprisingly, the clinical manifestations overlap greatly with more common airway diseases such as asthma and COPD, and patients are commonly misdiagnosed for many years before the correct diagnosis is made by pathologic examination.

Inflammatory bowel disease is currently considered a systemic inflammatory process, and the lungs may be involved in addition to the gut. Involvement of the lung can manifest as a wide variety of inflammatory, suppurative and granulomatous conditions, analogous to involvement of the gut. Most patients are young adults who develop lung symptoms in the setting of established gastrointestinal disease. In a small minority of cases, pulmonary disease is a harbinger of gastrointestinal tract involvement. Severe acute and chronic bronchiolitis in patients with Crohn's disease and ulcerative colitis often manifests itself after colectomy, when therapy is typically reduced or stopped. The specter of bronchiolitis related to inflammatory bowel disease is generally raised when infiltrates, nodules or masses are discovered in patients with known inflammatory bowel disease without an obvious explanation. The symptoms of inflammatory bowel disease-associated pulmonary disease are non-specific, and overlap greatly with other infectious and inflammatory lung diseases. Symptoms are often attributable to large or small airway involvement.

Diffuse panbronchiolitis has been reported mainly (but not exclusively) in individuals of Asian descent. The average age is in the 40s. Concurrent chronic sinusitis is common, and there is a tendency for *Hemophilus* and *Pseudomonas* to be recovered from the sputum. The presence of these organisms as well as several other features overlap considerably with idiopathic bronchiectasis. It is conceivable, therefore, that diffuse panbronchiolitis is simply a small airway manifestation of bronchiectasis.

Radiologic findings

The main radiologic features of bronchiolitis are centrilobular opacities, centrilobular nodules and tree-in-bud opacities. Adjacent ground-glass opacities may be present. Inflammatory

347

bowel disease-associated bronchiolitis shows similar findings, and large foci of suppuration can mimic the radiologic appearance of abscesses.

Differential diagnosis

- Severe acute and chronic bronchiolitis is a frequent finding in bronchiectasis. Such changes can be identical to those of bronchiolitis occurring without concurrent large airway disease. Radiologic review is helpful in order to exclude the possibility that the bronchiolitis is simply a manifestation of distal bronchiectasis.
- Inflammation and peribronchiolar fibrosis can occasionally mimic interstitial lung disease clinically and radiologically. The predominant involvement of small airways and sparing of the alveolar septa should easily distinguish bronchiolitis from interstitial lung disease in most instances. However, on rare occasions, inflammation and fibrosis of the bronchioles and peribronchiolar interstitium can cause interstitial lung disease. Peribronchiolar metaplasia – that is, replacement of alveolated epithelium in peribronchiolar alveoli by ciliated columnar epithelial cells – appears to be a common finding in such cases. Many different terms have been applied to the resultant pathologic appearance, including peribronchiolar metaplasia–interstitial lung disease, airway-centered interstitial fibrosis and idiopathic bronchiolocentric interstitial pneumonia. These conditions do not appear to represent a discrete pathologic entity. Rather, some appear to represent the residuum of prior bronchiolocentric infections, while others overlap with UIP.
- Before assuming that chronic bronchiolitis is a non-specific finding, every attempt should be made to identify a treatable etiology. The most important of these is infection. A careful search for findings that indicate an infectious etiology, such as necrosis, granulomas, necrotic acute inflammatory exudates and, of course, microorganisms, should be performed in all cases.
- In small transbronchial or endobronchial biopsies, sampling error is always a consideration. Larger specimens may show findings that will clarify the diagnosis.

Treatment and prognosis

Therapy for bronchiolitis varies depending upon the perceived underlying cause. Infectious causes of bronchiolitis are treated with antibiotics. Inflammatory bowel disease-associated bronchiolitis may respond to corticosteroid therapy. Diffuse panbronchiolitis may respond dramatically to macrolides such as erythromycin. The prognosis depends on the underlying etiology.

Sample diagnosis on pathology report

Lung, left lower lobe, surgical biopsy – Chronic bronchiolitis (See comment).

Asthma

Asthma is a common disorder of the airways characterized by bronchial hyper-responsiveness accompanied by recurrent episodes of wheezing or cough. The diagnosis is made on the basis of clinical features. Although pathology currently plays a limited role in the diagnosis, surgical pathologists should know what features to expect when a patient with asthma undergoes a lung biopsy. Familiarity with the pathologic findings of asthma is also helpful in the assessment of eosinophilic granulomatosis with polyangiitis (EGPA, Churg–Strauss) and allergic bronchopulmonary aspergillosis, which constitute the so-called *asthma-plus syndromes*. These diseases are thus named because they occur as superimposed complications in patients with a history of asthma.

Major diagnostic findings

There is no single pathognomonic histologic finding. Asthma is currently a clinically defined entity, and there is no defined role of pathologic findings in the diagnosis. The most common findings are listed below. It is reasonable to raise the possibility of asthma if one or more of these features are seen in a lung specimen. Also, in patients with a known or suspected clinical diagnosis of asthma, the presence of these features can support the diagnosis.

Variable pathologic findings

- The histologic findings commonly seen in asthmatics include thickening of the basement membrane, hyperplasia of goblet cells in the surface epithelium, denudation of surface epithelial cells, squamous metaplasia, hyperplasia of mucous glands in the submucosal salivary-type glands, smooth muscle hyperplasia, and mucin in the lumen (Figure 9.6). The luminal mucin in asthma lacks the layered appearance typical of mucoid impaction of bronchi.
- Eosinophils are prominent in the mucosal inflammatory infiltrate, but other cells including lymphocytes and mast cells may also be present.
- There may be no significant pathologic abnormalities in the airways between attacks and during mild attacks.
- Features of the asthma-plus syndromes may be superimposed on these findings. Histologic features that should suggest a diagnosis other than uncomplicated asthma include layered mucin, granulomas, vasculitis and eosinophilic pneumonia.

Diagnostic work-up

By definition, asthma is a clinical diagnosis. Pathologists seldom (if ever) diagnose asthma without knowledge of the clinical findings. No special stains are required.

Clinical profile

The clinical diagnosis of asthma is based on the presence of typical symptoms, history of atopy, family history of asthma, history of environmental triggers, and evidence of reversible airflow obstruction. The validity of the clinical diagnosis is somewhat weakened by the absence of a well-defined

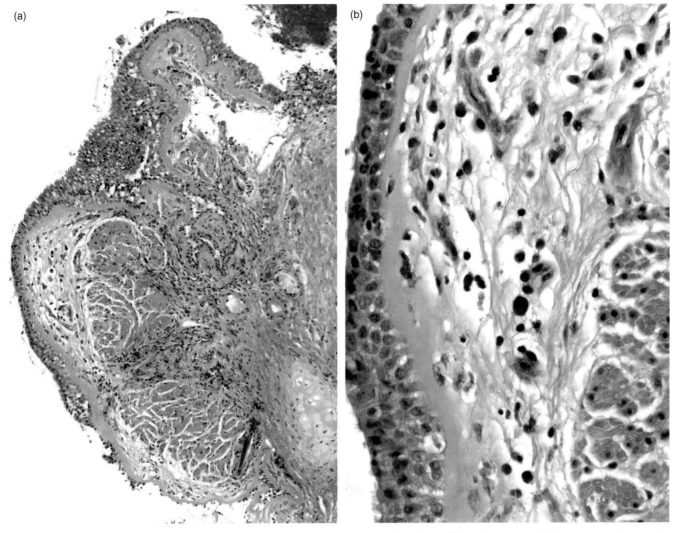

(a)

(b)

Figure 9.6. Bronchial asthma. (a) Endobronchial biopsy specimen showing a fragment of bronchial wall. Note thick eosinophilic basement membrane and prominent smooth muscle. **(b)** There are several eosinophils in the mucosa.

pathologic gold standard. Typical symptoms include wheezing, dyspnea, cough and chest tightness. The symptoms tend to reverse spontaneously or with treatment. They are often seasonal, recurrent and/or nocturnal. Cough may be the only manifestation of asthma (cough variant asthma). None of these symptoms is specific for the diagnosis of asthma, however, and patients may be completely asymptomatic at the time of initial evaluation.

Radiologic findings

Chest radiographs are not required for the diagnosis. When performed, they show either no abnormalities or mild hyperinflation.

Differential diagnosis

- Chronic bronchiolitis can show histologic overlap with asthma. Although evidence for the value of pathologic evaluation is lacking, the presence of eosinophils in the mucosa and a thick basement membrane should raise the possibility of asthma.

- Pathologic findings are perhaps most helpful in the diagnosis of complications in patients with a known history of asthma, the so-called *asthma-plus syndromes*. The presence of additional pathologic findings such as allergic mucin, granulomas, vasculitis or eosinophilic pneumonia (in transbronchial biopsies) should raise concern for these conditions, the best characterized of which are allergic bronchopulmonary aspergillosis and eosinophilic granulomatosis with polyangiitis (EGPA, Churg–Strauss).

- There is considerable scope for clinical overlap between asthma and COPD. For example, patients with asthma may also be smokers, or patients with COPD may happen to have a family history of asthma, challenging the simplistic diagnostic schemes currently in existence. Unfortunately, attempts to distinguish between COPD and asthma using pathologic findings on endobronchial biopsies have failed. At the very least, pathologic findings in these studies did not correlate with current clinical definitions of asthma and COPD. It is unclear why these clinically defined entities do not correspond to precise pathologic findings.

Treatment and prognosis

Bronchodilators and inhaled corticosteroids are the mainstays of therapy. Bronchial thermoplasty is being tried for some patients with severe asthma who are unresponsive to medical therapy; surgical pathologists may see endobronchial biopsies performed in the course of this type of therapy.

Sample diagnosis on pathology report

Lung, right middle lobe carina, endobronchial biopsy – Fragments of bronchial wall with severe basement membrane thickening and increased eosinophils consistent with bronchial asthma (See comment).

Mucoid impaction of bronchi

Mucoid impaction of bronchi is an unusual but distinctive clinicopathologic entity characterized by dilatation and filling of bronchi by a distinctive form of mucin known as *allergic mucin*. The word "impaction" refers to the fact that the mucus appears to be stuck (impacted) within the affected bronchi. This condition is usually encountered in asthmatic individuals, and is often – but not always – a manifestation of allergic bronchopulmonary aspergillosis. It may also occur in isolation, and without demonstrable evidence of *Aspergillus* hyphae. Some cases have been reported in the setting of chronic bronchitis or cystic fibrosis.

Major diagnostic findings

Mucoid impaction of bronchi can occur as an isolated finding or as a component of allergic bronchopulmonary aspergillosis. Identification of allergic mucin is central to the diagnosis. In endobronchial biopsies, the fact that the mucin is derived from the lumen of a bronchus may not be immediately apparent, especially in cases where the mucin is plucked out or debulked from the bronchial lumen. The location is more obvious in surgically resected specimens, where allergic mucin can be seen filling dilated bronchi. Allergic mucin is composed of a mix of eosinophils, fibrin, cell debris and mucin (Figure 9.7–9.9).

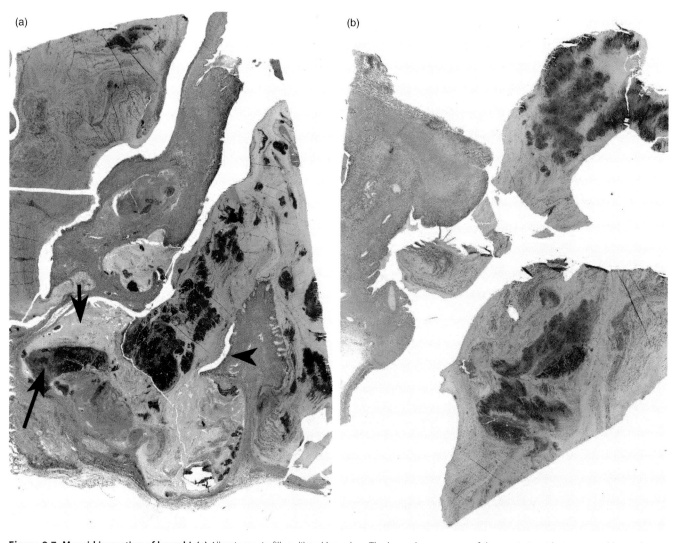

(a)

(b)

Figure 9.7. Mucoid impaction of bronchi. (a) Allergic mucin fills a dilated bronchus. The layered appearance of the mucin is evident even at this very low magnification. Arrowhead: bronchial wall, short arrow: lighter layer, long arrow: darker layer. **(b)** Another area, showing layered mucin within a dilated bronchial lumen. The patient was a young woman who underwent lobectomy for a pulmonary mass. Case courtesy of Dr. AV Arrossi.

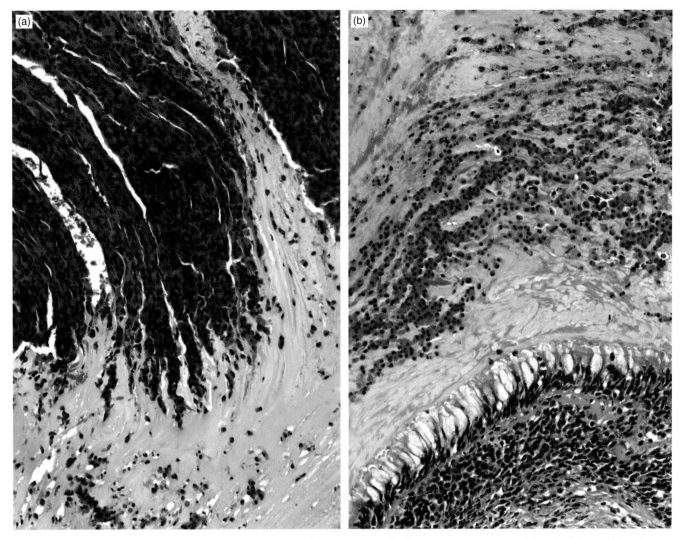

Figure 9.8. Mucoid impaction of bronchi. (a) Layered appearance of allergic mucin. Darker layers at top contain eosinophils and cell debris, while pale-staining mucin predominates in the lighter area at bottom. **(b)** Allergic mucin at top, bronchial wall at bottom. Note goblet cell hyperplasia and eosinophils in bronchial mucosa, both of which are pathologic features of asthma.

Eosinophils are usually numerous. They may be viable, but more often they are degenerated or necrotic. Degenerated eosinophils may lose their usual binucleation and granularity, and are commonly misinterpreted as neutrophils or histiocytes. A characteristic feature of allergic mucin recognizable at low magnification is its layered (*laminated* or *lamellated*) appearance. The lighter layers are composed mainly of mucin, while the darker layers contain a mix of fibrin, clusters of eosinophils and numerous Charcot–Leyden crystals. Charcot–Leyden crystals are eosinophilic, bipyramidal or compass needle-shaped structures derived from the breakdown products of degenerating eosinophils. They are discussed further in the section on allergic bronchopulmonary aspergillosis in Chapter 2 (p. 79).

Variable pathologic findings

- In surgical specimens, small areas of eosinophilic pneumonia may be identifiable in alveoli adjacent to the impacted bronchi. The bronchial mucosa may show the usual features of asthma, including thick basement membranes and goblet cell hyperplasia. Inflammatory changes in the bronchial wall may also be evident, including eosinophils, granulomas (so-called bronchocentric granulomatosis), chronic inflammation and squamous metaplasia.
- Fungal hyphae may be found within the allergic mucin in some cases. This finding is diagnostic of allergic bronchopulmonary fungal disease. The organisms are usually found within clusters of eosinophils rather than in the mucin.
- Foci of organizing pneumonia may be present in the adjacent lung.
- Grossly, the mucus plugs of mucoid impaction are firm and rubbery and vary from white to tan-brown to greenish-gray. Lamination is not always visible to the naked eye. They have been described as hard or putty-like. Bronchoscopists describe the secretions as thick or tenacious.

351

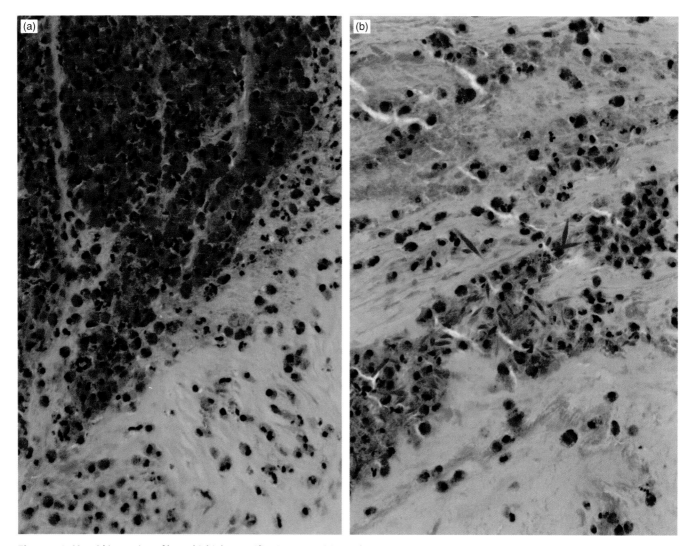

Figure 9.9. Mucoid impaction of bronchi, high magnification. (a) Dark layer of allergic mucin, top, contains innumerable eosinophils, many of which are degenerating. Light layer of allergic mucin is at bottom. It has fewer eosinophils and more mucin than the dark layer. **(b)** Charcot–Leyden crystals in allergic mucin.

Diagnostic work-up

Multiple blocks of allergic mucin should be stained with GMS in an attempt to identify fungal hyphae. Fungi are often sparse, degenerated and difficult to find.

Clinical profile

Patients with mucoid impaction of bronchi may be asymptomatic, or may present with symptoms of pneumonia such as fever and cough. Malaise, pleuritic pain and hemoptysis have also been reported. Cases have been reported in adults as well as children. Clinical features of an underlying disease – most commonly bronchial asthma – may also be present. Thick, branching, tenacious mucus plugs may be expectorated.

Cultures of the mucus plugs are positive for *Aspergillus* in some but not all cases. The inescapable conclusion – as pointed out in Jelihovsky's meticulous study of bronchial plugs in 1983 – is that the fungus is non-viable in some cases, as are the eosinophils.

Radiologic findings

Mucoid impaction of bronchi shows a predilection for bronchi in the central lung and upper lobes. The radiologic findings reflect the presence of impacted mucus plugs within dilated bronchi. Chest X-rays may show V- or Y-shaped densities with distal collapse or consolidation, the *finger-in-glove* sign, mass-like opacities, or a *cluster of grapes* appearance. Occasionally, mucoid impaction of bronchi presents as a solitary lung density, nodule or mass, prompting bronchoscopy or surgical resection.

Differential diagnosis

- Allergic bronchopulmonary aspergillosis enters the differential diagnosis since mucoid impaction of bronchi is one of its cardinal features. As mentioned earlier, identification of fungal hyphae within allergic mucin is diagnostic of allergic bronchopulmonary aspergillosis. In the absence of fungal hyphae, the distinction between mucoid impaction of bronchi and allergic bronchopulmonary aspergillosis rests mainly on clinical and radiologic findings.

- As summarized in Figure 9.2, other types of mucin and mucus plugs must be differentiated from mucoid impaction of bronchi. The usual mucus seen in asthmatic individuals often contains well-preserved eosinophils or even Charcot–Leyden crystals but does not show the layered pattern that characterizes allergic mucin. The rare entity known as *plastic bronchitis* is characterized clinically by the formation and occasional expectoration of peculiar tenacious mucus plugs similar to mucoid impaction of bronchi. Grossly, these plugs branch in a tree-like fashion since they are a perfect cast of the bronchial tree. Microscopically, they are relatively acellular. They usually contain cell debris and proteinaceous exudate but no eosinophils or Charcot–Leyden crystals. They also lack the layered appearance of mucoid impaction of bronchi. Mucin accumulating secondary to airway inflammation or proximal obstruction is usually admixed with an acute inflammatory exudate or other cellular debris. There are typically few if any eosinophils, and no Charcot–Leyden crystals. Plastic bronchitis has been reported in individuals with sickle cell disease, congenital heart disease, prior cardiac surgery or lymphatic obstruction. Altered vascular or lymphatic flow seems to be a common denominator of these conditions, although the exact mechanism of mucus plug formation remains unknown.

Treatment and prognosis

Removal of the mucus plug by spontaneous expectoration or aided by a mucolytic such as acetylcysteine is curative, but bronchoscopy or surgical excision is required in some cases.

Sample diagnosis on pathology report

Lung, right lower lobe, excision – Allergic mucin consistent with mucoid impaction of bronchi (See comment).

Tracheobronchial amyloidosis

Tracheobronchial amyloidosis, characterized by the presence of amyloid deposits within the walls of the trachea and/or bronchi, is one of the three major forms in which amyloid deposits within the lung, the others being alveolar septal amyloidosis and nodular amyloidosis. Alveolar septal amyloidosis is an interstitial process, discussed in Chapter 5. Nodular amyloidosis is addressed in Chapter 6. The three forms of amyloidosis are compared and contrasted in Table 9.4.

Table 9.4. The three major forms of amyloid deposition in the lung

	Tracheobronchial amyloidosis	Nodular amyloidosis	Alveolar septal amyloidosis
Site of amyloid deposition	Airways	Lung parenchyma	Lung parenchyma
Usual type of amyloid	AL (immunoglobulin-derived)	AL (immunoglobulin-derived)	AL (immunoglobulin-derived)
Predominant type of light chain	Lambda	Kappa	Lambda
Clinical presentation	Dyspnea, wheezing, hoarseness, hemoptysis, cough, recurrent pneumonia	Mostly an incidental finding	Symptoms related to systemic amyloidosis (dyspnea due to congestive heart failure, or peripheral neuropathy)
Radiology	Airway thickening, luminal narrowing, calcified wall	Lung nodule or nodules	Interstitial lung disease, signs of systemic amyloidosis (pleural effusions, cardiomegaly)
Pathologic features	Amyloid in airway wall, occasional giant cells, often foci of calcification or ossification	Amyloid-forming nodule in lung parenchyma, often giant cells	Amyloid diffusely deposited in alveolar septa, mimics interstitial fibrosis
Association with or progression to systemic amyloidosis	No	No	Yes
Treatment	No cure. Bronchoscopic stenting, forceps debulking, laser resection, external beam radiation	No treatment required in most cases	Chemotherapy
Prognosis	Variable (some patients remain stable, others die due to bronchial obstruction)	Excellent	Dismal, mostly due to cardiac involvement in systemic amyloidosis; death seldom due to lung disease

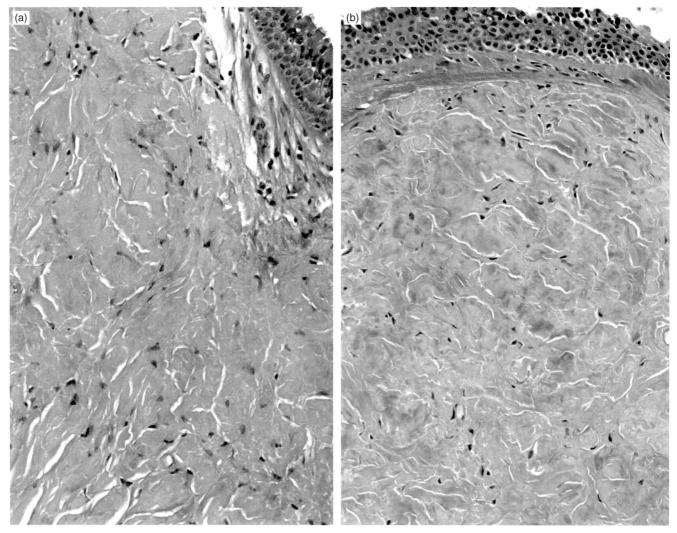

Figure 9.10. Tracheobronchial amyloidosis. (a) Amyloid in the tracheal wall. **(b)** The material is amorphous and eosinophilic.

In contrast to systemic amyloidosis, in which deposits of amyloid are present in various tissues throughout the body, tracheobronchial amyloidosis is a *limited* or *localized* form of amyloidosis unassociated with systemic amyloid deposition. In this respect, tracheobronchial amyloidosis is similar to nodular amyloidosis, which is also a localized form of amyloidosis. It is thought that limited forms of amyloidosis result from small clones of plasma cells that produce and deposit amyloid locally.

Tracheobronchial amyloidosis is mostly encountered by pathologists in endobronchial biopsies of bronchoscopically evident tracheal lesions.

Major diagnostic findings

The main finding is the presence of amyloid deposits in the walls of the trachea or bronchi (Figures 9.10 to 9.13). As in other forms of amyloidosis, the deposits are amorphous, eosinophilic and homogeneous. They are found in the subepithelial stroma ("mucosa" or "submucosa"). By definition, amyloid is positive for Congo red, i.e., it stains salmon-pink and shows apple-green birefringence when viewed under polarized light.

Variable pathologic findings

- Variable numbers of plasma cells may be present. Chromogenic in situ hybridization (CISH) or immunohistochemistry may show evidence of light chain restriction. A few lymphocytes may also be present.
- Foci of metaplastic calcification or ossification within the amyloid deposits are common.
- Multinucleated giant cells may be present in some cases.

Diagnostic work-up

- Congo red staining is the gold standard for the identification of amyloid deposits.
- Beyond confirmation that the deposited material is amyloid, further pathologic work-up is of unclear value. Amyloid subtyping is often claimed to be of critical importance, but since the vast majority of cases of tracheobronchial amyloidosis are localized and immunoglobulin light chain derived (AL type), the clinical

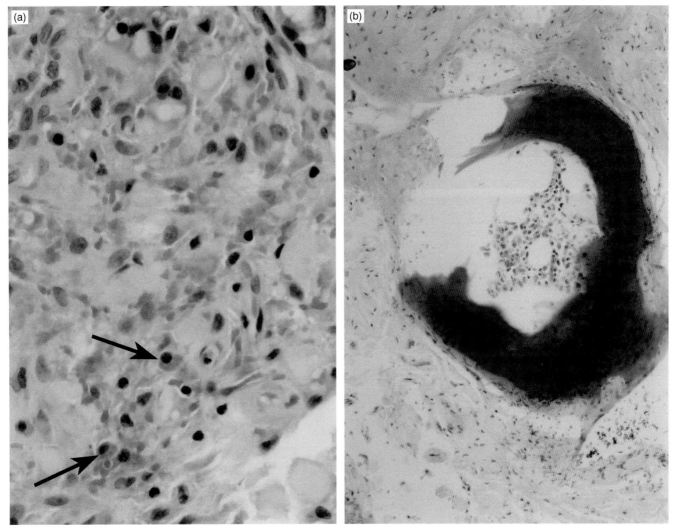

Figure 9.11. Tracheobronchial amyloidosis. (a) A few plasma cells are present within the amyloid deposits (arrows). **(b)** A focus of metaplastic ossification contains bone marrow elements.

value of an expensive work-up can be legitimately questioned.

- If lymphocytes or plasma cells are present in appreciable numbers, light chain restriction may be demonstrable by chromogenic in situ hybridization (CISH), which tends to be "cleaner" than immunohistochemistry.

- Traditional techniques for subtyping amyloid, such as potassium permanganate pre-treatment (AL amyloid is "resistant") and immunohistochemistry (difficult to interpret because of a "dirty" background) have been supplanted in many large referral centers by liquid chromatography and tandem mass spectrometry (MS). This technique uses amyloid obtained by laser capture microdissection from formalin-fixed paraffin-embedded tissues and identifies several amyloid-associated proteins within the deposits. Identification of kappa or lambda light chains allows classification of the amyloid as *AL amyloidosis*. In contrast, identification of serum amyloid-associated (SAA) protein indicates *AA amyloidosis* and identification of transthyretin indicates

TTR amyloidosis (senile or hereditary). Mass spectrometry also identifies other amyloid-associated proteins such as the serum amyloid P component (SAP), providing further confirmation of the diagnosis.

Clinical profile

Tracheobronchial amyloidosis most commonly occurs in elderly individuals of either gender. Most patients present with symptoms attributable to large airway disease, such as cough, wheezing, hoarseness or shortness of breath. Recurrent pneumonias are also common, most likely due to bronchial occlusion. Hemoptysis and stridor are less common. Flow volume curves usually show fixed airway obstruction. The diagnosis should be considered in patients with refractory asthma or chronic cough of unknown etiology. Diagnostic material is usually obtained by bronchoscopy, where amyloid deposits characteristically appear as plaques or nodules. These may be solitary or multiple, and are often described as yellow or waxy. Other bronchoscopic appearances, including polyps, mucosal irregularities, edema and redness, have also been

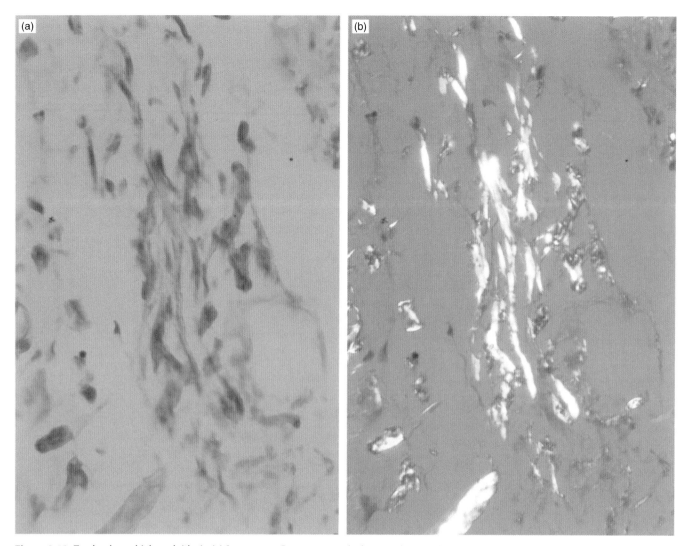

Figure 9.12. Tracheobronchial amyloidosis. (a) Same case as Figure 9.11. Amyloid stains salmon-pink with Congo red. **(b)** The Congo red-stained deposits show apple-green birefringence under polarized light.

described. In contrast to systemic amyloidosis, clinical work-up reveals no evidence of amyloid deposition in other organs or tissues. Such investigations may include serum protein electrophoresis, 24-hour urine analysis, rectal, fat pad or bone marrow biopsies, and echocardiography.

Radiologic findings

CT scans of the chest show multinodular eccentric protrusions into the tracheal lumen, or diffuse circumferential wall thickening with luminal narrowing. Calcification and ossification are common. Concentric disease that includes the posterior wall of the airways is used to differentiate tracheobronchial amyloidosis from tracheobronchopathia osteochrondroplastica, which is thought to spare the posterior wall.

Differential diagnosis

- Light chain deposition disease. Non-amyloid immunoglobulin light chain deposits can appear amyloid-like on H&E but are Congo red negative.

- Fibrosis. Since amyloid is eosinophilic and acellular, it can be easily missed, or misinterpreted as collagen, especially if the material is scant or staining is suboptimal. Failure to consider the possibility of amyloid is the major cause of misdiagnosis.

- *Tracheobronchopathia osteochondroplastica* (tracheobronchopathia osteoplastica) is an entity rarely seen by pathologists but well known to pulmonologists and radiologists. It is characterized by nodular lesions composed of cartilage and bone that protrude into the lumen of the trachea and bronchi. Similar intraluminal protrusions can occur in tracheobronchial amyloidosis, and the frequent occurrence of metaplastic calcification and ossification in amyloid deposits creates further overlap between the two entities. Clinically, tracheobronchopathia osteochondroplastica typically spares the posterior wall, whereas tracheobronchial amyloidosis is usually concentric. By definition, the presence of amyloid on pathologic examination excludes tracheobronchopathia osteochondroplastica.

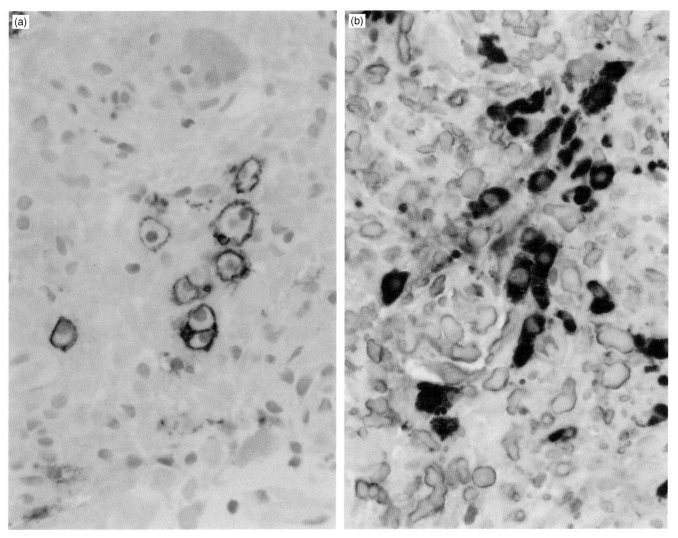

Figure 9.13. Tracheobronchial amyloidosis. Same case as Figure 9.11. The plasma cells are positive for CD138 **(a)** and express predominantly lambda light chains by immunohistochemistry **(b)**.

Treatment and prognosis

There is no cure for tracheobronchial amyloidosis. Bronchoscopic mechanical debulking of amyloid deposits from the tracheobronchial tree has been the approach to ameliorate symptoms in most cases, and appears effective, at least in the short term. Laser ablation has also been used. Post-operative bleeding and re-stenosis requiring additional interventions have been reported after debulking. After bronchoscopic interventions, some patients remain stable for years while others go on to develop recurrent obstruction, respiratory failure and pneumonia. Deaths due to disease have been reported. Novel approaches to therapy include external beam radiation and rituximab. Overall, the prognosis is variable, but still considerably better than the uniformly dismal prognosis associated with alveolar septal amyloidosis.

Sample diagnosis on pathology report

Lung, bronchus intermedius, endobronchial biopsy – Extensive amyloid deposition consistent with tracheobronchial amyloidosis. (See comment).

Obliterative bronchiolitis (constrictive bronchiolitis)

Obliterative bronchiolitis is a fibrosing disorder that narrows or obliterates the lumens of small membranous (non-respiratory) bronchioles. It is also known as *constrictive bronchiolitis*, constrictive bronchiolitis obliterans or *bronchiolitis obliterans*. The terminology, clinical features, radiologic findings and pathologic features of this condition are discussed at length in Chapter 11 (transplant pathology) since the disorder is seen by pathologists mainly in the setting of lung transplantation. This section addresses obliterative bronchiolitis that occurs in settings other than lung transplantation.

Outside of the transplant setting, obliterative bronchiolitis can occur (1) without a well-defined cause, (2) in the setting of a pre-existing disease such as rheumatoid arthritis, (3) after exposure to fumes or toxic gases (e.g., diacetyl fumes produced during the manufacture of microwave popcorn or ammonia), (4) after viral infections, the best known of which is adenovirus, and (5) due to ingestion of the juice of *Sauropus androgynus*, a vegetable cultivated in some parts of Asia. In 1995, the

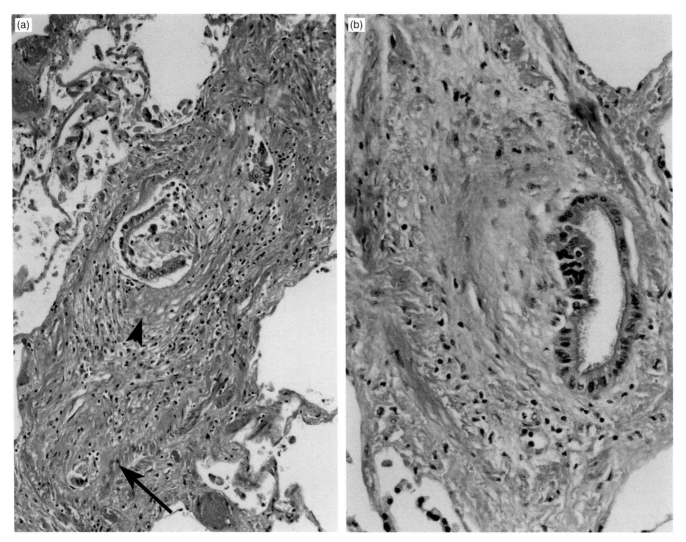

Figure 9.14. Constrictive bronchiolitis (obliterative bronchiolitis). (a) The lumen of this bronchiole is narrowed by extrinsic fibrosis (arrowhead). A few inflammatory cells are also present. The fibrous tissue is extraluminal. It occupies and expands the space between the smooth muscle (arrow) and the luminal epithelium. **(b)** Another example at high magnification, showing a mix of collagen and a few fibroblasts. The lumen is narrowed but not obliterated (also see Figures 11.11–11.16, Chapter 11).

consumption of *Sauropus androgynus* in large quantities for weight loss was associated with an outbreak of histologically documented obliterative bronchiolitis in Taiwan. A few cases were also reported from Japan in 2005.

Obliterative bronchiolitis is rare in non-transplant settings, especially from the surgical pathologist's perspective. Most cases are diagnosed clinically. Obliterative bronchiolitis can be diagnosed on the basis of pathologic findings in transbronchial biopsies, but surgical lung biopsies are more likely to sample diagnostic areas.

Major diagnostic findings

The hallmark of obliterative bronchiolitis is fibrosis or scarring that narrows or completely obliterates bronchiolar lumens by extrinsic compression (Figure 9.14; also see Figures 11.11–11.16, Chapter 11). The fibrosis may consist of collagen or fibroblasts or both, and typically expands the space between the bronchiolar epithelium and the surrounding smooth muscle.

In the non-transplant setting, the diagnosis has also been made in cases where chronic inflammation severely narrows bronchiolar lumens. We prefer to give a descriptive diagnosis in such cases, and restrict the term obliterative bronchiolitis to cases in which fibrosis is the predominant finding.

Variable pathologic findings

See Chapter 11.

Diagnostic work-up

An elastic stain such as EVG, or a combination of trichrome and elastic stains (Movat pentachrome), is very helpful (see Figures 11.11, 11.12 and 11.14 in Chapter 11).

Clinical profile

Obliterative bronchiolitis can occur at any age. Post-infectious obliterative bronchiolitis occurs mainly in children with prior adenovirus infection. Rheumatoid arthritis-associated obliterative bronchiolitis mainly affects middle-aged or elderly women with long-standing rheumatoid arthritis. Cryptogenic cases also occur mainly in women. Most patients present with progressive dyspnea or persistent cough that is unresponsive to bronchodilators or corticosteroids. The duration of symptoms at diagnosis ranges from a few months to several years. Pulmonary function tests typically show fixed obstruction and reduced diffusing capacity.

Radiologic findings

Chest radiographs are often normal or near-normal. The main findings on high-resolution chest CT are mosaic perfusion (mosaic attenuation), air trapping that is accentuated on expiratory views, and hyperinflation of lung parenchyma. However, none of these findings is specific for obliterative bronchiolitis.

Differential diagnosis

The differential diagnosis with organizing pneumonia (formerly bronchiolitis obliterans-organizing pneumonia) and non-specific bronchiolitis is discussed in detail in Chapter 11.

Treatment and prognosis

There is no effective therapy, and the long-term outcome is poor. Progressive airflow limitation may result in death.

Sample diagnosis on pathology report

Lung, right middle lobe, surgical biopsy – Obliterative (constrictive) bronchiolitis (See comment).

References

Bronchiectasis

Chalmers JD, Smith MP, McHugh BJ, Doherty C, Govan JR, Hill AT. Short- and long-term antibiotic treatment reduces airway and systemic inflammation in non-cystic fibrosis bronchiectasis. *Am J Respir Crit Care Med* 2012;**186**:657–65.

Goeminne P, Dupont L. Non-cystic fibrosis bronchiectasis: diagnosis and management in 21st century. *Postgrad Med J* 2010;**86**:493–501.

Kang EY, Miller RR, Müller NL. Bronchiectasis: comparison of preoperative thin-section CT and pathologic findings in resected specimens. *Radiology* 1995;**195**:649–54.

Li AM, Sonnappa S, Lex C, *et al.* Non-CF bronchiectasis: does knowing the aetiology lead to changes in management? *Eur Respir J* 2005;**26**:8–14.

Nicotra MB, Rivera M, Dale AM, Shepherd R, Carter R. Clinical, pathophysiologic characterization of bronchiectasis in an aging cohort. *Chest* 1995;**108**:955–61.

O'Donnell AE. Bronchiectasis. *Chest* 2008;**134**:815–23.

Pasteur MC, Bilton D, Hill AT; British Thoracic Society Bronchiectasis non-CF Guideline Group. British Thoracic Society guideline for non-CF bronchiectasis. *Thorax* 2010;**65** Suppl1:i1–58.

Pasteur MC, Helliwell SM, Houghton SJ, *et al.* An investigation into causative factors in patients with bronchiectasis. *Am J Respir Crit Care Med* 2000;**16**:1277–84.

Whitwell F. A study of the pathology and pathogenesis of bronchiectasis. *Thorax* 1952;**7**:213–39.

Yap VL, Metersky ML. New therapeutic options for noncystic fibrosis bronchiectasis. *Curr Opin Infect Dis* 2015;**28**:171–6.

Bronchiolitis

Couture C, Colby TV. Histopathology of bronchiolar disorders. *Semin Respir Crit Care Med* 2003;**24**:489–98.

Edwards C, Cayton R, Bryan R. Chronic transmural bronchiolitis. A non-specific lesion of small airways. *J Clin Pathol* 1992;**45**:993–8.

Howling SJ, Hansell DM, Wells AU, Nicholson AG, Flint JDA, Muller NL. Follicular bronchiolitis: thin-section CT and histologic findings. *Radiology* 1999;**212**:637–42.

Iwata M, Colby TV, Kitaichi M. Diffuse panbronchiolitis: diagnosis and distinction from various pulmonary diseases with centrilobular interstitial foam cell accumulations. *Hum Pathol* 1994;**25**:357–63.

Kraft M, Mortenson RL, Colby TV, Newman L, Waldron JA, King TE Jr. Cryptogenic constrictive bronchiolitis: a clinicopathologic study. *Am Rev Respir Dis* 1993;**148**:1093–101.

Macklem PT, Thurlbeck WM, Fraser RO. Chronic obstructive disease of small airways. *Ann Intern Med* 1971;**74**:167–77.

Nicholson AG, Wotherspoon AC, Diss TC, *et al.* Reactive pulmonary lymphoid disorders. *Histopathology* 1995;**26**:405–12.

Ryu JH, Myers JL, Swensen SJ. Bronchiolar disorders. *Am J Respir Crit Care Med* 2003;**168**:1277–92.

Schlesinger C, Meyer CA, Veeraraghavan S, Koss MN. Constrictive (obliterative) bronchiolitis: diagnosis, etiology, and a critical review of the literature. *Ann Diagn Pathol* 1998;**2**:321–34.

Visscher DW, Myers JL. Bronchiolitis. The pathologist's perspective. *Proc Am Thorac Soc* 2006;**3**:41–7.

Asthma

Aikawa T, Shimura S, Sasaki H, Ebina M, Takishima T. Marked goblet cell hyperplasia with mucus accumulation in the airways of patients who died of severe acute asthma attack. *Chest* 1992;**101**:916–21.

Barrios RJ, Kheradmand F, Batts L, Corry DB. Asthma. Pathology and pathophysiology. *Arch Pathol Lab Med* 2006;**130**:447–51.

Bourdin A, Serre I, Flamme H, *et al.* Can endobronchial biopsy analysis be recommended to discriminate between asthma and COPD in routine practice? *Thorax* 2004;**9**:488–93.

Djukanovic R, Roche WR, Wilson JW, *et al.* Mucosal inflammation in asthma. *Am Rev Respir Dis* 1990;**142**:434–57.

Dunnill MS. The pathology of asthma, with special reference to changes in the bronchial mucosa. *J Clin Pathol* 1960;**13**:27–33.

James AL, Pare PD, Hogg JC. The mechanics of airway narrowing in asthma. *Am Rev Respir Dis* 1989;**139**:242–6.

Jeffery PK, Wardlaw AJ, Nelson FC, Collins JV, Kay AB. Bronchial biopsies in asthma. An ultrastructural, quantitative study and correlation with hyperreactivity. *Am Rev Respir Dis* 1989;**40**:1745–53.

Ordonez CL, Khashayar R, Wong HH, *et al.* Mild and moderate asthma is associated with airway goblet cell hyperplasia and abnormalities in mucin gene expression. *Am J Respir Crit Care Med* 2001;**163**:517–23.

Salvato G. Quantitative and morphological analysis of bronchial biopsy specimens from asthmatic and non-asthmatic subjects. *Thorax* 2001;**56**:902–6.

Wahidi MM, Kraft M. Bronchial thermoplasty for severe asthma. *Am J Respir Crit Care Med* 2012;**185**:709–14.

Mucoid impaction of bronchi

Anderson WM. Mucoid impaction of upper lobe bronchi in the absence of proximal bronchiectasis. *Chest* 1990;**98**:1023–5.

Carlson V, Martin JE, Keegan JM, Dailey JE. Roentgenographic features of mucoid impaction of the bronchi. *Am J Roentgenol Radium Ther Nucl Med* 1966;**96**:947–52.

Irwin RS, Thomas HM 3rd. Mucoid impaction of the bronchus. Diagnosis and treatment. *Am Rev Respir Dis* 1973;**108**:955–9.

Jelihovsky T. The structure of bronchial plugs in mucoid impaction, bronchocentric granulomatosis and asthma. *Histopathology* 1983;**7**:153–67.

Morgan AD, Bogomoletz W. Mucoid impaction of the bronchi in relation to asthma and plastic bronchitis. *Thorax* 1968;**23**:356–69.

Moser C, Nussbaum E, Cooper DM. Plastic bronchitis and the role of bronchoscopy in the acute chest syndrome of sickle cell disease. *Chest* 2001;**120**:608–13.

Richard S, De Blic J, Pfister A, Lellouch-Tubiana A, Scheinmann P, Da Lage C. Mucoid impaction of bronchi. A scanning electron microscopic study. *Virchows Arch A Pathol Anat Histopathol* 1985;**406**:489–94.

Seear M, Hui H, Magee F, Bohn D, Cutz E. Bronchial casts in children: a proposed classification based on nine cases and a review of the literature. *Am J Respir Crit Care Med* 1997;**155**:364–70.

Shaw RR. Mucoid impaction of the bronchi. *J Thorac Surg* 1951;**29**:149–63.

Spotnitz M, Overholt EL. Mucoid impaction of the bronchi associated with aspergillus. Report of a case. *Dis Chest* 1967;**52**:92–6.

Tracheobronchial amyloidosis

Alloubi I, Thumerel M, Bégueret H, Baste J-M, Velly J-F, Jougon J. Outcomes after bronchoscopic procedures for primary tracheobronchial amyloidosis: *Pulm Med* 2012;**352719**:1–4.

Berk JL, O'Regan A, Skinner M. Pulmonary and tracheobronchial amyloidosis. *Semin Respir Crit Care Med* 2002;**23**:155–65.

Borie M, Danel C, Molinier-Frenkel V, *et al.* Tracheobronchial amyloidosis: evidence for local B-cell clonal expansion. *Eur Respir J* 2012;**39**:1042–5.

Capizzi SA, Betancourt E, Prakash UBS. Tracheobronchial amyloidosis. *Mayo Clin Proc* 2000;**75**:1148–52.

Cordier JF, Loire R, Brune J. Amyloidosis of the lower respiratory tract. Clinical and pathologic features in a series of 21 patients. *Chest* 1986;**90**:827–31.

Hui AN, Koss MN, Hochholzer L, Wehunt WD. Amyloidosis presenting in the lower respiratory tract. Clinicopathologic, radiologic, immunohistochemical and histochemical studies on 48 cases. *Arch Pathol Lab Med* 1986;**110**:212–8.

Neben-Wittich MA, Foote RL, Kalra S. External beam radiation therapy for tracheobronchial amyloidosis. *Chest* 2007;**132**:262–7.

O'Regan A, Fenlon HM, Beamis JF Jr, Steele MP, Skinner M, Berk JL. Tracheobronchial amyloidosis. The Boston University experience from 1984 to 1999. *Medicine (Baltimore)* 2000;**79**:69–79.

Piazza C, Cavaliere S, Foccoli P, Toninelli C, Bolzoni A, Peretti G. Endoscopic management of laryngo-tracheobronchial amyloidosis: a series of 32 patients. *Eur Arch Otorhinolaryngol* 2003;**260**:349–54.

Utz JP, Swensen SJ, Gertz MA. Pulmonary amyloidosis. The Mayo Clinic experience from 1980 to 1993. *Ann Intern Med* 1996;**124**:407–13.

Obliterative bronchiolitis (constrictive bronchiolitis)

Chang H, Wang JS, Tseng HH, Lai RS, Su JM. Histopathological study of *Sauropus androgynus*-associated constrictive bronchiolitis obliterans: a new cause of constrictive bronchiolitis obliterans. *Am J Surg Pathol* 1997;**21**:35–42.

Couture C, Colby TV. Histopathology of bronchiolar disorders. *Semin Respir Crit Care Med* 2003;**24**:489–98.

Gosink BB, Friedman PJ, Liebow AA. Bronchiolitis obliterans. Roentgenologic-pathologic correlation. *Am J Roentgenol Radium Ther Nucl Med* 1973;**117**:816–32.

Kraft M, Mortenson RL, Colby TV, Newman L, Waldron JA, King TE Jr. Cryptogenic constrictive bronchiolitis: a clinicopathologic study. *Am Rev Respir Dis* 1993;**148**:1093–101.

Kreiss K, Gomaa A, Kullman G, Fedan K, Simoes EJ, Enright PL. Clinical bronchiolitis obliterans in workers at a microwave-popcorn plant. *N Engl J Med* 2002;**347**:330–8.

Lai RS, Chiang AA, Wu MT, *et al.* Outbreak of bronchiolitis obliterans associated with consumption of *Sauropus androgynus* in Taiwan. *Lancet* 1996;**348**:83–5.

Meyer KC, Raghu G, Verleden GM, *et al.* An international ISHLT/ATS/ERS clinical practice guideline: diagnosis and management of bronchiolitis obliterans syndrome. *Eur Respir J* 2014;**44**:1479–503.

Ryu JH, Myers JL, Swensen SJ. Bronchiolar disorders. *Am J Respir Crit Care Med* 2003;**168**:1277–92.

Schlesinger C, Meyer CA, Veeraraghavan S, Koss MN. Constrictive (obliterative) bronchiolitis: diagnosis, etiology, and a critical review of the literature. *Ann Diagn Pathol* 1998;**2**:321–34.

Visscher DW, Myers JL. Bronchiolitis. The pathologist's perspective. *Proc Am Thorac Soc* 2006;**3**:41–7.

Chapter 10

Pathologic abnormalities of pulmonary blood vessels

This chapter discusses non-neoplastic pathologic findings in blood vessels. Some of these conditions are shown in Figure 10.1, and an algorithmic approach to non-neoplastic vascular disease in the lung is suggested in Figure 10.2. Pearls and pitfalls related to vascular abnormalities are listed in Table 10.1.

Pulmonary hypertension

Pulmonary hypertension is defined as a *resting mean pulmonary artery pressure of ≥ 25 mmHg*. The diagnosis is suspected on the basis of clinical, electrocardiographic, radiologic and echocardiographic findings, and confirmed by measurement of pulmonary artery pressures by right heart catheterization. The most common causes are left heart failure and parenchymal lung disease.

The role of the surgical pathologist in the diagnosis is limited mainly to confirmation and classification of parenchymal lung disease. In children, grading of pulmonary hypertension has been used to determine potential surgical reversibility of pulmonary hypertensive changes in congenital heart disease. Rarely, pathologic findings help to confirm unusual causes of pulmonary hypertension such as pulmonary veno-occlusive disease, pulmonary capillary hemangiomatosis, talc granulomatosis or tumor emboli. However, histologic examination is rarely if ever required for *diagnosis* of pulmonary hypertension. This is because pathologic abnormalities in pulmonary arteries do not reliably correlate with pulmonary artery pressures. The exception to this general rule is in cases where changes of severe pulmonary hypertension are the only significant pathologic abnormalities in an otherwise normal lung specimen.

Pulmonary hypertension is caused by impedance to blood flow at any point distal to the right ventricle, including pulmonary arteries, alveolar septal capillaries, pulmonary veins or the left heart. Cases in which the presumed site of obstruction is proximal to the alveolar septal capillary bed are known as *pre-capillary*, whereas those in which the obstruction is distal to the capillaries are classified as *post-capillary*. Pre-capillary causes of pulmonary hypertension include *pulmonary arterial hypertension*, and pulmonary artery obstruction by thrombi, emboli, malignant cells or foreign bodies. Post-capillary obstruction can occur in small veins (venules) in the interstitium, larger veins in the interlobular septa and the main pulmonary veins that drain from the lungs into the left atrium. Venules and veins within the lungs can be obstructed in *pulmonary veno-occlusive disease* (PVOD). Outside the lungs,

pulmonary veins can be obstructed by mediastinal masses such as tumors, cysts or fibrosing (sclerosing) mediastinitis, or by scar tissue formed after ablation of the pulmonary vein ostium for treatment of atrial fibrillation. Obstruction to outflow of blood can also occur as a result of mitral stenosis or tumors of the left heart.

Cases of pulmonary hypertension with an elevated pulmonary artery wedge pressure (PAWP) and unknown etiology have traditionally been referred to as *primary pulmonary hypertension* (PPH), whereas those with known underlying causes have been lumped together as *secondary pulmonary hypertension*. Current classification schemes do not use the pre-capillary vs. post-capillary or primary vs. secondary nomenclature. Instead, the various conditions causing pulmonary hypertension are grouped on the basis of shared clinical findings, pathologic manifestations, hemodynamic characteristics and management. In the latest classification scheme, primary pulmonary hypertension is known as *idiopathic pulmonary arterial hypertension* (Table 10.2).

The remainder of this section will focus mainly on pulmonary arterial hypertension. Pulmonary veno-occlusive disease (PVOD) is addressed in detail in the next section.

Pulmonary artery abnormalities are most commonly seen by surgical pathologists in lung biopsies for interstitial lung disease. The most common of these is UIP, but abnormal arteries can also be seen in combined pulmonary fibrosis and emphysema (CPFE), diffuse alveolar damage (DAD), connective tissue disease-related interstitial lung disease, and other forms of fibrosing interstitial lung disease. Lung biopsies in these conditions often show marked thickening of pulmonary arteries characterized by smooth muscle hypertrophy, intimal fibrosis or both. It is well known that these findings do not necessarily correlate with measurement of pulmonary artery pressures by right heart catheterization. Therefore, arterial thickening should be ignored when encountered in the context of interstitial lung disease. Arterial changes suggestive of pulmonary hypertension only assume diagnostic significance when they are seen in otherwise normal lungs.

Major diagnostic findings

- Hypertrophy of smooth muscle in the media of pulmonary arteries is the most common pathologic finding in pulmonary hypertension. Unfortunately, it is also the least specific. It is characterized by an increase in the number of smooth muscle layers in pulmonary arteries (Figure 10.3). It is seen in muscularized medium-sized and small

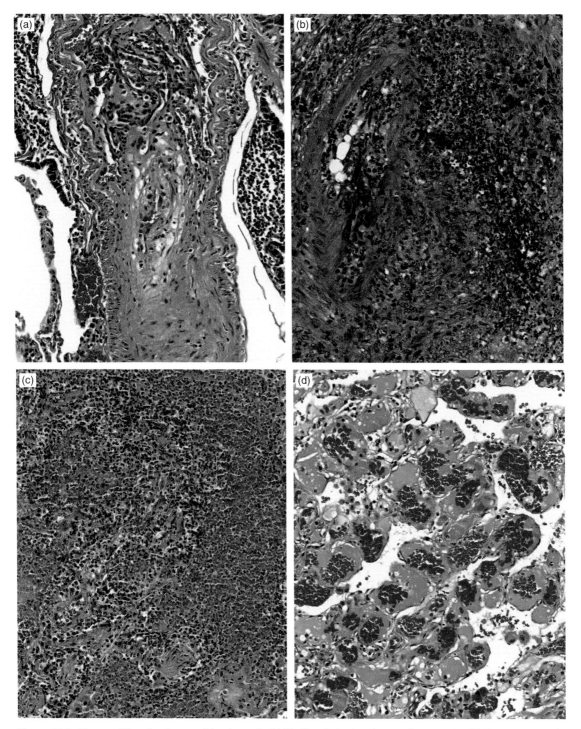

Figure 10.1. Abnormalities of pulmonary blood vessels. (a) Plexiform lesion in pulmonary hypertension. **(b)** Necrotizing vasculitis in granulomatosis with polyangiitis (Wegener's). **(c)** Capillaritis with alveolar hemorrhage in granulomatosis with polyangiitis (Wegener's). **(d)** Capillary congestion in a case of pulmonary vein obstruction caused by fibrosing mediastinitis. All pictures are at identical magnification.

pulmonary arteries. Usually, a qualitative assessment of arterial thickening suffices, but quantitative measurements of muscular artery thickness can also be provided. In general, the normal medial thickness in pulmonary arteries is less than 10% of the diameter of the artery. Medial thickness greater than 15% is considered abnormal.

- Arterioles are almost always prominent in the alveolar septa in pulmonary hypertension, whereas they are inconspicuous and indistinguishable from venules in normal lungs. The arteriolar prominence in pulmonary hypertension is caused by smooth muscle hypertrophy – a phenomenon known as *muscularization of arterioles* (Figure 10.4).

Variable pathologic findings

- *Intimal thickening, fibrosis or fibroelastosis* is characterized by expansion of the intima by stromal cells, fibroblasts or

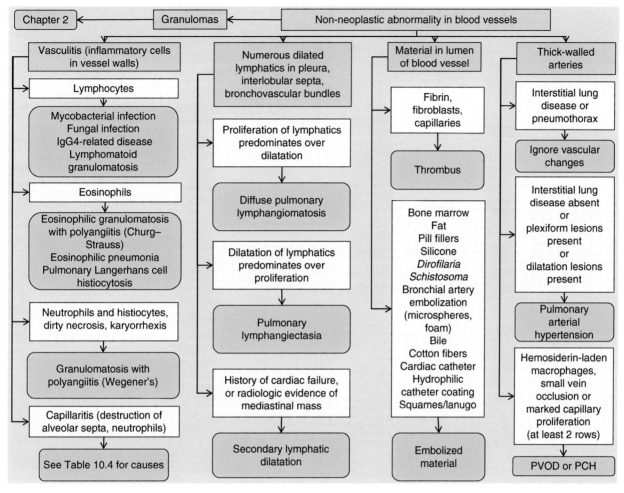

Figure 10.2. Algorithmic approach to non-neoplastic changes in blood vessels of the lung.

collagen. The tip-off to the presence of intimal involvement is the characteristic pale-staining nature of the lesion and the fact that it is located internal to the smooth muscle (Figure 10.5). The pale appearance has been referred to as fibroelastosis. Intimal thickening may be concentric or eccentric.

- *Plexiform lesions* are thought to be a histologic marker of sustained, irreversible pulmonary hypertension. Unfortunately, they are not always present, especially in mild cases. They are characterized by focal disruption of the elastic tissue of muscularized pulmonary arteries by glomeruloid proliferations of endothelium-lined vascular channels (Figures 10.6 and 10.7). They are usually seen in dilated muscular arteries. Disruption of the elastic lamina helps to separate these lesions from organizing thrombi. Occasionally, the connection to an artery may not be apparent.
- *Dilatation lesions* consist of dilated, thin-walled, congested capillary-sized vascular channels. They are closely related to plexiform lesions but as the name suggests they are composed of capillaries that are significantly dilated. Whether they are a variant or a consequence of plexiform lesions is unclear. Some authors refer to dilatation lesions as *angiomatoid lesions*. Plexiform lesions and dilatation

lesions are often found in close association with each other, supporting the contention that they are related (Figure 10.8). Both are reliable markers of pulmonary hypertension. In addition to idiopathic pulmonary arterial hypertension, they also occur in cardiac left-to-right shunts such as septal defects.

- Necrotizing arteritis and other forms of vasculitis containing either lymphocytes or polymorphonuclear leukocytes have been described in severe pulmonary hypertension.
- The *Heath–Edwards grading system* has been traditionally used for grading the severity of pulmonary hypertension in patients with left-to-right shunts due to congenital cardiac septal defects (Table 10.3). Grades 1 and 2 are thought to be potentially reversible, while Grades 3 through 6 are considered irreversible. This grading system was created to provide guidance to surgeons regarding potential reversibility of pulmonary hypertension with surgical repair of the underlying cardiac anomaly. However, it was gradually transposed onto pulmonary arterial hypertension, where its utility is questionable. First, it is unclear that progression from grade 1 to grade 6 occurs. Second, it has never been established that Heath–Edwards grading correlates with

Table 10.1. Pearls and pitfalls in vascular disease of the lung

Arteries can be alarmingly thick in usual interstitial pneumonia (UIP), other interstitial lung diseases, and specimens from patients with pneumothorax. This finding does not correlate with pulmonary artery pressures measured clinically and should not be diagnosed as pulmonary hypertension

Plexiform lesions and dilatation lesions are pathognomonic of pulmonary hypertension

Always consider the possibility of pulmonary veno-occlusive disease when you see hemosiderin-laden macrophages within the airspaces, especially in cases with thick pulmonary arteries or alveolar septal perivascular calcification

Significant lymphocytic vasculitis has a limited differential diagnosis, including granulomatous mycobacterial and fungal infections, lymphomatoid granulomatosis and IgG4-related lung disease

Capillaritis is a major cause of life-threatening alveolar hemorrhage. The pathologic findings can be very subtle because the affected capillaries are completely destroyed

Capillaritis can be very difficult to distinguish from acute bronchopneumonia. The characteristic mix of neutrophils, histiocytes and karyorrhectic debris within alveolar septa is a clue to the diagnosis, as is the presence of blood and hemosiderin-laden macrophages

The most common cause of capillaritis is granulomatosis with polyangiitis (Wegener's)

severity or duration of pulmonary hypertension. Third, there is no evidence that it has prognostic significance, especially in the setting of idiopathic pulmonary arterial hypertension. For these reasons, many pulmonary pathologists no longer use the Heath–Edwards grading system. In practice, a good description of the vascular lesions is sufficient to indicate the severity of the process.

Diagnostic work-up

Special stains such as Movat pentachrome or Verhoeff–Van Gieson can be very helpful to identify disruption of the elastic lamina, highlight medial hypertrophy and intimal fibrosis, and distinguish arteries from veins.

Clinical profile

The following discussion pertains mainly to pulmonary arterial hypertension. The mean age of onset was traditionally in the 30s, but with increasing diagnosis in elderly individuals, the mean age at diagnosis in current registries is between 50 and 65 years. The condition is slightly more common in women. Most patients present with non-specific symptoms such as dyspnea on exertion, syncope, fatigue, chest pain, dizziness, hemoptysis or Raynaud's phenomenon. Physical examination may show signs of right heart failure, including jugular vein distension, prominent right ventricular impulse, accentuated

P2, right-sided third heart sound (S3), tricuspid insufficiency murmur, hepatomegaly and peripheral edema.

Chest imaging can be helpful in demonstrating evidence of pulmonary artery enlargement or right heart failure. It may also show evidence of an underlying cause such as left heart failure or interstitial lung disease. An electrocardiogram may show signs of right ventricular hypertrophy such as tall R waves or right axis deviation. Once pulmonary hypertension is suspected, transthoracic echocardiography is the most important diagnostic tool with the potential to simultaneously detect pulmonary hypertension and exclude underlying cardiac disease. The gold standard for diagnosis is right heart catheterization with measurement of pulmonary artery pressures.

Radiologic findings

The main radiologic findings of pulmonary arterial hypertension are central pulmonary artery enlargement, sharply tapered or pruned peripheral vessels, and right ventricular hypertrophy and dilatation. A mosaic pattern of lung attenuation has been reported on high-resolution CT scans. Radiologic findings are also helpful in detecting or excluding pulmonary and cardiac causes of pulmonary hypertension.

Differential diagnosis

- The main pitfall in the histologic diagnosis of pulmonary hypertension is over-interpretation of vascular changes in interstitial lung disease. This error can be avoided by disregarding thick pulmonary arteries in patients with underlying interstitial lung disease.
- Pulmonary veno-occlusive disease and obstruction of pulmonary veins by mediastinal masses such as fibrosing mediastinitis enter the differential diagnosis since they can be associated with marked pulmonary arterial medial hypertrophy and intimal thickening. Pathologists should remember that *chronic congestion, hemosiderin deposition and hemorrhagic (venous) infarcts are not features of pulmonary arterial hypertension*; rather, they are histologic clues to the presence of venous/post-capillary obstruction to blood flow. The diagnosis of pulmonary veno-occlusive disease requires demonstration of occluded or recanalized small veins or venules within the lung parenchyma. Obstruction of pulmonary veins in the mediastinum can be detected by CT scans, and surgical pathologists can play an important role in diagnosing the precise cause in biopsies of mediastinal lesions.

Treatment and prognosis

Idiopathic pulmonary arterial hypertension is very difficult to treat and is usually irreversible. Treatment options include anticoagulants, calcium channel blockers, endothelin receptor antagonists such as bosentan, ambrisentan and macitentan, phosphodiesterase type 5 (PDE5) inhibitors such as sildenafil and tadalafil, and prostacyclin analogues such as epoprostenol, iloprost and treprostinil. A guanylate cyclase stimulator named riociguat has also recently become available. Lung

Table 10.2. Clinical classification of pulmonary hypertension (simplified version of Nice classification, Simonneau *et al* 2013)

Main category	Examples	Notes
Pulmonary arterial hypertension	Idiopathic pulmonary arterial hypertension Heritable pulmonary arterial hypertension Drug and toxin-associated pulmonary arterial hypertension Miscellaneous causes of pulmonary arterial hypertension (HIV infection, portopulmonary hypertension, congenital heart diseases and schistosomiasis)	Heritable causes include mutations in bone morphogenic protein receptor 2 (*BMPR2*), caveolin-1, endoglin, activin-like receptor kinase-1 (ALK$_1$) and SMAD9 Examples of drugs or toxins that cause pulmonary arterial hypertension include aminorex, fenfluramine, dexfenfluramine, toxic rapeseed oil, and benfluorex
Pulmonary veno-occlusive disease and/or pulmonary capillary hemangiomatosis	Pulmonary veno-occlusive disease (PVOD) Pulmonary capillary hemangiomatosis (PCH)	May require pathologic diagnosis
Persistent pulmonary hypertension of the newborn	Persistent pulmonary hypertension of the newborn	Most often seen in neonates Diagnosis requires demonstration of right-to left shunt, absence of congenital heart disease (echocardiography) Pulmonary artery pressure measurement not required
Pulmonary hypertension due to left heart disease	Systolic dysfunction Diastolic dysfunction Valvular disease Outflow tract obstruction Congenital inflow–outflow tract obstruction	Diagnosed on the basis of clinical and radiologic findings
Pulmonary hypertension due to lung disease and/or hypoxia	COPD Interstitial lung disease Other lung diseases with mixed restrictive and obstructive pattern Sleep-disordered breathing Alveolar hypoventilation disorders Chronic exposure to high altitude Developmental lung diseases	Surgical pathologists often play a role in diagnosing interstitial lung disease, but the associated pulmonary hypertension remains a clinical diagnosis
Chronic thromboembolic pulmonary hypertension (CTEPH)	Chronic or recurrent pulmonary embolism	Diagnosed by ventilation/perfusion scintigraphy Treated with pulmonary endarterectomy; emboli located in distal arteries may be inoperable
Unclear mechanisms	Hematologic disorders (sickle cell disease, myeloproliferative diseases) Sarcoidosis Langerhans cell histiocytosis Lymphangioleiomyomatosis Storage disorders Outflow tract obstruction by tumors or fibrosing mediastinitis	Pathologists play a key role in diagnosing many of these conditions

transplantation is an option for patients who do not respond to medical therapy.

Overall, the prognosis is exceedingly poor, with mortality rates of 5 to 10% per year. Complications of pulmonary hypertension include right heart failure (cor pulmonale) and sudden death. For untreated cases, estimated 3-year survival is approximately 41%. With intravenous prostacyclin therapy, 3-year survival increases to approximately 63%.

Recently, in some registries, 3-year survival of up to 83% has been reported.

Sample diagnosis on pathology report

Lung, right, explant pneumonectomy – Severe pulmonary hypertensive arteriopathy with plexiform lesions, consistent with pulmonary arterial hypertension (See comment).

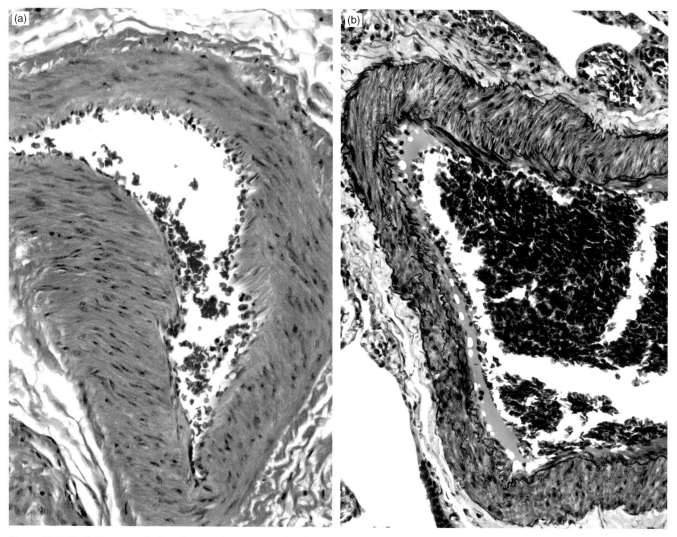

Figure 10.3. Medial hypertrophy in pulmonary hypertension. (a) The media is markedly thickened by smooth muscle hyperplasia. **(b)** A Movat pentachrome stain highlights the smooth muscle hyperplasia and also shows two distinct elastic tissue layers on both sides of the thickened media, confirming that the vessel is an artery. The images are from an explanted lung from a 56-year-old woman who underwent lung transplantation for idiopathic pulmonary arterial hypertension.

Pulmonary veno-occlusive disease

Pulmonary veno-occlusive disease (PVOD) is a rare cause of pulmonary hypertension characterized by *occlusion of veins within the lung*. The rarity of the disease is demonstrated by the fact that only 150 cases were reported in the first 66 years (1934–2000) after its description. Since veins are the source of obstruction in PVOD, it is classified as a post-capillary cause of pulmonary hypertension. The entire spectrum of clinical and histologic manifestations of PVOD is a consequence of venous occlusion, which leads to increased pressure in upstream blood vessels, i.e., capillaries and pulmonary arteries. Increased pressure in alveolar septal capillaries leads to congestive changes in the lung, and increased pressure in the pulmonary arteries manifests as pulmonary hypertension.

The cause of PVOD is unknown in the majority of cases. However, it has been hypothesized that infection, autoimmune insults or other types of injuries lead to thrombosis and subsequent occlusion of veins. Several potential etiologies have been proposed, including chemotherapeutic agents, connective tissue diseases and genetic mutations. The most commonly implicated chemotherapeutic agents are alkylating agents such as cisplatin, carmustine (BCNU), bleomycin, mitomycin-C, cytarabine and antimetabolites such as vincristine. A recent review claimed that cyclophosphamide was the most frequently responsible agent. Approximately 78% of cases of chemotherapy-associated PVOD occur within 1 year of therapy. Connective tissue disease has been implicated as a cause of PVOD because some patients with PVOD have a history of systemic lupus erythematosus, CREST syndrome (limited variant of progressive systemic sclerosis) or rheumatoid arthritis. Elevated antinuclear antibody (ANA), rheumatoid factor (RF) or anti-cardiolipin antibody titers have been found in some patients. Among genetic factors, a recent finding is mutation of *EIF2AK4*, a gene that is mutated in virtually all familial cases of PVOD and approximately one-fourth of sporadic cases. This gene is also mutated in pulmonary capillary hemangiomatosis. Mutation of the bone morphogenetic

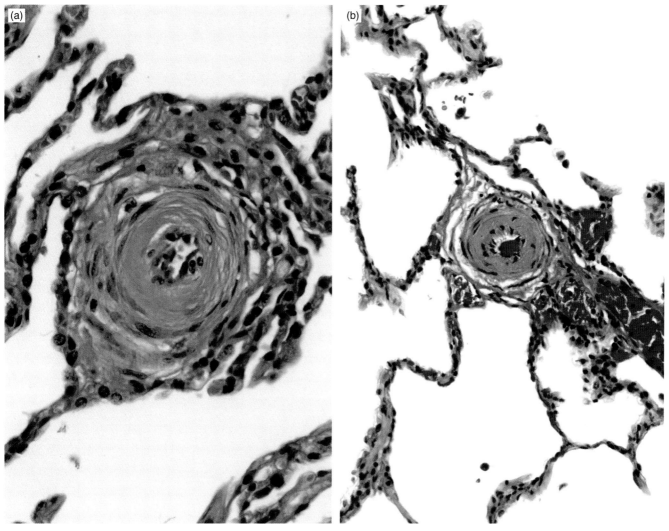

Figure 10.4. Thick and prominent arterioles in pulmonary hypertension. (a) Prominent arteriole from a case of idiopathic pulmonary arterial hypertension. Note thick, muscularized wall. **(b)**. Another prominent arteriole within the alveolar septa. Arterioles of this thickness do not occur in normal lungs.

protein receptor 2 (*BMPR2*) has also been described in PVOD. The reader will recall from the previous section that *BMPR2* is the most common mutation in heritable pulmonary arterial hypertension.

Major diagnostic findings

- The main pathologic finding in PVOD is narrowing or occlusion of small intrapulmonary veins (Figure 10.9). Medium or larger-sized veins may also be occluded. The occlusion is patchy and extremely difficult to find. The narrowing may be caused by concentric or eccentric intimal fibrosis. Some authors claim that recanalized thrombi are frequently a component of PVOD, but this has not been our experience.
- Chronic congestive changes in the lung are common in PVOD, and are far more obvious and prominent than obstruction of small veins. They are characterized by the presence of numerous hemosiderin-laden macrophages within alveoli (Figure 10.10). This is thought to be a reflection of hemorrhage, presumably due to rupture of

congested alveolar septal capillaries. Other evidence of long-standing alveolar hemorrhage may also be present in the form of so-called *endogenous pneumoconiosis* (Figure 10.10). This odd tissue reaction can be found in long-standing alveolar hemorrhage due to any cause, including congestive heart failure and vasculitis. It consists of encrustation of iron and calcium on elastic tissue layers of small pulmonary blood vessels, often accompanied by a foreign-body type giant cell type reaction. The term is a misnomer since this phenomenon is completely unrelated to pneumoconiosis.

- Arterial changes of mild to moderate pulmonary hypertension are seen in virtually all cases of PVOD. The most common finding is medial hypertrophy, but intimal fibrosis is also common.

Variable pathologic findings

- Patchy lymphatic dilatation is said to be more prominent in PVOD than in other causes of post-capillary pulmonary hypertension and can serve as a clue to the diagnosis.

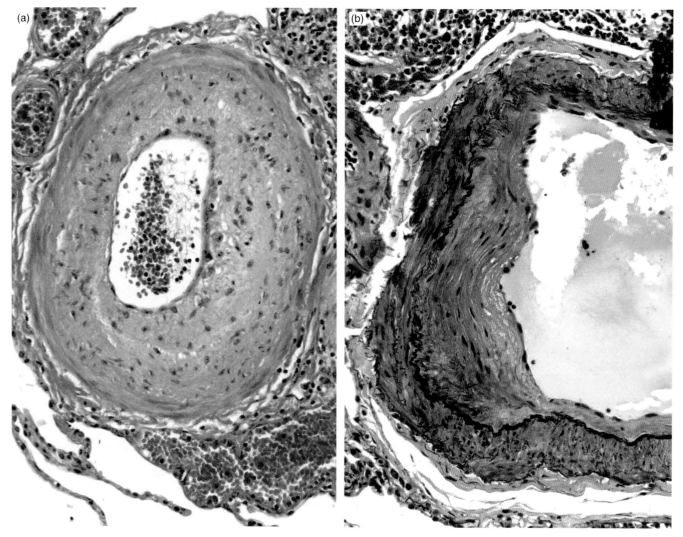

Figure 10.5. Intimal thickening in pulmonary hypertension. (a) Cells within a pale-staining background expand the intima. Note that the pale area is internal to smooth muscle cells. **(b)** Movat pentachrome stain greatly facilitates recognition of intimal fibrosis, which appears as a green area internal to the black internal elastic lamina.

- Arterial thrombi are usually absent in PVOD. When present, they are not prominent. There are only rare cases in which pulmonary arterial thrombosis was a prominent feature in PVOD.
- Other variable findings include heavy and congested lungs, prominent bronchial veins within bronchovascular bundles, interlobular septal edema, small hemorrhagic infarcts adjacent to interlobular septa (so-called "venous infarcts"), extension of smooth muscle cells from the media into the intima, and intra-vascular septa within pulmonary veins.

Diagnostic work-up

The most useful stain in the pathologic work-up of PVOD is an elastic stain or the Movat pentachrome stain. The latter highlights loose fibroblast-rich fibrosis, collagen-type fibrosis and normal elastic tissue, all in one stain. Several studies have highlighted the utility of this stain in the diagnosis of PVOD. Occlusion of small veins, which is very difficult to see on

H&E, is relatively easy to see on a Movat stain. On Movat and other elastic stains, veins usually have one elastic lamina while arteries have two. Arterialization of veins is a frequent finding in PVOD, resulting in multiple elastic laminae. Another clue to the diagnosis is the absence of normal-appearing small veins.

Clinical profile

PVOD can occur at virtually any age. The age in reported cases has ranged from 9 days to 67 years. However, most patients are less than 50 years of age and approximately one-third are children. An important observation that several authors have made is that the predilection of pulmonary arterial hypertension for young adult women is not seen in PVOD, where the sex ratio is equal or slightly favors men. The most common clinical symptom is progressive dyspnea. Other symptoms include chest pain, hemoptysis, cyanosis, cough and syncope. Signs of right heart failure may be present, including jugular vein distension, a third heart sound, a right ventricular heave

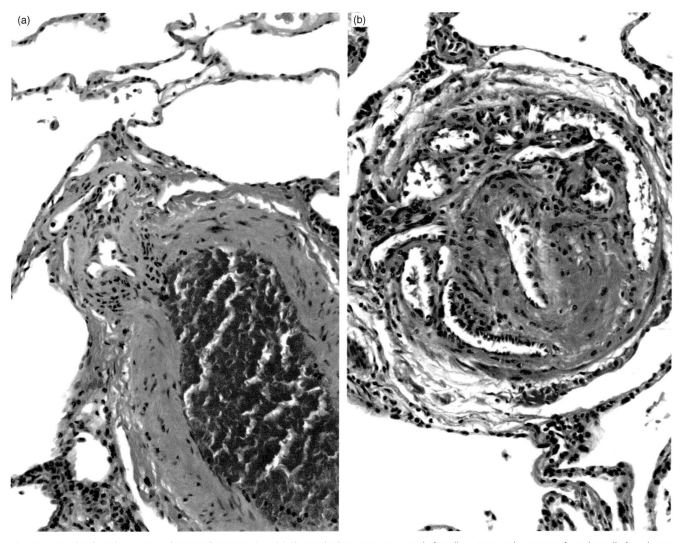

Figure 10.6. Plexiform lesions in pulmonary hypertension. (a) Glomeruloid structure composed of capillary-size vessels emanates from the wall of a pulmonary artery. **(b)** Another plexiform lesion, shown at higher magnification. The resemblance to a glomerulus is striking. The disrupted artery is in the center of the lesion. Plexiform lesions are diagnostic of pulmonary hypertension.

or lower extremity edema. Clubbing and rales are clinical clues that favor PVOD over pulmonary arterial hypertension.

Clinical investigations usually show evidence of increased pulmonary artery pressure consistent with pulmonary hypertension. Pulmonary artery wedge pressure in PVOD is controversial. Most authors state that the pulmonary artery wedge pressure in PVOD is normal to low (the normal range is 2 to 15 mmHg). In contrast, in left heart failure the pulmonary artery wedge pressure is usually in excess of 20 mmHg. Others state that the characteristic feature of PVOD is the failure to obtain a pulmonary artery wedge pressure tracing.

Radiologic findings

The main radiologic features of PVOD are enlargement of the pulmonary arteries along with signs of venous congestion such as interstitial edema, Kerley B lines and pleural effusions (rare in pulmonary arterial hypertension). Since congestion in PVOD results from intrapulmonary venous

obstruction rather than heart failure, radiologic studies show pulmonary edema in the *absence* of heart failure, left atrial dilatation or large pulmonary vein dilatation. CT scans of the chest may show intralobular septal thickening or smooth septal lines in addition to diffuse or mosaic ground-glass opacities. Ventilation profusion scans may be normal or show changes consistent with low probability for pulmonary embolism.

Before making a diagnosis of PVOD, imaging studies should be carefully re-examined to exclude left ventricular failure, mitral valve disease, left atrial myxoma, pulmonary vein obstruction by lung cancer or other mediastinal masses, anomalous pulmonary vein drainage, fibrosing (sclerosing) mediastinitis, cor triatriatum or pulmonary vein obstruction due to prior catheter ablation for atrial fibrillation. Recognition of prior catheter ablation is extremely important, since pulmonary vein stenosis mimicking PVOD can develop after ablation of the pulmonary vein ostia, which is often used as a treatment for atrial fibrillation.

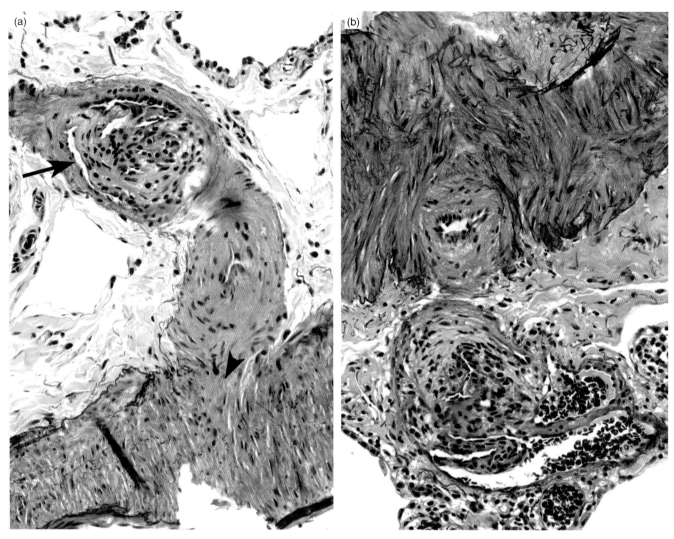

Figure 10.7. Plexiform lesions in pulmonary hypertension (Movat pentachrome stain). **(a)** Glomeruloid structure (arrow) focally disrupts elastic tissue as it emanates from a pulmonary artery (arrowhead). **(b)** In this example, the disrupted artery is at top, and the plexiform lesion is at bottom.

Differential diagnosis

- Occlusion of pulmonary veins in the mediastinum can produce lung parenchymal changes histologically indistinguishable from those of PVOD. These include the presence of numerous hemosiderin-laden macrophages within the airspaces, striking congestion of alveolar septal capillaries, hemorrhagic infarcts, endogenous pneumoconiosis, dilatation of lymphatics and marked thickening of pulmonary arteries. The key to the diagnosis is careful radiologic evaluation of the mediastinum to exclude the possibility of a mediastinal mass compressing the pulmonary veins. Pathologists should be aware of this phenomenon since radiologists may not necessarily recognize that the parenchymal changes are causally related to pulmonary vein obstruction. In our experience, fibrosing mediastinitis is the most common cause of this underappreciated phenomenon.
- PVOD and pulmonary capillary hemangiomatosis (PCH) share many features, including pulmonary hypertension,

occurrence in young individuals, *EIF2AK4* mutations, hemosiderin-laden macrophages, pulmonary artery thickening and capillary proliferation. Given these similarities, it is not surprising that these disorders are often thought to be part of an overlapping spectrum. Some have suggested that PCH is simply a consequence of PVOD, and given the difficulty in finding obstructed veins in PVOD, this is certainly plausible. Histologic findings that favor PCH over PVOD include increased capillary proliferation (widening of alveolar septa by multiple layers of capillaries, which may have a sheet-like growth pattern), invasion of blood vessels by capillaries, the presence of patchy nodular lesions, and the presence of nodular lesions on imaging studies.
- Idiopathic pulmonary hemosiderosis causes abundant hemosiderin deposition in the lung parenchyma, without accompanying vascular changes. The presence of small pulmonary vein obstruction or medial hypertrophy in the pulmonary arteries helps to exclude this possibility. Another helpful differentiating feature is that idiopathic

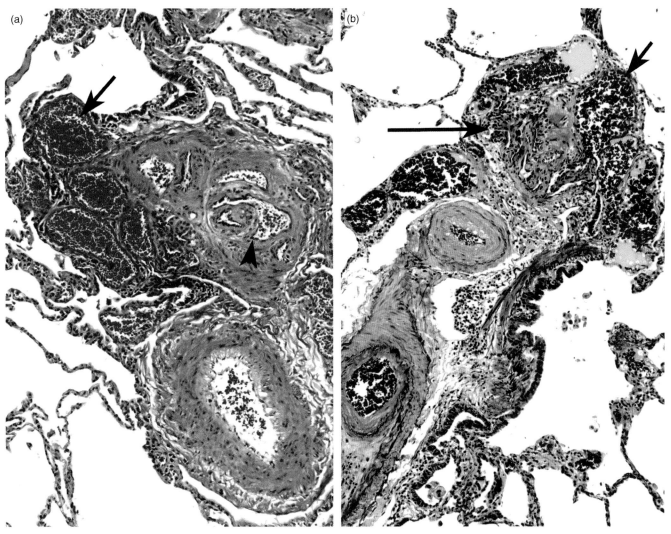

Figure 10.8. Dilatation lesions in pulmonary hypertension. (a) A cluster of dilated, congested, thin-walled vascular spaces is a dilatation lesion (arrow). A plexiform lesion is present nearby (arrowhead). An artery showing medial hypertrophy is at bottom right. **(b)** Movat pentachrome stain. Short arrow indicates dilatation lesion, and long arrow points to a plexiform lesion. Artery with medial hypertrophy and intimal fibrosis is at bottom left.

pulmonary hemosiderosis is usually accompanied by anemia, whereas PVOD is sometimes accompanied by polycythemia.

- Pulmonary arterial hypertension is usually the first consideration when the pulmonary arteries are found to be markedly thickened. However, in the absence of underlying left heart failure or venous occlusion, pulmonary arterial hypertension does not show evidence of capillary congestion, hemosiderin-laden macrophages or hemorrhagic infarcts. Conversely, the presence of plexiform lesions or dilatation lesions excludes PVOD.
- PVOD is unlikely to be confused with alveolar hemorrhage caused by small-vessel vasculitis (capillaritis) on clinical grounds. However, histologically both entities feature intra-alveolar hemosiderin-laden macrophages and endogenous pneumoconiosis. Evidence of venous occlusion or pulmonary hypertension argues against capillaritis, while the presence of a mixed neutrophilic–histiocytic infiltrate with karyorrhexis in the alveolar septa excludes PVOD.

Treatment and prognosis

- Treatment options for PVOD are extremely limited, especially because drugs used in pulmonary arterial hypertension such as calcium channel blockers or epoprostenol have been shown to cause life-threatening pulmonary edema when used in PVOD. In fact, the development of pulmonary edema in patients with pulmonary hypertension after treatment with calcium channel blockers or epoprostenol is virtually diagnostic of PVOD. The only intervention that has been shown to prolong survival in PVOD is lung transplantation. Survival of as long as 11 years after lung transplantation has been reported. Overall, the prognosis of PVOD is extremely poor. Most patients die within 2 years of diagnosis. There are only rare reports of longer survival.

Sample diagnosis on pathology report

Lung, left, explant pneumonectomy – Pulmonary veno-occlusive disease (See comment).

Table 10.3. Heath–Edwards grading system of pulmonary hypertensive changes

Grade	Media and arterioles	Intimal reaction
1	Medial hypertrophy in arteries and arterioles	None
2	Medial hypertrophy in arteries and arterioles	Cellular intimal proliferation
3	Medial hypertrophy in arteries and arterioles Early generalized vascular dilatation	Intimal fibrosis
4	Medial hypertrophy in arteries and arterioles Progressive generalized vascular dilatation Dilatation lesions	Intimal fibrosis and fibroelastosis Plexiform lesions
5	Medial hypertrophy in arteries and arterioles Generalized vascular dilatation Dilatation lesions Hemosiderin deposition	Intimal fibrosis Plexiform lesions
6	Medial hypertrophy in arteries and arterioles Generalized vascular dilatation Dilatation lesions Necrotizing arteritis	Intimal fibrosis Plexiform lesions

Pulmonary capillary hemangiomatosis

Pulmonary capillary hemangiomatosis (PCH) is an extremely rare cause of pulmonary hypertension, first described in 1978 by Wagenvoort and colleagues. Attesting to its rarity is the fact that only 37 cases had been reported by 2002. As the name suggests, the cardinal feature of this disease is proliferation of capillaries within the lung. PCH has many clinical and pathologic features in common with PVOD, and controversy persists to this day as to whether the two entities are actually different manifestations of the same process. The recent discovery of mutations of the eukaryotic translation initiation factor 2α kinase 4 (*EIF2AK4*) in both PCH and PVOD support the contention that they are related, if not identical. In PCH, *EIF2AK4* mutations have been reported in 2 affected brothers and 2 of 10 unrelated individuals with no family history of PCH.

Surgical pathologists may rarely see this entity in surgical lung biopsies, explant pneumonectomies or autopsies.

Major diagnostic findings

The main pathologic finding in PCH is proliferation of congested capillary-size blood vessels within alveolar septa. The proliferating blood vessels are usually distributed in a patchy,

nodular fashion, separated by intervening areas of relatively normal lung. They typically form two or more layers in the alveolar septa in less involved areas, and sheets of back-to-back vessels in severely involved areas (Figure 10.11). Extension of the process into the walls of arteries, veins, venules/arterioles and bronchioles is common. Plexiform lesions and dilatation lesions, which are features of idiopathic or shunt-related pulmonary arterial hypertension, are absent.

Variable pathologic findings

- Manifestations of chronic congestion, such as intra-alveolar hemosiderin-laden macrophages and mild capillary congestion are common but not invariable. Infarcts have been reported in some cases.
- A more diffuse, interstitial pneumonia-like appearance has also been described. There is generally no appreciable interstitial fibrosis.
- Atypia in the form of mild hyperchromasia of the nuclei has been described in the endothelial cells of the proliferating capillaries.
- Arterial changes attributable to pulmonary hypertension such as medial hypertrophy and intimal thickening are almost invariably present.

Diagnostic work-up

As in PVOD, a Movat stain or other elastic stains can be very helpful in the differential diagnosis. Reticulin staining has also been suggested as being helpful in outlining the architecture of the proliferating blood vessels.

Clinical profile

The age range in reported cases of PCH is wide (9 months to 71 years). Unlike idiopathic pulmonary arterial hypertension, there is a slight male preponderance. The mean age is approximately 30 years. Most patients present with dyspnea. In contrast to PVOD, hemoptysis is relatively common, occurring in more than a third of patients. Cough, fatigue and weight loss have also been reported. As in other conditions that cause pulmonary hypertension, there may be hypoxia, cyanosis, hypotension, edema, ascites, hepatomegaly, hepatojugular reflex and a right parasternal heave.

As in PVOD, a characteristic finding observed during right heart catheterization is a combination of elevated pulmonary arterial pressure and low or normal *pulmonary capillary wedge pressure*. It is important to note that, contrary to its name, the pulmonary capillary wedge pressure does not measure the pressure in capillaries per se, but instead measures pressure distal to the small veins, and reflects the pressure in the large pulmonary veins and the left atrium, rather than the pressure in the pulmonary capillary bed itself.

Radiologic findings

Chest radiographs may be normal or may show bilateral interstitial infiltrates. Findings common to any cause of pulmonary hypertension – such as cardiomegaly and pulmonary artery

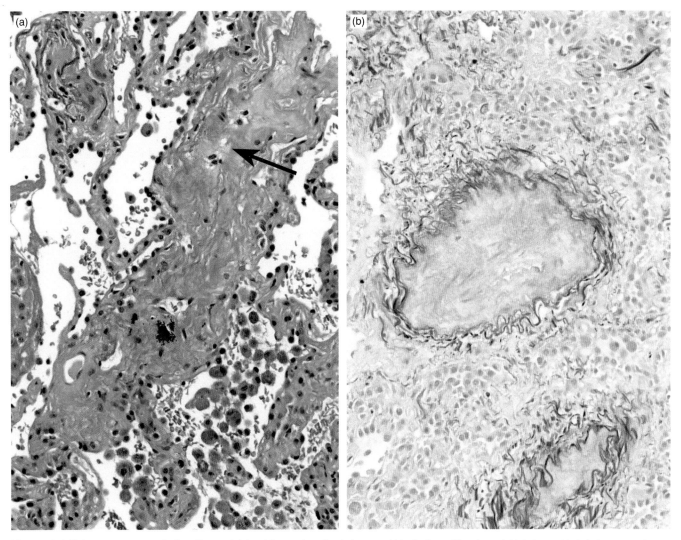

Figure 10.9. Pulmonary veno-occlusive disease. (a) An obliterated small vein is seen within the interstitium (arrow). Note hemosiderin-laden macrophages within airspaces at bottom right, and "endogenous pneumoconiosis" at top left. **(b)** Verhoeff–Van Gieson (VVG) stain from same case shows a small vein with near-total occlusion of the lumen.

enlargement – may be present. Pleural effusions in the setting of pulmonary hypertension are a clue to the diagnosis. High-resolution CT scans often show bilateral or diffuse reticulo-nodular or micronodular opacities. Septal lines may be present but are less prominent than in PVOD. Ill-defined centrilobular nodules and ground-glass opacities are common.

Differential diagnosis

- Pulmonary veno-occlusive disease (PVOD) is the main lesion in the differential diagnosis. Since PVOD and PCH share so many clinical, radiologic and pathologic features, it has been suggested that they represent the same entity. Some authors suggest that PCH is simply a consequence of PVOD, reflecting revascularization secondary to venous occlusion. An alternative view is that PCH is a separate entity in which capillary proliferation is the primary event, with secondary invasion and obstruction of veins. Currently, PCH persists as an entity because in practice rare cases show

capillary proliferation without demonstrable evidence of venous obstruction, despite exhaustive sampling. It has been argued that the distribution and morphology of the capillary proliferation in PCH is not consistent with a pure post-obstructive compensatory capillary proliferation. Clinically, 30% of patients with PCH have hemoptysis, whereas hemoptysis is rare in PVOD. Also, hemorrhagic pleural effusions are seen in a third of cases of PCH but not in PVOD. Pathologically, loop-like dilatation of the capillary vessels is common in PVOD, whereas the presence of multiple back-to-back rows of proliferating capillaries favors PCH. Identification of small veins occluded by fibrosis or recanalizing thrombi establishes a diagnosis of PVOD, whereas vascular occlusion in PCH is usually caused by proliferating capillaries.

- Chronic congestion can show some of the findings seen in PCH, including hemosiderin-laden macrophages and prominent capillaries within the interstitium. The features

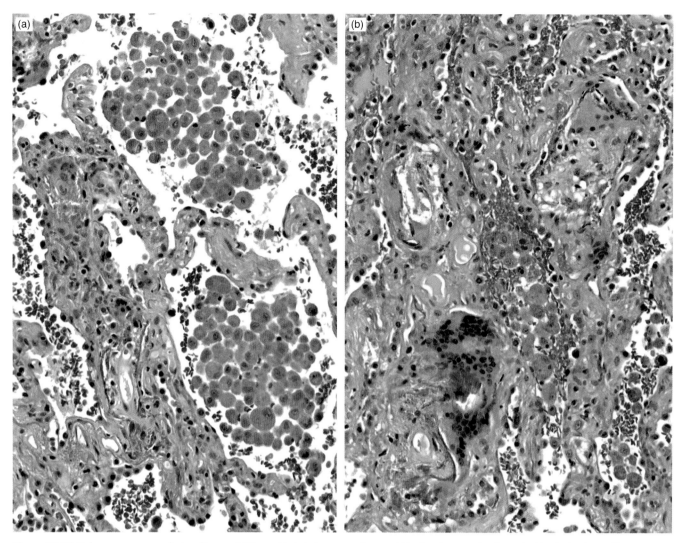

Figure 10.10. Pulmonary veno-occlusive disease. (a) Hemosiderin-laden macrophages within the airspaces dominate the histologic picture. Note calcification around small vessels in alveolar septa at left. **(b)** Alveolar septal perivascular calcification elicits a foreign-body-type giant cell reaction. This phenomenon can be seen in any cause of long-standing alveolar hemorrhage, and has been termed "endogenous pneumoconiosis". The term is a misnomer.

that distinguish PCH from chronic congestion are the nodular nature of the capillary proliferation, the presence of infiltrative growth into arteries and veins, and features of pulmonary hypertension in the arteries.

- Artifactual prominence of capillaries is an under-recognized phenomenon. PCH-like changes can be seen in a variety of lung specimens including lobectomy specimens, explant pneumonectomies and autopsies. The cause is unknown, but excessive inflation with formalin may be contributory in some cases. The capillary proliferation can be very striking and may show all the histologic features of true PCH other than vascular invasion. The absence of clinical evidence of pulmonary hypertension helps to avoid misdiagnosis of PCH.

Treatment and prognosis

Treatments that have been tried in PCH include diuretics, oxygen, warfarin, recombinant interferon α-2a and doxycycline. The prostaglandin epoprostenol is widely used in idiopathic pulmonary arterial hypertension but is contraindicated in PCH because it has been associated with pulmonary edema and worsening of hypoxemia. Currently, a combination of antiangiogenic therapy and lung transplantation is offered to most patients with PCH. The condition is slowly progressive and eventually leads to death due to right heart failure or hemoptysis. Sudden death occurs in some patients. The median survival is approximately 3 years from the initial clinical symptoms.

Sample diagnosis on pathology report

Lung, right, explant pneumonectomy – Pulmonary capillary hemangiomatosis (see comment).

Diffuse pulmonary lymphangiomatosis and lymphangiectasis

Diffuse pulmonary lymphangiomatosis and pulmonary lymphangiectasis are two closely related disorders

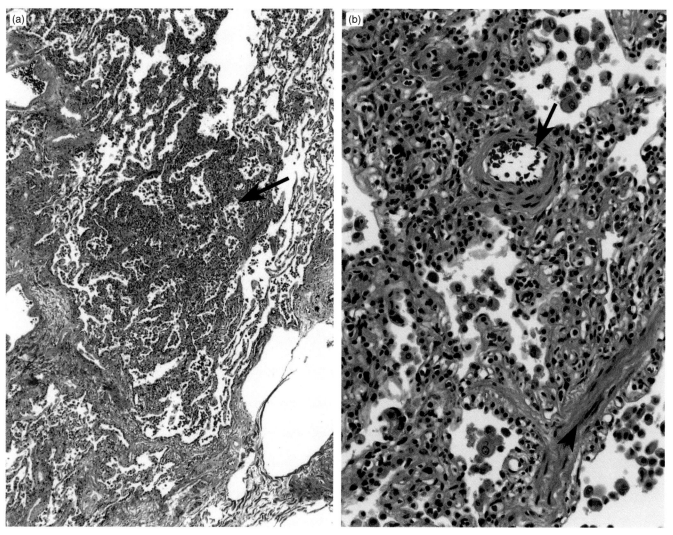

Figure 10.11. Pulmonary capillary hemangiomatosis. (a) A vaguely nodular area of interstitial thickening is seen at low magnification, mimicking interstitial lung disease. The area indicated by the arrow is shown at high magnification in b. **(b)** The interstitial widening is caused by proliferating capillaries. The capillaries form sheets (top left) and surround a small blood vessel (arrow) and an alveolar duct (arrowhead).

characterized by the presence of numerous prominent dilated lymphatics throughout the interstitium of the lung. The purported difference between the two is the relative predominance of dilatation vis-a-vis proliferation/complexity of the lymphatic channels. Both diseases are rare. They typically occur in childhood but have also been reported in adults. Their recognition is important because they can mimic interstitial lung disease clinically and radiologically, and can be missed or misinterpreted by pathologists. The lymphatic abnormalities in these diseases may be limited to the lungs, or may be part of multi-system disease. Extrapulmonary sites that may be involved include the mediastinum, thoracic duct, spleen, bone and chest wall. In some cases, multi-system lymphatic abnormalities may be associated with Down syndrome, Turner syndrome or Noonan syndrome.

Diffuse lymphatic disorders of the lung are usually recognized by pathologists in surgical lung biopsies. Prominent lymphatic dilatation may be recognizable in transbronchial or endobronchial biopsies but the diffuse distribution of the changes cannot be appreciated in such samples.

Major diagnostic findings

- The key pathologic finding is the presence of prominent dilated lymphatics along bronchovascular bundles, interlobular septa and the pleura (Figure 10.12). The reader will recall that this distribution is referred to as "lymphangitic" or peri-lymphatic, since it reflects the normal distribution of lymphatics in the lung. In normal lungs, lymphatics are generally indistinct or invisible.
- The diagnosis requires clinical and radiologic exclusion of cardiac failure and obstruction to lymphatic flow by mediastinal masses, both of which can cause secondary lymphatic dilatation in the lung.

Variable pathologic findings

- The walls of the dilated spaces may be muscularized. Mild fibrosis may surround the dilated lymphatics.
- In some cases, compressed slit-like vascular channels have been observed, an appearance described as "Kaposiform".

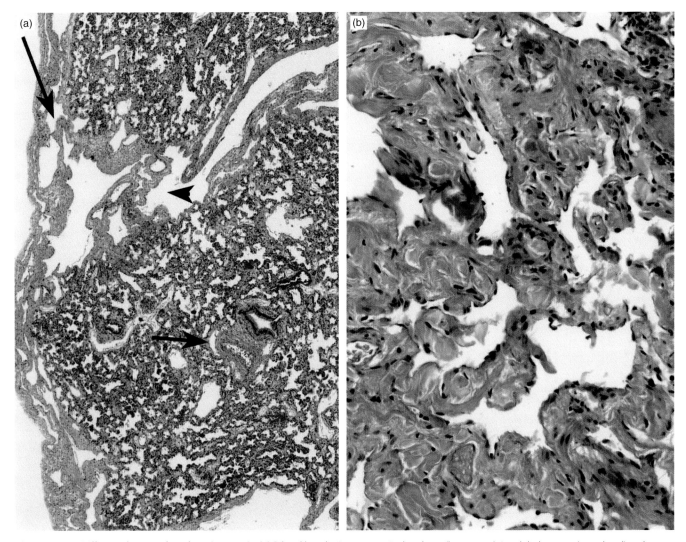

Figure 10.12. Diffuse pulmonary lymphangiomatosis. (a) Dilated lymphatics are seen in the pleura (long arrow), interlobular septa (arrowhead) and bronchovascular bundles (short arrow). This image is from an autopsy of a 2-week-old neonate. **(b)** Typical irregular contours of lymphatics in diffuse pulmonary lymphangiomatosis. Note similarity to alveoli. This picture is from a surgical lung biopsy from a 26-year-old man.

- The histologic appearance can be deceptively normal at first glance because dilated lymphatics mimic alveoli. Therefore, diffuse pulmonary lymphatic disease should always be considered in the differential diagnosis of a normal-appearing lung.

Diagnostic work-up

Immunohistochemical staining for D2–40 is very helpful for confirming that the vascular spaces are lymphatics, and for highlighting their number and distribution. CD34 and CD31 are less specific because they also mark other types of blood vessels.

Clinical profile

Diffuse pulmonary lymphangiomatosis and pulmonary lymphangiectasis have been reported in newborns, infants, older children and adults up to 65 years of age. Both sexes are affected. The condition usually presents in the neonatal period or childhood, but rare cases presenting in adulthood are well documented. Only 18 cases (ages 19 to 65) had been reported in adults by 2014. The most common presenting symptoms are cough and dyspnea. Other manifestations include chest tightness, hemoptysis, bronchial casts, bronchorrhea, milky sputum, fever, recurrent bronchitis or pneumonia, and progressive hypoxic respiratory failure. Some patients are asymptomatic. Children often present with wheezing that is misdiagnosed as asthma. Symptoms may be present for up to 20 years prior to the correct diagnosis, and may date back to childhood. Pleural effusion and chylothorax are clues to the diagnosis, as are signs of systemic lymphatic disease such as lymphedema. Exclusion of underlying heart failure and mediastinal masses is mandatory before lymphatic dilatation in the lungs is considered a primary abnormality.

Pulmonary function tests often show restrictive changes. Bronchoscopy may demonstrate endobronchial vesicles. Lymphangiography and lymphoscintigraphy can help to confirm the diagnosis in some cases.

Radiologic findings

Chest radiographs may be normal or may show increased interstitial or bronchovascular markings in both lungs. The abnormalities are often more prominent in the lower lung fields. On CT scans, the most common finding is diffuse thickening along the interlobular septa and bronchovascular bundles. The thickening may occasionally be nodular or micronodular. Other common findings include diffuse pleural thickening, bilateral pleural effusion, patchy bilateral ground-glass opacities and low-attenuation infiltration of the hilum or mediastinum. The radiologic differential diagnosis includes lymphangitic carcinoma, lymphoma and PVOD. Therefore, histologic confirmation is necessary for the diagnosis.

Differential diagnosis

- Differentiation between diffuse pulmonary lymphangiomatosis and pulmonary lymphangiectasis rests on a subjective assessment as to whether dilatation or proliferation/complexity is the predominant pathologic abnormality. There is no evidence that this arbitrary distinction is reproducible, and it is difficult to apply in practice.
- Lymphangioma is a localized mass-forming lesion, and should not pose problems in diagnosis if the radiologic context is provided to the pathologist.
- Lymphangioleiomyomatosis occasionally causes confusion to clinicians, but only because it sounds similar to lymphangiomatosis. In reality, there is little or no similarity between lymphangioleiomyomatosis and diffuse lymphatic lesions of the lung. Lymphangioleiomyomatosis manifests as bilateral lung cysts while diffuse lymphatic lesions do not. Histologically, diffuse lymphatic lesions are composed of lymphatics while the cysts of lymphangioleiomyomatosis are not.

Treatment and prognosis

There is no established therapy for lymphangiomatosis or lymphangiectasis of the lung. Treatments that have been tried include low-fat medium-chain triglycerides, interferon α, radiation, corticosteroids, medroxyprogesterone acetate, tamoxifen, chemotherapy, somatostatin, propranolol and surgical ligation of the thoracic duct. Patients with minimal or no symptoms have been observed without treatment.

In neonates, mortality is high, frequently resulting in stillborn infants. In adults, the condition appears to be more indolent, although there are too few cases reported for any meaningful conclusions to be drawn.

Sample diagnosis on pathology report

Lung, right lower lobe, surgical biopsy – Diffuse pulmonary lymphangiomatosis (See comment).

Vasculitis and capillaritis

Vasculitis of the lung – defined by the presence of inflammatory cells within vessel walls – is most commonly seen as a secondary phenomenon in granulomatous infections and sarcoidosis. However, true primary vasculitis is overwhelmingly related to the ANCA-associated vasculitides, which are discussed in detail in Chapter 2 and contrasted in Table 2.3 of that chapter. The main causes of vasculitis in the lung that are likely to be seen by surgical pathologists are listed in Table 10.4.

In contrast to the processes mentioned above, which mainly involve small and medium-sized arteries and veins, *capillaritis*, also known as *acute necrotizing capillaritis*, is a *small-vessel vasculitis* that involves and destroys alveolar septal capillaries. Conceptually and histologically, capillaritis is the pulmonary counterpart of *leukocytoclastic vasculitis* of the skin. It is the single most important cause of diffuse alveolar hemorrhage identified by surgical pathologists in lung biopsies. Most cases of capillaritis are a manifestation of ANCA-related vasculitides, especially granulomatosis with polyangiitis (Wegener's). The causes of capillaritis are shown in Table 10.5.

Large-vessel vasculitides such as Takayasu arteritis and giant cell arteritis, and other medium-vessel vasculitides such as polyarteritis nodosa and Kawasaki disease are vanishingly rare in surgical pathology of the lung and will not be addressed here.

Capillaritis is most commonly diagnosed in surgical lung biopsies or at autopsy. The diagnosis can be made in small biopsies, but sampling considerations greatly limit the yield.

Major diagnostic findings

- The most important diagnostic finding in capillaritis is patchy destruction of alveolar septa by an inflammatory infiltrate composed of neutrophils and histiocytes (Figures 10.13 and 10.14). The neutrophils are often necrotic, and the histiocytes typically have squiggly nuclei. Karyorrhectic nuclear debris is a tip-off to the diagnosis. In most cases, alveolar septal destruction is very focal, subtle and difficult to find. The majority of the alveolar septa and capillaries in the rest of the lung are intact.
- The inflammatory infiltrate is accompanied by red blood cells and numerous hemosiderin-laden macrophages within the alveoli (Figure 10.15a).

Variable pathologic findings

- In most cases of capillaritis, classic features of granulomatosis with polyangiitis (Wegener's) such as dirty necrosis, necrotizing vasculitis and necrotizing granulomas are absent. However, in some cases, these features may co-exist with foci of capillaritis.
- Hemosiderin-laden macrophages may occasionally be present within the interstitium.
- Fibrinoid necrosis may be seen in the alveolar septa. Fibrinous exudates may be present within airspaces along with red blood cells and hemosiderin-laden macrophages.

Table 10.4. Causes of vasculitis in the lung

Diagnosis	Main histologic feature	Where to find the entity in this book	Notes
Granulomatous myco-bacterial and fungal infections	Necrosis associated with epithelioid histiocytes	Chapter 2 Figures 2.21, 2.22	Typically a few lymphocytes in walls of a few blood vessels (secondary phenomenon) Can be very striking in immunocompromised individuals No necrosis in vessel wall
Sarcoidosis	Non-necrotizing granulomas	Chapter 2 Figure 2.45	Non-necrotizing granulomas infiltrate vessel walls (secondary phenomenon) Usually no necrosis Typical features of sarcoidosis in background lung
Granulomatosis with polyangiitis (Wegener's)	Necrotizing granulomas with dirty, basophilic necrosis Necrotizing vasculitis with destruction of vessel wall, often focal and difficult to find	Chapter 2 Figure 2.39	Mix of histiocytes and neutrophils in involved vessels with karyorrhectic debris Vasculitis often "eccentric" See Table 2.3 in Chapter 2
Eosinophilic granulomatosis with polyangiitis (Churg–Strauss)	Necrotizing granulomas with numerous eosinophils Eosinophilic pneumonia	Chapter 2 Figure 2.41a	Mix of histiocytes and eosinophils in involved vessels with focal necrosis Vasculitis may be "eccentric" See Table 2.3 in Chapter 2
Capillaritis	Blood and hemosiderin-laden macrophages within alveoli Destruction of alveolar septa by mixed histiocytic–neutrophilic inflammatory infiltrate	This chapter Figures 10.13, 10.14	Usually bilateral ground-glass opacities ANCA serology most helpful See Table 10.5 for causes of capillaritis
Langerhans cell histiocytosis	Stellate interstitial nodules containing sheets of Langerhans cells	Chapter 5 Figure 5.61	Eosinophils may occasionally infiltrate vessel walls (secondary phenomenon)
IgG4-related lung disease	Fibrosis and chronic inflammation with numerous IgG4-positive plasma cells	Chapter 6	Vascular infiltration common Necrotizing vasculitis rare

- The term *diffuse alveolar hemorrhage* is often used by clinicians because the alveolar hemorrhage in capillaritis is often radiologically diffuse and bilateral. However, at the microscopic level, the hemorrhage is usually quite patchy. Some of the airspaces may be filled with red blood cells in a vaguely nodular pattern while adjacent areas of lung are completely uninvolved.

- Elastic tissue in small blood vessels adjacent to areas of long-standing hemorrhage can become encrusted with a mix of calcification and hemosiderin producing linear blue-purple lines that follow the contours of elastic tissue. This encrustation is often accompanied by a foreign-body giant cell reaction. This phenomenon has been termed "endogenous pneumoconiosis" (Fig 10.15b). It should be clear from the preceding discussion that this process is not a pneumoconiosis. Although it is a useful marker of long-standing hemorrhage and hemosiderin deposition, it is of no further diagnostic utility, since it is also seen in other entities that enter the differential

diagnosis of hemosiderin-laden macrophages, including pulmonary veno-occlusive disease and congestive heart failure.

- Capillaritis is a difficult diagnosis to make because the vasculitis is most often patchy, focal and subtle, and is frequently overshadowed by the presence of abundant blood and numerous hemosiderin-laden macrophages within the airspaces. Identification of vasculitis in such cases can be painstaking and time-consuming. The involved capillaries and alveolar septa are often completely destroyed, leaving behind an inflammatory infiltrate that closely mimics acute bronchopneumonia or margination of neutrophils. Clues to the correct diagnosis are the alveolar septal-centered nature of the inflammatory infiltrate, the relative sparing of the center of the airspaces, the presence of karyorrhectic nuclear debris and the characteristic mix of neutrophils and squiggly histiocytes. Identifying occasional alveolar septa that are involved but not completely destroyed is helpful in making the diagnosis.

Table 10.5. Causes of capillaritis in the lung

Cause	How to establish the diagnosis
Granulomatosis with polyangiitis (Wegener's)	Concurrent necrotizing granulomas in lung or elsewhere (not necessary for diagnosis) Known pre-existing diagnosis of granulomatosis with polyangiitis (Wegener's) ANCA positivity (c-ANCA > p-ANCA) See Table 2.3 in Chapter 2
Microscopic polyangiitis	No granulomatous inflammation Hematuria or proteinuria with pauci-immune glomerulonephritis on renal biopsy Leukocytoclastic vasculitis on skin biopsy ANCA positivity (p-ANCA > c-ANCA) See Table 2.3 in Chapter 2
Isolated pauci-immune pulmonary capillaritis (rare)	No clinical features of underlying systemic disorder ANCA negative Very rare (8 cases by 2015)
Primary antiphospholipid syndrome (rare)	High titers of antiphospholipid antibodies (anticardiolipin antibodies) or positive testing for lupus anticoagulant (prolonged partial thromboplastin time (PTT) or dRVVT) Concurrent thrombosis or known history of antiphospholipid antibody syndrome
Systemic lupus erythematosus (SLE) (rare) – "acute lupus pneumonitis"	Usually occurs in patients with established diagnosis of SLE; rarely alveolar hemorrhage is the initial manifestation Concurrent nephritis; renal biopsy ANA, ds-DNA
Cryoglobulinemia (rare)	Serum cryoglobulin levels
Other connective tissue diseases (rare)	Polymyositis, rheumatoid arthritis, scleroderma, mixed connective tissue disease
Miscellaneous conditions (rare)	Henoch–Schönlein purpura, Behçet syndrome, ulcerative colitis, bone marrow transplant, lung transplant
Drugs (rare)	Propylthiouracil, phenytoin, retinoic acid, sulfonamides

Clinical profile

The clinical presentation of vasculitis varies greatly depending on the underlying cause. The clinical features of granulomatosis with polyangiitis (Wegener's) and eosinophilic granulomatosis with polyangiitis (Churg–Strauss) are discussed in Chapter 2. Alveolar hemorrhage due to Goodpasture's syndrome is addressed in Chapter 4.

Diffuse alveolar hemorrhage due to capillaritis usually presents with cough, fever, dyspnea, or chest pain with or without hemoptysis. One-third of patients lack hemoptysis. Some are asymptomatic. Clinical clues to the diagnosis include signs of extrapulmonary involvement such as purpuric rashes, uveitis, sinus or ocular symptoms, arthritis or mononeuritis multiplex.

Laboratory findings include anemia, reflecting intrapulmonary blood loss. The diagnosis is supported by BAL fluid that demonstrates a progressively bloody return and contains hemosiderin-laden macrophages. The latter may be detectable in BAL fluid for weeks to months after active hemorrhage has ceased.

Radiologic findings

Capillaritis with alveolar hemorrhage typically manifests as diffuse bilateral ground-glass opacities or extensive consolidation. The findings are occasionally focal or unilateral rather than diffuse and bilateral. Cavitary nodules may be present in cases with concurrent granulomatous inflammation.

Differential diagnosis

- Acute bronchopneumonia may also feature a mix of neutrophils and histiocytes, and there may be evidence of acute and old hemorrhage. The distinction from capillaritis in such cases can be extremely challenging, and hinges on demonstration of alveolar septal destruction by the inflammatory infiltrate.
- Congestive heart failure can be associated with blood and hemosiderin-laden macrophages but inflammatory infiltrates are not a feature.
- Margination of neutrophils from capillaries results in the presence of neutrophils within alveolar septa, and is often over-interpreted as capillaritis. The diagnosis of capillaritis should not be made unless convincing destruction of alveolar septa is present. Karyorrhexis is a good indicator that the changes are not artifactual.

Treatment and prognosis

The first priority in the management of diffuse alveolar hemorrhage is cardiopulmonary stabilization. Subsequent

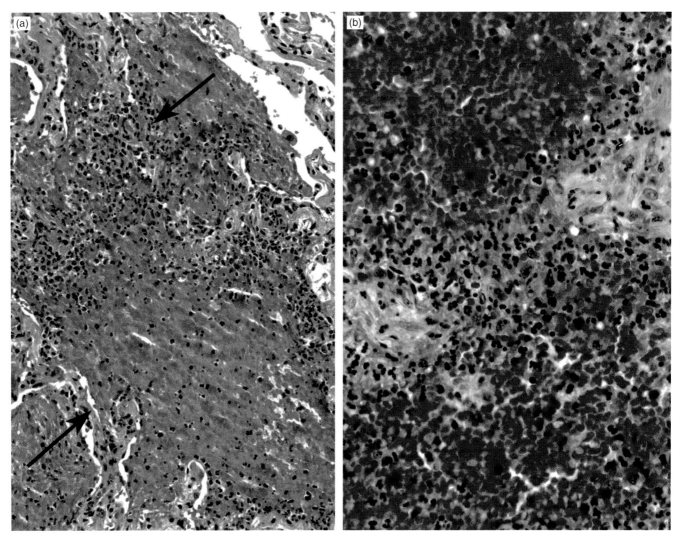

Figure 10.13. Capillaritis with alveolar hemorrhage. (a) Alveolar hemorrhage with capillaritis in a surgical lung biopsy. The alveoli are filled with red blood cells. Alveolar septa are focally destroyed by an inflammatory infiltrate rich in neutrophils (top arrow). Compare with relatively preserved alveolar septa at bottom (bottom arrow). The presence of karyorrhectic debris is a clue to the diagnosis. **(b)** Another field from the same case shown at higher magnification. Destroyed alveolar septum is in the center. Blood-filled airspaces are at top and bottom. Note that the inflammatory infiltrate is a mix of neutrophils and histiocytes.

treatment depends on the underlying etiology, details of which are outside the scope of this book. Depending on the underlying etiology, treatment options include high-dose corticosteroids, cyclophosphamide, rituximab and intravenous immunoglobulin, among others.

Diffuse alveolar hemorrhage caused by capillaritis is potentially life-threatening. It can rapidly cause respiratory failure and death. The mortality rate is high. However, some individuals do survive episodes of diffuse alveolar hemorrhage, especially if appropriate high-dose corticosteroid therapy is initiated in a timely fashion.

Sample diagnosis on pathology report

Lung, right middle lobe, surgical biopsy – Acute necrotizing capillaritis with extensive alveolar hemorrhage (See comment).

Pulmonary thrombosis and embolism

Thrombi and a variety of embolic materials may occasionally be found within the lumens of pulmonary arteries and other blood vessels in a wide variety of settings. The most common of these are thrombi, which are either formed in situ within the pulmonary vasculature, or are derived from embolism to the lungs from distant sources, most commonly the deep veins of the calves. Other common sources of emboli to the lungs include deep veins of the arms, veins of the periprostatic venous plexus and the right side of the heart; emboli to the lung can also originate from catheters. Other non-thrombotic emboli can also be found within the lung parenchyma, including silicone emboli, tumor emboli, filler material from injected pills, parasites (e.g., *Schistosoma*), fat, cotton, bile, cardiac catheter material and bone marrow emboli. The last is often found at autopsy or may be a consequence of bone trauma during

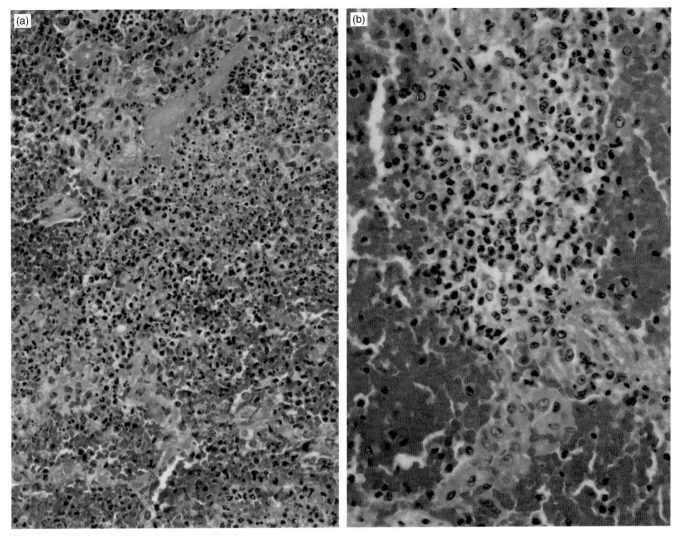

Figure 10.14. Capillaritis with alveolar hemorrhage. (a) Striking inflammatory infiltrate admixed with blood. The infiltrate contains neutrophils, histiocytes and karyorrhectic debris. **(b)** High magnification of another case, from an autopsy of a patient who died of granulomatosis with polyangiitis (Wegener's). The alveolar septum is completely destroyed by a neutrophilic-histiocytic inflammatory infiltrate. The adjacent airspaces are filled with blood.

surgical lung biopsies. Bronchial artery emboli can be encountered after therapeutic embolization of the bronchial arteries for hemoptysis.

Major diagnostic findings

The main finding in pulmonary thrombosis is at least partial filling of the lumen of an affected blood vessel by fibrin (acute thrombus) or fibrosis and vascular channels (organizing thrombus) (Figure 10.16). In other types of emboli, the morphology varies depending on the type of embolized material.

Variable pathologic findings

- Acute thrombi are most commonly formed by a combination of blood, fibrin, platelets and neutrophils. They are often found within dilated and thin-walled blood vessels.

- *Lines of Zahn* are the hallmark of an acute thrombus. They consist of alternating zones of platelets and fibrin and are indicative of in situ pre-mortem thrombosis. Embolized thrombi can also sometimes form lines of Zahn.
- After 2 to 3 days, the so-called organizing thrombus is formed. It is composed of fibroblasts and capillaries that grow into the thrombus.
- After 4 to 6 weeks, the thrombus is replaced by fibrosis and capillaries and is then referred to as an organized thrombus. After several weeks, recanalization of the thrombus occurs. At this stage, the thrombus is replaced by fibrous bands, multiple lumens and webs, findings that can also be seen grossly in autopsy specimens.
- Silicone emboli appear as transparent globules within alveolar septal capillaries (Figure 10.17). They are refractile, and may occasionally be surrounded by multinucleated giant cells. Bronchial artery embolization material appears

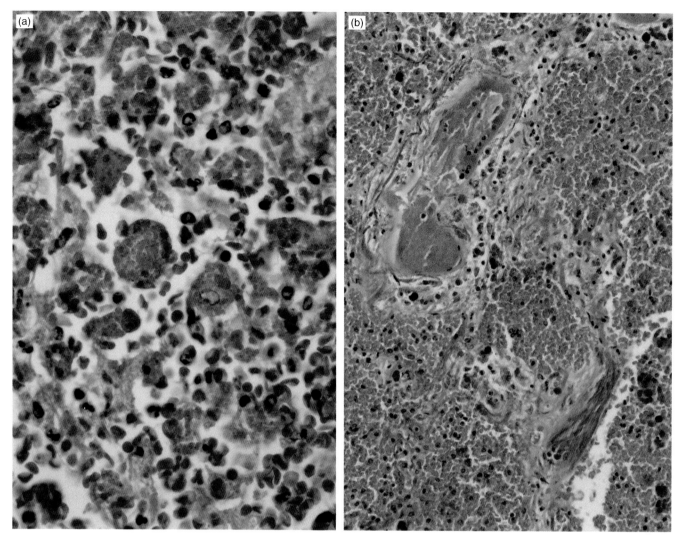

Figure 10.15. Other findings in alveolar hemorrhage due to capillaritis. (a) Red blood cells and hemosiderin-laden macrophages within the airspaces. **(b)** Calcification in the wall of blood vessels (so-called endogenous pneumoconiosis).

as blue microspheres found within bronchial arteries (Figure 10.17). It is used in the course of therapeutic bronchial artery embolization procedures to occlude bronchial arteries in an attempt to control intractable hemoptysis.

Diagnostic work-up

No special stains are required in most cases. Connective tissue stains such as elastic stains, trichrome stains and the Movat pentachrome stain can be helpful in evaluating pulmonary thrombi. These stains help to demonstrate that the involved structures are blood vessels and show the intraluminal nature of the process.

Clinical profile

- Thrombi are found in the lung in many of the same settings in which peripheral emboli are formed, including vascular stasis, obesity, congestive heart failure, thromboembolic disease and hypercoagulable states.

- Massive pulmonary emboli may cause acute symptoms and lead to sudden death. The most common symptoms are pleuritic pain, shortness of breath and hemoptysis.
- Patients with pulmonary embolism may be asymptomatic for several years (the honeymoon period) before they present with shortness of breath, dyspnea, productive cough, atypical chest pain, tachycardia, syncope or cor pulmonale. In patients with chronic thromboembolic pulmonary hypertension (CTEPH), arterial occlusion by thrombi leads to pulmonary hypertension.

Radiologic findings

The most common radiologic findings are filling defects within the pulmonary arteries.

Differential diagnosis

- Blood clots need to be distinguished from pulmonary thrombosis. This issue usually arises at autopsy, where

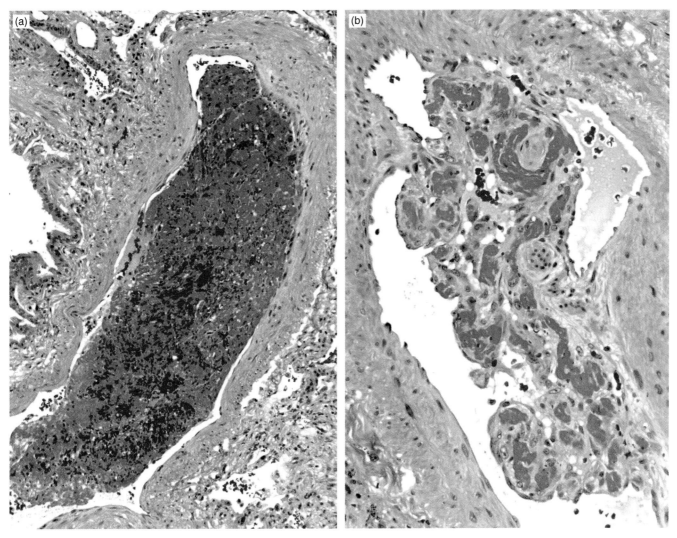

Figure 10.16. Thrombosis. (a) Acute (fresh) thrombus with minimal organization. **(b)** Organizing thrombus.

post-mortem blood clots can mimic thrombi grossly. While blood clots are shiny, soft and elastic, and show a characteristic "horse's tail" sign, thrombi characteristically show lines of Zahn, which indicate that they formed in situ and pre-mortem.

- Thromboses that form in situ cannot be distinguished histologically from emboli. The term *thrombotic arteriopathy* can be used for both these entities.

Treatment and prognosis

Treatment options in pulmonary embolism include anti-coagulation, thrombolysis, surgical embolectomy and placement of vena cava filters.

Sample diagnosis on pathology report

Lung, right lower lobe, surgical biopsy – Pulmonary thrombi and organized thromboemboli (See comment).

References

Pulmonary hypertension

Burke A, Virmani R. Mini-symposium: Pulmonary pathology – evaluation of pulmonary hypertension in biopsies of the lung. *Curr Diagn Pathol* 1996;**3**:14–26.

Frazier AA, Galvin JR, Franks TJ, Rosado-De-Christenson ML. From the Archives of the AFIP.

Pulmonary vasculature: Hypertension and infarction. *RadioGraphics* 2000;**20**:491–524.

Hoeper MM, Bogaard HJ, Condliffe R, *et al.* Definitions and diagnosis of pulmonary hypertension. *J Am Coll Cardiol* 2013;**62**: D42–50.

Palevsky HI, Schloo BL, Pietra GG, *et al.* Primary pulmonary hypertension. Vascular structure,

morphometry, and responsiveness to vasodilator agents. *Circulation* 1989;**80**:1207–21.

Pietra GG, Edwards WD, Kay JM, *et al.* Histopathology of primary pulmonary hypertension. A qualitative and quantitative study of pulmonary blood vessels from 58 patients in the National Heart, Lung, and Blood Institute, Primary Pulmonary Hypertension Registry. *Circulation* 1989;**80**:1198–206.

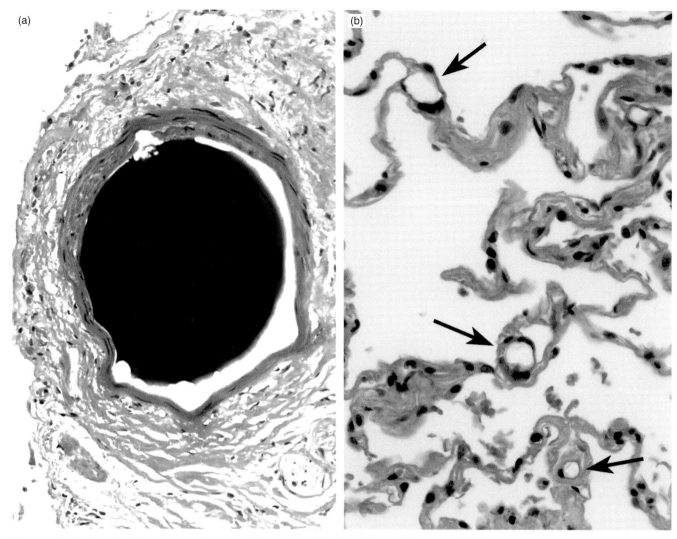

Figure 10.17. Emboli to pulmonary blood vessels. (a) Microsphere within bronchial artery. This patient had a history of bronchial artery embolization for hemoptysis. **(b)** Pale transparent silicone globules in pulmonary capillaries (arrows). The patient had a history of breast implants. Leakage of silicone into the mediastinum had formed a fibrotic mediastinal mass.

Pietra GG, Capron S, Stewart F, *et al.* Pathologic assessment of vasculopathies in pulmonary hypertension. *J Am Coll Cardiol* 2004;**43**:25S–32S.

Rosenkranz S. Pulmonary hypertension 2015: current definitions, terminology, and novel treatment options. *Clin Res Cardiol* 2015;**104**:197–207.

Simonneau G, Gatzoulis MA, Adatia I, *et al.* Updated clinical classification of pulmonary hypertension. *J Am Coll Cardiol* 2013;**62**: D34–41.

Wagenvoort CA, Yamaki S. Plexogenic pulmonary arteriopathy: significance of medial thickness with respect to advanced pulmonary vascular lesions. *Am J Pathol* 1981;**105**:70–5.

Wagenvoort CA, Wagenvoort N. Primary pulmonary hypertension. A pathologic study of the lung vessels in 156 clinically diagnosed cases. *Circulation* 1970;**42**:1163–84.

Pulmonary veno-occlusive disease

Carrington CB, Liebow AA. Pulmonary veno-occlusive disease. *Hum Pathol* 1970;**1**:322–4.

Holcomb BW, Jr., Loyd JE, Ely EW, Johnson J, Robbins IM. Pulmonary veno-occlusive disease. A case series and new observations. *Chest* 2000;**118**:1671–9.

Joselson R, Warnock M. Pulmonary veno-occlusive disease after chemotherapy. *Hum Pathol* 1982;**14**:88–91.

Katz DS, Katzenstein AA, Kohman LJ, Scalzetti EM. Pulmonary veno-occlusive disease presenting with thrombosis of pulmonary arteries. *Thorax* 1995;**50**:699–700.

Lantuéjoul S, Sheppard MN, Corrin B, Burke MM, Nicholson AG. Pulmonary veno-occlusive disease and pulmonary capillary hemangiomatosis. A clinicopathologic study of 35 cases. *Am J Surg Pathol* 2006;**30**:850–7.

Mandel J, Mark EJ, Hales CA. State of the art. Pulmonary veno-occlusive disease. *Am J Respir Crit Care Med* 2000;**162**:1964–73.

Montani D, Achouh L, Dorfmüller P, *et al.* Pulmonary veno-occlusive disease. Clinical, functional, radiologic and hemodynamic characteristics and outcome of 24 cases confirmed by histology. *Medicine* 2008;**87**:220–3.

Porres DV, Morenza OP, Pallisa E, Roque A, Andreu J, Martínez M. Learning from the pulmonary veins. *RadioGraphics* 2013;**33**:999–1022.

Ranchoux B, Günther S, Quarck R, *et al.* Chemotherapy-induced pulmonary hypertension. Role of alkylating agents. *Am J Pathol* 2015;**185**;356–71.

Wagenvoort CA, Wagenvoort N, Takahashi T. Pulmonary veno-occlusive disease: Involvement of pulmonary arteries and review of the literature. *Hum Pathol* 1985;**16**:1033–41.

Pulmonary capillary hemangiomatosis

Almagro P, Julià J, Sanjaume M, *et al.* Pulmonary capillary hemangiomatosis associated with primary pulmonary hypertension: report of 2 new cases and review of 35 cases from the literature. *Medicine* 2002;**81**:417–24.

Best DH, Sumner KL, Austin ED, *et al. EIF2AK4* mutations in pulmonary capillary hemangiomatosis. *Chest* 2014;**145**:231–6.

Erbersdobler A, Niendorf A. Multifocal distribution of pulmonary capillary hemangiomatosis. *Histopathology* 2002;**40**:88–91.

Faber CN, Yousem SA, Dauber JH, Griffith BP, Hardesty RL, Paradis IL. Pulmonary capillary hemangiomatosis. A report of 3 cases and a review of the literature. *Am Rev Respir Dis* 1989;**140**:808–13.

Frazier AA, Franks TJ, Mohammed TL, Ozbudak IH, Galvin JR. From the Archives of the AFIP: pulmonary veno-occlusive disease and pulmonary capillary hemangiomatosis. *RadioGraphics* 2007;**27**:867–82.

Ginns LC, Roberts DH, Mark EJ, Brusch JL, Marler JJ. Pulmonary capillary hemangiomatosis with atypical endotheliomatosis: successful antiangiogenic therapy with doxycycline. *Chest* 2003;**124**:2017–22.

Havlik DM, Massie LW, Williams WL, Crooks LA. Pulmonary capillary hemangiomatosis-like foci. An autopsy study of 8 cases. *Am J Clin Pathol* 2000;**113**:655–62.

Humbert M, Maitre S, Capron F, Rain B, Musset D, Simonneau G. Pulmonary edema complicating continuous intravenous prostacyclin in pulmonary capillary hemangiomatosis. *Am J Respir Crit Care Med* 1998;**157**:1681–5.

Lantuéjoul S, Sheppard MN, Corrin B, Burke MM, Nicholson AG. Pulmonary veno-occlusive disease and pulmonary capillary hemangiomatosis. A clinicopathologic study of 35 cases. *Am J Surg Pathol* 2006;**30**:850–7.

Tron V, Magee F, Wright JL, Colby T, Churg A. Pulmonary capillary hemangiomatosis. *Hum Pathol* 1986;**17**:1144–50.

Diffuse pulmonary lymphangiomatosis and lymphangiectasis

Boland JM, Tazelaar HD, Colby TV, Leslie KO, Hartman TE, Yi ES. Diffuse pulmonary lymphatic disease presenting as interstitial lung disease in adulthood. Report of 3 cases. *Am J Surg Pathol* 2012;**36**:1548–54.

El Hajj L, Mazières J, Rouquette I, *et al.* Diagnostic value of bronchoscopy, CT and transbronchial biopsies in diffuse pulmonary lymphangiomatosis: case report and review of the literature. *Clin Radiol* 2005;**60**:921–5.

Faul JL, Berry GJ, Colby TV, *et al.* Thoracic lymphangiomas, lymphangiectasis, lymphangiomatosis and lymphatic dysplasia syndrome. *Am J Respir Crit Care Med* 2000;**145**:231–6.

Lim H, Han J, Kim HK, Kim TS. A rare case of diffuse pulmonary lymphangiomatosis in a middle-aged woman. *Korean J Radiol* 2014;**15**:295–9.

Nobre LF, Müller NL, de Souza Júnior AS, Marchiori E, Souza IV. Congenital pulmonary lymphangiectasia. CT and pathologic findings. *J Thorac Imaging* 2004;**19**:56–9.

Swensen SJ, Hartman TE, Mayo JR, Colby TV, Tazelaar HD, Müller NL. Diffuse pulmonary lymphangiomatosis: CT findings. *J Comput Assist Tomogr* 1995;**19**:348–52.

Tazelaar HD, Kerr D, Yousem SA, Saldana MJ, Langston C, Colby TV. Diffuse pulmonary lymphangiomatosis. *Hum Pathol* 1993;**24**:1313–22.

Toyoshima M, Suzuki S, Kono M, Nakamura Y, Suda T. Mildly progressive pulmonary lymphangiectasis diagnosed in a young adult. *Am J Respir Crit Care Med* 2014;**189**:860–2.

Wagenaar SS, Swierenga J, Wagenvoort CA. Late presentation of primary pulmonary lymphangiectasis. *Thorax* 1978;**33**:791–5.

White JE, Veale D, Fishwick D, Mitchell L, Corris PA. Generalised lymphangiectasia: pulmonary presentation in an adult. *Thorax* 1995;**51**:767–8.

Vasculitis and capillaritis

Castañer E, Alguersuari A, Gallardo X, *et al.* When to suspect pulmonary vasculitis: radiologic and clinical clues. *RadioGraphics* 2010;**30**:33–53.

Deane KD, West SG. Antiphospholipid antibodies as a cause of pulmonary capillaritis and diffuse alveolar hemorrhage: a case series and literature review. *Semin Arthritis Rheum* 2005;**35**:154–65.

Krause ML, Cartin-Ceba R, Specks U, Peikert T. Update on diffuse alveolar hemorrhage and pulmonary vasculitis. *Immunol Allergy Clin North Am* 2012;**32**:587–600.

Lauque D, Cadranel J, Lazor R, *et al.* Microscopic polyangiitis with alveolar hemorrhage. A study of 29 cases and review of the literature. Gourp d'Etudes et de recherche sur les Maladies "Orphelines" Pulmonaires (GERM"O"P) *Medicine (Baltimore)* 2000;**79**:222–33.

Mukhopadhyay S, Hensley RG, Tazelaar HD. Cardiac involvement in Wegener granulomatosis diagnosed at autopsy. *Cardiovasc Pathol* 2010;**19**:312–5.

Myers JL, Katzenstein AL. Wegener's granulomatosis presenting with massive pulmonary hemorrhage and capillaritis. *Am J Surg Pathol* 1987;**11**:895–8.

Myers JL, Katzenstein AL. Microangiitis in lupus-induced pulmonary hemorrhage. *Am J Clin Pathol* 1986;**85**:552–6.

Schwarz MI, Sutarik JM, Nick JA, Leff JA, Emlen JW, Tuder RM. Pulmonary capillaritis and diffuse alveolar hemorrhage. A primary manifestation of polymyositis. *Am J Respir Crit Care Med* 1995;**151**:2037–40.

Thompson G, Specks U, Cartin-Ceba R. Isolated pauci-immune pulmonary capillaritis successfully treated with rituximab. *Chest* 2015;**147**:e134–6.

Zamora MR, Warner ML, Tuder R, Schwarz MI. Diffuse alveolar hemorrhage and systemic lupus erythematosus. *Medicine* 1997;**76**:192–202.

Pulmonary thrombosis and embolism

Blauwet LA, Edwards WD, Tazelaar HD, McGregor CGA. Surgical pathology of pulmonary thromboendarterectomy: A study of 54 cases from 1990 to 2001. *Hum Pathol* 2003;**34**:1290–8.

Chen YM, Lu CC, Perng RP. Silicone fluid-induced pulmonary embolism. *Am Rev Respir Dis* 1993;**147**:1299–302.

Dalen JE, Haffajee CI, Alpert JS 3rd, Howe JP, Ockene IS, Paraskos JA. Pulmonary embolism, pulmonary haemorrhage and pulmonary infarction. *N Engl J Med* 1977;**296**:1431–5.

Dorfman GS, Cronin JJ, Tupper DB, Messersmith RN, Denny DF, Lee CH. Occult pulmonary embolism: A common occurrence in deep venous thrombosis. *AJR Am J Roentgenol* 1987;**148**:263–6.

Frazier AA, Galvin JR, Franks TJ, Rosado-De-Christenson ML. From the Archives of the AFIP. Pulmonary vasculature: Hypertension and infarction. *RadioGraphics* 2000;**20**:491–524.

Huisman MV, Büller HR, ten Cate JW, *et al.* Unexpected high prevalence of silent pulmonary embolism in patients with deep venous thrombosis. *Chest* 1989;**95**:498–502.

Khalil A, Fartoukh M, Bazot M, Parrot A, Marsault C, Carette MF. Systemic arterial embolization in patients with hemoptysis: initial experience with ethylene vinyl alcohol copolymer in 15 cases. *AJR Am J Roentgenol* 2010;**194**:W104–10.

Morpurgo M, Schmid C. The spectrum of pulmonary embolism. Clinicopathologic correlations. *Chest* 1995;**107**:18S-20S.

Price EA, Schueler H, Perper JA. Massive systemic silicone embolism. A case report and review of literature. *Am J Forensic Med Pathol* 2006;**27**:97–102.

Wagenvoort CA. Pathology of pulmonary thromboembolism. *Chest* 1995;**107**:10S-17S.

Lung transplant pathology

This chapter addresses common pathologic abnormalities encountered in lung transplant pathology, with a focus on surveillance transbronchial biopsies of transplanted lungs. Figure 11.1 shows some of the common lesions encountered in transplant lung biopsies. Figure 11.2 suggests a simple algorithm for approaching transplant lung biopsies. Table 11.1 lists pertinent pearls and pitfalls.

At our transplant center, the most common indications for lung transplantation are idiopathic pulmonary fibrosis, emphysema (centrilobular/smoking-related) and cystic fibrosis. Less common indications include primary pulmonary hypertension, emphysema caused by α-1 antitrypsin deficiency, end-stage sarcoidosis and pulmonary veno-occlusive disease. Lung transplantation may also be performed for Eisenmenger syndrome, talc granulomatosis, lymphangioleiomyomatosis, and end-stage fibrosis caused by pneumoconioses and pulmonary Langerhans cell histiocytosis.

Acute cellular rejection

Acute cellular rejection is a cell-mediated immunologic response mounted by the recipient to antigens in the donor lung. It is estimated to develop in 36 to 75% of lung transplant recipients within the first year after transplantation. T-lymphocytes are the predominant cells involved in this response. Detection of acute cellular rejection is one of the main reasons for surveillance (protocol) transbronchial biopsies of transplanted lungs, and is by far the most common significant pathologic finding in these biopsies. Histologic demonstration of acute cellular rejection is valuable because clinical and radiologic features do not reliably detect it, and often fail to distinguish it from its mimics, including infection. The word *acute* in the term *acute cellular rejection* is misleading in two ways. First, it causes confusion for pathologists, who consider neutrophils to be the histologic hallmark of acute inflammation in most other settings. Second, it implies that the process occurs soon after transplantation, whereas in practice it can occur months to years later.

Acute cellular rejection is usually diagnosed in transbronchial biopsies of transplanted lungs. Five fragments of alveolated lung parenchyma are generally thought to be adequate for the evaluation of rejection.

Major diagnostic findings

Transbronchial lung biopsy is the gold standard for the diagnosis of acute cellular rejection. The pathologic hallmark is the presence of lymphocytic infiltrates in and around the walls of small blood vessels (arterioles/venules) in the alveolar septa (Figure 11.3, Figure 11.1a). The affected blood vessels are often described as venules, but as discussed in Chapter 1, these small blood vessels show overlapping features and cannot be reliably differentiated. The lymphocytic infiltrates form tight circumferential cuffs around the affected vessels. They involve the vessel wall as well as perivascular connective tissue. The striking predilection for small blood vessels is the most useful diagnostic feature of the process. In the vast majority of cases, the infiltrates do not extend beyond the perivascular interstitium. The lymphocytes are typically a mix of small, cytologically bland cells and a few larger cells with mildly enlarged nuclei, often described as "transformed" or "activated". The mix of small and large cells is a characteristic feature of acute cellular rejection, and helps to distinguish it from its mimics.

Variable pathologic findings

- Lymphocytes are the predominant inflammatory cells in acute cellular rejection, but small numbers of histiocytes are common, and an occasional plasma cell may also be present. A few scattered eosinophils are commonly present, especially in grades A2 and higher.
- The lymphocytic infiltrate may also involve bronchioles or bronchi. Bronchiolar involvement in acute cellular rejection is known as *lymphocytic bronchiolitis*. In the absence of specific findings of an alternative diagnosis such as microorganisms or aspirated particulate material, it is very difficult to determine whether airway inflammation is rejection-related, infection-related or non-specific, and a diagnosis of lymphocytic bronchiolitis is presumptive at best. Features that favor rejection-related airway inflammation include a mix of small and large cells, intraepithelial lymphocytosis and concurrent acute cellular rejection involving blood vessels.
- Hemosiderin-laden macrophages are commonly seen within airspaces in transplant lung biopsies. They are presumably a residuum of bleeding from prior biopsies, and should be considered an artifact.
- Multiple blood vessels may be involved by acute cellular rejection. However, in small transbronchial biopsies, it is not uncommon to find only a single involved blood vessel. Not surprisingly, the likelihood of finding multiple involved vessels depends on the number of pieces of alveolated lung in the sample.

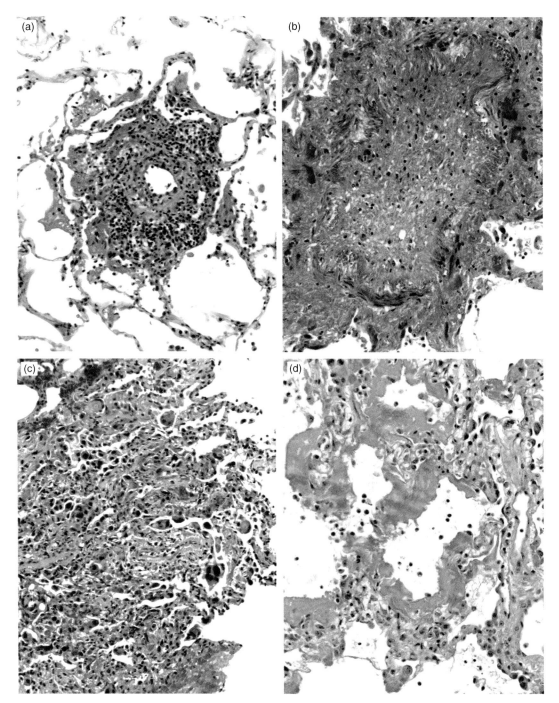

Figure 11.1. Common pathologic findings in lung transplant biopsies. (a) Acute cellular rejection. **(b)** Chronic airway rejection (constrictive bronchiolitis/obliterative bronchiolitis). **(c)** Cytomegalovirus pneumonia. **(d)** Diffuse alveolar damage.

- Grading of acute cellular rejection is based on the intensity of the lymphocytic infiltrate (Table 11.2). At our institution, we use the 2007 revision of the grading system first developed by the Lung Rejection Study Group (LRSG) of the International Society for Heart and Lung Transplantation (ISHLT). This system includes five categories for the vascular component of acute cellular rejection (designated A), four for the airway component (designated B) and two for chronic airway rejection, also known as obliterative bronchiolitis (designated C). Obliterative bronchiolitis is discussed in detail in the next section. The grades for each category are combined to give an overall LRSG Grade that is included in the final diagnosis (e.g., *LRSG Grade A0 B0 C1*). For the sake of brevity, in cases with no evidence of obliterative bronchiolitis, we omit the C component (e.g., *LRSG Grade A1 B0*). The histologic features of the various grades are

Table 11.1. Non-neoplastic findings in transplant lung biopsies: pearls and pitfalls

Most surveillance transplant transbronchial biopsies show no significant pathologic changes

Always look for abnormalities that will significantly impact management: acute cellular rejection, organisms, malignant cells

Acute cellular rejection is the most common pathologic diagnosis in transbronchial biopsies of transplanted lungs

The principal inflammatory cells in acute cellular rejection are lymphocytes, not neutrophils

Do not diagnose acute cellular rejection unless the inflammatory infiltrate forms a tight perivascular cuff centered on a small venule/arteriole; over-interpretation of non-specific chronic inflammation is a major pitfall

In the lung, antibody-mediated rejection is not a pathologic diagnosis, and the C4d immunostain is seldom helpful in practice

Obliterative bronchiolitis (chronic airway rejection) is very easy to miss; include an elastic stain or a Movat pentachrome stain in your routine evaluation of transplant biopsies

Acute cellular rejection is often clinically occult, but chronic rejection (obliterative bronchiolitis) is usually clinically evident

The most helpful clinical surrogate marker of obliterative bronchiolitis is a decrease in the forced expiratory volume in 1 second (FEV_1)

Never ignore necrosis in a transplant lung biopsy. Always request special stains for organisms if you see necrosis or granulomatous inflammation

Consider the possibility of post-transplant lymphoproliferative disorder (PTLD) if lymphoid infiltrates are dense or atypical, or are associated with necrosis

described in detail below. It should be obvious to the reader from the following description that the boundaries of these arbitrary grades are not always sharp.

- Grade A0: no evidence of acute cellular rejection. Most surveillance biopsies fall under this category, and show no significant pathologic changes other than variable numbers of hemosiderin-laden macrophages within the airspaces.
- Grade A1: minimal acute cellular rejection. This common finding is regarded as clinically insignificant by some authors and an indication for augmented immunosuppression by others. It consists of a few layers of lymphocytes arranged around small blood vessels in a circumferential pattern (Figure 11.4). Eosinophils and endothelialitis are not seen. Concurrent lymphocytic bronchiolitis is uncommon. There is considerable overlap in the number of layers of lymphocytes in the vessel wall in grades A1 and A2.
- Grade A2: mild acute cellular rejection. Mild acute cellular rejection is one of the most common diagnoses in transbronchial lung biopsies of transplanted lungs, and is widely regarded as clinically significant, especially in symptomatic patients. The incidence in surveillance biopsies ranges from 12 to 26%. The perivascular infiltrates in grade A2 are said to be unequivocal and readily recognizable at low or scanning magnification. The diagnosis can be made even if a single blood vessel shows a prominent and easily recognizable perivascular lymphocytic infiltrate (Figures 11.5 and 11.6). The infiltrates are generally confined to the wall of the involved blood vessel and

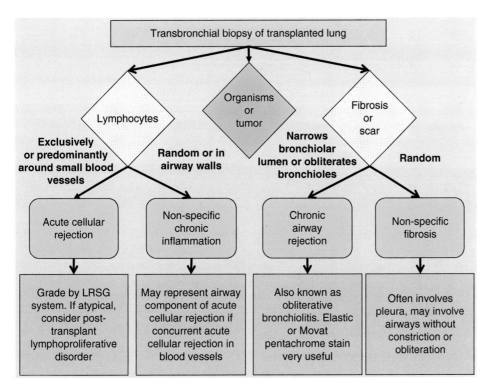

Figure 11.2. Algorithm: approach to transplant lung biopsies.

the potential space of the perivascular adventitia. There is no significant involvement of alveolar septa away from the involved vessel. Subendothelial infiltration by lymphocytes – also known as *endothelialitis* – is often present and may be associated with reactive

Table 11.2. Grading of pulmonary allograft rejection (adapted from the 2007 revision of the 1996 Working Formulation)

Category	Possible grades
A: Acute cellular rejection (vascular inflammation)	Grade 0 – none Grade 1 – minimal Grade 2 – mild Grade 3 – moderate Grade 4 – severe
B: Airway inflammation	Grade 0 – none Grade 1R – low grade Grade 2R – high grade Grade X – ungradeable
C: Chronic airway rejection – obliterative bronchiolitis	0 – absent 1 – present
D: Chronic vascular rejection – accelerated graft vascular sclerosis	Not applicable

endothelial changes. A few scattered eosinophils are frequently present and serve as a tip-off to the correct interpretation. Occasional plasma cells may also be seen but they are seldom prominent. Concurrent lymphocytic infiltrates may involve the small airways (lymphocytic bronchiolitis) or bronchi.

- Grade A3: moderate acute cellular rejection. This uncommon grade of acute cellular rejection is characterized by extension of perivascular lymphocytic infiltrates into adjacent alveolar septa and occasionally into airspaces (Figure 11.7). The airspaces may additionally contain macrophages and a fibrinous exudate. Type 2 pneumocytes may be prominent. Endothelialitis is present in most cases, and eosinophils are frequently admixed with the lymphocytic infiltrates.

- Grade A4: severe acute cellular rejection. This rare manifestation of acute cellular rejection allegedly manifests as diffuse alveolar damage, a form of severe acute injury with a wide range of possible etiologies (see Chapter 5). To complicate matters, diffuse alveolar damage is also a manifestation of antibody-mediated rejection. In practice, it is seldom possible to determine on histologic grounds whether diffuse alveolar damage in a transplant biopsy is a

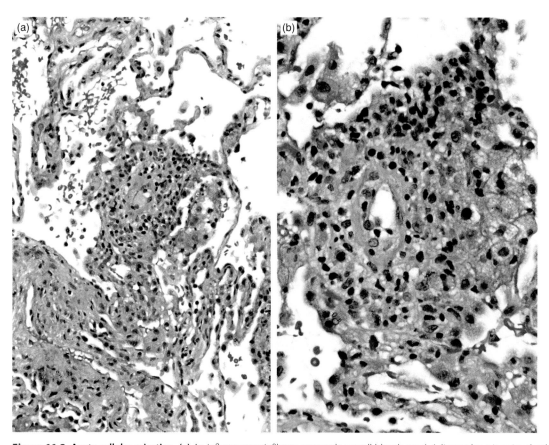

Figure 11.3. Acute cellular rejection. (a) An inflammatory infiltrate surrounds a small blood vessel. Adjacent lung is uninvolved. **(b)** At higher magnification, it is apparent that most of the inflammatory cells are lymphocytes. They are present in the vessel wall as well as in the connective tissue around it. There is a mix of small and large lymphocytes, and a few histiocytes are also present.

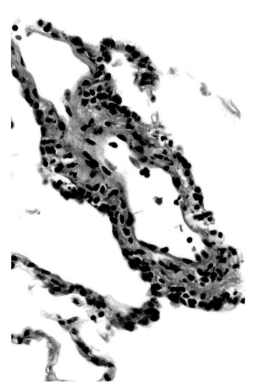

Figure 11.4. Acute cellular rejection, grade A1. A lymphocytic inflammatory infiltrate surrounds a small blood vessel. Note circumferential involvement, and absence of eosinophils or endothelialitis.

consequence of severe acute cellular rejection, antibody-mediated rejection or other infectious or non-infectious causes.

- Grade B0: no airway inflammation.
- Grade B1R: low-grade small airway inflammation. This finding, also known as lymphocytic bronchiolitis, is characterized by the presence of lymphocytes in the walls of small airways without epithelial damage or intraepithelial lymphocytosis. Occasional eosinophils may also be present.
- Grade B2R: high-grade small airway inflammation. This grade of lymphocytic bronchiolitis differs from low-grade small airway inflammation by featuring greater numbers of large lymphocytes in expanded bronchiolar walls accompanied by evidence of epithelial damage or intraepithelial lymphocytosis. Eosinophils and plasma cells are common, and neutrophils may also be present. In addition, the epithelial lining may be ulcerated (Figure 11.8).
- Grade BX: ungradeable due to sampling problems, tangential sectioning, infection, artifact, etc.
- Grade C1 (chronic airway rejection or obliterative bronchiolitis) is addressed in the next section.
- Grade D (so-called chronic vascular rejection) is characterized by fibrous thickening of the intima similar to coronary artery disease. It is rarely diagnosed in practice.

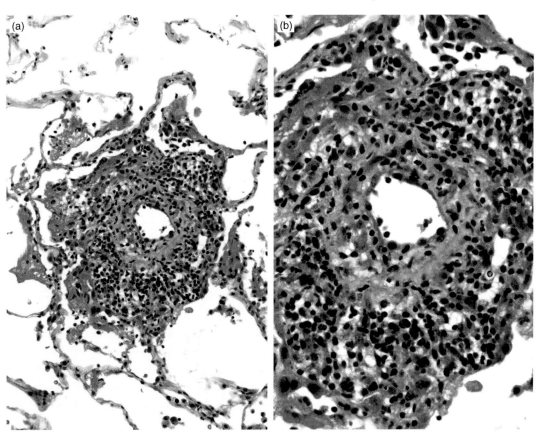

Figure 11.5. Acute cellular rejection, grade A2. (a) An inflammatory infiltrate centered on a small blood vessel is easily recognized at low magnification. Adjacent alveolar septa are uninvolved. **(b)** At higher magnification, the lymphocytic composition of the infiltrate is apparent. Compare the intensity and thickness of the process to Figure 11.4. Also note scattered eosinophils, and occasional lymphocytes in the endothelium (endothelialitis).

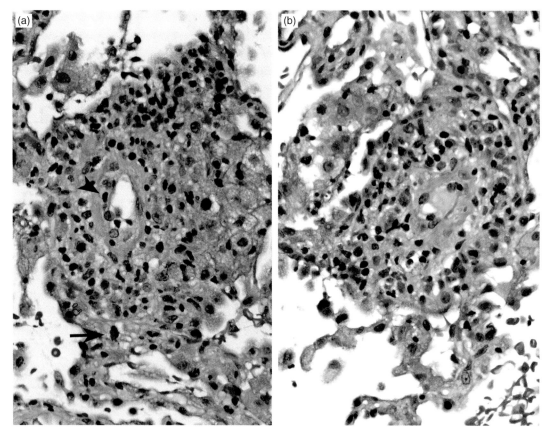

Figure 11.6. Acute cellular rejection, grade A2. (a) Perivascular inflammatory infiltrate composed mainly of lymphocytes. A few histiocytes are also present. Note endothelialitis (arrowhead) and single eosinophil (arrow).
(b) Another focus from the same biopsy. The infiltrate is polymorphous, containing small and large lymphocytes.

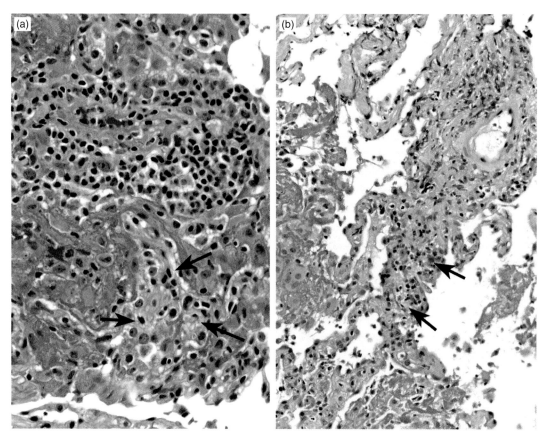

Figure 11.7. Acute cellular rejection, grade A3. (a) The perivascular lymphocytic infiltrate seen at top extends into adjacent alveolar septa (arrows). Note macrophages within nearby airspaces. **(b)** In this example, the perivascular infiltrate is at top right. Extension of the infiltrate into adjacent alveolar septa defines grade A3 (arrows).

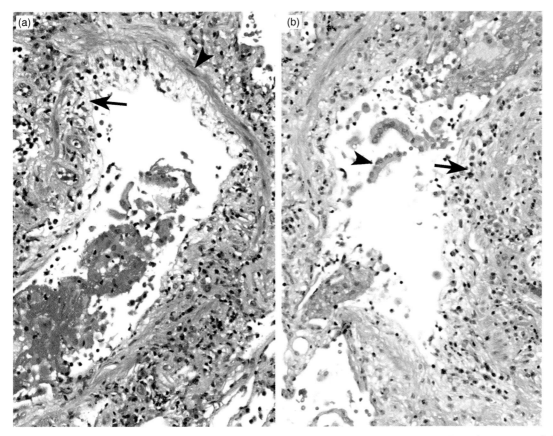

Figure 11.8. Lymphocytic bronchiolitis/high-grade small airway inflammation (B2R) in a case with moderate acute cellular rejection.
(a) This severely inflamed bronchiole is ulcerated. Note bronchiolar smooth muscle (arrowhead) and inflammatory infiltrate (arrow). **(b)** Another image from the same case shows detached epithelial cells (arrowhead) and a few eosinophils (arrow).

Diagnostic work-up

No special stains are required for the diagnosis. Deeper levels can help to detect or confirm perivascular infiltrates if findings on the original slides are equivocal. We routinely use a Movat pentachrome for our lung transplant biopsies, mainly to detect obliterative bronchiolitis. A side-benefit of this stain is that it highlights vascular involvement in acute cellular rejection (Figure 11.9). In situ hybridization for Epstein–Barr virus encoded RNA (EBER) can be very helpful when post-transplant lymphoproliferative disorder enters the differential diagnosis.

Clinical profile

The clinical features of acute cellular rejection are variable and non-specific. The condition is clinically silent in up to 40% of cases. Many patients are asymptomatic. In symptomatic patients, malaise, dyspnea, cough and low-grade fever are common. Decline in oxygenation or spirometric parameters are other non-specific findings. Peripheral leukocytosis may occur. Mild acute cellular rejection has been documented as early as 3 days after transplantation, and can occur as late as several years after transplantation. However, most cases of acute cellular rejection occur within the first year after surgery.

Radiologic findings

The radiologic findings lack sensitivity and specificity, a fact that comes as no surprise to pathologists given the microscopic and patchy nature of the inflammatory infiltrates. The most common findings on chest radiographs are perihilar and lower lobe alveolar and interstitial infiltrates. Findings on chest CT include ground-glass opacities, consolidation, septal thickening, pleural effusion, volume loss and peribronchovascular thickening. In one study based on thin-section CT scans, the combination of volume loss, pleural effusion and septal thickening was 100% specific but had very low sensitivity (8%). The overall accuracy of thin-section CT for the diagnosis of acute cellular rejection was 53%.

Differential diagnosis

- Non-specific chronic inflammation is the most common finding likely to be misinterpreted as acute cellular rejection. Non-specific inflammatory infiltrates tend to be randomly distributed, are often seen in airway walls or peribronchiolar parenchyma, and usually lack admixed large lymphocytes or eosinophils. In contrast, true acute cellular rejection is exquisitely centered on small blood vessels and almost invariably consists of a mix of small and large cells.
- Normal lymphoid aggregates in the lung (bronchus-associated lymphoid tissue, or BALT) may enter the

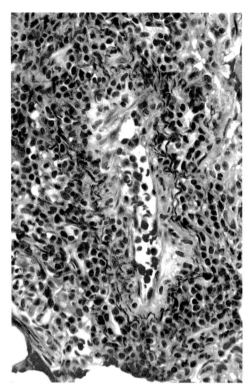

Figure 11.9. Acute cellular rejection, Movat pentachrome stain. The Movat stain highlights elastic tissue layers in this inflamed structure, supporting the impression that it is a blood vessel. Several lymphocytes are seen internal to the elastic layers, and there is evidence of endothelialitis.

differential diagnosis. These lymphoid aggregates are usually found in airway walls and can be distinguished from acute cellular rejection using the same features as listed above. In addition, because dendritic cells are often present in normal lymphoid aggregates, CD21 can be a helpful marker to exclude this possibility.

- Lymphoid infiltrates that are dense or sheet-like, distort lung architecture, contain numerous large and atypical lymphoid cells, numerous plasma cells, binucleated Reed–Sternberg-like cells or necrosis should raise the possibility of post-transplant lymphoproliferative disorder (PTLD). PTLD is an Epstein–Barr virus (EBV)-driven B-cell lymphoproliferative process that varies from polymorphous reactive lymphoid infiltrates to T-cell rich diffuse large B-cell lymphoma to monomorphous infiltrates of large cells easily recognizable as lymphoma. It often contains plasma cells, and is positive for EBV encoded RNA (EBER) by in situ hybridization. Radiologically, PTLD usually presents as lung nodules rather than infiltrates.

- Antibody-mediated rejection (AMR, humoral rejection) in the lung is typically suspected in cases that show clinical signs of acute graft dysfunction along with serologic evidence of de novo donor-specific anti-human leukocyte antigen (HLA) alloantibodies. The histologic features of this emerging entity remain controversial and poorly described. Early reports of

capillaritis as the main pathologic correlate have not been substantiated. A recent study reported that the majority of biopsies from lung transplant recipients with donor-specific HLA alloantibodies showed histologic features of acute cellular rejection (grades A2, A3 or A4). The others showed organizing acute lung injury or lymphocytic bronchiolitis. The role of C4d in confirming the diagnosis is currently debated, but in our experience this stain is not helpful in practice since most cases with clinical evidence of antibody-mediated rejection lack convincing C4d staining. There are no uniform criteria for what constitutes positive C4d staining, but strong doughnut-shaped staining of capillaries is accepted as positive in other organs. In the lung, such unequivocal C4d positivity is extremely rare and does not appear to correlate with any consistent clinical or pathologic abnormalities (Figure 11.10). At the present time, therefore, antibody-mediated rejection of the lung remains primarily a clinical diagnosis.

- Grade A1 vs. A2. Grade A2 acute cellular rejection is characterized by unequivocal lymphocytic infiltrates, endothelialitis, occasional eosinophils and associated lymphocytic bronchiolitis. In contrast, the infiltrates in grade A1 are subtle, lack eosinophils or endothelialitis, and only infrequently show concurrent lymphocytic bronchiolitis. Occasionally, there is overlap between these grades, and the distinction is arbitrary.

Treatment and prognosis

There is widespread agreement that acute cellular rejection graded as A3 or A4 requires therapy. The approach to grades A1 and A2 is more variable. Many centers including ours augment immunosuppression in most cases of grade A2, especially in symptomatic patients. This is achieved by increasing the dose of intravenous corticosteroids, usually in the form of a 3-day *pulse* dose of Solu-Medrol, often followed by a tapering course of prednisone. There is no uniform or standardized approach to therapy, however, and clinicians must constantly balance the benefit of treating acute cellular rejection against the risk of opportunistic infections. Treatment usually results in rapid resolution of symptoms and radiologic abnormalities, but follow-up biopsies show persistent rejection in 26% of patients.

The natural history of untreated, clinically silent grade A2 (mild) acute cellular rejection is not completely understood. In one study, subsequent transbronchial biopsies showed no evidence of disease and stable pulmonary function tests in nearly 40% of such patients. The remainder showed persistent or worsening acute cellular rejection on subsequent biopsies, or deterioration of pulmonary function tests. In the latter group, some showed obliterative bronchiolitis on subsequent biopsies, and died of chronic airway rejection (bronchiolitis obliterans syndrome). Based on these findings, it is speculated that mild acute cellular rejection, left untreated, leads to subsequent chronic airway

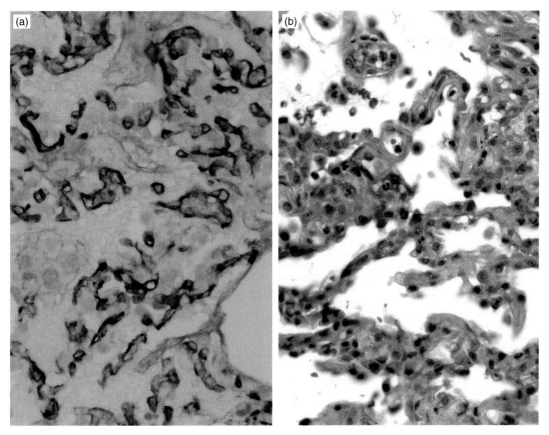

Figure 11.10. C4d staining in lung transplant biopsies. (a) Rare example of convincing doughnut-shaped staining of capillaries in a transplant lung biopsy. **(b)** The corresponding H&E appearance is underwhelming.

rejection. However, it is unclear how a cellular, predominantly perivascular process might progress to a fibrotic, airway-centered process.

The significance of a single perivascular focus of mild acute cellular rejection has also been studied. In such cases, if immunosuppression is not augmented, subsequent biopsies show progression to involvement of multiple vessels, or worsening of the grade of rejection, suggesting that they should be treated as equivalent to cases with multiple involved blood vessels.

The treatment of grade A1 (minimal) acute cellular rejection remains controversial. Asymptomatic patients have typically been observed without treatment, but data demonstrating progression to a higher grade in one-quarter of cases and an increased risk of bronchiolitis obliterans syndrome have challenged this approach.

Overall, the value of detecting and treating acute cellular rejection in symptomatic patients is widely accepted, whereas the importance of diagnosing and treating clinically occult acute cellular rejection remains unclear.

Sample diagnosis on pathology report

Lung, right lower lobe, transplant transbronchial biopsy – Mild acute cellular rejection (See comment).
– LRSG Grade A2 B0.

Obliterative bronchiolitis (chronic airway rejection, constrictive bronchiolitis)

Obliterative bronchiolitis is the most common cause of long-term failure of transplanted lungs. The diagnosis of this condition in non-transplant settings is discussed in Chapter 9. A number of similar-sounding terms have been applied to this process, creating considerable confusion. From a pathologic standpoint, the terms *obliterative bronchiolitis* and *constrictive bronchiolitis* are equivalent, and the former will be used when referring to pathologic changes in the rest of this section. The term *bronchiolitis obliterans*, used as a synonym for obliterative bronchiolitis in some publications, is best avoided in order to prevent confusion with *bronchiolitis obliterans-organizing pneumonia* (BOOP), a distinctive form of acute lung injury characterized by polyp-like fibroblast plugs within airspaces. To further reduce the likelihood of confusion, BOOP is currently known as *organizing pneumonia*. In the lung transplant setting, obliterative bronchiolitis is thought to be a manifestation of *chronic airway rejection* because its clinical manifestations usually appear over months to years, and reflect involvement of small airways. The term *chronic allograft rejection* encompasses all causes of long-term graft failure, the most common of which is obliterative bronchiolitis. Obliterative bronchiolitis is also the pathologic basis of the *bronchiolitis*

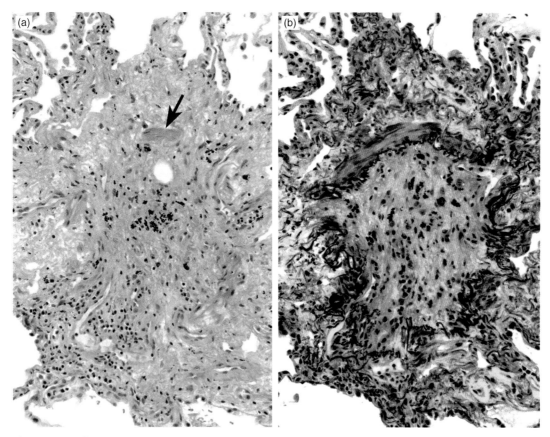

Figure 11.11. Chronic airway rejection/obliterative bronchiolitis. (a) The presence of residual smooth muscle (arrow) is a clue that this scarred focus is an obliterated bronchiole. Note pigment-laden macrophages within scar. **(b)** The Movat pentachrome stain is more compelling, as it highlights residual elastic tissue and smooth muscle fibers. The bronchiolar lumen is completely replaced by fibrosis.

obliterans syndrome (BOS), a condition defined on the basis of pulmonary function testing (reduced FEV_1) rather than histopathology. BOS develops in 50% or more of lung transplant recipients who survive for 5 years and 75% of those who survive for 10 years. The cause is unknown. However, it is speculated that BOS may be preceded by airway inflammation that occurs in the setting of acute cellular rejection. This hypothesis is based on studies that have documented an increased incidence of BOS in patients with prior episodes of acute cellular rejection. Other causes of airway injury such as repeated infection or aspiration may also contribute to its development.

Pathologists most commonly encounter obliterative bronchiolitis in surveillance transbronchial biopsies. It is also a common finding in autopsies of individuals who die after lung transplantation.

Major diagnostic findings

Obliterative bronchiolitis is characterized by fibrosis and scarring that narrows or obliterates the lumens of the affected bronchioles (Figures 11.11 and 11.12, Figure 11.1b). The fibrosis may be composed of collagen or fibroblasts or both. In early stages, fibrosis is seen in the subepithelial tissue between the bronchiolar epithelium and the surrounding smooth muscle. It may be eccentric or concentric, and causes narrowing of the

bronchiolar lumen by extrinsic compression (Figure 11.12). In later stages, the bronchiolar lumen is completely obliterated, leaving behind a scar that is barely recognizable as an airway (Figure 11.11). Occasional residual smooth muscle fibers are a clue to the nature of the scarred structure. Another helpful histologic finding is the presence of a pulmonary artery adjacent to the scar (Figure 11.13). Late stages of the process are often encountered in autopsies of patients who die several years after lung transplantation.

Variable pathologic findings

- Obliterative bronchiolitis is primarily a fibrotic process. However, a few inflammatory cells and capillaries may occasionally be present within the scar. The inflammatory cells may include a few lymphocytes, hemosiderin-laden macrophages and other pigment-filled macrophages. Bronchiolar scarring may be accompanied by smooth muscle hyperplasia.
- Lung parenchyma away from the affected bronchioles is normal, as are uninvolved bronchioles. The diagnosis of obliterative bronchiolitis should therefore be considered when one encounters a lung biopsy that is normal-appearing at first glance.
- The diagnosis can be challenging, even for experienced pathologists. The process is usually patchy and subtle.

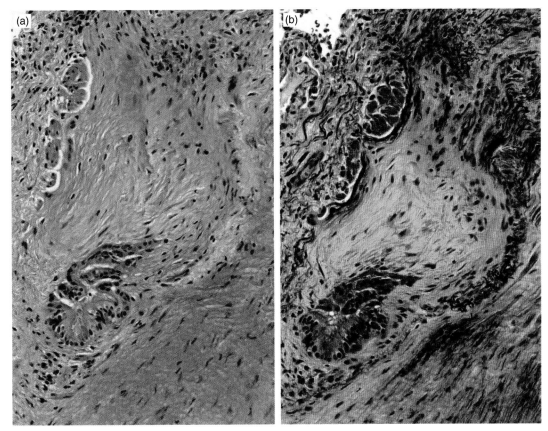

Figure 11.12. Obliterative bronchiolitis. (a) In this example, fibrosis narrows the lumen of a bronchiole but does not completely obliterate it. It is composed mainly of fibroblasts rather than collagen. The fibroblasts are internal to the smooth muscle but extrinsic to the lumen. Compare with organizing pneumonia, Chapter 5, Figure 5.34. Also note hemosiderin-laden macrophages at top. **(b)** The Movat pentachrome stain highlights elastic tissue and smooth muscle fibers, making the process easier to appreciate.

Bronchiolar lumens may be narrowed rather than completely obliterated, and in such cases the judgement as to whether the degree of luminal narrowing is significant is subjective. Since luminal narrowing and peribronchiolar fibrosis may be patchy, bronchioles elsewhere in the lung may be normal, and serial sections may be necessary to identify abnormal foci. Needless to say, diagnostic changes are more difficult to appreciate on transbronchial biopsies where involved bronchioles may not be sampled, or only part of a bronchiolar wall may be present, than in surgical lung biopsies or autopsies. Therefore, transbronchial biopsies are often non-diagnostic in patients with clinical evidence of obliterative bronchiolitis, and surgical lung biopsy may be the only means of obtaining pathologic confirmation of the diagnosis. Fortunately, the clinical diagnosis of bronchiolitis obliterans syndrome does not require pathologic confirmation.

Diagnostic work-up

We find the Movat pentachrome stain to be very helpful for detecting scarred bronchioles, and elastic stains such as EVG are essentially equivalent. The advantage of the Movat stain is that it simultaneously highlights fibrosis as well as elastic tissue and smooth muscle fibers in the obliterated bronchioles (Figures 11.11, 11.12 and 11.14).

Clinical profile

The bronchiolitis obliterans syndrome occurs within the first 2 years after transplant in one-third to one-half of cases. Most patients present with chronic dyspnea, cough, weight loss or recurrent purulent bronchitis. Pulmonary function tests typically show obstructive changes, often accompanied by an insidious or abrupt decline in FEV_1 or a reduction in diffusing capacity for carbon monoxide (DL_{CO}). The symptoms do not respond to bronchodilators or prednisone. In the lung transplant setting, the bronchiolitis obliterans syndrome is defined on the basis of spirometric parameters because of sampling difficulties inherent in transbronchial biopsies. Bronchiolitis obliterans syndrome is defined as a *persistent decline in FEV_1 to $\leq 80\%$ of the baseline post-transplant value for a minimum of 3 weeks* in the absence of confounding factors. Other potential reasons for a decline in FEV_1 include infection and restrictive allograft syndrome.

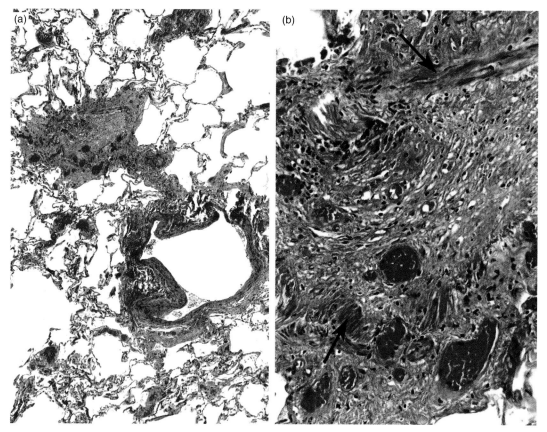

Figure 11.13. Obliterative bronchiolitis. (a) The scar at top left is quite unremarkable at low magnification, but the presence of a nearby artery hints at its significance. **(b)** At higher magnification, residual smooth muscle bundles are clearly visible (arrows), supporting the interpretation that the scar is a completely obliterated bronchiole.

Radiologic findings

Chest radiographs may be normal or near-normal. They are neither sensitive nor specific for the diagnosis. Features on chest CT include bronchiolar thickening, hyperinflation of the lung parenchyma and mosaic perfusion/mosaic attenuation. Infiltrates, opacities and nodules are not features of obliterative bronchiolitis, and should suggest an alternative diagnosis. The presence of air trapping on expiratory views and/or mosaic attenuation on high-resolution CT supports the diagnosis, but is neither perfectly sensitive (74 to 91%) nor completely specific (67 to 94%).

Differential diagnosis

- Bronchiolitis obliterans-organizing pneumonia (BOOP), currently known as organizing pneumonia, enters the differential diagnosis mainly because of similar-sounding terminology rather than pathologic similarity. In organizing pneumonia, polypoid fibroblast plugs mainly involve peribronchiolar alveoli rather than bronchioles, whereas obliterative bronchiolitis is limited to bronchioles, and does not extend distally into alveoli (Figure 11.15). There is some scope for misinterpretation because both obliterative bronchiolitis and organizing pneumonia

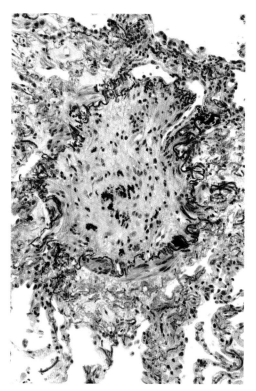

Figure 11.14. Movat pentachrome stain in obliterative bronchiolitis. The lumen of this bronchiole is completely obliterated by collagen (yellow) and some loose connective tissue (green). Note residual elastic fibers and smooth muscle.

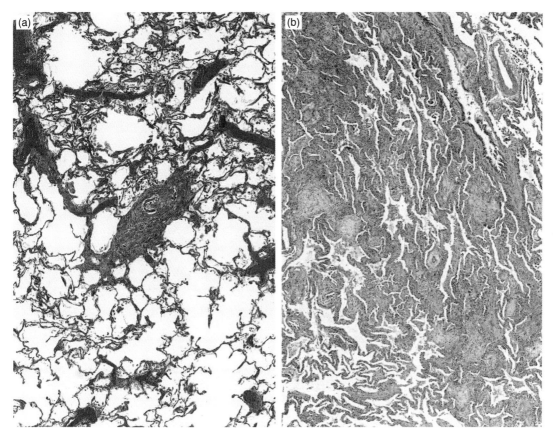

Figure 11.15. Obliterative bronchiolitis vs. organizing pneumonia. (a) Obliterative bronchiolitis. A scar obliterates a single bronchiole. The surrounding alveoli are unremarkable. **(b)** Organizing pneumonia. Numerous polypoid fibroblast plugs fill peribronchiolar alveoli. The bronchiole at top right is uninvolved.

involve bronchioles and are characterized by fibrosis. When bronchioles are involved, the fibrosis in obliterative bronchiolitis occurs *around* the bronchiolar lumen or obliterates it completely while in organizing pneumonia it occurs *within* the bronchiolar lumen, without complete obliteration (Figure 11.16). Also, the fibrosis in obliterative bronchiolitis is usually collagenous rather than fibroblastic, whereas organizing pneumonia is characterized by fibroblasts rather than collagen deposition. From a functional standpoint, both conditions cause dyspnea, but the extrinsic bronchiolar constriction that characterizes obliterative bronchiolitis causes significant and irreversible airway obstruction, while the fibroblast plugs of organizing pneumonia do not cause significant airway obstruction. Radiologically, obliterative bronchiolitis is characterized by air trapping, while organizing pneumonia manifests as infiltrates, opacities or nodules on imaging.

- Chronic bronchiolitis. This common non-specific finding is associated with several causes, including viral or bacterial infection, proximal bronchial obstruction, bronchiectasis and aspiration. In most cases seen by

pathologists, a definite cause is not demonstrable. The main difference between chronic bronchiolitis and obliterative bronchiolitis is that significant luminal narrowing or obliteration by fibrosis occurs only in the latter.

Treatment and prognosis

There is no effective medical therapy. Treatments that have been tried include macrolides such as azithromycin, tacrolimus, cytotoxic agents, anti-fibrotic drugs, statins and fundoplication. Some studies have shown a short-term improvement in FEV_1 with macrolide therapy. Re-transplantation is the only definitive intervention. It is recommended for patients who develop end-stage bronchiolitis obliterans syndrome refractory to other therapies.

The prognosis is poor. Most cases are progressive and irreversible. The condition is unresponsive to corticosteroids and other immunosuppressant or cytotoxic medications. In some patients the disease stabilizes, but complete return to normal function is unusual. In lung transplant patients, survival after development of the bronchiolitis obliterans syndrome is 51% at 3 years and 13% at 5 years. Median survival from diagnosis varies from 1.5 to 2.5 years.

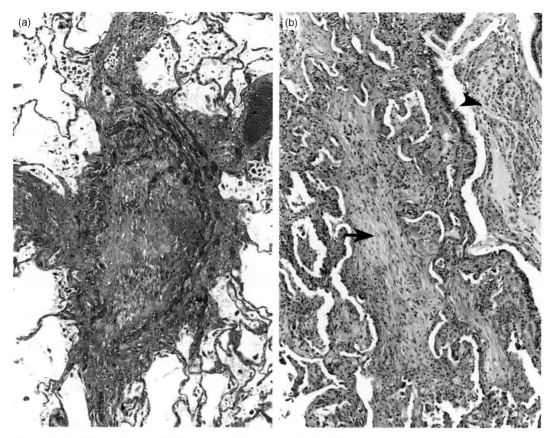

Figure 11.16. Obliterative bronchiolitis vs. organizing pneumonia. (a) Obliterative bronchiolitis. The scar obliterating this bronchiole is composed mainly of collagen. **(b)** Organizing pneumonia. This polypoid lesion within peribronchiolar alveoli is composed of fibroblasts (arrow). The adjacent bronchiole contains mucin but is uninvolved by fibroblast plugs (arrowhead).

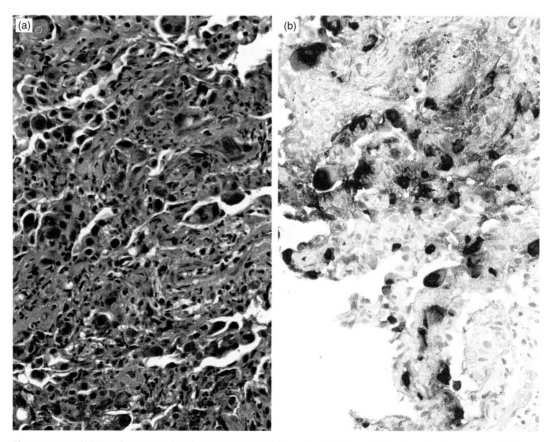

Figure 11.17. CMV in a lung transplant biopsy. (a) Typical intranuclear inclusions within enlarged cells accompanied by interstitial chronic inflammation. **(b)** Immunohistochemistry for CMV shows nuclear as well as cytoplasmic positivity. Case courtesy of Dr. AV Arrossi.

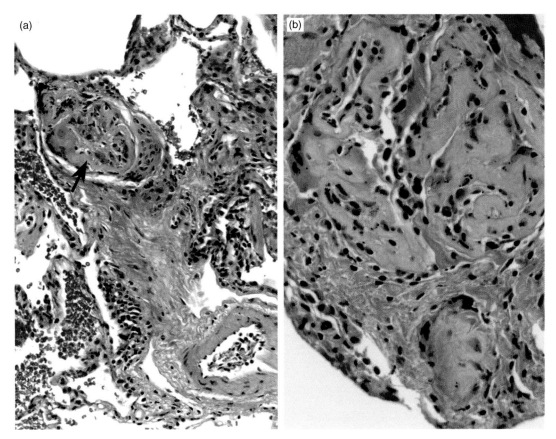

Figure 11.18. Particulate matter aspiration in transbronchial biopsies of transplanted lungs. (a) Markedly degenerated vegetable fragment (arrow). Clues to the correct interpretation are the peribronchiolar location (nearby partner artery is at lower right) and few multinucleated giant cells attached to the particle. **(b)** Similar degenerated particles from another case, shown at higher magnification.

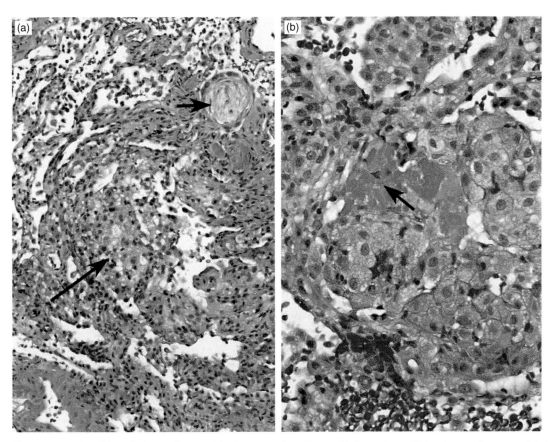

Figure 11.19. Possible amiodarone lung toxicity in a transplant biopsy. (a) Macrophages fill the airspaces (long arrow). A tiny focus of fibroblast proliferation suggests a component of organizing acute lung injury (short arrow). **(b)** The foamy nature of the macrophage cytoplasm is apparent at higher magnification. Note focal fibrinous exudate in the airspaces, also a sign of concurrent acute lung injury. The patient was on amiodarone for atrial fibrillation and had ground-glass opacities. Amiodarone was discontinued after the biopsy findings.

Table 11.3. Miscellaneous non-neoplastic pathologic findings in lung transplant biopsies

Pathologic findings	Notes
Cytomegalovirus (CMV)	Most common infection in lung transplant biopsies, yet overall quite rare with modern prophylaxis (Chapter 3) Typical inclusions (Figure 11.17, Figure 11.1c) Often clinically apparent May present as endobronchial polyps
Aspergillus	Uncommon in lung transplant biopsies May cause anastomotic infections Aspergilloma, tracheobronchitis, invasive aspergillosis (Chapter 3)
Candida	Uncommon in lung transplant biopsies May cause anastomotic infections
Herpes	Uncommon in lung transplant biopsies with adequate prophylaxis Necrosis, inclusions (Chapter 3)
Adenovirus	Uncommon in lung transplant biopsies with adequate prophylaxis Necrosis, inclusions (Chapter 3)
Pneumocystis	Very uncommon in lung transplant biopsies with adequate prophylaxis Rarely reported with typical frothy exudate (Chapter 3)
Bacterial organisms	Uncommon Acute bronchitis, acute bronchopneumonia Limited role of biopsy; bacteria may be detectable but must defer to cultures for classification
Aspiration pneumonia	Particulate matter aspiration is quite common, usually clinically occult Degenerating vegetable particles, not necessarily in bronchioles; easy to overlook (Figure 11.18, and Chapter 2) May be associated foreign-body granulomas
Diffuse alveolar damage	Hyaline membranes in acute stage (Chapter 5, Figure 5.1d) Fibroblasts and edema in interstitium in organizing stage Cause usually cannot be determined by histology
Organizing pneumonia	Fibroblast plugs within airspaces (Chapter 5) Cause usually cannot be determined by histology
Organizing acute lung injury	Fibroblast proliferation that cannot be clearly categorized as diffuse alveolar damage or organizing pneumonia
Graft vs. host disease (GVHD)	Four histologic patterns: (1) diffuse alveolar damage, (2) lymphocytic bronchitis/bronchiolitis with regenerative epithelium, and cellular chronic interstitial pneumonia, (3) organizing pneumonia, (4) obliterative bronchiolitis Most cases have evidence of GVHD in skin or gastrointestinal tract Other causes such as infection and drug toxicity need to be excluded
Respiratory bronchiolitis	Smoker's macrophages in airspaces Incidental finding
Drug toxicity	The combination of foamy macrophages and acute lung injury may be suggestive of amiodarone toxicity, but definitive diagnosis requires response to cessation of therapy (Figure 11.19)
Pulmonary alveolar proteinosis	Unclear etiology
Recurrence of original disease	Sarcoidosis (nearly a quarter of patients within first year; most are transient, with no impact on survival, Chapter 2) Lymphangioleiomyomatosis (derived from recipient cells, Chapter 7) Pulmonary Langerhans cell histiocytosis (up to 20%, does not appear to affect survival, Chapter 5)

Sample diagnosis on pathology report

Lung, right lower lobe, transplant transbronchial biopsy – Chronic airway rejection (obliterative bronchiolitis) (See comment).

- No evidence of acute cellular rejection.
- LRSG Grade A0 B0 C1.

Infections and other non-neoplastic findings in transplanted lungs

A wide range of other non-neoplastic pathologic findings can be encountered in transplanted lungs, either in surveillance biopsies, biopsies of symptomatic patients, or explant pneumonectomies. These will not be discussed in detail here since they are either very rare in practice, or because they are not unique to the transplant setting. For example, diffuse alveolar damage and organizing pneumonia are fairly common findings in transplant biopsies, but their features in this setting are identical to those in non-transplant settings, discussed in detail in Chapter 5. Table 11.3 lists some of these miscellaneous findings.

References

Acute cellular rejection

Gotway MB, Dawn SK, Sellami D, et al. Acute rejection following lung transplantation: limitations in accuracy of thin-section CT for diagnosis. *Radiology* 2001;**221**:207–12.

Hasegawa T, Iacono AT, Yousem SA. The anatomic distribution of acute cellular rejection in the allograft lung. *Ann Thorac Surg* 2000;**69**:1529–31.

Kim DW, Dacic S, Iacono A, Grgurich W, Yousem SA. Significance of a solitary perivascular mononuclear infiltrate in lung allograft recipients with mild acute cellular rejection. *J Heart Lung Transplant* 2005;**24**:152–5.

Kotloff RM, Thabut G. Lung transplantation. *Am J Respir Crit Care Med* 2011;**184**:159–71.

Martinu T, Pavlisko EN, Chen DF, Palmer S. Acute allograft rejection: cellular and humoral processes. *Clin Chest Med* 2011;**32**:295–310.

Stewart S, Fishbein MC, Snell GI, et al. Revision of the 1996 working formulation for the standardization of nomenclature in the diagnosis of lung rejection. *J Heart Lung Transplant* 2007;**26**:1229–42.

Yousem SA. Lymphocytic bronchitis/bronchiolitis in lung allograft recipients. *Am J Surg Pathol* 1993;**17**:491–6.

Yousem SA. Significance of clinically silent untreated mild acute cellular rejection in lung allograft recipients. *Hum Pathol* 1996;**27**:269–73.

Yousem SA, Randhawa P, Locker J, et al. Posttransplant lymphoproliferative disorders in heart-lung transplant recipients. Primary presentation in the allograft. *Hum Pathol* 1989;**20**:361–9.

Yousem SA, Zeevi A. The histopathology of lung allograft dysfunction associated with the development of donor-specific HLA alloantibodies. *Am J Surg Pathol* 2012;**36**:987–92.

Obliterative bronchiolitis (chronic airway rejection, constrictive bronchiolitis)

Abernathy EC, Hruban RH, Baumgartner WA, Reitz BA, Hutchins GM. The two forms of bronchiolitis obliterans in heart-lung transplant recipients. *Hum Pathol* 1991;**22**:1102–10.

Bankier AA, Muylem AV, Knoop C, Estenne M, Gevenois PA. Bronchiolitis obliterans syndrome in heart-lung transplant recipients: diagnosis with expiratory CT. *Radiology* 2001;**218**:533–9.

Burke CM, Theodore J, Dawkins KD, et al. Post-transplant obliterative bronchiolitis and other late lung sequelae in human heart-lung transplantation. *Chest* 1984;**86**:824–9.

Estenne M, Maurer JR, Boehler A, et al. Bronchiolitis obliterans syndrome 2001: an update of the diagnostic criteria. *J Heart Lung Transplant* 2002;**21**:297–310.

Kotloff RM, Thabut G. Lung transplantation. *Am J Respir Crit Care Med* 2011;**184**:159–71.

Kraft M, Mortenson RL, Colby TV, Newman L, Waldron JA, King TE Jr. Cryptogenic constrictive bronchiolitis: a clinicopathologic study. *Am Rev Respir Dis* 1993;**148**:1093–101.

Meyer KC, Raghu G, Verleden GM, et al. An international ISHLT/ATS/ERS clinical practice guideline: diagnosis and management of bronchiolitis obliterans syndrome. *Eur Respir J* 2014;**44**:1479–503.

Stewart S, Fishbein MC, Snell GI, et al. Revision of the 1996 working formulation for the standardization of nomenclature in the diagnosis of lung rejection. *J Heart Lung Transplant* 2007;**26**:1229–42.

Visscher DW, Myers JL. Bronchiolitis. The pathologist's perspective. *Proc Am Thorac Soc* 2006;**3**:41–7.

Yousem SA, Burke CM, Billingham ME. Pathologic pulmonary alterations in long-term human heart-lung transplantation. *Hum Pathol* 1985;**16**:911–23.

Infections and other non-neoplastic findings in transplanted lungs

Banga A, Sahoo D, Lane CR, Farver CF, Budev MM. Disease recurrence and acute cellular rejection episodes during the first year after lung transplantation among patients with sarcoidosis. *Transplantation* 2015;**99**:1940–5.

Chemaly RF, Yen-Lieberman B, Castilla EA, et al. Correlation between viral loads of cytomegalovirus in blood and bronchoalveolar lavage specimens from lung transplant recipients determined by histology and immunohistochemistry. *J Clin Microbiol* 2004;**42**:2168–72.

Dauriat G, Mal H, Thabut G, et al. Lung transplantation for pulmonary Langerhans cell histiocytosis. *Transplantation* 2006;**81**:746–50.

Johnson BA, Duncan SR, Ohori NP. Recurrence of sarcoidosis in pulmonary allograft recipients. *Am Rev Respir Dis* 1983;**148**:1373–7.

Karbowniczek M, Astrinidis A, Balsara BR, et al. Recurrent lymphangiomyomatosis after transplantation. Genetic analyses reveal a metastatic mechanism. *Am J Respir Crit Care Med* 2003;**167**:976–82.

Mehrad B, Paciocco G, Martinez FJ, Ojo TC, Iannettoni MD, Lynch JP III. Spectrum of *Aspergillus* infection in lung transplant recipients. Case series and review of the literature. *Chest* 2001;**119**:169–75.

Naber JM, Palmer SM, Howell DN. Cytomegalovirus infection presenting as bronchial polyps in lung transplant recipients. *J Heart Lung Transplant* 2005;**24**:2109–13.

Trulock EP, Ettinger NA, Brunt EM, Pasque MK, Kaiser LR, Cooper JD. The role of transbronchial biopsy in the treatment of lung transplant recipients. An analysis of 200 consecutive procedures. *Chest* 1992;**102**: 1049–54.

Yousem SA. The histological spectrum of pulmonary graft-vs-host disease in bone marrow transplant recipients. *Hum Pathol* 1995;**26**:668–75.

Yousem SA, Ducan SR, Griffith BP. Interstitial and airspace granulation tissue reactions in lung transplant recipients. *Am J Surg Pathol* 1992;**16**:877–84.

Index

Figures and tables are denoted in bold typeface.

405